D0077202

An Invitation to Health

Taking Charge of Your Health, Brief Edition

Dianne Hales

11th Edition

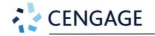
CENGAGE

Australia • Brazil • Mexico • Singapore • United Kingdom • United States

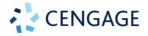

An Invitation to Health: Taking Charge of Your Health, Brief Edition, **11th Edition**
Dianne Hales

VP, Product Management: Thais L. Alencar

Product Manager: Courtney Heilman

Product Assistant: Hannah Shinn

Marketing Manager: Shannon Hawkins

Senior Content Manager: Lianne Ames

IP Analyst: Ann Hoffman

IP Project Manager: Nick Barrows

Production Service/Compositor: Lori Hazzard, MPS Limited

Art Director: Sarah Cole

Text Designer: Liz Harasymczuk

Cover Designer: Sarah Cole

Cover Image: Klaus Vedfelt/DigitalVision/Getty Images

© 2021, 2018, 2016 Cengage Learning, Inc.

Unless otherwise noted, all content is © Cengage.

ALL RIGHTS RESERVED. No part of this work covered by the copyright herein may be reproduced or distributed in any form or by any means, except as permitted by U.S. copyright law, without the prior written permission of the copyright owner.

> For product information and technology assistance, contact us at
> **Cengage Customer & Sales Support, 1-800-354-9706 or support.cengage.com.**
>
> For permission to use material from this text or product, submit all requests online at **www.cengage.com/permissions.**

Library of Congress Control Number: 2019921257

Student Edition:
ISBN: 978-1-337-91940-1
Loose-leaf Edition:
ISBN: 978-1-337-91941-8

Cengage
200 Pier 4 Boulevard
Boston, MA 02210
USA

Cengage is a leading provider of customized learning solutions with employees residing in nearly 40 different countries and sales in more than 125 countries around the world. Find your local representative at **www.cengage.com.**

Cengage products are represented in Canada by Nelson Education, Ltd.

To learn more about Cengage platforms and services, register or access your online learning solution, or purchase materials for your course, visit **www.cengage.com.**

Printed in the United States of America
Print Number: 01   Print Year: 2020

Brief Contents

Contents

Key Features

Preface

To the Student: Starting Now

College prepares you for the future. But when it comes to health, your future starts *now*! Every day you make choices and take actions that may or may not have long-term consequences, but they do have effects on how you feel now. Here are some examples:

- You stay up late and get less than 5 hours' sleep. The next day you feel groggy, your reflexes are off, and you find it harder to concentrate.

- You scarf down a double cheeseburger with bacon, a supersized side of fries, and a milkshake. By the time you're done with your meal, harmful fats are coursing through your bloodstream.

- You chug a combo of Red Bull and vodka and keep partying for hours. Even before you finish your first drink, your heart is racing and your blood pressure is rising. If you keep drinking, you'll reach dangerous levels of intoxication—probably without realizing how inebriated you are.

- Too tired to head to the gym, you stream videos for hours. Your metabolism slows; your unexercised muscles weaken.

- Just this once, you have sex without a condom. You wake up the next morning worrying about a sexually transmitted infection (STI) or a possible pregnancy.

- You don't have time to get to the student health center for a flu shot. Then your roommate comes down with the flu.

- You text while driving—and don't notice that the traffic light is changing.

There are countless other little things that can have very big consequences on your life today as well as through all the years to come. But they don't have to be negative. Consider these alternatives:

- Get a solid night's sleep after studying and you'll remember more course material and probably score higher on a test.

- Eat a meal of a low-fat protein, vegetables, and grains and you'll feel energized.

- Limit your alcohol intake and you'll enjoy the evening and feel better the morning after.

- Go for a 10-minute walk or bike ride and you'll feel less stressed and weary.

- Consistently practice safe sex and you won't have to wonder if you've jeopardized your sexual health.

- Keep up with your vaccinations and you lower your odds of serious illnesses.

- Pay attention to the road when you drive and you can avoid accidents.

In addition to their immediate effects, the impact of health behaviors continues for years and decades to come. Consider these facts:

- More than 40 percent of college students are already overweight or obese.

- One in four college students may have at least one risk factor for cardiovascular disease.

- Nine in 10 college students report feeling stressed.

- One in three college students reports binge drinking at least once in the previous 2 weeks.

Such risky behaviors take a toll. According to an international study, young Americans are less likely than their peers in other developed nations to survive until age 55. Those who do live to middle age and beyond are more likely to suffer serious chronic diseases and disabilities.

You do not have to be among them. *An Invitation to Health: Taking Charge of Your Health* shows you how to start living a healthier, happier, and fuller life now and in the years to come.

To the Instructor

You talk to your students about their future because it matters. But in the whirl of undergraduates' busy lives, today matters more. As recent research has documented, payoffs in the present are more powerful motivators for healthful behaviors than future rewards. Individuals exercise more, choose healthier foods, quit smoking, and make positive changes when immediate actions yield short-term as well as long-term benefits.

An Invitation to Health: Taking Charge of Your Health incorporates this underlying philosophy throughout its chapters. As you can see in the Preface for students, we consistently point out the impact that everyday choices have on their health now and in the future. Each chapter highlights specific, practical steps that make a difference in how students feel and function. The "Health Now!" feature gives students step-by-step guidance on how to apply what they're learning in their daily lives. The "Taking Charge of Your Health" checklist at each chapter's end reinforces key behavioral changes that can enhance and safeguard health.

Each chapter's "check-in" feature engages students as they read by posing questions that relate directly to their lives, experiences, and perspectives. After the definitions of wellness in Chapter 1, for instance, a "check-in" asks "What does wellness mean to you?" In the section on healthy habits, another "check-in" instructs students to rate their own health habits. As they learn about behavioral changes, this feature prompts them to identify a health-related change they want to make and their stage of readiness for change.

As an instructor, you can utilize the "check-in" features in different ways. For instance, you might suggest that students use them to test their comprehension of the material in the chapter. Or you might draw on the "check-ins" to spark classroom discussion and increase student engagement.

This textbook is an invitation to you as an instructor. I invite you to share your passion for education and to enter into a partnership with the editorial team at Cengage Learning. We welcome your feedback and suggestions. Please let us hear from you at www.cengage.com/health. I personally look forward to working with you toward our shared goal of preparing a new generation for a healthful future.

What's New in *An Invitation to Health, Brief: Taking Charge of Your Health*

Some things don't change: as always, this *Invitation* presents up-to-date, concise, research-based coverage of all the dimensions of health. It also continues to define health in the broadest sense of the word—not as an entity in itself, but as an integrated process for discovering, using, and protecting all possible resources within the individual, family, community, and environment.

What is new is the theme that threads through every chapter: providing students with practical knowledge and tools they can apply immediately to take charge of their health. One of the keys to doing so is behavioral change, which has always been fundamental to *An Invitation to Health*. The one feature that has appeared in every edition—and that remains the most popular—is "Your Strategies for Change."

Each chapter begins with "What Do You Think?" questions to have the reader think about his or her personal experience and knowledge with regard to concepts in the chapter. At the end of the chapter the "What Did You Decide?" questions ask the reader to reflect on how his or her answers to these questions may have changed after reading the chapter and follows the questions with a reflection that invites the reader to consider next steps to take, based on their reading.

Every chapter concludes with "Taking Charge of Your Health," a checklist that students can use to assess their current status and work toward specific goals, whether by creating better relationships (Chapter 7), getting in better shape (Chapter 6), or taking charge of their alcohol and tobacco intake (Chapter 13). Chapter 4, Personal Nutrition, is updated with information on applying federal dietary guidelines and the benefits and risks of dietary supplements. Chapter 11, Consumer Health, contains updated information on the Affordable Care Act as well as ways to prepare for a medical exam, get quality traditional and alternative health care, and navigate the health-care system.

Throughout this edition, the focus is on students, with real-life examples, the latest statistics on undergraduate behaviors and attitudes, and coverage of relevant health issues including alcohol mixed with energy drinks (AmEDs), the dangers of vaping, the opioid epidemic, the #MeToo movement on campuses, and cyberbullying.

An interactive feature, "On Campus Now," showcases the latest research on student behavior, including their sleep habits (Chapter 2), stress levels (Chapter 3), weight (Chapter 5), and sexual experiences (Chapter 8). "Health Now!" presents practical, ready-to-use tips related to real-life issues such as recognizing substance abuse (Chapter 12) and how to avoid date rape (Chapter 14).

Other popular features that have been retained and updated include "Health on a Budget" and "Consumer Alert." End-of-chapter resources include a "Self-Survey" and "Review Questions." At the end of the book is a full Glossary as well as complete chapter references.

Because health is an ever-evolving field, this edition includes many new topics, including insomnia's effect on quality of life, managing money to reduce financial stress, first-generation and minority students, student athletes and military veterans; coping techniques such as mindfulness; gluten-free diets; sugar-sweetened beverages; the obesity epidemic; ethnic differences in eating; "screen time" and physical activity in college students; the impact of exercise on the brain, including mood, symptoms of depression and anxiety, and cognitive functioning at different ages; online and mobile dating; a new and expanded section on The Gender Spectrum, including the LGBTQIA community; hooking-up (prevalence, pros, cons); updated section on STIs on Campus; updates on risks and benefits of contraceptives; new section on Digital Birth Control (Fertility awareness apps); fertility issues for transgender individuals; newly recognized risk factors for cardiometabolic diseases; controversy over vaccinating children; the boom in mHealth apps and devices; medical marijuana legalization; mobile phone use and neck pain; gun violence and campus shootings; new section on Sexual Victimization and Violence; changing the college sexual culture and #MeToo; new section on Green Space; fatal drug overdoses as an increasing cause of death in young adults; suicides among the young; and factors influencing cognitive decline and Alzheimer's disease.

All the chapters have been updated with the most current research, including many citations published in 2019, and with the latest available statistics. The majority come from primary sources, including professional books; medical, health, and mental health journals; health education periodicals; scientific meetings, federal agencies, and consensus panels; publications from research laboratories and universities; and personal interviews with specialists in a number of fields. In addition, "What's Online" presents reliable Internet addresses where students can turn for additional information.

As I tell students, *An Invitation to Health, Brief: Taking Charge of Your Health* can serve as an owner's manual to their bodies and minds. By using this book and taking the course, they can acquire a special type of power—the power to make good decisions, to assume responsibility, and to create and follow a healthy lifestyle. This textbook is our invitation to them to live what they learn and make the most of their health—now and in the future.

An Overview of Changes and Updates

Below is a chapter-by-chapter listing of some of the key topics that have been added, expanded, or revised for this edition.

Chapter 1: Taking Charge of Your Health
Updated statistics on health in America; updated statistics on college students' health; new research on older students and health care issues related to age, race, sex, and living arrangements; new section on "Informing Yourself," including guidance on evaluating online health information, evidence-based medicine, outcomes research, and practice guidelines.

Chapter 2: Psychological and Spiritual Well-Being
Latest findings from the science of subjective well-being; expanded coverage of student self-care; review of research on the benefits and components of happiness; impact of growing up in a religious family; science linking gratitude and health; insomnia's effects on quality of life; sleep health on college campuses; latest research on student mental health; mental health disparities among college students of color; mental health issues for LGBTQIA students; mental health issues for athletes and veterans; impact of depression on health; depression, anxiety, and attention disorders on campus; suicidal thoughts and behaviors among students; campus counseling after student deaths.

Chapter 3: Stress Management
Updated statistics on student stress from the ACHA National College Health Assessment; latest findings from the American Psychological Association's Stress in America survey; new section on Managing

Your Money, including behavioral strategies such as organizing financial files, making a budget, frugal living, banking basics, avoiding debit and credit card stress, and digital financial management; expanded coverage of stress for specific student groups, including first-generation students, minority students, student athletes, and military veterans; updated research on student vulnerability to stress and on coping techniques such as mindfulness.

Chapter 4: Personal Nutrition

Recommendations for most recent dietary guidelines; updated research on college students' food choices and diets; comprehensive review of research on the benefits of fiber; new findings on vitamin D, fish oil supplements, and calcium; gluten-free diets; latest research on the health benefits of the Mediterranean diet; coverage of "food insecurity" on campus; impact of sugar-sweetened beverages; update on nutrition labels; recent findings on benefits of organic food; update on use of dietary supplements.

Chapter 5: Weight Management and the Obesity Epidemic

New section and focus on the obesity epidemic; most recent statistics on overweight and obesity in the United States; updated research on the causes of obesity; updated statistics on college students' weights; new section on body composition; new research on the efficacy of various diets; latest findings on nonsugar sweeteners; coverage of ethnic differences in eating disorders among young women.

Chapter 6: Physical Activity and Fitness

New section on the dangers of inactivity and excess sitting; findings on "screen time" and physical activity in college students; updated statistics on exercise on campus; updated, expanded coverage of the recently revised federal Physical Activity Guidelines; official definitions of types of recommended exercises; updates on latest research on the benefits of various levels of physical activity and exercise; comparison of benefits of aerobic, resistance, and combination training; new findings on the health benefits of resistance and strength training; new coverage of the "extreme exercise hypothesis"; new research on the impact of exercise on the brain, including mood, symptoms of depression and anxiety, and cognitive functioning at different ages; new section on smartwatches as fitness trackers; update on performance-enhancing supplements; update on nutrition for athletes.

Chapter 7: Communicating and Connecting

New chapter on "communicating and connecting"; updated statistics on student loneliness, shyness, social anxiety; new research on the digital life of college students; positive and negative impact of Facebook and social networks; new section on "online and mobile dating"; cyberbullying on college campuses; impact of problematic Internet/smartphone use on college students; how falling in love affects the immune system; intimate partner violence and depression; impact of parental divorce on college students; need for financial aid and child care for students with young children.

Chapter 8: Sexual Health

Updated statistics on the sex lives of college students; new and expanded section on the Gender Spectrum, including the latest on the LGBTQIA community; new section on Sex on Campus, including the latest on hooking up (prevalence, pros, cons) and friends with benefits; latest research on treatments for premenstrual syndrome; new research on benefits of circumcision; new research on prevalence and treatment of erectile dysfunction in young men;

latest statistics on STI incidence globally and nationally; newest recommendations for screening for STIs; updated section on STIs on Campus; update on HPV, including vaccinations and outcomes; updated coverage of herpes, chlamydia, gonorrhea, and syphilis; extensively revised and updated sections on HIV/AIDS, including latest statistics, stages of infection, and advances such as PrEP and PEP.

Chapter 9: Reproductive Options

New statistics on contraception on campus; update on ACA coverage of birth control and related state legislations; latest CDC report on contraception in the United States; updates on risks and benefits of contraceptives; expanded coverage of LARCs; new section on Digital Birth Control (Fertility awareness apps); new section on fertility issues for transgender individuals; update on state restrictions on abortions.

Chapter 10: Diseases and Disorders

Updated statistics on major diseases; updated statistics on college students diagnosed with various diseases; importance of physical activity for cardiometabolic health of young people; latest research on enhancing cardiometabolic health; newly recognized risk factors for cardiometabolic diseases; new guidelines on high blood pressure diagnosis and treatment; latest findings on the impact of supplements, blood fats, and active and passive smoking on cardiovascular health; updated statistics on cancer in America, including cancer rates, survival, and deaths; new coverage of male breast cancer; latest findings on skin cancer risks and prevention; asthma update; updated statistics on infectious diseases in America; updated data on vaccinations of college students; latest recommendation for immunizations of various age groups and for adults in general; coverage of controversy over vaccinating children; updated statistics on influenza; latest findings and recommendations on meningitis vaccinations; latest findings and recommendations for hepatitis A, B, and C; updates on Zika and Lyme disease.

Chapter 11: Consumer Health

The most recent available status of the Affordable Care Act; controversial provisions in the ACA; the boom in mHealth apps and devices; research on benefits of mHealth for consumers and patients; increase in cosmetic surgery among young adults and minorities; growth of interest in and use of CAM; risks and cautions related to yoga.

Chapter 12: Addictive Behaviors and Drugs

New section on the Opioid Epidemic; updated statistics on drug use on campus; trends in drug use in America; caffeine and health; impact of medical marijuana legalization; new research on gambling disorders; new section on CBD; update on treatment options for drug addiction.

Chapter 13: Alcohol and Tobacco

Updated statistics on alcohol in America; newest data on drinking in college; impact of social norms on student drinking; drinking behavior through the college years; social anxiety as a motive for student drinking; secondhand dangers of alcohol for students; long-term impact of college drinking after graduation; alcohol and cardiovascular health; alcohol's impact on women; latest statistics on smoking in America; update on smoking on campus; new section on "Electronic Cigarettes and Vaping"; dangers of electronic cigarette smoke; patterns of e-cigarette use; vaping and use of illicit drugs; college students' beliefs about e-cigarettes; updates on hookah use; cigar smoking prevalence; medications for quitting.

Chapter 14: Protecting Yourself and Your Environment

Updates on statistics on motor vehicle accidents and safety; new data on drowsy driving; effect of texting-while-driving bans on emergency department visits; preventing musculoskeletal disorders in the workplace; impact of sit-stand stations on activity and health; mobile phone use and neck pain; new section on gun violence; updated statistics on campus shootings; impact of concealed carry laws on campus crime; updated data on intimate partner and sexual violence; new section on Sexual Victimization and Violence; cyberbullying research; definition of sexual harassment; sexual violence on campus; revictimization of college student sexual violence survivors; risk factors for sexual violence in dating relationships; campus sexual violence statistics; new coverage of changing the college sexual culture and #MeToo; college services for sexual assault survivors; new Student Snapshot: How Students View Climate Change; updated sections on climate change and global warming; updated coverage of health risks of climate change; updated coverage of air pollution; health risks of outdoor exercise in polluted air; new section on Green Space; updated coverage of household air pollution and its impact on health; environmental tobacco smoke and cardiovascular disease; heavy metal and nanoplastic contamination; health risks of mobile phone use; updated coverage of hearing loss.

Chapter 15: A Lifetime of Health

Updated statistics on longevity and life expectancy; fatal drug overdoses as an increasing cause of death in young adults; increase in suicides among the young; functional impairment and decline in middle age; impact of healthy behaviors on life expectancy; benefits of high-intensity exercise for older adults; anxiety and depression in perimenopause; treatments for menopause symptoms; changes in immunity over time; cognitive training for the aging brain; preventing/treating frailty in the elderly; factors influencing cognitive decline and Alzheimer's disease; calcium supplements for bone health; low-dose and transdermal hormone therapy for osteoporosis; where people die; new Student Snapshot data on Causes of Death in Young Adults.

Supplemental Resources

MindTap for *An Invitation to Health Brief: Taking Charge of Your Health*

MindTap is an outcomes-driven application that propels students from memorization to mastery. MindTap is the platform that gives you complete control of your course—to craft unique learning experiences that challenge students, build confidence, and elevate performance. cengage.com/mindtap

Cengage Unlimited

Cengage Unlimited saved students over $60 million in its first year. One subscription includes access to every Cengage online textbook and platform, along with study tools and resources that help students explore careers and gain the skills employers want. cengage.com/unlimited/instructor

Diet & Wellness Plus

Diet & Wellness Plus helps you understand how nutrition relates to your personal health goals. Track your diet and activity, generate reports, and analyze the nutritional value of the food you eat. Diet & Wellness Plus includes over 82,000 foods as well as custom food and recipe features. The Behavior Change Planner helps you identify risks in your life and guides you through the key steps to make positive changes. Diet & Wellness Plus can also be accessed from the app dock in MindTap.

Instructor Companion Site

Everything you need for your course in one place! This collection of book-specific lecture and class tools is available online via www.cengage.com/login. Access and download PowerPoint presentations, images, an instructor's manual, and more.

Cengage Learning Testing Powered by Cognero

This flexible online system allows the instructor to edit and manage test bank content from multiple Cengage Learning solutions; create multiple test versions in an instant; and deliver tests from an LMS, a classroom, or wherever the instructor wants.

Acknowledgments

One of the joys of writing each edition of *An Invitation to Health* is the opportunity to work with a team I consider the best of the best in textbook publishing. I thank Courtney Heilman, product manager, for her enthusiasm and support; Paula Dohnal, learning designer, for her work on the textbook and MindTap; and Sarah Cole, art director, for providing the evocative cover.

I thank Hannah Shin, our product assistant, for her invaluable aid; Lianne Ames, senior content manager, for expertly shepherding this edition and the MindTap from conception to production; Liz Harasymczuk for the vibrant new design; and Lori Hazzard of MPS Limited for her supervision of the production process. Ann Hoffman and Nick Barrows managed the overall permissions process. My thanks also to Shannon Hawkins, marketing manager.

Finally, I would like to thank the reviewers whose input has been so valuable through these many editions. I thank the following for their comments and helpful assistance on the current edition:

Kelly Adam, *Big Sandy Community and Technical College*
James Bath, *Harrisburg Area Community College*
Thomas Brennan, *Macomb Community College*
Shane Callahan, *Lewis & Clark Community College*
Ari Fisher, *Louisiana State University-Baton Rouge*
Heather Grimm, *King's College*
Jessica Lowery, *Coastal Carolina University*
Christopher Malone, *Penn State*
Jennifer Sandke, *Rowan Cabarrus Community College*

For their help with earlier editions, I offer my gratitude to:

Ghulam Aasef, *Kaskaskia College*
Andrea Abercrombie, *Clemson University*
Daniel Adame, *Emory University*
Dr. Lisa Alastuey, *University of Houston*
Carol Allen, *Lone Community College*
Lana Arabas, *Truman State University*
Joseph Bails, *Parkland College*
Judy Baker, *East Carolina University*
Marcia Ball, *James Madison University*
Dr. Jeremy Barnes, *Southeast Missouri State University*
Rick Barnes, *East Carolina University*
Lois Beach, *SUNY-Plattsburg*
Liz Belyea, *Cosumnes River College*
Christina L. Benjamin, *Montgomery College*
Betsy Bergen, *Kansas State University*
Nancy Bessette, *Saddleback College*
Carol Biddington, *California University of Pennsylvania*
David Black, *Purdue University*
Jill M. Black, *Cleveland State University*
Cynthia Pike Blocksom, *Cincinnati Health Department*
Nikki Bonnani, M.S., CPT, CES, *Ithaca College*
Laura Bounds, *Northern Arizona University*
James Brik, *Willamette University*
Mitchell Brodsky, *York College*
Jodi Broodkins-Fisher, *University of Utah*

Elaine D. Bryan, *Georgia Perimeter College*
James G. Bryant, Jr., *Western Carolina University*
Conswella Byrd, *California State University East Bay*
Marsha Campos, *Modesto Junior College*
Richard Capriccioso, *University of Phoenix*
James Lester Carter, *Montana State University*
Jewel Carter-McCummings, *Montclair State University*
Peggy L. Chin, *University of Connecticut*
Olga Comissiong, *Kean University*
Patti Cost, *Weber State University*
Maxine Davis, *Eastern Washington University*
Maria Decker, *Marian Court College*
Laura Demeri, *Clark College*
Lori Dewald, *Shippensburg University of Pennsylvania*
Julie Dietz, *Eastern Illinois University*
Peter DiLorenzo, *Camden County College*
Robert Dollinger, *Florida International University College of Medicine*
Dr. Rachelle D. Duncan, *Oklahoma State University*
William E. Dunscombe, *Union County College*
Rachelle D. Duncan, *Oklahoma State University*
Sarah Catherine Dunsmore, *Idaho State University*
Gary English, *Ithaca College*
Alicia M. Eppley, *Theil College*
Victoria L. Evans, *Hendrix College*
Melinda K. Everman, *Ohio State University*
Michael Felts, *East Carolina University*
Lynne Fitzgerald, *Morehead State University*
Matthew Flint, *Utah Valley University*
Kathie C. Garbe, *Kennesaw State College*
Gail Gates, *Oklahoma State University*
Dawn Graff-Haight, *Portland State University*
Carolyn Gray, *New Mexico State University*
Mary Gress, *Lorain County Community College*
Janet Grochowski, *University of St. Thomas*
Jack Gutierrez, *Central Community College*
Autumn R. Hamilton, *Minnesota State University*
Amanda J. Harvey M.S., CHES, *Eastern Illinois University*
Christy D. Hawkins, *Thomas Nelson Community College*
Stephen Haynie, *College of William and Mary*
Amy Hedman, *Mankato State University*
Ron Heinrichs, *Central Missouri State University*
Candace H. Hendershot, *University of Findlay*
Michael Hoadley, *University of South Dakota*
Debbie Hogan, *Tri County Community College*
Margaret Hollinger, *Reading Area Community College*
Harold Horne, *University of Illinois at Springfield*
Linda L. Howard, *Idaho State University*
Mary Hunt, *Madonna University*
Kim Hyatt, *Weber State University*
Bill Hyman, *Sam Houston State University*
Dee Jacobsen, *Southeastern Louisiana University*
John Janowiak, Ph.D., *Appalachian State University*
Peggy Jarnigan, *Rollins College*
Jim Johnson, *Northwest Missouri State University*
Ches Jones, *University of Arkansas*
Herb Jones, *Ball State University*
Jane Jones, *University of Wisconsin, Stevens Point*
Lorraine J. Jones, *Muncie, Indiana*
Walter Justice, *Southwestern College*
Becky Kennedy-Koch, *The Ohio State University*
Margaret Kenrick, *Los Medanos College*
Anthony F. Kiszewski, *Bentley University*
Mark J. Kittleson, *Southern Illinois University*
Darlene Kluka, *University of Central Oklahoma*
John Kowalczyk, *University of Minnesota, Duluth*
Debra A. Krummel, *West Virginia University*
Roland Lamarine, *California State University, Chico*
David Langford, *University of Maryland, Baltimore County*
Terri Langford, *University of Central Florida*
Beth Lanning, *Baylor University*
Norbert Lindskog, *Harold Washington College*

Loretta Liptak, *Youngstown State University*
Raymond A. Lomax, *Kean University*
Michelle Lomonaco, *The Citadel*
David G. Lorenzi, *West Liberty State College*
S. Jack Loughton, *Weber State University*
Rick Madson, *Palm Beach Community College*
Ashok Malik, *College of San Mateo*
Michele P. Mannion, *Temple University*
Jerry Mayo, *Hendrix College*
Wajeeha Mazhar, *California Polytechnic State University–Pomona*
Jessica Middlebrooks, *University of Georgia*
Claudia Mihovk, *Georgia Perimeter College*
Kim H. Miller, *University of Kentucky*
Susan Milstein, *Montgomery College*
Esther Moe, *Oregon Health Sciences University*
Kris Moline, *Lourdes College*
Richard Morris, *Rollins College*
Rosemary Moulahan, *High Point University*
Sophia Munro, *Palm Beach Community College*
John W. Munson, *University of Wisconsin–Stevens Point*
Jeannie M Neiman, *Edmonds Community College*
Ray Nolan, *Colby Community College*
Shannon Norman, *University of South Dakota*
Anne O'Donnell, *Santa Rosa Junior College*
Terry Oehrtman, *Ohio University*
Shanyn Olpin, *Weber State University*
David Oster, *Jefferson College*
Randy M. Page, *University of Idaho*
Carolyn P. Parks, *University of North Carolina*
Anthony V. Parrillo, *East Carolina University*
Lorraine Peniston, *Hartford Community College*
Miguel Perez, *University of North Texas*
Pamela Pinahs-Schultz, *Carroll College*
Dena Block Pistor, *Rollins College*
Rosanne Poole, *Tallahassee Community College*
Jennifer Pridemore, *Parkland College*
Thomas Roberge, *Norwich University*
Keisha Tyler Robinson, *Youngstown State University*
Joel Rogers, *West Hills Community College District*
Linda J. Romaine, M.S., MBA, B.S., *Raritan Valley Community College*
Pamela Rost, *Buffalo State College*
Karla Rues, M.S., *Ozarks Technical Community College*
Veena Sallan, *Owensboro Community and Technical College*
Sadie Sanders, *University of Florida*
Steven Sansone, *Chemeketa Community College*
Debra Secord, *Coastline College*
Behjat Sharif, *California State University–Los Angeles*
Andrew Shim, *Southwestern College*
Agneta Sibrava, *Arkansas State University*
Steve Singleton, *Wayne State University*
Larry Smith, *Scottsdale Community College*
Teresa Snow, *Georgia Institute of Technology*
Sherm Sowby, *Brigham Young University*
Stephen P. Sowulewski, *Reynolds Community College*
Carl A. Stockton, *Radford University*
Linda Stonecipher, *Western Oregon State College*
Ronda Sturgill, *Marshall University*
Jacob W. Surratt, *Gaston College*
Rosemarie Tarara, *High Point University*
Laurie Tucker, *American University*
Julia VanderMolen, *Davenport University*
Emogene Johnson Vaughn, *Norfolk State University*
Jennifer Vickery, *Winthrop College*
Andrew M. Walker, *Georgia Perimeter College*
David M. White, *East Carolina University*
Sabina White, *University of California–Santa Barbara*
Robert Wilson, *University of Minnesota*
Roy Wohl, *Washburn University*
Martin L. Wood, *Ball State University*
Sharon Zackus, *City College of San Francisco*

About the Author

Dianne Hales is a widely published and esteemed journalist and author. In addition to more than 30 editions of college textbooks related to health, she is the author of 16 trade books, including *La Passione: How Italy Seduced the World*; *Mona Lisa: A Life Discovered; La Bella Lingua; Just Like a Woman;* and *Caring for the Mind*. Her books have been translated into many languages, including Chinese, Japanese, Italian, French, Spanish, Portuguese, German, Dutch, Swedish, Danish, and Korean.

Hales is a former contributing editor for *Parade*, *Ladies' Home Journal*, *Working Mother*, and *American Health,* and she has written more than 1,000 articles for national publications. She has received writing awards from the American Psychiatric Association and the American Psychological Association; an EMMA (Exceptional Media Merit Award) for health reporting from the National Women's Political Caucus and Radcliffe College; three EDI (Equality, Dignity, Inclusion) awards for print journalism from the National Easter Seal Society; the National Mature Media Award; and awards from the Arthritis Foundation, California Psychiatric Association, CHADD (Children and Adults with Attention-Deficit/Hyperactivity Disorder), Council for the Advancement of Scientific Education, and New York Public Library.

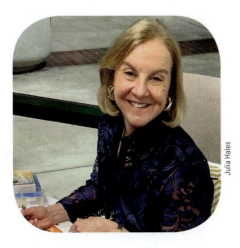

Julia Hales

An Invitation
to Health

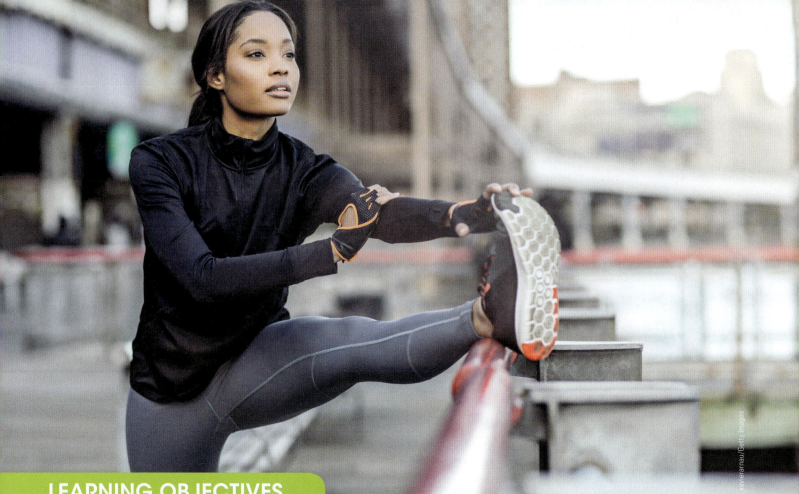

Getty Images

LEARNING OBJECTIVES

After reading this chapter, you should be able to:

1.1 Define health and wellness.

1.2 Outline the dimensions of health.

1.3 Assess the current health status of Americans.

1.4 Discuss health disparities based on sex and race.

1.5 Evaluate the health behaviors of undergraduates.

1.6 Describe the impact of habits formed in college on future health.

1.7 Evaluate health information for accuracy and reliability.

1.8 Explain the influences on behavior that support or impede healthy change.

1.9 Identify the stages of change.

WHAT DO YOU THINK?

• What does "health" mean to you?

• How healthy are today's college students?

• Is online health information generally accurate?

• Can people successfully change their health behaviors?

1

Taking Charge of Your Health

Keisha always thought of health as something you worry about when you get older. Then her twin brother developed a health problem she'd never heard of: prediabetes (discussed in Chapter 12), which increased his risk of diabetes and heart disease. At a health fair on campus, she found out that her blood pressure was higher than normal. She also learned that young adults with high blood pressure could be at greater risk of heart problems in the future.[1]

"Maybe I'm not too young to start thinking about my health," Keisha concluded. Neither are you, whether you're a traditional-age college student or, like an ever-increasing number of undergraduates, years older.

An Invitation to Health is both **about** and **for** you; it asks you to go beyond thinking about your health to taking charge and making healthy choices for yourself and your future. This book includes material on your mind and your body, your spirit and your social ties, your needs and your wants, your past and your potential. It will help you explore options, discover possibilities, and find new ways to make your life worthwhile.

What you learn from this book and in this course depends on you. You have more control over your life and well-being than anything or anyone else does. Through the decisions you make and the habits you develop, you can take charge of your health and influence how well—and how long—you will live.

Simple changes in your lifestyle can add more than a decade to your life expectancy—and enhance your well-being through all the years of your life.[2]

The time to start is **now**. Every day, you make choices that have short- and long-term consequences for your health. Eat a high-fat meal, and your blood chemistry changes. Spend a few hours slumped in front of the television, and your metabolism slows. Chug a high-caffeine energy drink, and your heart races. Have yet another beer, and your reflexes slow. Text while driving, and you may weave into another lane. Don't bother with a condom, and your risk of sexually transmitted infection (STI) skyrockets.

Sometimes making the best choices demands making healthy changes in your life. This chapter shows you how—and how to live more fully, more happily, and more healthfully. This is an offer that you literally cannot afford to refuse. Your life may depend on it— starting now. <

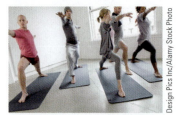

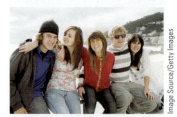

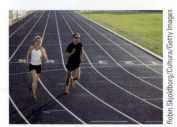

Health is the process of discovering, using, and protecting all the resources within our bodies, minds, spirits, families, communities, and environment.

Health and Wellness

By simplest definition, **health** means being sound in body, mind, and spirit. The World Health Organization defines *health* as "not merely the absence of disease or infirmity" but "a state of complete physical, mental, and social well-being." Health involves discovering, using, and protecting all the resources within your body, mind, spirit, family, community, and environment.

Health has many dimensions: physical, psychological, spiritual, social, intellectual, environmental, occupational, and financial. This book integrates these aspects into a *holistic* approach that looks at health and the individual as a whole rather than part by part.

Your own definition of health may include different elements, but chances are you and your classmates would include at least some of the following:

- A positive, optimistic outlook.
- A sense of control over stress and worries, time to relax.
- Energy and vitality, freedom from pain or serious illness.
- Supportive friends and family, and a nurturing intimate relationship with someone you love.
- A personally satisfying job or intellectual endeavor.
- A clean, healthful environment.

✓**check-in** How would you define health?

Wellness can be defined as purposeful, enjoyable living or, more specifically, a deliberate lifestyle choice characterized by personal responsibility and optimal enhancement of physical, mental, and spiritual health. In the broadest sense, wellness is:

- A decision you make to move toward optimal health.
- A way of life you design to achieve your highest potential.
- A process of developing awareness that health and happiness are possible in the present.
- The integration of body, mind, and spirit.
- The belief that everything you do, think, and feel has an impact on your state of health and the health of the world.

✓**check-in** What does wellness mean to you?

health A state of complete well-being, including physical, psychological, spiritual, social, intellectual, and environmental dimensions.

wellness A deliberate lifestyle choice characterized by personal responsibility and optimal enhancement of physical, mental, and spiritual health.

The Dimensions of Health

By learning more about the dimensions of health, you gain insight into the complex interplay of factors that determine your level of wellness. The following are the most commonly recognized dimensions of health and wellness, but some models treat emotional, cultural, or financial health as separate categories rather than aspects of psychological, social, or occupational health.

✓**check-in** What do you consider the most important or relevant dimensions of health?

Physical Health The 1913 *Webster's Dictionary* defined *health* as "the state of being hale, sound, or whole, in body, mind, or soul, especially the state of being free from physical disease or pain." More recent texts define physical health as an optimal state of well-being, not merely the absence of disease or infirmity. Health is not a static state but a process that depends on the decisions we make and the behaviors we practice every day. To ensure optimal physical health, we must feed our bodies nutritiously, exercise them regularly, avoid harmful behaviors and substances, watch for early signs of sickness, and protect ourselves from accidents.

Psychological Health Like physical well-being, psychological health, discussed in Chapter 2, encompasses our emotional and mental states—that is, our feelings and our thoughts. It involves awareness and acceptance of a wide range of feelings in oneself and others, as well as the ability to express emotions, to function independently, and to cope with the challenges of daily stressors.

Spiritual Health Spiritually healthy individuals identify their own basic purpose in life; learn how to experience love, joy, peace, and fulfillment; and help themselves and others achieve their full potential. As they devote themselves to others' needs more than their own, their spiritual development produces a sense of greater meaning in their lives.

Social Health Social health refers to the ability to interact effectively with other people and the social environment, to develop satisfying interpersonal relationships, and to fulfill social roles. It involves participating in and contributing to your community, living in harmony with fellow human beings, developing positive interdependent relationships, and practicing healthy sexual behaviors (see Chapter 7).

Intellectual Health

Every day, you use your mind to gather, process, and act on information; to think through your values; to make decisions; set goals; and figure out how to handle a problem or challenge. Intellectual health refers to your ability to think and learn from life experience, your openness to new ideas, and your capacity to question and evaluate information. Throughout your life, you'll use your critical thinking skills, including your ability to evaluate health information, to safeguard your well-being.

Environmental Health

You live in a physical and social setting that can affect every aspect of your health. Environmental health refers to the impact your world has on your well-being. It involves protecting yourself from dangers in the air, water, and soil, as well as in products you use—and working to preserve the environment itself (see Chapter 14).

Occupational and Financial Health

Even a part-time job can have an impact on your health. Freshmen who work more than 10 hours a week are more likely to smoke and drink than those who aren't employed.[3] However, they may be gaining valuable experience in managing their time, setting priorities, and finding a healthy balance in their lives.

After graduation, you will devote much of your time and energy to your career. Ideally, you will contribute your unique talents and skills to work that is rewarding in many ways—intellectually, emotionally, creatively, and financially. College provides the opportunity for you to choose and prepare for a career that is consistent with your personal values and beliefs and to learn how to manage your money and safeguard your financial well-being.

Community Health

Educators have expanded the traditional individualistic concept of health to include the complex interrelationships between one person's health and the health of the community and environment. This change in perspective has given rise to a new emphasis on **health promotion**, which educators define as "any planned combination of educational, political, regulatory, and organizational supports for actions and conditions of living conducive to the health of individuals, groups, or communities."[4] Examples on campus include establishing smoke-free policies for all college buildings, residences, and dining areas; prohibiting tobacco advertising and sponsorship of campus social events; ensuring safety at parties; and enforcing alcohol laws and policies.

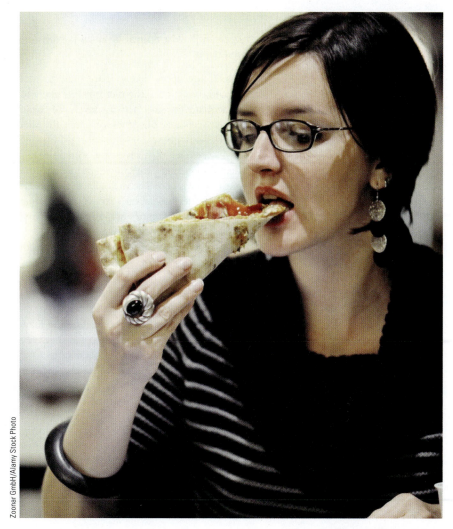

Zoonar GmbH/Alamy Stock Photo

Your choices and behaviors during your college years can influence how healthy you will be in the future.

Health in America

✓**check-in** Do you exercise regularly? Eat nutritious meals? Maintain a healthy weight? Avoid smoking? If you answer yes to all four questions, you're among the 2.7 percent of Americans who do so.

According to a national survey of more than 4,700 people, 97.3 percent get a failing grade in healthy lifestyle habits. For the minority who do adapt these health guidelines, the payoff includes a lower risk of many health problems, including type 2 diabetes, heart disease, and cancer. Although few Americans get a perfect health-habit score, a significant number report at least one healthy habit:

- 71 percent do not smoke.

- 46 percent get sufficient amounts of physical activity.

health promotion Any planned combination of educational, political, regulatory, and organizational supports for actions and conditions of living conducive to the health of individuals, groups, or communities.

- 38 percent eat a healthy diet.
- 10 percent have a normal body fat percentage (see Chapter 6).

Women are more likely than men to not smoke and to eat a healthy diet but less likely to have adequate physical activity levels. Mexican Americans are more likely to eat a healthy diet than blacks or whites.[5]

Life expectancy at birth in the United States has declined recently to 76.1 years in men and 81.1 years in women. The major factors contributing to the decline in life expectancy among younger Americans are unintentional injury, including fatal drug overdoses, and suicide.[6]

The Americans experiencing the greatest health deficits and losing the most years to illness, disability, and premature death are not the elderly but young adults. As a young American, your probability of reaching your 50th birthday is lower than in almost every other high-income nation. The main reasons for the gap in life discrepancy between the United States and 12 comparable countries are motor vehicle accidents, firearm-related injuries, and drug poisonings and overdoses.[7]

Quality of life matters as much as quantity. Rather than focusing solely on life expectancy, experts are calculating healthy life expectancy (HALE), based on years lived without disease or disability. The average HALE for Americans is considerably shorter than their life expectancy: about 68 years.[8]

✓**check-in** How do you think your life expectancy and your healthy life expectancy (HALE) compare?

Healthy People 2020

Every decade since 1980, the U.S. Department of Health and Human Services (HHS) has published a comprehensive set of national public health objectives as part of the Healthy People Initiative. The government's vision is to create a society in which all people can live long, healthy lives. Its mission includes identifying nationwide health improvement priorities, increasing public awareness of health issues, and providing measurable objectives and goals.[9] These include:

- Eliminate preventable disease, disability, injury, and premature death.
- Achieve health equity, eliminate disparities, and improve the health of all groups.
- Create social and physical environments that promote good health for all.
- Promote healthy development and healthy behaviors across every stage of life.

✓**check-in** What are your personal health objectives?

Health Disparities

Americans who are members of certain racial and ethnic groups—including African Americans, American Indians, Alaska Natives, Asian Americans, Hispanics, Latinos, and Pacific Islanders—are more likely than whites to suffer disease and disability, including major depression, poor physical health, functional limitations, and premature death. However, there has been progress in some important areas, including less racial discrepancy in infant death rates, cesarean birth rates, and smoking among women.[10]

Genetic variations, environmental influences, and specific health behaviors contribute to health disparities, but poverty may be a more significant factor. A much higher percentage of blacks (26 percent) than non-Hispanic whites (10 percent) live below the federal poverty level and may be unable to get needed medical treatment.[11] This may be changing for young Americans. The expected lifespan for those under age 20 is less affected by whether they are rich or poor now than in the past.[12]

YOUR STRATEGIES FOR PREVENTION

If You Are at Risk

Certain health risks may be genetic, but behavior influences their impact. Here are specific steps you can take to protect your health:

- **Ask if you are at risk for any medical conditions or disorders based on your family history or racial or ethnic background.**

- **Find out if there are tests that could determine your risks.** Discuss the advantages and disadvantages of such testing with your doctor.

- **If you or a family member requires treatment for a chronic illness, ask your doctor whether any medications have proved particularly effective for your racial or ethnic background.**

- **If you are African American, you are significantly more likely to develop high blood pressure, diabetes, and kidney disease.** Being overweight or obese adds to the danger. The information in Chapters 6 through 8 can help you lower your risk by keeping in shape, making healthy food choices, and managing your weight.

- **Hispanics and Latinos have disproportionately high rates of respiratory problems, such as asthma, chronic obstructive lung disease, and tuberculosis.** To protect your lungs, stop smoking and avoid secondary smoke. Learn as much as you can about the factors that can trigger or worsen lung diseases.

If you are a member of a racial or ethnic minority, you need to educate yourself about your health risks, take responsibility for those within your control, and become a savvy, assertive consumer of health-care services. The federal Office of Minority Health and Health Disparities (www.cdc.gov/omhd), which provides general information and the latest research and recommendations, is a good place to start.

✓**check-in** Are you a member of a racial or ethnic minority? If so, do you think this status affects your health or health care?

Why Race Matters If, like many other Americans, you come from a racially mixed background, your health profile may be complex. Here are just some of the differences race makes[13]:

- Black Americans lose substantially more years of potential life to homicide (nine times as many), stroke (three times as many), and diabetes (three times as many) as whites.
- About 1 to 3 Hispanics has prediabetes; only about half of Hispanics with diabetes have it under control.[14]
- Caucasians are prone to osteoporosis (progressive weakening of bone tissue), cystic fibrosis, skin cancer, and phenylketonuria (PKU, a metabolic disorder that can lead to cognitive impairment).
- Native Americans, including those indigenous to Alaska, are more likely to die young than the population as a whole, primarily as a result of accidental injuries, cirrhosis of the liver, homicide, pneumonia, and complications of diabetes.
- The suicide rate among American Indians and Alaska Natives is 50 percent higher than the national rate. The rates of co-occurring mental illness and substance abuse (especially alcohol abuse) are also higher among Native American youth and adults.

Cancer Overall, black Americans are more likely to develop cancer than persons of any other racial or ethnic group.[15] As discussed in Chapter 10, medical scientists have debated whether the reason might be that treatments are less effective in blacks or whether many are not diagnosed early enough or treated rigorously enough.

Although blacks continue to have higher cancer death rates than whites, the disparity has narrowed for all cancers combined in men and women, and for lung and prostate cancers in men. However, the racial gap in death rates

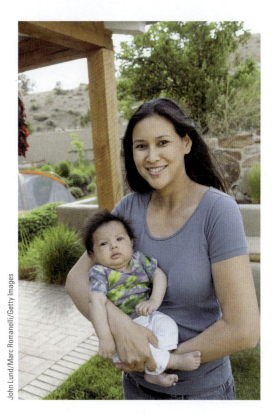

John Lund/Marc Romanelli/Getty Images

Heredity places this Pima Indian infant at higher risk of developing diabetes, but environmental factors also play a role.

has widened for breast cancer in women and remained level for colorectal cancer in men.[16]

- African American women are more than twice as likely to die of cervical cancer as are white women, and are more likely to die of breast cancer than are women of any racial or ethnic group except Native Hawaiians.
- Native Hawaiian women have the highest rates of breast cancer. Women from many racial minorities, including those of Filipino, Pakistani, Mexican, and Puerto Rican descent, are more likely to be diagnosed with late-stage breast cancer than white women.
- Cancer has surpassed heart disease as the leading cause of death among Hispanics in the United States.

Cardiovascular Disease Heart disease and stroke are the leading causes of death for all racial and ethnic groups in the United States, but mortality rates of death from these diseases are higher among African American adults than among white adults. African Americans also have higher rates of high blood pressure (hypertension), develop this problem earlier in life, suffer more severe hypertension, and have higher rates of stroke.

Diabetes American Indians and Alaska Natives, African Americans, and Hispanics are twice as likely to be diagnosed with diabetes as are non-Hispanic whites.

Infant Mortality African American, American Indian, and Puerto Rican infants have higher death rates than white infants.

Mental Health American Indians and Alaska Natives suffer disproportionately from depression and substance abuse. Minorities have less access to mental health services and are less likely to receive needed high-quality mental health services.[17] The prevalence of dementia varies significantly among Americans of different racial and ethnic groups, with the highest rates among blacks and American Indians/Alaskan Natives and the lowest among Asian Americans. Hispanics and whites have intermediate rates.[18]

Infectious Disease Asian Americans and Pacific Islanders have much higher rates of hepatitis B than other racial groups. Black teenagers and young adults become infected with hepatitis B three to four times more often than those who are white. Black people also have a higher incidence of hepatitis C infection than white people. Almost 80 percent of reported cases affect racial and ethnic minorities.

HIV and Sexually Transmitted Infections Although African Americans and Hispanics represent only about one-quarter of the U.S. population, they account for about two-thirds of adult AIDS cases and more than 80 percent of pediatric AIDS cases.[19]

Sex, Gender, and Health

Medical scientists define sex as a classification, generally as male or female, according to the reproductive organs and functions that derive from the chromosomal complement. *Gender* refers to a person's self-representation as male or female or how social institutions respond to a person on the basis of the individual's gender presentation. Gender is rooted in biology and shaped by environment and experience.

The experience of being male or female in a particular culture and society can and does have an effect on physical and psychological well-being. In fact, sex and gender may have a greater impact than any other variable on how our bodies function, how long we live, and the symptoms, course, and treatment of the diseases that strike us (see Figure 1.1).

Here are some health differences between men and women:

- Boys are more likely to be born prematurely, to suffer birth-related injuries, and to die before their first birthdays than girls.

- Men around the world have shorter lifespans than women and higher rates of cancer, heart disease, stroke, lung disease, kidney disease, liver disease, and HIV/AIDS.[20] They are four times more likely to take their own lives or to be murdered than women.

- Cardiovascular disease is the leading cause of death for women in the United States, yet

He:

- averages 12 breaths a minute
- has lower core body temperature
- has a slower heart rate
- has more oxygen-rich hemoglobin in his blood
- is more sensitive to sound
- produces twice as much saliva
- has a 10 percent larger brain
- is 10 times more likely to have attention deficit disorder
- as a teen, has an attention span of 5 minutes
- is more likely to be physically active
- is more prone to lethal diseases, including heart attacks, cancer, and liver failure
- is five times more likely to become an alcoholic
- has a life expectancy of 76.2 years

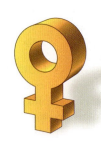

She:

- averages 9 breaths a minute
- has higher core body temperature
- has a faster heart rate
- has higher levels of protective immunoglobulin in her blood
- is more sensitive to light
- takes twice as long to process food
- has more neurons in certain brain regions
- is twice as likely to have an eating disorder
- as a teen, has an attention span of 20 minutes
- is more likely to be overweight
- is more vulnerable to chronic diseases, like arthritis and autoimmune disorders, and age-related conditions like osteoporosis
- is twice as likely to develop depression
- has a life expectancy of 81.1 years

FIGURE 1.1 Some of the Many Ways Men and Women Are Different

only about one-third of clinical trial subjects in cardiovascular research have been female.

- Lung cancer is the leading cause of cancer death among women, with increased rates particularly among young female nonsmokers.
- Women are 70 percent more likely than men to suffer from depression over the course of their lifetimes.

✓**check-in** How do you think your gender affects your health?

Among the reasons that may contribute to the health and longevity gap between the sexes are the following:

- **Biological factors.** For example, women have two X chromosomes and men only one, and men and women have different levels of sex hormones (particularly testosterone and estrogen).
- **Social factors.** These include work stress, hostility levels, and social networks and supports.
- **Behavioral factors.** Men and women differ in risky behavior, aggression, violence, smoking, and substance abuse.
- **Health habits.** The sexes vary in terms of regular screenings, preventive care, and minimizing symptoms.

Sexual orientation can also affect health. LGBTQIA (lesbian, gay, bisexual, transgender, queer or questioning, intersex, and asexual) individuals are more likely to encounter health disparities linked to social stigma, discrimination, and denial of their human and civil rights.[21] Gender-based discrimination increases the risk of psychiatric disorders, substance abuse, and suicide. On campus, transgender students may face similar issues, as well as particular stigma over so-called bathroom bills that require them to use public facilities corresponding with the sex designated on their birth certificates.[22] The *Healthy People 2020* initiative has made improvements in LGBTQIA health one of its new goals.

Health on Campus

As one of an estimated 19.9 million college students in the United States, you are part of a remarkably diverse group. Today's undergraduates come from every age group and social, racial, ethnic, economic, political, and religious background. Some 12 million are female; 9 million, male. You may have served in the military, started a family, or emigrated from another country. You might be enrolled in a two-year college, a four-year university, or a technical school. Your classrooms might be in a busy city or a small town—or they might exist solely as a virtual campus. Although the majority of undergraduates are "traditional" age (between 18 and 24 years), more of you than ever before—8 million—are over age 25.[23]

Today's college students are both similar to and different from previous generations in many ways. Among the unique characteristics of current traditional-age undergraduates are the following:

- They are the first generation of "digital natives," who've grown up in a wired world.
- They are the most diverse in higher education history. About 15 percent are black; an equal percentage are Hispanic.
- They are both more connected and more isolated than their predecessors, with a "tribe" of friends, family, and acquaintances in constant contact through social media but with weak interpersonal, communications, and problem-solving skills.
- More students are working, working longer hours, taking fewer credits, requiring more time to graduate, and leaving college with large student loan debts.
- They face a future in which the pace and scale of change will constantly accelerate.

✓**check-in** A recent analysis of community college students identified four types of undergraduates: dreamers, drifters, passengers, and planners. Here is some specific advice for each type:
- If you're a dreamer, seek guidance to fill in the details of your "big picture" goal for college.
- If you're a drifter, focus on developing specific strategies to reach your educational goals.
- If you're a passenger, find a mentor or advisor to help you interpret what you learn.
- If you're a planner, look for help in applying the information you've gathered to your unique situation.[24]

College and Health

Although the words "college health" often appear together, they are, in fact, two different things that profoundly influence each other. Healthier students get better grades and are more likely to graduate. A college education boosts health status, income, and community engagement later in life.[25] Yet the transition from high school to college is considered an at-risk period for health and healthy behaviors.

As studies in both the United States and Europe have documented, from their final year of high school to the second year of college, students are likely to:

- Gain weight, generally an average of 6 pounds.
- Cut back on their participation in sports—perhaps because they move away from local teams or they lack free time.
- Decrease some sedentary behaviors, such as streaming videos and playing computer games, but increase others, such as social media and studying.
- Eat fewer fruits and vegetables.
- Consume more alcohol.[26]

Although healthier than individuals of the same age who are not attending college, undergraduates have significant health issues that can affect their overall well-being and ability to perform well in an academic environment[27]:

- More than half report common acute illnesses, such as colds and flus, that interfere with their studies.
- A significant proportion report symptoms of depression, anxiety, and other mental disorders.
- For many, poor sleep has an impact on academic performance.
- They are more likely to use alcohol and drugs than nonstudents their age.
- College students experience higher rates of interpersonal violence.
- On the positive side, college students are less likely to be overweight or obese, to smoke, to consume high-fat and low-fiber foods, to have high cholesterol levels, and to engage in high-risk sexual behavior than young adults who are not attending college.
- Compared to those at four-year colleges, students at community colleges and technical schools are less likely to binge-drink but more likely to speed, consume more sodas, and report lower family satisfaction.[28]

College represents a rite of passage, when undergraduates typically engage in "adult" behaviors such as drinking, getting involved in intimate relationships, and taking personal responsibility for health behaviors (e.g., sleep schedules and nutrition) that their parents may have previously supervised. Students cramming for a big exam may decide not to sleep and accept the short-term consequences on their health. Others, thinking ahead to future goals, may consciously choose to avoid behaviors, such as unsafe sex or drug use, that may jeopardize their plans.

✓**check-in** Do you feel that today's undergraduates face unique pressures that can take a toll on physical and psychological health?

How Healthy Are Today's Students?

In the American College Health Association's National College Health Assessment (ACHA-NCHA) survey, about half of college students—54.9 percent of men and 45 percent of women—rate their health as very good or excellent (see Snapshot: On Campus Now).[29] Here are some details about the health and habits of undergraduates:

- Forty percent of undergraduates have a body mass index (BMI) indicating they are overweight or obese (see Chapter 6).[30]
- Fewer than half (46.2 percent) of undergraduates get the recommended amounts of physical activity (see Chapter 7).[31]
- Of those engaging in vaginal intercourse, about half of college men report having used a condom most of the time or always (see Chapter 9).[32]
- About half of students report drinking alcohol at least once in the previous month; twenty percent report having consumed five or more drinks in a single sitting at least once within the past 2 weeks (see Chapter 16).[33]
- About 5 percent smoked a cigarette at least once in the past month. A growing number are trying e-cigarettes, which they perceive as less risky and addictive than conventional cigarettes, but which increase the likelihood of cigarette smoking (see Chapter 17).
- One in five used marijuana in the previous month (see Chapter 15).[34]
- Many undergraduates use prescription stimulants because they believe the drugs can

Student Health

Percentage of students who describe their health as good, very good, or excellent:

Men	Women	Average
85.2	81.9	82.4

Top Ten Health Problems	Percent
1. Allergies	19.2
2. Sinus infection	15.2
3. Back pain	13.2
4. Strep throat	9.6
5. Urinary tract infection	10.2
6. Asthma	9.5
7. Migraine headache	9.5
8. Ear infection	6.8
9. Broken bone/fracture/sprain	5.8
10. Bronchitis	5.6

Proportion of college students who reported being diagnosed or treated for these health problems in the past year.

Source: American College Health Association. American College Health Association-National College Health Assessment II: Undergraduate Student Reference Group Executive Summary. Hanover, MD: American College Health Association; Spring 2018.

provide academic benefits, but longitudinal studies have found no detectable improvements in grades[35] (see Chapter 15).

- In a recent sample of college students, 9.5 percent reported misuse of prescription opioid drugs at some time in their lives, primarily to relieve physical or emotional pain, "feel good/get high," or experiment[36] (see Chapter 15).

- Only 11 percent of students say they get enough sleep to feel rested in the morning 6 or more days a week; 12 percent never feel rested (see Chapter 2).

- College athletes have lower health-related quality of life than their same-age peers who did not or no longer play college sports.[37]

- About one in three undergraduates have been tested for HIV in the past year.

✓**check-in** How do you think your current health behaviors may affect your future?

Colleges and universities have tried various interventions to improve students' health choices and habits. Do they work? In a meta-analysis of 41 studies, most conducted in the United States, 34 yielded significant improvements in one of several key outcomes, including the following:

- **Physical activity:** more steps per day, more time in vigorous and/or moderate exercise, greater maximum oxygen consumption, and improved muscle strength, endurance, and flexibility.

- **Nutrition:** lower calorie intake, more fruits and vegetables, reduced fat consumption, more macronutrients, and better overall diet quality.

- **Weight:** improved weight, lower body fat, and healthier waist circumference and waist-to-hip ratio.

The most effective interventions spanned a semester or less, targeted only nutrition rather than multiple behaviors, and were imbedded within college courses. As the researchers

- To lower your risk of heart disease, get your blood pressure and cholesterol checked. Don't smoke. Stay at a healthy weight. Exercise regularly.

- To lower your risks of major diseases, get regular check-ups. Make sure you are immunized against infectious illnesses.

- To lower your risks of substance abuse and related illnesses and injuries, don't drink, or limit how much you drink. Avoid illegal drugs.

- To lower your risk of sexually transmitted infections or unwanted pregnancy, abstain from sex. If you engage in sexual activities, protect yourself with contraceptives, condoms, and spermicides.

- To prevent car accidents, stay off the road in hazardous circumstances, such as bad weather. Wear a seat belt when you drive and use defensive driving techniques.

Identify your top preventive health priority—lowering your risk of heart disease, for instance, or avoiding accidents. Write down a single action you can take this week that will reduce your health risks. As soon as you take this step, write a brief reflection in your online journal.

social norm A behavior or an attitude that a particular group expects, values, and enforces.

prevention Information and support offered to help healthy people identify their health risks, reduce stressors, prevent potential medical problems, and enhance their well-being.

protection Measures that an individual can take when participating in risky behavior to prevent injury or unwanted risks.

noted, "Universities and colleges are an ideal setting for implementation of health promotion programs." Why?

- They reach a large student population during a crucial life transition.

- They offer access to world-class facilities, technology, and highly educated staff in various health disciplines.

- They reach young adults at an age "where health behaviors that impact on health later in life can be provided."[38]

The Future Starts Now

The choices you make today have an immediate impact on how you feel as well as long-term consequences, including the following:

- Individuals who begin using tobacco or alcohol in their teens and 20s are more likely to continue to do so as they get older.

- Obese children often grow into obese adolescents and obese adults, with ever-increasing risks of diabetes and cardiovascular disease.

- People in their 20s who have even mildly elevated blood pressure face an increased risk of clogged heart arteries by middle age.

- Young adults who acquire an STI may jeopardize both their future fertility and their health.

At any age, health risks are not inevitable. As recent research has shown, young adults with high aerobic fitness (discussed in Chapter 7) have a reduced risk of cardiovascular disease later in life.[39] Simple steps such as those listed in Health Now! can get you started in the right direction now!

Student Health Norms

Psychologists use the term *norm*, or **social norm**, to refer to a behavior or an attitude that a particular group expects, values, and enforces. Norms influence a wide variety of human activities, including health habits. However, perceptions of social norms are often inaccurate. Only anonymous responses to a scientifically designed questionnaire can reveal what individuals really do—the actual social norms—as compared to what they may say they do to gain social approval.

Undergraduates are particularly likely to misjudge what their peers are—and aren't—doing. In recent years, colleges have found that publicizing research data on behaviors such as drinking, smoking, and drug use helps students get a more accurate sense of the real health norms on campus.

The gap between students' misperceptions and accurate health norms can be enormous. For example, undergraduates in the ACHA survey estimate that only 13 percent of students had never smoked cigarettes. In fact, 70 percent never had. Students guessed that only 4 percent of their peers never drank alcohol. In reality, 21 percent never did.[40] Providing accurate information on drinking norms on campus has proven effective in changing students' perceptions and in reducing alcohol consumption by both men and women.

✓**check-in** Do you think your peers have better or worse health habits than you?

The Promise of Prevention

Although you may think you are too young to worry about serious health conditions, many chronic problems begin early in life:

- Two percent of college-age women already have osteoporosis, a bone-weakening disease; another 15 percent have osteopenia, a low bone density that puts them at risk of osteoporosis.

- Many college students have several risk factors for heart disease, including high blood pressure and high cholesterol. Others increase their risk by eating a high-fat diet and not exercising regularly. The time to change is now.

No medical treatment, however successful or sophisticated, can compare with the power of **prevention**. Two out of every three deaths and 1 in 3 hospitalizations in the United States could be prevented by changes in six main risk factors: tobacco use, alcohol abuse, accidents, high blood pressure, obesity, and gaps in screening and primary health care.

Prevention remains the best weapon against cancer and heart disease. One of its greatest successes has come from the antismoking campaign, which in the past 40 years has prevented 8 million premature deaths in the United States, giving these ex-smokers an average of nearly 20 additional years of life.[41]

Protecting Yourself

There is a great deal of overlap between prevention and **protection**. Some people might think of immunizations as a way of preventing illness; others see them as a form of protection against dangerous diseases. Unfortunately, many adults are not getting the immunizations they need—and are putting their health in jeopardy as a result. (See Chapter 10 to find out which vaccinations you should receive.)

You can prevent STIs or unwanted pregnancy by abstaining from sex. But if you decide to engage in sexual activities, you can protect yourself with condoms and spermicides. Similarly, you can prevent many automobile accidents by not driving when road conditions are hazardous. But if you do have to drive, you can protect yourself by wearing a seat belt and using defensive driving techniques.

✓**check-in** What steps are you taking to protect your health?

Informing Yourself

More than ever, consumers need clear, concise, and accurate information, not just on specific health conditions but also on factors such as the effectiveness of a particular treatment. By learning how to maintain your health, evaluate medical information, and spot early signs of a problem, you are more likely to get the best possible care.

✓**check-in** Where do you turn for health information?

Which sources do you consider the most reliable?

Evaluating Online Health Information

Millions of Americans turn to the Internet to diagnose health problems. If you go online for medical information, here are some guidelines for evaluating websites:

- Check the creator. Websites are produced by health agencies, health support groups, school health programs, health product advertisers, health educators, and health education organizations. Read site headers and footers carefully to distinguish biased commercial advertisements from unbiased sites created by scientists and health agencies.
- If you are looking for the most recent research, check the date the page was created and last updated, as well as the links. Several nonworking links signal that the site isn't carefully maintained or updated.

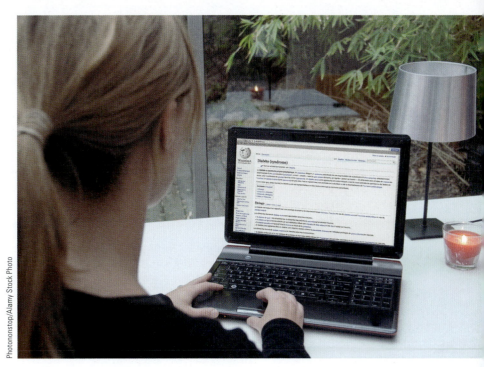

Photononstop/Alamy Stock Photo

- Check the references. As with other health education materials, Web documents should provide the reader with references. Unreferenced suggestions may be scientifically unsound and possibly unsafe.
- Consider the author. Is the author recognized in the field of health education or otherwise qualified to publish a health-information Web document? Does the author list his or her occupation, experience, and education?
- Look for possible bias. Websites may attempt to provide health information to consumers, but they also may attempt to sell a product. Many sites are merely disguised advertisements. (See Table 1.1 for physician-endorsed websites.)

✓**check-in** Which websites have you used to find health information? Which ones do you trust?

Which ones don't you trust?

Getting Medical Facts Straight
Cure! Breakthrough! Medical miracle! When you see headlines like these, keep in mind that although medical breakthroughs do occur, most scientific progress is made one small step at a time. Rather than trust the most recent report or the hottest trend, try to gather as much background information and as many opinions as you can.

When reading a newspaper or magazine story or listening to a radio or television report about a

Millions of Americans go online to learn about medical problems and treatments and to chat with others who have similar conditions.

TABLE 1.1 Doctor-Recommended Websites

National Library of Medicine: MedlinePlus	(www.nlm.nih.gov/medlineplus/)
MedlinePlus contains links to information on hundreds of health conditions and issues. The site also includes a medical dictionary, an encyclopedia with pictures and diagrams, and links to physician directories.	
FDA Center for Drug Evaluation and Research	(www.fda.gov)
Click on Drugs@FDA for information on approved prescription drugs and some over-the-counter medications.	
WebMD	(www.webmd.com)
WebMD is full of information to help you manage your health. The site's quizzes and calculators are a fun way to test your medical knowledge. Get diet tips, find information on drugs and herbs, and check out special sections on men's and women's health.	
Mayo Clinic	(www.mayoclinic.com)
The renowned Mayo Clinic offers a one-stop health resource website. Use the site's Health Decision Guides to make decisions about prevention and treatment. Learn more about complementary and alternative medicine, sports medicine, and senior health in the Healthy Living Centers.	
Centers for Disease Control and Prevention	(www.cdc.gov)
Stay up to date on the latest public health news and get the CDC's recommendations on travelers' health, vaccines and immunizations, and protecting your health in case of a disaster.	
Medscape	(www.medscape.com)
Medscape delivers news and research specifically tailored to your medical interests. The site requires (free) registration.	

medical advance, look for answers to the following questions:

- Who are the researchers? Are they recognized, legitimate health professionals? What are their credentials? Are they affiliated with respected medical or scientific institutions? Be wary of individuals whose degrees or affiliations are from institutions you've never heard of, and be sure that a person's educational background is in a discipline related to the area of research reported.

- Where did the researchers report their findings? The best research is published in peer-reviewed professional journals, such as the *New England Journal of Medicine and the Journal of the American Medical Association*. Research findings also may be reported at meetings of professional societies.

- Is the information based on personal observations? Does the report include testimonials from cured patients or satisfied customers? If the answer to either question is yes, be wary.

- Does the article, report, or advertisement include words like "amazing," "secret," or "quick"? Does it claim to be something the public has never seen or been offered before? Such sensationalized language is often a tipoff that the treatment is dubious.

- Is someone trying to sell you something? Manufacturers that cite studies to sell a product may embellish the truth. Although they may sound scientific, direct-to- consumer advertisements for medications, treatments, hospitals, and health-care providers are well-packaged sales pitches.[42]

- Does the information defy all common sense? Be skeptical. If something sounds too good to be true, it probably is.

Understanding Risky Behaviors

Today's students face different—and potentially deadlier—risks than undergraduates did a generation or two ago. The problem is not that students who engage in risky behavior feel invulnerable or do not know the danger. Young people, according to recent research, actually overestimate the risk of some outcomes. However, they also overestimate the benefit of immediate pleasure when, for instance, engaging in unsafe sex, and they underestimate the negative consequences, such as an STI.

College-age men are more likely than women to engage in risky behaviors—to use drugs and alcohol, to have unprotected sex, and to drive

$ HEALTH ON A BUDGET

Invest in Yourself

Trying to save money in the short term by doing without needed health care can cost you a great deal—financially and physically—in the long term. Here are some ways to keep medical costs down without sacrificing your good health:

- **Stay healthy**. Use this book to learn the basics of a healthy lifestyle and then live accordingly. By eating nutritiously, exercising, getting enough sleep, not smoking, and getting regular immunizations, you'll reduce your risk of conditions that require expensive treatments.

- **Build a good relationship with a primary care physician**. Although your choices may be limited, try to schedule appointments with the same doctor. A physician who knows you, your history, and your concerns can give you the best advice on staying healthy.

- **Don't go to a specialist without consulting your primary care provider**, who can help you avoid overtesting and duplicate treatments.

- **If you need a prescription, ask if a generic form is available**. Brand names cost more, and most insurers charge higher copayments for them.

- **Take medications as prescribed**. Skipping doses or cutting pills in two may seem like easy ways to save money, but you may end up spending more for additional care because the treatment won't be as effective.

- **Don't go to an emergency department unless absolutely necessary**. Call your doctor for advice or go to the student health service. Emergency departments are overburdened with caring for the very ill and for injured people, and their services are expensive.

dangerously. Men are also more likely to be hospitalized for injuries and to commit suicide. Three-fourths of the deaths in the 15- to 24-year-old age range are men.

Drinking has long been part of college life and, despite efforts across U.S. college campuses to curb alcohol abuse, two out of five students engage in binge drinking—consumption of five or more drinks at a single session for men or four for women. Heavy drinking increases the likelihood of other risky behaviors, such as smoking cigarettes, using drugs, and having multiple sexual partners. New trends, such as drinking caffeinated alcoholic beverages and vaping (Chapter 12) and using dangerous stimulants called "bath salts" (Chapter 11), present new risks.

✓**check-in** What is the greatest health risk you've ever taken?

Making Healthy Changes

If you would like to improve your health behavior, you have to realize that change isn't easy. Between 40 and 80 percent of those who try to kick bad health habits lapse back into their unhealthy ways within 6 weeks (see Health on a Budget). Fortunately, our understanding of change has itself changed. Thanks to decades of research, we now know what sets the stage for change, the way change progresses, and the keys to lasting change. We also know that personal change is neither mysterious nor magical but rather a methodical science that anyone can master.

✓**check-in** What health-related change would you like to make?

Understanding Health Behavior

Three types of influences shape behavior: predisposing, enabling, and reinforcing factors (Figure 1.2).

Predisposing Factors **Predisposing factors** include knowledge, attitudes, beliefs, values, and perceptions. Unfortunately, knowledge isn't enough to cause most people to change their behavior; for example, people fully aware of the grim consequences of smoking often continue to puff away. Nor is attitude—one's likes and dislikes—sufficient; an individual may dislike the smell and taste of cigarettes but continue to smoke anyway.

Beliefs are more powerful than knowledge and attitudes, and researchers report that people

predisposing factors The beliefs, values, attitudes, knowledge, and perceptions that influence our behavior.

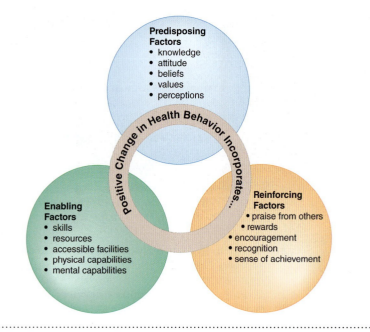

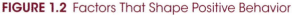

FIGURE 1.2 Factors That Shape Positive Behavior

A decision to change a health behavior should stem from a permanent, personal goal, not from a desire to please or impress someone else. If you lose weight for the homecoming dance, you're almost sure to regain pounds afterward. But if you shed extra pounds because you want to feel better about yourself or get into shape, you're far more likely to keep off the weight.

✓**check-in** What goal would motivate you to change?

How People Change

Change can simply happen. You get older. You put on or lose weight. You have an accident. Intentional change is different: A person consciously, deliberately sets out either to change a negative behavior, such as chronic procrastination, or to initiate a healthy behavior, such as daily exercise. For decades, psychologists have studied how people intentionally change, and have developed various models that reveal the anatomy of change.

In the *moral model*, you take responsibility for a problem (such as smoking) and its solution; success depends on adequate motivation, while failure is seen as a sign of character weakness. In the *enlightenment model*, you submit to strict discipline to correct a problem; this is the approach used in Alcoholics Anonymous. The *behavioral model* involves rewarding yourself when you make positive changes. The *medical model* sees the behavior as caused by forces beyond your control (e.g., a genetic predisposition to being overweight) and employs an expert to provide advice or treatment. For many people, the most effective approach is the *compensatory model*, which doesn't assign blame but puts responsibility on individuals to acquire whatever skills or power they need to overcome their problems.

Health Belief Model Psychologists developed the **health belief model (HBM)** about 50 years ago to explain and predict health behaviors by focusing on the attitudes and beliefs of individuals. (Remember that your attitudes and beliefs are predisposing influences on your capacity for change.) According to this model, people will take a health-related action (e.g., use condoms) if they:

- Feel susceptible to a possible negative consequence, such as a sexually transmitted infection (STI).

are most likely to change health behavior if they hold three beliefs:

- **Susceptibility.** They acknowledge that they are at risk for the negative consequences of their behavior.

- **Severity.** They believe that they may pay a very high price if they don't make a change.

- **Benefits.** They believe that the proposed change will be advantageous in some way. For example, they may quit smoking primarily for their health or for social acceptance, depending on their attitudes and self-esteem.[43]

Enabling Factors

Enabling factors include skills, resources, accessible facilities, and physical and mental capacities. Before you initiate a change, assess the means available to reach your goal. No matter how motivated you are, you'll become frustrated if you keep encountering obstacles. Breaking down a task or goal into step-by-step strategies is very important in behavioral change.

Reinforcing Factors

Reinforcing factors may be praise from family members and friends, rewards from teachers or parents, or encouragement and recognition for meeting a goal. Although these help a great deal in the short run, lasting change depends not on external rewards but on an internal commitment and sense of achievement. To make a difference, reinforcement must come from within.

enabling factors The skills, resources, and physical and mental capabilities that shape our behavior.

reinforcing factors Rewards, encouragement, and recognition that influence our behavior in the short run.

health belief model (HBM) A model of behavioral change that focuses on the individual's attitudes and beliefs.

- Perceive the consequence as serious or dangerous.
- Think that a particular action (using a condom) will reduce or eliminate the threat (of STIs).
- Feel that they can take the necessary action without difficulty or negative consequences.
- Believe that they can successfully do what's necessary—for example, use condoms comfortably and confidently.

Readiness to act on health beliefs, in this model, depends on how vulnerable individuals feel, how severe they perceive the danger to be, the benefits they expect to gain, and the barriers they think they will encounter. Another key factor is self-efficacy, confidence in their ability to take action.

In a study that tested the relationship between college students' health beliefs and cancer self-examinations, women were more likely to examine their breasts than men were to perform testicular exams. However, students of both sexes were more likely to do self-exams if they felt susceptible to developing cancer, if they felt comfortable and confident doing so, and if they were given a cue to action (such as a recommendation by a health professional).[44]

Self-Determination Theory
This approach, developed several decades ago by psychologists Edward Deci and Richard Ryan, focuses on whether an individual lacks motivation, is externally motivated, or is intrinsically motivated. Someone who is "amotivated" does not value an activity, such as exercise, or does not believe it will lead to a desired outcome, such as more energy or lower weight. Individuals who are externally motivated may engage in an activity like exercise to gain a reward or avoid a negative consequence (such as a loved one's nagging). Some people are motivated by a desired outcome; for instance, they might exercise for the sake of better health or longer life. Behavior becomes self-determined when someone engages in it for its own sake, such as exercising because it's fun.

Numerous studies have evaluated self-determination as it relates to health behavior. In research on exercise, individuals with greater self-determined motivation are less likely to stop exercising; they have stronger intentions to continue exercise, higher physical self-worth, and lower social anxiety related to their physique.

Motivational Interviewing
Health professionals, counselors, and coaches use motivational interviewing, developed by psychologists William Miller and Stephen Rollnick, to inspire individuals, regardless of their enthusiasm for

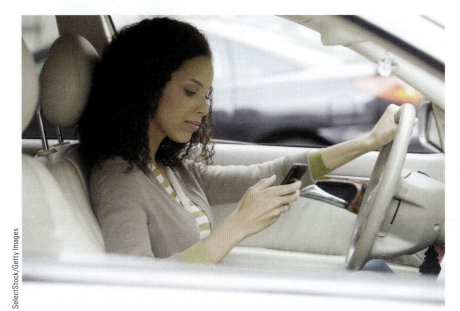

SelectStock/Getty Images

change, to move toward improvements that could make their lives better. The U.S. Public Health Service, based on its assessment of current research, recommends motivational interviewing as an effective way to increase all tobacco users' willingness to quit. Building a collaborative partnership, the therapist does not persuade directly but uses empathy and respect for the patient's perspective to evoke recognition of the desirability of change.

Self-Affirmation Theory
Affirmations, discussed in Chapter 2, can improve integrity, problem solving, self-worth, and self-regulation. They are also effective in encouraging behavioral change. According to self-affirmation theory, thinking about core personal values, important personal strengths, or valued relationships can provide reassurance and reinforce self-worth. Repeating an affirmation is one of the fastest ways to restructure thought patterns, develop new pathways in the brain, and make individuals less defensive about changing health behaviors.[45]

Recent neuroimaging studies have revealed how self-affirmations may increase the effectiveness of many health interventions. Using functional magnetic resonance imaging (fMRI), scientists were able to visualize changes in the brains of volunteers as they were reciting affirmations in their minds. These internal messages produced more activity in a region of the brain associated with positive responses.[46]

✓**check-in** Some common self-affirmations are "I am strong" and "I can handle this challenge."

Your stated knowledge-based belief may be that distracted driving can cause accidents. Your actual belief is that it won't happen to you.

What would you say to yourself to encourage a behavioral change?

Transtheoretical Model Psychologist James Prochaska and his colleagues, by tracking what they considered to be universal stages in the successful recovery of drug addicts and alcoholics, developed a way of thinking about change that cuts across psychological theories. Their **transtheoretical model** focuses on universal aspects of an individual's decision-making process rather than on social or biological influences on behavior.

The transtheoretical model has become the foundation of programs for smoking cessation, exercise, healthy food choices, alcohol cessation, weight control, condom use, drug use cessation, mammography screening, and stress management. Recent studies have demonstrated that it is more effective in encouraging weight loss than physical activity.[47]

The following sections describe these key components of the transtheoretical model:

- **Stages of change**—a sequence of stages to make a change.

- **Processes of change**—cognitive and behavioral activities that facilitate change.

- **Self-efficacy and locus of control**—the confidence people have in their ability to cope with challenge.

transtheoretical model A model of behavioral change that focuses on the individual's decision making; it states that an individual progresses through a sequence of six stages as he or she makes a change in behavior.

The Stages of Change. According to the transtheoretical model of change, individuals progress through a sequence of stages as they make a change (Figure 1.3). No one stage is more important than another, and people often move back and forth between them. Most people "spiral" from stage to stage, slipping from maintenance to contemplation or from action to precontemplation, before moving forward again.

People usually cycle and recycle through the stages several times. Smokers, for instance, report making three or four serious efforts to quit before they succeed.

The six stages of change are as follows:

1. **Precontemplation.** You are at this stage if you, as yet, have no intention of making a change. You are vaguely uncomfortable, but this is where your grasp of what is going on ends. You may never think about exercise, for instance, until you notice that it's harder to zip up your jeans or that you get winded walking up stairs. Still, you don't quite register the need to do anything about it.

   During precontemplation, change remains hypothetical, distant, and vague. Yet you may speak of something bugging you and wish that things were somehow different.

2. **Contemplation.** In this stage, you still prefer not to have to change, but you start to realize that you can't avoid reality. Maybe none of your jeans fit anymore, or you feel sluggish and listless. In this stage, you may alternate between wanting to take action and resisting it.

✓**check-in** Are you contemplating change? You may be if you find yourself thinking

- "I hate it that I keep…"
- "I should…"
- "Maybe I'll do it someday—not tomorrow, but someday."

3. **Preparation.** At some point, you stop waffling, make a clear decision, and feel a burst of energy. This decision heralds the preparation stage. You gather information, make phone calls, do research online, and look into exercise classes at the gym. You begin to think and act with change specifically in mind. If you were to eavesdrop on what you're saying to yourself, you would hear statements such as, "I am going to do this."

4. **Action.** You are actively modifying your behavior according to your plan. Your resolve is strong, and you know you're on your way to a better you. You may be getting up 15 minutes earlier to make time for a healthy breakfast or to walk to class rather than take the shuttle. In a relatively short time, you acquire a sense of comfort and ease with the change in your life.

5. **Maintenance.** This stabilizing stage, which follows the flurry of specific steps taken in the

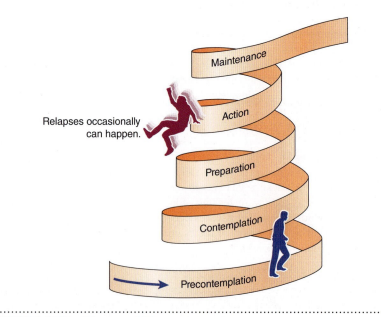

Relapses occasionally can happen.

action stage, is absolutely necessary to retain what you've worked for and to make change permanent. In this stage, you strengthen, enhance, and extend the changes you've initiated. Among college students, those in the maintenance stage of an exercise program display greater self-motivation to work out and a greater engagement in the experience.[48]

6. **Relapse.** It's not unusual for people to slip backward at any stage. However, a relapse is simply a pause, an opportunity to regroup and regain your footing so you can keep moving forward. After about two to five years, a behavior becomes so deeply ingrained that you can't imagine abandoning it.

Research on college students has shown that attitudes and feelings are related to stages of change. Smokers who believe that continuing to smoke would have only a minor or no impact on their health remain in the precontemplation stage; those with respiratory symptoms move on to contemplation and preparation.

✓**check-in** Do you want to change a health behavior? If so, what stage of change are you in?

The Processes of Change. Anything you do to modify your thinking, feeling, or behavior can be called a *change process*. The processes of change included in the transtheoretical model are as follows:

- **Consciousness-raising.** This most widely used change process involves increasing knowledge about yourself or the nature of your problem. As you learn more, you gain understanding and feedback about your behavior.

    Example: Reading Chapter 5 on making healthy food choices.

- **Social liberation.** In this process, you take advantage of alternatives in the external environment that can help you begin or continue your efforts to change.

    Example: Spending as much time as possible in nonsmoking areas.

- **Emotional arousal.** This process, also known as dramatic relief, works on a deeper level than consciousness-raising and is equally important in the early stages of change. Emotional arousal means experiencing and expressing feelings about a problem behavior and its potential solutions.

    Example: Resolving never to drink and drive after the death of a friend in a car accident.

- **Self-reevaluation.** This process requires a thoughtful reappraisal of your problem, including an assessment of the person you might be once you have changed the behavior.

    Example: Recognizing that you have a gambling problem and imagining yourself as a nongambler.

- **Commitment.** In this process, you acknowledge—first privately and then publicly—that you are responsible for your behavior and are the only one who can change it.

    Example: Joining a self-help or support group.

- **Rewards.** In this process, you reinforce positive behavioral changes with self-praise or small gifts.

    Example: Getting a massage after a month of consistent exercise.

- **Countering.** Countering, or counterconditioning, involves substituting healthy behaviors for unhealthy ones.

    Example: Chewing gum rather than smoking.

- **Environmental control.** This is an action-oriented process in which you restructure your environment so you are less likely to engage in a problem behavior.

    Example: Getting rid of your stash of sweets.

- **Helping relationships.** In this process, you recruit individuals—family, friends, therapist, coach—to provide support, caring, understanding, and acceptance.

    Example: Finding an exercise buddy.

Self-Efficacy and Locus of Control. Do you see yourself as master of your fate, asserting control over your destiny? Or do so many things happen in your life that you just hang on and hope for the best? The answers to these questions reveal two important characteristics that affect your health: your sense of **self-efficacy** (the belief in your ability to change and to reach a goal) and your **locus of control** (the sense of being in control of your life).

Your confidence in your ability to cope with challenge can determine whether you can and will succeed in making a change. In his research on self-efficacy, psychologist Albert Bandura of

self-efficacy Belief in one's ability to accomplish a goal or change a behavior.

locus of control An individual's belief about the sources of power and influence over his or her life.

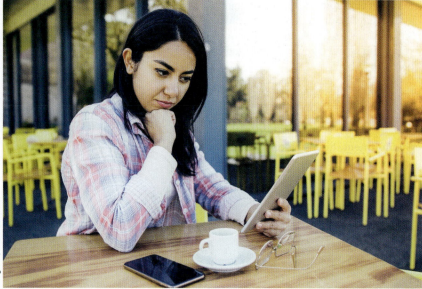

Do you picture yourself as master of your own destiny? You are more likely to achieve your health goals if you do.

begin an exercise program, those with lower self-efficacy are more likely to drop out.

✓**check-in** How "internal" or "external" do you rate your locus of control?

If you believe that your actions will make a difference in your health, your locus of control is internal. If you believe that external forces or factors play a greater role, your locus of control is external. Hundreds of studies have compared people who have these different perceptions of control:

- "Internals," who believe that their actions largely determine what happens to them, act more independently, enjoy better health, are more optimistic about their future, and have lower mortality rates.

- "Externals," who perceive that chance or outside forces determine their fate, find it harder to cope with stress and feel increasingly helpless over time. When it comes to weight, for instance, they see themselves as destined to be fat. However, social support has proven effective in helping students meet physical activity guidelines, particularly for muscle-strengthening workouts.[49]

Stanford University found that the individuals most likely to reach a goal are those who believe they can. The stronger their faith in themselves, the more energy and persistence they put into making a change. The opposite is also true, especially for health behaviors: Among people who

WHAT DID YOU DECIDE?

- What does "health" mean to you?
- How healthy are today's college students?
- Can you believe health information you find online?
- Can people successfully change their health behaviors?

Reflection

Consider how your answers changed after reading this chapter. Identify one way you might apply what you've learned about health in your daily life—starting now.

TAKING CHARGE OF YOUR HEALTH

Making Healthy Changes

Ultimately, you have more control over your health than anyone else. Use this course as an opportunity to zero in on at least one less-than-healthful behavior and improve it. Here are some suggestions for small steps that can have a big payoff. Check those that you commit to making today, this week, this month, or this term. Indicate "t," "w," "m," or "term," and repeat this self-evaluation throughout the course.

____ **Use seat belts.** In the past decade, seat belts have saved more than 40,000 lives and prevented millions of injuries.

____ **Eat an extra fruit or vegetable every day.** Adding more fruits and vegetables to your diet can improve your digestion and lower your risk of several cancers.

____ **Get enough sleep.** A good night's rest provides the energy you need to make it through the following day.

____ **Take regular stress breaks.** A few quiet minutes spent stretching, looking out the window, or simply letting yourself unwind are good for body and soul.

____ **Lose a pound.** If you're overweight, you may not think a pound will make a difference, but it's a step in the right direction.

____ **If you're a woman, examine your breasts regularly.** Get in the habit of performing a breast self-examination every month after your period (when breasts are least swollen or tender).

____ If you're a man, **examine your testicles regularly.** These simple self-exams can help you spot signs of cancer early, when it is most likely to be cured.

____ **Get physical.** Just a little exercise will do some good. A regular workout schedule will be good for your heart, lungs, muscles, and bones—even your mood.

____ **Drink more water.** You need eight glasses a day to replenish lost fluids, prevent constipation, and keep your digestive system working efficiently.

____ **Do a good deed.** Caring for others is a wonderful way to care for your own soul and connect with others.

SELF-SURVEY

Are You in Control of Your Health?

To test whether you are the master of your fate, asserting control over your destiny, or just hanging on, hoping for the best, take the following test. Depending on which statement you agree with, check either (a) or (b).

1. a. Many of the unhappy things in people's lives are partly due to bad luck. _____
   b. People's misfortunes result from mistakes they make. _____

2. a. One of the major reasons why we have wars is that people don't take enough interest in politics. _____
   b. There will always be wars, no matter how hard people try to prevent them. _____

3. a. In the long run, people get the respect they deserve in this world. _____
   b. Unfortunately, an individual's worth often passes unrecognized no matter how hard he or she tries. _____

4. a. The idea that teachers are unfair to students is nonsense. _____
   b. Most students don't realize the extent to which their grades are influenced by accidental happenings. _____

5. a. Without the right breaks, one cannot be an effective leader. _____
   b. Capable people who fail to become leaders have not taken advantage of their opportunities. _____

6. a. No matter how hard you try, some people just don't like you. _____
   b. People who can't get others to like them don't understand how to get along with others. _____

7. a. I have often found that what is going to happen will happen. _____
   b. Trusting to fate has never turned out as well for me as making a decision to take a definite course of action. _____

8. a. In the case of the well-prepared student, there is rarely, if ever, such a thing as an unfair test. _____
   b. Oftentimes exam questions tend to be so unrelated to course work that studying is really useless. _____

9. a. Becoming a success is a matter of hard work; luck has little or nothing to do with it. _____
   b. Getting a good job depends mainly on being in the right place at the right time. _____

10. a. The average citizen can have influence in government decisions. _____
    b. This world is run by the few people in power, and there is not much the little guy can do about it. _____

11. a. When I make plans, I am almost certain that I can make them work. _____
    b. It is not always wise to plan too far ahead because many things turn out to be a matter of luck anyway. _____

12. a. In my case, getting what I want has little or nothing to do with luck. _____
    b. Oftentimes, we might just as well decide what to do by flipping a coin. _____

13. a. What happens to me is my own doing. _____
    b. Sometimes I feel that I don't have enough control over the direction my life is taking. _____

Scoring

Give yourself 1 point for each of the following answers:
1a, 2b, 3b, 4b, 5a, 6a, 7a, 8b, 9b, 10b, 11b, 12b, 13b
You do not get any points for other choices.

Add up the totals. Scores can range from 0 to 13. A high score indicates an external locus of control, the belief that forces outside yourself control your destiny. A low score indicates an internal locus of control, a belief in your ability to take charge of your life.

Source: Based on J.B. Rotter, "Generalized Expectancies for Internal versus External Control of Reinforcement," *Psychological Monographs*, Vol. 80, Whole No. 609 (1966).

If you turned out to be external on this self-assessment quiz, don't accept your current score as a given for life. If you want to shift your perspective, you can. People are not internal or external in every situation. At home you may go along with your parents' or roommates' preferences and let them call the shots. In class you might feel confident and participate without hesitation.

Take inventory of the situations in which you feel most and least in control. Are you bold on the basketball court but hesitant on a date? Do you feel confident that you can resolve a dispute with your friends but throw up your hands when a landlord refuses to refund your security deposit? Look for ways to exert more influence in situations in which you once yielded to external influences. See what a difference you can make.

REVIEW QUESTIONS

(LO 1.1) 1. The World Health Organization defines *health* as _____.
a. access to appropriate medicines
b. the absence of disease or infirmity
c. whatever brings personal satisfaction
d. a state of complete physical, mental, and social well-being

(LO 1.2) 2. Learning from life experience and the capacity to question and evaluate information requires _____ health.
a. psychological
b. intellectual
c. social
d. spiritual

(LO 1.3) 3. Which age group of Americans experiences the greatest health deficits?
a. Children
b. Teenagers
c. Young adults
d. The elderly

(LO 1.4) 4. Which of the following statements is true of the health differences between gender and/or race?
a. Women are more likely than men to not smoke and to eat a healthy diet, but less likely to have adequate physical activity levels.
b. As a young American, your probability of reaching your 50th birthday is higher than in almost every other high-income nation.
c. About 1 to 6 Hispanics has prediabetes; most Hispanics with diabetes have it under control.
d. Overall, black Americans are less likely to develop cancer than persons of any other racial or ethnic group.

(LO 1.5) 5. Which of the following is one of the health issues that undergraduate college students in particular experience?
a. Athletes have higher health-related quality of life than their same-age peers who do not or no longer play college sports.
b. They are less likely to use alcohol and drugs than nonstudents their age.

c. A significant proportion report symptoms of depression, anxiety, and other mental disorders.
d. Undergraduates typically lose weight.

(LO 1.6) 6. Which of the following statements is true about the impact of unhealthy choices on young Americans?
a. Obese children often grow into obese adults, with risks of diabetes and cardiovascular disease.
b. A mild rise in blood pressure during young adulthood does not increase the risk of clogged heart arteries by middle age.
c. Young adults who begin using tobacco or alcohol in their teens and 20s are less likely to continue to do so as they get older.
d. Aerobic fitness has little impact on the cardiovascular health of individuals in later years.

(LO 1.7) 7. In searching the Internet for information about a question you have regarding your health, which one of these is NOT a key concern?
a. Potential author bias
b. Researcher credentials
c. Date the page was created and/or updated
a. The web browser used

(LO 1.8) 8. Factors that influence health behavior that include knowledge, attitudes, beliefs, values, and perceptions are _____ factors.
a. predisposing
b. enabling
c. risk
d. reinforcing

(LO 1.9) 9. According to which theory or model of personal change do people take a health-related action if they feel susceptible to a possible negative consequence?
a. Moral
b. Behavioral
c. Compensatory
d. Health belief

Answers to these questions can be found on page 531.

Phovoir/Shutterstock.com

After reading this chapter, you should be able to:

2.1   Identify the components of psychological health.

2.2   Discuss the ways in which positive psychology enhances quality of life.

2.3   Review the relationship between sleep and health.

2.4   Describe the key factors related to depressive disorders, their symptoms, and treatments.

2.5   Summarize four categories of anxiety disorders.

2.6   Outline the patterns of attempting or committing suicide among Americans.

2.7   List treatment options available for mental disorders.

WHAT DO YOU THINK?

• How do depression and anxiety affect students?

• What are the keys to a happy, satisfying, and meaningful life?

• What are some of the reasons that college students commit suicide?

• How important is a good night's sleep?

2

Psychological and Spiritual Well-Being

For years, Travis put on his "happy face" around his friends and family. Popular and athletic in high school, he never let anyone know how desperately unhappy he actually felt. "Whatever I was doing during the day, nothing was on my mind more than wanting to die," he recalls. On a perfectly ordinary day in his senior year, Travis tried to kill himself with an overdose of pills. Rushed to a hospital, Travis recovered, resumed his studies, and entered college. By the middle of his freshman year, he was struggling once more with feelings of hopelessness. This time he realized what was happening and sought help from a therapist.

"I thought college was supposed to be the happiest time of your life," he said. "What went wrong?" This is a question many young people might ask. Although youth can seem a golden time, when body and mind glow with potential, the process of becoming an adult is a challenging one in every culture and country. Psychological health can make the difference between facing this challenge with optimism and confidence or feeling overwhelmed by expectations and responsibilities. <

Emotional and Mental Well-Being

"A sound mind in a sound body" was, according to the ancient Roman poet Juvenal, something all should strive for. This timeless advice still holds. Almost 2,000 years later, we understand on a much more scientific level that physical and mental health are interconnected in complex and vital ways.

Over the past two decades research has produced more than 170,000 articles and books, as well as new terms to identify specific aspects of emotional and psychological health. These include:

- **Well-being:** a general term for how well individuals are doing in life, including social, physical, financial, and subjective (self-evaluated) dimensions

- **Subjective well-being:** a general term for the various ways individuals evaluate their lives, including thoughtful analysis and psychological feelings

- **Psychological well-being:** a combination of desirable psychological characteristics and positive social relationships

- **Emotional well-being:** high levels of positive moods and emotions as well as low levels of negative moods and emotions, reflecting not only momentary enjoyment but also resilience after bad events, movement toward significant goals, and ability to express emotions appropriate to various situations

- **Life satisfaction:** people's explicit and conscious evaluations of their lives, often based on factors that each individual deems relevant
- **Happiness:** a commonly used word that can be confusing because it means different things to different people (see discussion on page 28).[1]

✓**check-in** How would you describe your subjective well-being?

Unlike physical health, psychological well-being cannot be measured, tested, x-rayed, or dissected. Yet psychologically healthy men and women generally share certain characteristics:

- They value themselves and strive toward happiness and fulfillment.
- They establish and maintain close relationships with others.
- They accept the limitations as well as the possibilities that life has to offer.
- They feel a sense of meaning and purpose that makes the gestures of living worth the effort required.

✓**check-in** How many of these characteristics do you have?

Psychological health encompasses both our emotional and mental states—that is, our feelings and our thoughts. **Emotional health** generally refers to feelings and moods, both of which are discussed later in this chapter. Characteristics of emotionally healthy persons include the following:

- Determination and effort to be healthy.
- Flexibility and adaptability to a variety of circumstances.
- Development of a sense of meaning and affirmation of life.
- An understanding that the self is not the center of the universe.
- Compassion for others.
- The ability to be unselfish in serving or relating to others.
- Increased depth and satisfaction in intimate relationships.
- A sense of control over the mind and body that enables the person to make health-enhancing choices and decisions.

emotional health The ability to express and acknowledge one's feelings and moods and exhibit adaptability and compassion for others.

mental health The ability to perceive reality as it is, respond to its challenges, and develop rational strategies for living.

culture The set of shared attitudes, values, goals, and practices of a group that are internalized by an individual within the group.

Mental health describes our ability to perceive reality as it is, to respond to its challenges, and to develop rational strategies for living. A mentally healthy person doesn't try to avoid conflicts and distress but can cope with life's transitions, traumas, and losses in a way that allows for emotional stability and growth. The characteristics of mental health include:

- The ability to function and carry out responsibilities.
- The ability to form relationships.
- Realistic perceptions of the motivations of others.
- Rational, logical thought processes.
- The ability to adapt to change and to cope with adversity.

✓**check-in** How would you assess yourself on each of these characteristics?

Culture also helps define psychological health. In one culture, men and women may express feelings with great intensity, shouting in joy or wailing in grief, while in another culture, such behavior might be considered abnormal or unhealthy. In our diverse society, many cultural influences affect Americans' sense of who they are, where they came from, and what they believe. Cultural rituals help bring people together, strengthen their bonds, reinforce the values and beliefs they share, and provide a sense of belonging, meaning, and purpose.

To find out where you are on the psychological well-being scale, take the Self-Survey: How Satisfied Are You with Your Life? at the end of this chapter.

The Lessons of Positive Psychology

Positive psychology (the scientific study of ordinary human strengths and virtues) and positive psychiatry (which promotes positive psychosocial development in those with or at high risk of mental or physical illness) focus on the aspects of human experience that lead to happiness and fulfillment—in other words, on what makes life worthwhile.[2] This perspective has expanded the definition of psychological well-being.

According to psychologist Martin Seligman, who popularized the positive psychology movement, everyone, regardless of genes or fate, can achieve a happy, gratifying, meaningful life. The goal is not simply to feel good momentarily or to avoid bad experiences but to build positive strengths and virtues that enable us to find meaning and purpose in life. The core philosophy is to add a "build what's strong" approach to the "fix what's wrong" focus of traditional psychotherapy.[3]

Among the positive psychology interventions that have proven effective in enhancing emotional, cognitive, and physical well-being; easing depression; lessening disease and disability; and even increasing longevity are:

- Counting one's blessings.
- Savoring experiences.
- Practicing kindness.
- Pursuing meaning.
- Setting personal goals.
- Expressing gratitude.
- Building compassion for oneself and for others.
- Identifying and using one's strengths (which may include traits such as kindness or perseverance).
- Visualizing and writing about one's best possible self at a time in the future.[4]

Neuroscientists, using sophisticated imaging techniques, have been able to identify specific areas in the brain associated with positive emotions, such as love, hope, and enthusiasm. As people age, the processing of emotions in the brain appears to change, with older adults responding more to positive information and filtering out irrelevant negative stimuli.

✓check-in Practice positive psychology:

- The next time you think, "I've never tried that before," also say to yourself, "This is an opportunity to learn something new."

- When something seems too complicated, remind yourself to tackle it from another angle.

- If you get discouraged and feel that you're never going to get better at some new skill, tell yourself to give it another try. (See Health Now! for more suggestions.)

Develop Self-Compassion

Self-compassion is a healthy form of self-acceptance and self-care that enhances wellness

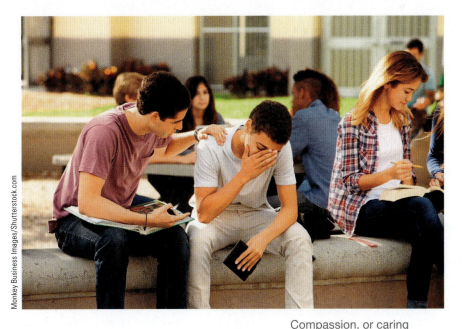

Monkey Business Images/Shutterstock.com

and strengthens resilience.[5] Some psychologists describe it as being kind to yourself in the face of suffering and practicing a "reciprocal golden rule," in which you treat yourself with the kindness usually reserved for others.

Individuals high in self-compassion tend to:

- Be understanding toward themselves when they make mistakes.
- Recognize that all humans are imperfect.
- Not ruminate about their errors in judgment or behavior.
- When feeling inadequate, engage in soothing and positive self-talk.
- Not exaggerate the significance of painful thoughts (though they're mindful of them).
- Manage frustration by quelling self-pity and melodrama.
- Accept their flaws.
- Let go of regrets, illusions, and disappointments.
- Seek psychological help when needed.[6]
- Take responsibility for actions that may have harmed others without feeling a need to punish oneself.[7]

In contrast, individuals low in self-compassion are extremely critical of themselves, believe they are unique in their imperfection, and obsessively fixate on their mistakes.

After a traumatic life event, self-compassion may help individuals recognize the need to care for themselves, reach out for social support, engage in less self-blame and self-criticism, and look back on the time as an emotionally difficult event rather than an experience

Compassion, or caring about others, is a characteristic of an emotionally healthy person.

self-compassion A healthy form of self-acceptance in the face of perceived inadequacy or failure.

HEALTH NOW!

Count Your Blessings

Gratitude has proven as effective in brightening mood and boosting energy as the standard, well-studied techniques used in psychotherapy. The following are some simple steps to cultivate and express gratitude.

- Every day, write down 10 new things for which you are grateful. You can start with this list and keep adding to it: your bed, your cell phone and every person whose efforts led to its development, every road you take, your toothbrush, your toes, the sky, ice cream, etc.

- Record the ways you express gratitude. How do you feel when doing so?

- Create a daily practice of appreciation. This may be as simple as saying a few words of thanks before each meal (if only to yourself) or writing down your feelings of gratitude.

- Make a list of 10 people—teachers, coaches, neighbors, and relatives—to whom you owe a debt of gratitude. Write a one- to two-page letter to each of them, stating your appreciation of what he or she has contributed to you and your well-being. You do not have to send the letters. What is important is that you focus deeply on the contribution of each person and allow feelings of gratitude to come as they may.

emotional intelligence The ability to monitor and use emotions to guide thinking and actions.

self-actualization A state of wellness and fulfillment that can be achieved once certain human needs are satisfied; living to one's full potential.

that defines or changes them.[8] Therapists have developed specific cognitive treatments that can increase the attributes of compassion for self and others, and alleviate feelings of anxiety and depression.

✓**check-in** How do you practice self-compassion?

Boost Emotional Intelligence

A person's intelligence quotient (IQ) was once considered the leading predictor of achievement. However, psychologists have determined that another "way of knowing," dubbed **emotional intelligence**, makes an even greater difference in personal and professional success.

Emotional quotient (EQ) is the ability to monitor and use emotions to guide thinking and actions. Neuroscientists have mapped the brain regions involved in emotional intelligence, which overlap significantly with those involved in general intelligence. Among the emotional competencies that most benefit students are focusing on clear, manageable goals and identifying and understanding emotions rather than relying on "gut" feelings.

✓**check-in** How emotionally intelligent do you think you are?

People with high EQ are more likely to enjoy good mental and physical health, and are more productive at work and happier at home. They're also less prone to stress, depression, and anxiety, and they bounce back more quickly from serious illnesses.

Meet Your Needs

Newborns are unable to survive on their own. They depend on others for the satisfaction of their physical needs for food, shelter, warmth, and protection, as well as their less tangible emotional needs. In growing to maturity, children take on more responsibility and become more independent.

No one, however, becomes totally self-sufficient. As adults, we easily recognize our basic physical needs, but we often fail to acknowledge our emotional needs. Yet they, too, must be met if we are to be as fulfilled as possible.

Humanist theorist Abraham Maslow believed that human needs are the motivating factors in personality development. First, we must satisfy basic physiological needs, such as those for food,

shelter, and sleep. Only then can we pursue fulfillment of our higher needs—for safety and security, love and affection, and self-esteem. Few individuals reach the state of **self-actualization**, in which they function at the highest possible level and derive the greatest possible satisfaction from life (Figure 2.1).

Pursue Happiness

"Imagine a drug that causes you to live eight or nine years longer, to make $15,000 more a year, to be less likely to get divorced," says Martin Seligman, the "father" of positive psychology. "Happiness seems to be that drug." As a meta-analysis of long-term studies has shown, happiness even reduces the risk of dying—both in healthy people and in those with diagnosed diseases. But even if just about everyone might benefit from smiling more and scowling less, can almost anyone learn to live on the brighter side of life?

Skeptics who dismiss "happichondria" as the latest feel-good fad are dubious. However, happiness researchers, backed by thousands of scientific studies, cite mounting evidence suggesting that happiness is, to a significant degree, something anyone can nurture. (See Health on a Budget.) Among 5,000 students in 280 countries around the world who completed a massive online open course (MOOC) on happiness, positive feelings kept going up as the course progressed. The students registered progressively less sadness, anger, and increasing fear and more amusement, enthusiasm, and affection.[9]

The Roots of Happiness Psychological research has identified several factors that contribute to a sense of well-being:

- Your happiness set point—a genetic component that contributes about 50 percent to individual differences in contentment.

- Life circumstances such as income or marital status, which account for about 10 percent.

- Thoughts, behaviors, beliefs, and goal-based activities, which may account for up to 40 percent of individual variations.[10]

- In addition to genes and personal beliefs and experiences, happiness also is influenced by social and cultural factors, including living in a country that ensures its citizens' safety and human rights.[11]

Education may protect against mental disorders, but it doesn't guarantee happiness. Asked if they were "feeling good and functioning well," people with varying levels of education had similar odds of high levels of emotional well-being.[12] As studies with apps to monitor activity have shown, individuals who are more physically active are happier in general—and feel even happier when they are physically active.[13]

Intelligence, gender, and race do not matter much for happiness. Men and women in global surveys report similar levels of life satisfaction and happiness.[14] Health has a greater impact on happiness than income, but pain and anxiety take an even greater toll. People seem to be less able to adapt to the unpredictability of certain health conditions than they are to others. The well-being of individuals who can no longer walk after an accident, for example, typically returns to its pre-accident levels, while many diagnosed with epilepsy face a lifetime of uncertainty about the occurrence of seizures. Surveys of various nations indicate that happiness levels remain stable through most of the lifespan, although the sense of well-being typically decreases in the period of decline before death.[15]

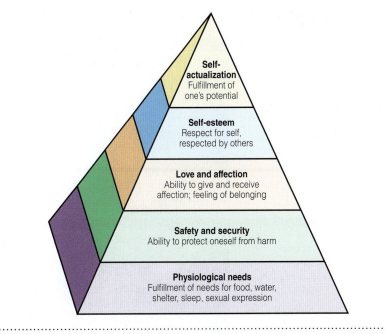

FIGURE 2.1 The Maslow Pyramid

To attain the highest level of psychological health, you must first satisfy your needs for safety and security, love and affection, and self-esteem.

Source: Maslow, Abraham H., Frager, Robert D., Fadiman, James, Motivation and Personality, 3rd Edition, © 1987. Reprinted by permission of Pearson Education, Inc., Upper Saddle River, NJ.

What Does and Doesn't Make Us Happy

Many people assume that they can't be happy unless they get into a certain school, earn a certain grade, get a certain job, make a certain income, find a perfect mate, or look a certain way. But according to psychologist Sonja Lyubomirsky, author of *The Myths of Happiness*, such notions are false. "People find a way to be happy in spite of unwanted life circumstances," she notes, "and many people who are blessed

$ HEALTH ON A BUDGET

Happiness for Free!

Money can't buy happiness. As long as you have enough money to cover the basics, you don't need more wealth or more possessions for greater joy. Even people who win a fortune in a lottery return to their baseline of happiness within months. So rather than spend money on lottery tickets, try these ways to put a smile on your face:

- **Make time for yourself.** It's impossible to meet the needs of others without recognizing and fulfilling your own.

- **Boost your appreciation quotient.** Regularly take stock of all the things for which you are grateful. To deepen the impact, write a letter of gratitude to someone who's helped you along the way.

- **String beads.** Think of every positive experience during the day as a bead on a necklace. This simple exercise focuses you on positive experiences, such as a cheery greeting from a cashier or a funny e-mail from a friend, and encourages you to act more kindly toward others.

- **Create a virtual DVD.** Visualize several of your happiest memories in as much detail as possible. Smell the air. Feel the sun. Hear the sea. Play this video in your mind when your spirits slump.

- **Fortify optimism.** Whenever possible, see the glass as half-full. Keep track of what's going right in your life. Imagine and write down your vision for your best possible future and track your progress toward it.

- **Immerse yourself.** Find activities that delight and engage you so much that you lose track of time. Experiment with creative outlets. Look for ways to build these passions into your life.

- **Seize the moment.** Rather than wait to celebrate big birthday-cake moments, savor a bite of cupcake every day. Delight in a child's cuddle, a glorious sunset, a lively conversation. Cry at the movies. Cheer at football games. This life is your gift to yourself. Open it!

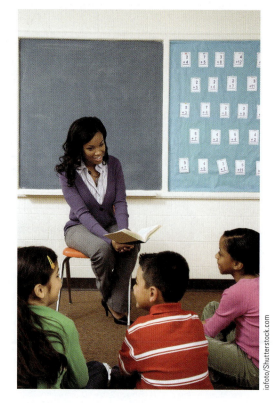
iofoto/Shutterstock.com

Positive activities, such as reading to children, can enhance happiness and self-esteem.

The Benefits of Happiness

Two decades of research on happy people have found that they:

- tend to be healthier and live longer.

- have stronger immune systems and better cardiovascular health.

- practice healthier behaviors, such as wearing seat belts and using sunscreen.

- report better social relationships and more friends.

- are more likely to marry and remain married.

- rate their marriages as better than those of less happy individuals.

- are more involved in groups, organizations, and other social networks.

- are more successful at work.[22]

✓**check-in** What are the greatest sources of happiness in your life?

Become Optimistic

Mental health professionals define **optimism** as the "extent to which individuals expect favorable outcomes to occur." Studies have established "significant relationships" between optimism and cardiovascular health, recovery from heart attack,[23] stroke risk, immune function, cancer prognoses, physical symptoms, pain, and mortality rates.[24] As a recent review concluded, "individuals with greater optimism and hope seek to engage in healthier behaviors"—which can protect from disease and aid in recovery.[25]

For various reasons—because they believe in themselves, because they trust in a higher power, because they feel lucky—optimists expect positive experiences from life. When bad things happen, they tend to see setbacks or losses as specific, temporary incidents, which fortifies their resilience.[26] In their eyes, a disappointment is "one of those things" that happens every once in a while rather than the latest in a long string of disasters. Even when depressed, individuals able to envision a brighter future are more optimistic and regain optimism more quickly over time.[27]

In terms of health, optimists not only expect good outcomes—for instance, that a surgery will be successful—but also take steps to increase this likelihood. Pessimists, expecting the worst, are more likely to deny or avoid a problem, sometimes through drinking or other destructive behaviors. In a longitudinal study of more than

by wealth and good fortune aren't any happier than those who lack these fortunes."[16] Individuals with enough cash in their checking and savings accounts so they don't have to worry about money report more positive perceptions of their financial well-being and overall life satisfaction.

People are generally happier in richer countries than poor ones, although this may reflect factors such as safety and stability as well as income.[17] In a global study, happiness peaked at an income of the equivalent of about $100,000 and began to reverse above $250,000.[18]

What does make us happier? According to recent research:

- Focusing on time leads to greater happiness than focusing on money.

- Spending time and money on others rather than oneself increases happiness.

- Spending time and money to acquire experiences rather than possessions boosts happiness.[19]

- Moral judgments influence self-assessments of happiness.[20] Simply put, doing good makes us feel good.

- Having a happy partner may enhance health as much as striving to being happy oneself.[21]

optimism The tendency to seek out, remember, and expect pleasurable experiences.

70,000 women, those who ranked highest in optimism were at much lower risk of dying of cancer, heart disease, stroke, infection, respiratory disease, or other causes than those who ranked the lowest. [28]

Individuals aren't born optimistic or pessimistic. Researchers have documented changes over time in the ways that individuals view the world and what they expect to experience in the future.[29] Cognitive-behavioral techniques (discussed later in this chapter) have proven effective in helping pessimists become more positive.

✓**check-in** Do you usually anticipate the best or the worst possible outcome?

Manage Your Moods

Feelings come and go within minutes. A **mood** is a more sustained emotional state that colors our view of the world for hours or days. Most people experience a range of moods but respond to them differently. When struggling with a bad mood, men typically try to distract themselves (a partially successful strategy) or use alcohol or drugs (an ineffective tactic). Women are more likely to talk to someone (which can help) or to ruminate on why they feel bad (which doesn't help).

The most effective way to banish a sad or bad mood is by changing what caused it in the first place—if you can figure out what made you upset and why. The questions to ask are: What can I do to fix the failure? What can I do to remedy the loss? Is there anything under my control that I can change? If there is, take action and solve it. Ask to take a makeup exam. Apologize to the friend whose feelings you hurt. Tell your parents you feel bad about the argument you had. If there's nothing you can do, accept what happened and focus on doing things differently next time. As studies have shown, resolving to try harder can be as effective in improving mood as taking specific actions.[30]

Learning effective mood-boosting, mood-regulating strategies can help both men and women pull themselves up and out of an emotional slump. You also can try to think about what happened in a different way and put a positive spin on it. This technique, known as *cognitive reappraisal*, or *reframing*, helps you look at a setback in a new light: What lessons did it teach you? What would you have done differently? Could there be a silver lining or hidden benefit?

✓**check-in** Track your moods

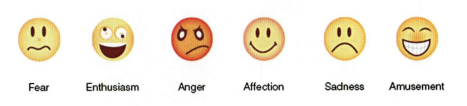

| Fear | Enthusiasm | Anger | Affection | Sadness | Amusement |

Every day, rate how much each emoji matches how you have been feeling on a scale of 1 to 10. At the end of the week, average your daily ratings into a collective score. Track how your feelings change throughout the term.

Spiritual Health

Whatever your faith, whether or not you belong to any formal religion, you are more than a body of a certain height and weight occupying space on the planet. You have a mind that equips you to learn and question. And you have a spirit that animates everything you say and do. **Spiritual health** refers to this breath of life and to our ability to identify our basic purpose in life and experience the fulfillment of achieving our full potential. Spiritual readings or practices can increase calmness, inner strength, and meaning; improve self-awareness; and enhance your sense of well-being. Religious support has also been shown to help lower depression and increase life satisfaction beyond the benefits of social support from friends and family.

Spirituality is a belief in what some call a higher power, in someone or something that transcends the boundaries of self. It gives rise to a strong sense of purpose, values, morals, and ethics. Throughout life you make choices and decide to behave in one way rather than another because your spirituality serves as both a compass and a guide.

The terms *religiosity* and *religiousness* refer to various spiritual practices. That definition may seem vague, but one thing is clear. According to thousands of studies on the relationship between religious beliefs and practices and health, religious individuals are less depressed, less anxious, and better able to cope with crises such as illness or divorce than are nonreligious ones. It doesn't matter if your beliefs are Christian,

mood A temporary feeling or state of mind.

spiritual health The ability to identify one's basic purpose in life and to achieve one's full potential.

spirituality A belief in someone or something that transcends the boundaries of self.

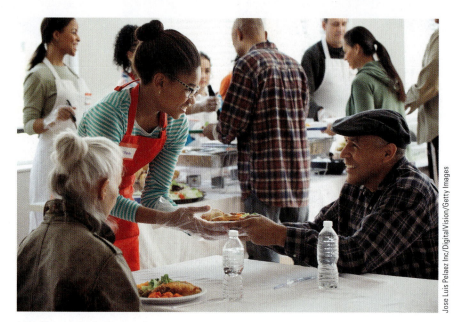

Like these students serving meals at a shelter for the homeless, you can enrich your spiritual life by giving of yourself.

Jewish, Muslim, Buddhist, or any other religion. The more that believers incorporate spiritual practices—such as prayer, meditation, or attending services—into daily life, the less likely they are to experience symptoms of mental disorders, anxiety, and stress.[31]

Religious beliefs and practices are generally passed from parents to children. In research on Catholic, Christian, Jewish, and Muslim families, about 60 percent of parents who attend religious services at least weekly have children who continue to participate frequently in religious services as adults.[32]

Did you grow up in a religious family? If so, you may benefit in various ways. In a recent study that followed teenagers through young adulthood, those who had attended religious services regularly reported greater life satisfaction, fewer symptoms of depression, more positive emotions and character strengths, lower rates of smoking or use of illicit drugs, later age at sexual initiation, and fewer lifetime sexual partners than those who did not attend these services.[33]

✓**check-in** How would you describe your spiritual self?

Spirituality and Physical Health

A growing body of scientific evidence indicates that faith and spirituality can enhance health—and perhaps even extend life. Individuals[34] who pray and experience spiritual well-being consistently describe themselves as enjoying greater psychological and overall well-being. Various studies have found that religiosity reduces alcohol

use disorders,[35] binge drinking,[36] vulnerability to eating disorders, and symptoms of depression. Among Latino men and women, those who are more spiritual are also significantly less sedentary—an important boost for good health.[37]

Church attendance may account for an additional 2 to 3 years of life (by comparison, exercise may add 3 to 5 extra years), according to researchers' calculations. The reason may be the sense of community or support, or that people feel less depressed when they join in religious services. Prayer and other religious experiences, including meditation, may actually change the brain for the better. Using neuroimaging techniques, scientists have documented alterations in various parts of the brain that are associated with stress and anxiety. This effect may slow down the aging process, reduce psychological symptoms, and increase feelings of security, compassion, and love. Increasingly, physicians are recognizing the importance of spiritual engagement for individuals at the end of life and their families.[38]

Deepen Your Spiritual Intelligence

Mental health professionals have recognized the power of **spiritual intelligence**, which some define as "the capacity to sense, understand, and tap into the highest parts of ourselves, others, and the world around us." Spiritual intelligence, unlike spirituality, does not center on the worship of a God above, but on the discovery of a wisdom within.

All of us are born with the potential to develop spiritual intelligence, but most of us aren't even aware of it—and do little or nothing to nurture it. Part of the reason is that we confuse spiritual intelligence with religion, dogma, or old-fashioned morality. "You don't have to go to church to be spiritually intelligent; you don't even have to believe in God," says Rev. Paul Edwards, a retired Episcopalian priest and therapist. "It is a scientific fact that when you are feeling secure, at peace, loved, and happy, you see, hear, and act differently than when you're feeling insecure, unhappy, and unloved. Spiritual intelligence allows you to use the wisdom you have when you're in a state of inner peace. And you get there by changing the way you think, basically by listening less to what's in your head and more to what's in your heart."[39]

Clarify Your Values

Your **values** are the criteria by which you evaluate things, people, events, and yourself; they represent what's most important to you. In a world

spiritual intelligence The capacity to sense, understand, and tap into ourselves, others, and the world around us.

values The criteria by which one makes choices about one's thoughts, actions, goals, and ideals.

of almost dizzying complexity, values can provide guidelines for making decisions that are right for you. If understood and applied, they help give life meaning and structure.

When you confront a situation in which you must choose different paths or behaviors, follow these steps:

1. Carefully consider the consequences of each choice.

2. Choose freely from among all the options.

3. Publicly affirm your values by sharing them with others.

4. Act out your values.

Values clarification is not a once-in-a-lifetime task but an ongoing process of sorting out what matters most to you. Values are more than ideals we'd like to attain; they should be reflected in the way we live day by day.

✓**check-in** Do you put your values into action? If you believe in protecting the environment—for instance, do you shut off lights or walk rather than drive in order to conserve energy? Do you recycle newspapers, bottles, and cans?

Enrich Your Spiritual Life

Whatever role religion plays in your life, you have the capacity for deep, meaningful spiritual experiences that can add great meaning to everyday existence. You don't need to enroll in theology classes or commit to a certain religious preference. The following simple steps can start you on an inner journey to a new level of understanding:

- **Sit quietly.** The process of cultivating spiritual intelligence begins in solitude and silence. "There is an inner wisdom," says Dr. Dean Ornish, the pioneering cardiologist who incorporates spiritual health into his mind–body therapies, "but it speaks very, very softly."[40] To tune into its whisper, turn down the volume in your busy, noisy, complicated life and force yourself to do nothing at all. This may sound easy; it's anything but.

- **Start small.** Create islands of silence in your day. Don't reach for the radio dial as soon as you get in the car. Leave your ear buds on as you walk across campus but turn off the music. Shut the door to your room, take a few huge deep breaths, and let them out very, very slowly. Don't worry if you're too busy to

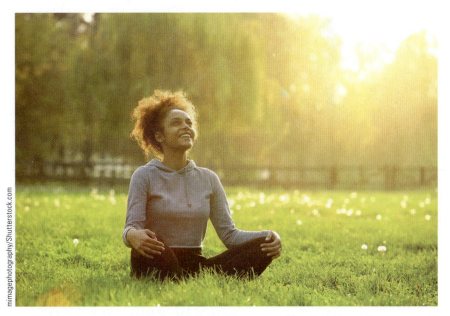

mimagephotography/Shutterstock.com

Simply taking a few moments to stop and enjoy the day can help quiet your mind and soothe your spirit.

carve out half an hour for quiet contemplation. Even 10 minutes every day can make a difference.

- **Step outside.** For many people, nature sets their spirit free. Being outdoors, walking by the ocean, or looking at the hills puts the little hassles of daily living into perspective. As you wait for the bus or for a traffic light to change, let your gaze linger on silvery ice glazing a branch or an azalea bush in wild bloom. Follow the flight of a bird; watch clouds float overhead. Gaze into the night sky and think of the stars as holes in the darkness, letting the light of heaven shine through.

- **Use activity to tune into your spirit.** Spirituality exists in every cell of the body, not just in the brain. As a student, you devote much of your day to mental labor. To tap into your spirit, try a less cerebral activity, such as singing, chanting, dancing, or drumming. Alternative ways of quieting your mind and tuning into your spirit include gardening, walking, arranging flowers, listening to music that touches your soul, or immersing yourself in a simple process like preparing a meal.

- **Ask questions of yourself.** Some people use their contemplative time to focus on a line of scripture or poetry. Others ask open-ended questions, such as: What am I feeling? What are my choices? Where am I heading?

- **Trust your spirit.** While most of us rely on gut feelings to alert us to danger, our inner spirits usually nudge us not away from but toward some action that will somehow lead to a greater good—even if we can't see it at the time. You may suddenly feel the urge to call or e-mail a friend you've lost touch with—only to discover that he just lost a loved one and was grateful for the comfort of your caring.

- **Develop a spiritual practice:**
  - **If you are religious:** Deepen your spiritual commitment through prayer, more frequent church attendance, or participation in a prayer group.
  - **If you are not religious:** Keep an open mind about the value of religion or spirituality. Consider visiting a church or synagogue. Read the writings of inspired people of deep faith, such as Rabbi Harold Kushner and Rev. Martin Luther King Jr.
  - **If you are not unsure of religion:** Try nonreligious meditation or relaxation training. Focusing the mind on a single sound or image can slow heart rate, respiration, and brain waves; relax muscles; and lower stress-related hormones—responses similar to those induced by prayer.

✓**check-in** Live your legacy. Write a one-page essay detailing your legacy as if you were a biographer recounting a long, fruitful life. Consider traits, accomplishments, and behaviors that you hope to be remembered for. Then consider what you do on an average day and how these activities align with the legacy you'd like to leave behind.

Consider the Power of Prayer

Prayer, a spiritual practice of millions, is the most commonly used form of complementary and alternative medicine. However, only in recent years has science launched rigorous investigations of the healing power of prayer. As research has documented, people who pray regularly have significantly lower blood pressure and stronger immune systems, are hospitalized less often, and are less likely to smoke heavily or abuse alcohol than those who are less religious. However, praying for others, regardless of the type of prayer or religion, has not been shown to improve either symptoms or recovery of patients undergoing various medical procedures.

✓**check-in** Do you pray? Is there a specific reason why or why not?

Cultivate Gratitude

A grateful spirit brightens mood, boosts energy, and infuses daily living with a sense of glad abundance. Although giving thanks is an ancient virtue, only recently have researchers focused on the "trait" of gratitude—appreciation not just for a special gift but for everything that makes life a bit better. Feelings of gratitude are associated with better mood, relief of depression in individuals with chronic illnesses,[41] improved sleep, less fatigue, recovery from posttraumatic stress,[42] healthier eating behaviors,[43] and lower risk of heart failure.[44] Here are some of its psychological effects:

- More frequent and intense positive emotions.
- More positive views of the social environment.
- More productive coping strategies.
- Greater appreciation of life and possessions.

In addition to its benefits on psychological well-being, gratitude also may enhance physical health. Researchers have reported that "gratitude interventions," such as writing gratitude lists (see Health Now), may lower blood pressure, improve sleep, and decrease symptoms of chronic diseases.[45]

Among the most popular "gratitude interventions"—techniques for increasing appreciation—is keeping a diary and recording three things you are grateful for every day. In clinical studies, this approach has proven as effective as the rigorously developed and tested techniques used in psychotherapy. However, a recent meta-analysis of gratitude studies found that such interventions are most effective in inducing feelings of thankfulness rather than relieving anxiety and that other regular activities involving self-discipline may also promote psychological well-being.[46]

✓**check-in** Three Good Things
Every night, write down three good things that happened during the day. They can be big or small but should be specific (e.g., "having a great dinner with close friends" rather than "having great friends").
As you train yourself to notice and remember the little things that make a difference, you'll feel their impact more.

Forgive

Being angry, harboring resentments, or reliving hurts over and over again is bad for your health in general and your heart in particular. The word *forgive* comes from the Greek for "letting go," and that's what happens when you forgive: You let go of all the anger and pain that have been demanding your time and draining your energy.

People may feel more in control and more powerful when they're filled with anger, but forgiving instills a much greater sense of power. Forgiving a friend or family member may be more difficult than forgiving a stranger because the hurt occurs in a context in which people deliberately make themselves vulnerable. Forgiving yourself may be even harder.

When you forgive, you reclaim your power to choose. It doesn't matter whether someone deserves to be forgiven; you deserve to be free. However, forgiveness isn't easy. It's not a one-time thing but a process that takes a lot of time and work, and involves both the conscious and the unconscious mind.

✓**check-in** Is there someone in your life you haven't forgiven—yet?

YOUR STRATEGIES FOR CHANGE

How to Forgive

- **Compose an apology letter.** Address it to yourself and write it from someone who's hurt you. This simple task enables you to get a new perspective on a painful experience.

- **Leap forward in time.** In a visualization exercise, imagine that you are very old, meet a person who hurt you long ago, and the two of you sit down together on a park bench on a beautiful spring day. You talk until everything that needs to be said is finally said. This allows you to benefit from the perspective time brings without having to wait years to achieve it.

- **Talk with "safe" people.** Vent your anger or disappointment with a trusted friend or a counselor, without the danger of saying or doing anything you'll regret later. And if you can laugh about what happened with a friend, the laughter helps dissolve the rage.

- **Forgive the person, not the deed.** In themselves, abuse, rape, murder, and betrayal are beyond forgiveness. But you can forgive people who couldn't manage to handle their own suffering, misery, confusion, and desperation.

Sleep and Health

You stay up late cramming for a final. You drive through the night to visit a friend at another campus. You get up for an early class during the week but stay in bed until noon on weekends. And you wonder: "Why am I so tired?" The answer: You're not getting enough sleep. You're hardly alone. According to the Centers for Disease Control and Prevention (CDC):

- About 35 percent of U.S. adults sleep less than 7 hours a night, which puts them at risk of obesity, type 2 diabetes, high blood pressure, heart disease, stroke, mental distress, and death.[47]

- Women are more likely than men to report not getting enough sleep.

- African Americans report getting less sleep compared with all other ethnic groups.

✓**check-in** Are you getting enough sleep? The National Sleep Foundation recommends 7 to 9 hours for men and women ages 18 to 25. How do you compare?

Sleepless on Campus

College students are notorious for their erratic sleep schedules and late bedtimes. According to the CDC, about a third of young adults between ages 18 and 24 get the recommended 7 to 9 hours of sleep. Among college students, 60 percent describe themselves as poor sleepers; while about a third report short sleep.[48]

In the American College Health Association–National College Health Assessment (ACHA-NCHA) survey, 22 percent of college students said that sleep difficulties have affected their academic performance, ranking behind stress and anxiety.[49] (See Snapshot: On Campus Now.)

In one recent study, about 75 percent of students reported having tiredness, fatigued, or daytime sleepiness, while 88 percent reported getting less than 8 hours of sleep a night. More than 40 percent reported snoring. About one in three reported mild to moderate psychological distress.[50] Alcohol compounds many students' sleep problems.[51] Poor-quality sleepers report drinking more alcohol than good sleepers and are twice as likely to use alcohol to induce sleep as are better sleepers. Students who drink more alcohol go to bed later, sleep less, and show greater differences between weekday and weekend sleep timing and duration.[52] In general, students who do not adhere to a regular bedtime and rising schedule are more likely to be poor sleepers. In a recent analysis, other factors that contributed to poor sleep health among college students include experiencing discrimination, not being able to afford or obtain balanced nutritious meals, skipping or reducing meal size, and greater psychological distress.[53]

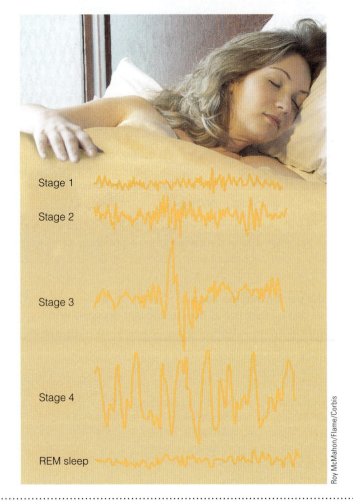

Stage 1

Stage 2

Stage 3

Stage 4

REM sleep

Roy McMahon/Flame/Corbis

FIGURE 2.2 The Stages of Sleep

A good night's sleep consists of a sequence of different brain rhythms.

On average, college students go to bed 1 to 2 hours later and sleep 1 to 1.6 hours less than students of a generation ago. Their sleep quality declines with increasing levels of stress or alcohol/cigarette use and with decreasing levels of general health. Fortunately, college students can learn to practice good "sleep hygiene" to improve the quality of their sleep—as well as their moods and overall feelings of well-being.[54] One important step: turning off digital devices, since "screen time" can delay and disrupt sleep, impair thinking, and increase stress and anxiety.[55]

How Much Sleep Do You Need?

Over the past century, we have cut our average nightly sleep time by 20 percent. More than half of us try to get by with less than 7 hours of shut-eye a night. College students are no exception, with an average sleep time slightly less than

7 hours, with little difference between men and women.

No formula can say how long a good night's sleep should be. In various studies, short sleep duration has been associated with increased mortality, diabetes, hypertension, obesity, and cardiovascular diseases.[56] Normal sleep times range from 5 to 10 hours; the average is 7.5 hours. About one or two people in every hundred can get by with just 5 hours; another small minority needs twice that amount. Each of us seems to have an innate sleep *appetite* that is as much a part of our genetic programming as hair color and skin tone.

✓**check-in** Do you use an electronic device before bedtime? If so, it may be disrupting your sleep. Smartphone users need more time to fall asleep and get less sleep compared to nonusers.[57]

To figure out your sleep needs, keep your wakeup time the same every morning and vary your bedtime. Are you groggy after 6 hours of shut-eye? Does an extra hour give you more stamina? What about an extra 2 hours? Since too much sleep can make you feel sluggish, don't assume that more is always better. Listen to your body's signals, and adjust your sleep schedule to suit them.

Sleep's Impact on Health

The following are some of the key ways in which your nighttime sleep affects your daytime well-being:

- **Learning and memory.** When you sleep, your brain helps "consolidate" new information, so you are more likely to retain it in your memory. Are you better off pulling an all-nighter before a big test or closing the books and getting a good night's sleep? According to researchers, that depends on the nature of the exam. If it's a test of facts—Civil War battles, for instance—cramming all night works. However, if you will have to write analytical essays in which you compare, contrast, and make connections, you need to sleep to make the most of your reasoning abilities.

- **Academic performance.** Poor sleep can affect academic performance. In a recent study, students who felt tired, fatigued, or sleepy during the day had mean GPAs of 3.04, compared to 3.24 among those who did not report these symptoms. Students who slept

Sleepy Students

Over the past 7 days, students getting enough sleep to feel rested in the morning:

	Percent (%)		
	Male	Female	Average
0 days	10.4	12.6	12.2
1–2 days	27.7	32.9	31.3
3–5 days	47.2	44.5	45.1
6+ days	14.6	10.0	11.3

Students often feeling tired, dragged out, or sleepy during the day:

	Percent (%)		
	Male	Female	Average
0 days	12.8	6.4	8.3
1–2 days	34.1	27.6	29.2
3–5 days	40.1	46.0	44.3
6+ days	13.0	20.0	18.2

Impact of sleepiness on daytime activities:

	Percent (%)		
	Male	Female	Average
No problem	13.9	7.9	9.7
A little problem	49.1	46.4	46.9
More than a little problem	22.7	26.2	25.3
A big problem	10.2	13.7	12.8
A very big problem	4.1	5.8	6.4

Source: American College Health Association. American College Health Association-National College Health Assessment II: Reference Group Executive Summary Spring 2018. Silver Spring, MD: American College Health Association, 2018.

8 or more hours during the week averaged GPAs of 3.17; those who slept less had lower GPAs, averaging 3.08.[58]

- **Metabolism and weight.** Chronic sleep deprivation may cause weight gain by altering metabolism (e.g., changing the way individuals process and store carbohydrates) and by stimulating excess stress hormones. Loss of sleep also reduces levels of the hormones that regulate appetite.

- **Safety.** People who don't get adequate nighttime sleep are more likely to fall asleep during the daytime. Daytime sleepiness can cause falls, medical errors, air traffic mishaps, and road accidents.

- **Mood/quality of life.** Too little sleep—whether just for a night or two or for longer periods—can cause psychological symptoms, such as irritability, impatience, inability to concentrate, lack of motivation, moodiness, and lowered long-term life satisfaction.

- **Immunity.** Sleep deprivation alters immune function, including the activity of the body's killer cells. If you get less than 7 hours of sleep a night, you're three times more likely to catch a cold. And if you sleep poorly, you're five times more susceptible.

- **Mental disorders.** Disturbed sleep can be an early sign of mental illness; sleep loss may trigger or may be an early sign of a manic episode (see the discussion of bipolar disorder in Chapter 3).[59] Too much (10 or more hours a night) or too little (5 or fewer hours) sleep, according to recent research, can increase the risk of depression.

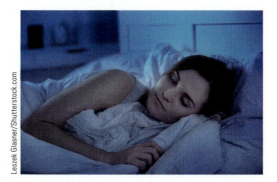

Leszek Glasner/Shutterstock.com

A good night's sleep enhances physical and psychological well-being.

ⓘ CONSUMER ALERT

Sleeping Pill Precautions

Chances are you've taken some form of sleep medication. After aspirin, they are the most widely used drugs in the United States. If sleeping pills seem the best option at a certain time in your life, use them with caution.

Facts to Know

- **Sleeping pills** are not a long-term solution to a sleep problem, but they can be helpful if travel, injury, or illness interfere with your nightly rest.

- **Prescription and over-the-counter sleep aids** can interact with other medications or a medical condition, so always check with your doctor before taking them.

- **If taken too often** or for more than several nights, some sleeping pills may cause rebound insomnia—sleeplessness that returns in full force when you stop taking the medication.

Steps to Take

- **Read carefully.** Take time to read through the informational materials and warnings on pill containers. Make sure you understand the potential risks and the behaviors to avoid.

- **If you are a woman, take half the standard dose.** The Food and Drug Administration (FDA) has found that women metabolize sleeping medications much more slowly than men so their effects linger longer.

- **Avoid alcohol.** Never mix alcohol and sleeping pills. Alcohol increases the sedative effects of the pills. Even a small amount of alcohol combined with sleeping pills can make you feel dizzy, confused, or faint.

- **Quit carefully.** When you're ready to stop taking sleeping pills, follow your doctor's instructions or the directions on the label. Some medications must be stopped gradually.

- **Watch for side effects.** If you feel sleepy or dizzy during the day, talk to your doctor about changing the dosage or discontinuing the pills.

- **Alcohol use.** Poor sleep can contribute to increased alcohol-related consequences among heavy-drinking college students. In research on college students, adequate sleep proved crucial in preventing heavy drinking, perhaps by enhancing the ability to plan ahead and anticipate the consequences of one's behavior.[60]

- **Major diseases and death.** Serious sleep disorders such as insomnia and sleep apnea have been linked to hypertension, increased stress hormone levels, irregular heartbeats, and increased inflammation (which, as discussed in Chapter 10, may play a role in heart attacks). Inadequate sleep has also been linked to higher overall death rates.

- **Sexuality.** In a study of college women, those who slept longer were more likely to engage in sexual activity the following day. On average the women slept 7 hours and 22 minutes, with each hour of sleep increasing the women's sexual desire and likelihood of sexual activity.[61] Young men and women report sleeping better with a partner, regardless of where they sleep.[62]

Getting a Better Night's Sleep

Individuals with insomnia—a lack of sleep so severe that it interferes with functioning during the day—may toss and turn for an hour or more when they get into bed, wake frequently in the night, wake up too early, or not be able to sleep long enough to feel alert and energetic the next day. Most often insomnia is transient, typically occurring before or after a major life event (such as a job interview) and lasting for three or four nights. During periods of prolonged stress (such as a marriage breakup), short-term insomnia may continue for several weeks. Chronic, or long-term, insomnia, which can begin at any age, may persist for long periods. About three-fourths of insomniacs struggle to sleep more for at least 1 year and almost half, for 3 years.

For about a third of those with chronic insomnia, the underlying problem is a mental disorder, most often depression or an anxiety disorder. Many substances, including alcohol, medications, and drugs of abuse, often disrupt sleep. Caffeine in coffee or other beverages and foods can increase problems falling asleep and interfere with quality of sleep.[63]

About 15 percent of those seeking help for chronic insomnia suffer from "learned" or "behavioral" insomnia. While a life crisis may trigger their initial sleep problems, each night they try harder and harder to get to sleep, but they cannot—although they often doze off while reading or watching a movie.

Sleeping Pills

The use of prescription sleeping pills has more than doubled in the past decade, and increasing numbers of teenagers and young adults use these medications either occasionally or regularly. An even greater number buy nonprescription or over-the-counter (OTC) sleep inducers. Others rely on herbal remedies, antihistamines, and other medications to get to sleep. Here is what you need to know about them:

- **OTC medications.** Various OTC sleeping pills, sold in any pharmacy or supermarket, contain antihistamines, which induce drowsiness by working against the central nervous system chemical histamine. They may help for an occasional sleepless night, but the more often you take them, the less effective they become.

- **Dietary supplements.** The most widely publicized dietary supplement is the hormone melatonin, which may help control your body's internal clock. The melatonin supplements most often found in health food stores and pharmacies are synthetic versions of the natural hormone. Although these supplements may help some people fall asleep or stay asleep and may sometimes help prevent jet lag, there are many unanswered questions about melatonin. Reported side effects include drowsiness, headaches, stomach discomfort, confusion, decreased body temperature, seizures, and drug interactions. The optimal dose isn't certain, and the long-term effects are unknown. Other supplements—such as valerian, chamomile, and kava—have yet to be fully studied for safety or effectiveness in relieving insomnia.

- **Prescription medications.** Current sleep drugs—nonbenzodiazepine hypnotic medications such as Lunesta (eszopiclone), Ambien/Ambien CR (zolpidem), and Sonata (zaleplon)—quiet the nervous system, which helps induce sleep. They're metabolized quickly, which helps reduce the risk of side effects the next day. These medications, which can interact with other medications, are mainly intended for short-term or intermittent use.

Understanding Mental Health

Mentally healthy individuals value themselves, perceive reality as it is, accept their limitations and possibilities, carry out their responsibilities, establish and maintain close relationships, pursue work that suits their talent and training, and feel a sense of fulfillment that makes the efforts of daily living worthwhile.

The state of mental health around the world is far from ideal. Psychiatric illness and substance abuse affect 450 million people worldwide and cause more premature deaths than any other factor.

The most common psychiatric conditions are depression, alcohol dependence and abuse, bipolar disorder, schizophrenia, Alzheimer's and other forms of dementia, panic disorder, and drug dependence and abuse. An estimated 17.3 million Americans—7.1 percent adults of the United States--have had at least one major depressive episode. Individuals between ages 18 and 25 have the highest rates.[64]

Across the globe, depression is the leading cause of years of health lost to disease in both men and women. The worldwide rate of depression among women is 50 percent

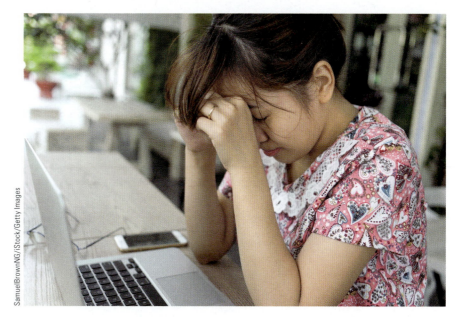

higher than in men, and women and girls have higher rates of anxiety disorders, migraine, and Alzheimer's disease. Men's rates of alcohol and substance abuse are nearly seven times higher than women's.

Despite public education campaigns, the level of prejudice and discrimination against people with a serious mental illness has changed little over the last 10 years. More people now attribute problems like depression and substance abuse to neurobiological causes—and are more likely to favor providing treatment. Preventive steps can help maintain and enhance your psychological health, just as similar actions boost physical health.

What Is a Mental Disorder?

While laypeople may speak of "nervous breakdowns" or "insanity," these are not scientific terms. The U.S. government's official definition states that a serious mental illness is "a diagnosable mental, behavioral, or emotional disorder that interferes with one or more major activities in life, like dressing, eating, or working."

About one in four adults in the United States suffers from mental illness at some point in life. Psychiatrists define a **mental disorder** as a clinically significant behavioral or psychological syndrome or pattern that is associated with present distress (a painful symptom) or disability (impairment in one or more important areas of functioning) or with a significantly increased risk of suffering death, pain, disability, or an important loss of freedom.[65]

Factors that can contribute to feelings of distress among college students include stressful events, poor academic performance, loneliness, and relationship problems.

mental disorder A behavioral or psychological syndrome associated with distress or disability or with a significantly increased risk of suffering death, pain, disability, or loss of freedom.

✓**check-in** Do you feel that your mental health affects your physical well-being—and vice versa?

Mental Health on Campus

Although the lives of college students hold great promise, many struggle—to be healthy, to find and grow into themselves, to launch their adult lives with confidence and competence, to make decisions that will affect their futures as well as the future of others.[66]

Mental health professionals have identified an "epidemic of serious psychiatric disturbances" in college students.[67] The number of students seeking psychological services has increased, and the problems they report—drug use, alcohol abuse, sexual assaults, self-injury, and suicidal thoughts and behaviors—are more severe than in the past.[68] However, among all students with apparent mental disorders, only 40 percent receive treatment.[69]

Here is a statistical snapshot of mental health among today's undergraduates[70]:

- About 18 percent have been diagnosed with or treated for depression over the past 12 months.

- Incoming students rated their emotional health at the lowest point in the last two decades.

- Some schools report that the number of students diagnosed with depression or anxiety has more than doubled in recent years.

- Students who live off campus are more likely to be depressed or anxious, perhaps because of the added stress of dealing with rent, household expenses, and housekeeping tasks.

- In a recent study of more than 40,000 undergraduates, including 13,000-plus students of color, found that Arab/Arab American students had the highest prevalence of mental health problems.[71]

- Transfer students score higher in anxiety than other undergraduates, while depression, anxiety, and stress ratings typically increase as students progress through college and are higher in upperclassmen than underclassmen.

- Students who are veterans or currently serving in the military are more likely to report depressive symptoms and suicidal ideas on screening tests—and to perceive stigma about seeking help.

✓**check-in** Do you feel that more undergraduates today are experiencing mental health issues than in the past?

Students at Risk According to the ACHA-NCHA survey, about one in three undergraduates has been diagnosed or treated for a mental disorder[72] (see Snapshot: On Campus Now). Despite having access to campus mental health providers and insurance to cover services, many college students do not receive necessary services. In a recent survey of California students, about one in five reported serious psychological distress in the past 30 days; slightly more than 1 in 10 experienced significant mental health-related impairment in the past year.[73]

- **History of a mental disorder**. Many undergraduates arrive on campus with a history of psychological problems. Medications for common disorders such as depression and attention-deficit/hyperactivity (ADHD) disorder have made it possible for young people who might otherwise not have been able to function in a college setting to pursue higher education.

- **Ongoing psychiatric issues**. Some undergraduates are dealing with ongoing issues such as bulimia, self-cutting, and childhood sexual abuse.

- **Breakup**. Many students become distressed following a romantic breakup or loss. In the survey, about one in eight individuals reported a breakup in the previous year. Their odds of having a psychiatric disorder are significantly higher than those who hadn't been through a breakup.

- **Financial pressures**. Student loans amount to a staggering $1 trillion, with the average graduate owing $23,300. Student loan debt may not only induce stress and worry but also increase stress in other ways, such as forcing students to delay marriage or parenthood or to forgo home ownership or other life goals.[74]

- **Discrimination**. Racial discrimination may be experienced more intensely than other forms of discrimination and may have a more ominous impact on mental and physical well-being. As research in psychology, sociology, and epidemiology has confirmed, the harmful effects of racial discrimination on African Americans include distress, depression, anxiety, and psychiatric symptoms.[75] Among African American students, a sense of hopelessness can contribute to or intensify symptoms of depression and anxiety.[76]

- **Minority status**. Mental health problems and psychological distress are more prevalent among ethnic, sexual, and gender minority students than among their peers.[77]

Student Mental Health

Within the past 12 months, students diagnosed or treated by a professional for the following:

	Percent (%)		
	Male	**Female**	**Total**
Anorexia	0.9	1.9	1.7
Anxiety	11.5	26.3	22.0
Attention-deficit/hyperactivity disorder	7.4	6.1	6.7
Bipolar disorder	1.7	2.1	2.1
Bulimia	0.8	1.4	1.3
Depression	9.7	20.1	17.3
Insomnia	3.3	5.6	5.1
Other sleep disorder	2.4	2.4	2.5
Obsessive–compulsive disorder	2.5	3.7	3.4
Panic attacks	4.6	13.5	11.0
Phobia	1.1	1.6	1.6
Schizophrenia	0.9	0.3	0.6
Substance abuse or addiction	1.7	1.1	1.4
Other addiction	1.1	0.8	1.0
Other mental health condition	2.6	4.3	4.1
Students reporting none of the above	79.6	65.6	69.5
Students reporting only one of the above	8.3	9.9	9.4
Students reporting both depression and anxiety	7.2	17.0	14.3
Students reporting any two or more of the above excluding the combination of depression and anxiety	5.7	10.6	9.5

Source: American College Health Association. American College Health Association-National College Health Assessment II: Reference Group Executive Summary Spring 2018. Silver Spring, MD: American College Health Association, 2018.

Among LGBTQIA students, interpersonal microaggressions (defined as subtle derogatory expressions) increase the likelihood of depression and attempted suicide.[78] Transgender students are at increased risk of harassment as well as discrimination.[79]

- **Athletics**. Student-athletes often encounter specific challenges, including balancing athletic and academic demands, stereotyping, navigating dual identities as students and athletes, group pressures, and individual factors such as perfectionism and body image concerns.[80]

✓**check-in** Has a psychological or emotional problem ever affected your ability to study or your academic performance?

The Impact of Mental Disorders

Psychological and emotional problems can affect every aspect of a student's life, including physical health, overall satisfaction, and relationships. Students who struggle with symptoms of anxiety or depression, which can interfere with concentration, study habits, classroom participation, and testing, commonly report struggling with academics. Students diagnosed with a mental health disorder in the previous 12 months are more likely to report unhealthy behaviors, including smoking, binge-drinking, substance abuse, poor dietary habits, and little or no physical activity.[81]

In the ACHA-NCHA's national survey, 26.5 percent of students reported that anxiety had impaired their ability to learn and earn higher grades; 18.7 percent said that depression had affected their academic performance.[82] Some estimate that 5 percent of undergraduates may not complete their degrees because of psychological problems.

Yet only a minority of troubled students seek or receive treatment.[83] Among the reasons that college students don't seek help with psychological problems are the following:

- **Lack of time.** With classes to attend, papers to write, tests to study for, and new relationships to form, students—even those so distressed that they are contemplating suicide—often say they can't find time to seek help.[84]

- **Stigma.** Students worry that others will think them "crazy" if they seek mental health services, especially if they come from families or cultures that view psychological problems and treatments negatively. Asian and Asian American students are the least likely to seek help, largely because of personal and cultural stigma, with 80 percent of those in need never receiving help.[85]

- **Underestimating the severity of the problem.** Many students who would benefit from treatment believe that they don't need professional help. Regardless of race or ethnicity, women are more likely than men to say, "I prefer to deal with issues on my own."[86]

- **Access.** Regardless of whether or not they have health insurance, cost remains a barrier to many students in need of mental health treatment. Other obstacles are lack of transportation and difficulty in scheduling appointments.[87]

In a report on students diagnosed with mental illness, 25 percent received psychiatric drugs; 20 percent, outpatient psychotherapy; and 4 percent inpatient care. Non-Hispanic blacks, Asians, and Hispanics were less likely than non-Hispanic whites to receive outpatient mental health services or psychotropic medications.[88]

The impact of mental health problems extends beyond an individual student to roommates, friends, classmates, family, and instructors. Suicides or suicide attempts affect all members of the campus community, who may experience profound sadness and grief. (See the discussion of suicide later in this chapter.) Although serious mental disorders may begin or worsen during young adulthood, 18- to 24-year-olds are less likely to seek and receive mental health care than any other age group.[89]

Depressive Disorders

Depression, the most common mental ailment worldwide, affects more than 13 million adults in the United States every year and costs billions of dollars in treatment and lost productivity and lives.

Those most likely to have major depression are:

- Women.
- Racial and ethnic minorities.
- Those without a high school education.
- Divorced or never-married individuals.
- Those without jobs.
- Those without health insurance.

Depression in Students

An estimated 15 to 40 percent of college students under age 25 may develop depression, but the number may be rising. About one in five college students report that depression has had a negative impact on their academic performance.[90] Although more students seek treatment for anxiety, they are more often likely to be diagnosed with a depressive disorder.[91]

Key contributors to depression in college students are:

- **Stress**. As they adjust to campus life, undergraduates face the ongoing stress of forging a new identity and finding a place for themselves in various social hierarchies. This triggers the release of the so-called stress hormones, which can change brain activity. A lack of social support can increase stress and depressive symptoms in first-year students.[92] Drugs and alcohol, widely used on campus, also affect the brain in ways that make managing stress even harder.

- **Too little sleep**. Computers, the Internet, around-the-clock television, and the college tradition of pulling all-nighters can contribute to sabotaging rest and increasing vulnerability to depression.

- **Academic and athletic pressures**. Depression has been linked to poorer academic performance and increased likelihood of dropping out before graduation. Students engaged in intercollegiate sports, according to a recent study, are twice as likely to be depressed as nonathletes. The reasons may include overtraining, injury, pressure to perform, lack of free time, and the stress of juggling athletics and schoolwork. Concussions may increase the risk of depression as well as academic problems in some college athletes.

The impacts of depression on college students include:

- Poorer academic performance.
- Increased risk of dropping out.
- Greater anxiety.
- Decreased physical activity.
- Medical symptoms and illnesses.
- Unsafe sexual behavior.
- Greater likelihood of smoking.
- Alcohol and drug dependence.
- Poorer quality of life.
- Self-harming behaviors.
- Increased risk of suicide.[93]

✓check-in Can you identify any factors that might increase your risk of depression?

Sex and Depression

Female Depression Depression is twice as common in women as in men. However, this gender gap decreases or disappears in studies of men and women in similar socioeconomic situations, such as college students, civil servants, and the Amish community.

Black women are much less likely to report suffering from depression than white women are. About 10 percent of black women report struggling with the mental health disorder at some point in their lives, compared with 21 percent of white women. The reason may be that they have developed resources and coping strategies to deal with stressful circumstances, such as supportive social ties, religious participation, group identity, and a strong sense of mastery and self-esteem.[94]

Women may not necessarily be more likely to develop depression, this research suggests, but may have an underlying predisposition that puts them at greater risk under various social stressors.

Brain chemistry and sex hormones may play a role in the following ways:

- Women produce less of certain metabolites of serotonin, a messenger chemical that helps regulate mood.
- Women's brains register sadness much more intensely than men's.
- Women, more sensitive to changes in light and temperature, are at least four times more likely than men to develop seasonal affective disorder (SAD) and to become depressed in the dark winter months.
- Some women also seem more sensitive to their own hormones or to the changes in them that occur at puberty, during the menstrual cycle, after childbirth, or during perimenopause and menopause.

The *Diagnostic and Statistical Manual of Mental Disorders*, Fifth Edition (*DSM-5*) classifies premenstrual dysphoric disorder (PDD), which is not the same as premenstrual syndrome (PMS), discussed in Chapter 8, as a depressive disorder. In the final week before onset of menstruation, an estimated 1.8 to 5.8 percent of women experience the characteristic symptoms of PDD[95]:

- Marked mood swings, tearfulness, sadness, or sensitivity to rejection.
- Marked irritability, anger, or conflicts with others.
- Marked depressed moods, hopelessness, or self-deprecating thoughts.
- Marked anxiety, tension, or feelings of being on edge.

✓check-in If you are a woman, have you ever experienced any symptoms of premenstrual dysphoric disorder?

Symptoms start to improve within a few days after menstruation begins and end or become minimal in the following week.

Pregnancy, contrary to what many people assume, does not "protect" a woman from depression, and women who discontinue treatment when they become pregnant are at risk of a relapse. Women and their psychiatrists must carefully weigh the risks and benefits of psychiatric medications during pregnancy.

Male Depression More than 6 million men in the United States—1 in every 14—suffer from this insidious disorder, many without recognizing what's wrong. Experts describe male depression as an "under" disease: underdiscussed, underrecognized, underdiagnosed, and undertreated.

Depression "looks" different in men than in women in the following ways:

- Irritability or tremendous fatigue rather than sadness.
- A sense of being dead inside, of worthlessness, hopelessness, helplessness, of losing their life force.
- Physical symptoms such as headaches, pain, and insomnia.
- Attempts to "self-medicate" with alcohol or drugs.

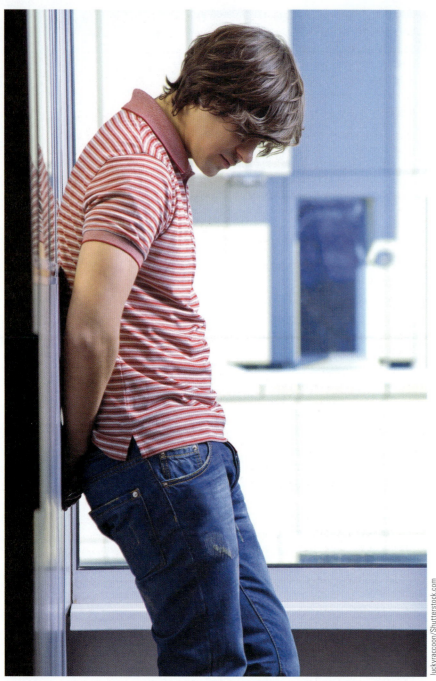

Many men don't realize that a sense of hopelessness, worthlessness, helplessness, or feeling dead inside can be a symptom of depression.

major depressive disorder
Sadness that does not end; ongoing feelings of utter helplessness.

antidepressants Drugs used primarily to treat symptoms of depression.

luckyraccoon/Shutterstock.com

Genes may make some men more vulnerable than others, but chronic stress of any sort plays a major role in male depression, possibly by raising levels of the stress hormone cortisol and lowering testosterone. Men are also more likely than women to become depressed following divorce, job loss, or a career setback.

Whatever its roots, male depression alters brain chemistry in potentially deadly ways. Four times as many men as women kill themselves; depressed men are two to four times more likely to take their own lives than are depressed women.

Major Depressive Disorder

An estimated 20 to 30 percent of college students may develop a **major depressive disorder**, which can simply be defined as sadness that does not end.[96] Food, friends, sex, or any form of pleasure no longer appeals. It is impossible to concentrate on work and responsibilities. Unable to escape a sense of utter hopelessness, depressed individuals may fight back tears throughout the day and toss and turn through long, empty nights. Thoughts of death or suicide may push into their minds.

The characteristic symptoms of major depression include:

- **Feeling depressed**, sad, empty, discouraged, or tearful most of the day, nearly every day.
- **Losing interest** or pleasure in once-enjoyable activities.
- **Eating more or less** than usual and either gaining or losing a significant amount of weight.
- **Having trouble sleeping** or sleeping much more than usual.
- **Feeling slowed down** or restless and unable to sit still.
- **Lacking energy** or fatigue nearly every day.
- **Feeling helpless**, hopeless, worthless, inadequate, or inappropriately guilty.
- **Difficulty thinking or concentrating**; indecisiveness.
- **Persistent thoughts of death** or suicide.

As many as half of major depressive episodes are not recognized because the symptoms are "masked." Rather than feeling sad or depressed, individuals may experience low energy, insomnia, difficulty concentrating, and physical symptoms.

Treating Depression

The American Psychiatric Association's guidelines for treating depression call for an individualized approach tailored to each patient's symptoms. Specific treatments might include medication, healthy behaviors, exercise (proven to reduce depressive symptoms, especially in older adults and those with chronic medical problems), and psychotherapy. Complementary approaches, such as imagining positive events in the future, may help by boosting optimism.[97]

The rate of depression treatment, particularly with **antidepressants**, has increased in the past decade. Medication has become the most common approach, while fewer patients receive psychotherapy than in the past, possibly because of limited insurance coverage. A combination of psychotherapy and medication is considered the most effective approach for most patients (see Consumer Alert).

Psychotherapy helps individuals pinpoint the life problems that contribute to their depression, identify negative or distorted thinking patterns, explore behaviors that contribute to depression, and regain a sense of control and pleasure in life. Various therapies, including cognitive-behavioral therapy and mindfulness-based therapy, have proved as helpful as antidepressant drugs, although they take longer than medication to achieve results.[98]

Even without treatment, depression generally lifts after 6 to 9 months. However, in more than 80 percent of people, it recurs, with each episode lasting longer and becoming more severe and difficult to treat.

Bipolar Disorder

Bipolar disorder, known as manic depression in the past, consists of mood swings that may take individuals from manic states of feeling euphoric and energetic to depressive states of utter despair. In episodes of full mania, they may become so impulsive and out of touch with reality that they endanger their careers, relationships, health, or even survival. Psychiatrists view bipolar symptoms on a spectrum that includes depression and states of acute irritability and distress.

During a manic episode, individuals may make grandiose plans, feel little need for sleep, talk more than usual, and get involved in activities with a high potential for painful consequences (such as buying sprees or sexual indiscretions). During a hypomanic episode, people may feel an elevated, expansive, or irritable mood and abnormally and persistently increased activity or energy along with symptoms similar to those of mania. Often those with bipolar disorder plunge from these exhilarating states into major depressive episodes, in which they may feel sad, hopeless, and helpless and develop other characteristic symptoms of depression.

Bipolar and related disorders affect approximately 4 percent of the population. Men tend to develop bipolar disorder earlier in life (between ages 16 and 25), but women have higher rates overall. About 50 percent of patients with bipolar illness have a family history of the disorder.[99]

The characteristic symptoms of bipolar disorder include the following:

- **Mood swings**—from happy to miserable, optimistic to despairing, and so on.

- **Changes in thinking**—thoughts speeding through one's mind, unrealistic self-confidence, difficulty concentrating, delusions, and hallucinations.

bipolar disorder Severe depression alternating with periods of manic activity and elation.

YOUR STRATEGIES FOR PREVENTION

How to Help Someone Who Is Depressed

- **Express your concern, but don't nag.** You might say, "I'm concerned about you. You are struggling right now. We need to find some help."

- **Don't be distracted by behaviors like drinking or gambling, which can disguise depression in men.**

- **Encourage the individual to remain in treatment** until symptoms begin to lift (which takes several weeks).

- **Provide emotional support.** Listen carefully. Offer hope and reassurance that with time and treatment, things will get better.

- **Do not ignore remarks about suicide.** Report them to the person's doctor or, in an emergency, call 911.

ⓘ CONSUMER ALERT

The Pros and Cons of Antidepressants

Millions of individuals have benefited from the category of antidepressant drugs called selective serotonin reuptake inhibitors (SSRIs). However, like all drugs, they can cause side effects that range from temporary physical symptoms, such as stomach upset and headaches, to more persistent problems, such as sexual dysfunction. The most serious—and controversial—risk is suicide. Some studies have shown an association between SSRIs and an increased risk of suicide, especially during the first months of treatment, but more recent reports have not confirmed this link in adults.

Facts to Know

- The FDA has issued a "black box" warning about the risk of suicidal thoughts, hostility, and aggression in both children and young adults.

- This risk of suicide while taking an antidepressant is about 1 in 3,000; the risk of a serious attempt is 1 in 1,000.

Steps to Take

- If you are younger than age 20, be aware of the increased suicide risk with the use of SSRIs. Talk these over carefully with a psychiatrist. Discuss alternative treatments, such as psychotherapy.

- For individuals older than age 20, the benefits of antidepressants have proved to outweigh their risks in most cases. Adults treated with SSRIs are 40 percent less likely to commit suicide than depressed individuals who do not receive this therapy.

- In patients initially treated with antidepressants, two approaches based on mindfulness (discussed in Chapter 3)—mindfulness-based cognitive therapy and mindfulness meditation—have proven as effective as continuing drug therapy in preventing a return of depression symptoms.

- Whatever your age, arrange for careful monitoring and follow-up with a psychiatrist when you start taking an antidepressant. Familiarize yourself with possible side effects, and seek help immediately if you begin to think about taking your own life.

- **Changes in behavior**—sudden immersion in plans and projects, talking very rapidly and much more than usual, excessive spending, impaired judgment, and impulsive sexual involvement.
- **Changes in physical condition**—less need for sleep, increased energy, and fewer health complaints than usual.

Professional therapy is essential in treating bipolar disorders. Bipolar disorder decreases the life expectancy of patients diagnosed at age 15 by 11 years or more.[100] An estimated 25 to 50 percent of bipolar patients attempt suicide at least once. About 1 percent take their own lives every year. Mood-stabilizing medications are the keystone of treatment, although psychotherapy plays a critical role in helping individuals understand their illness and rebuild their lives. Most individuals continue taking medication indefinitely after remission of their symptoms because the risk of recurrence is high.

Anxiety Disorders

Anxiety disorders, which affect an estimated 10 to 15 percent of psychiatric patients, are more common than depression (diagnosed in 7 to 10 percent of patients).[101] More than a quarter of college students report that anxiety has negatively affected their academic performance. About 22 percent—12 percent of college men and 26 percent of college women—have been diagnosed with an anxiety disorder in the previous year.[102]

Anxiety disorders may involve inordinate fears of certain objects or situations (**phobias**); episodes of sudden, inexplicable terror (**panic attacks**); chronic distress (generalized anxiety disorder [GAD]); or persistent, disturbing thoughts. These disorders can increase the risk of developing depression.

Over a lifetime, as many as one in four Americans may experience an anxiety disorder. More than 40 percent are never correctly diagnosed and treated. Yet most individuals who do get treatment, even for severe and disabling problems, improve dramatically.

anxiety disorders A group of psychological disorders involving episodes of apprehension, tension, or uneasiness, stemming from the anticipation of danger and sometimes accompanied by physical symptoms, which cause significant distress and impairment.

phobias Anxiety disorders marked by an inordinate fear of an object, a class of objects, or a situation, resulting in extreme avoidance behaviors.

panic attacks Short episodes characterized by physical sensations of light-headedness, dizziness, hyperventilation, and numbness of extremities, accompanied by an inexplicable terror, usually of a physical disaster such as death.

✓**check-in** Are you experiencing any of the following symptoms of anxiety?

_____ Apprehenson

_____ Panicky feelings

_____ Trembling

_____ Shakiness

_____ Dry mouth

_____ Difficulty breathing

_____ Pounding heart

_____ Sweaty palms

_____ Constant worrying about small or large concerns

Specific Phobia

Phobias—the most prevalent type of anxiety disorder—are out-of-the-ordinary, irrational, intense, persistent fears of certain objects or situations. About 2 million Americans develop such acute terror that they go to extremes to avoid whatever it is that they fear, even though they realize these feelings are excessive or unreasonable.

The most common phobias involve:

- Animals, particularly dogs, snakes, insects, and mice.
- The sight of blood.
- Closed spaces (*claustrophobia*).
- Heights (*acrophobia*).
- Air travel.
- Being in open or public places or situations from which one perceives it would be difficult or embarrassing to escape (*agoraphobia*).

Although various medications have been tried, the best approach is behavioral therapy, which consists of gradual, systematic exposure to the feared object (a process called *systematic desensitization*). Numerous studies have proved that exposure—especially *in vivo* exposure, in which individuals are exposed to the actual source of their fear rather than simply imagining it—is highly effective. Medical hypnosis—the use of induction of an altered state of consciousness—also can help.

✓**check-in** Does any particular object or situation make you fearful or anxious?

Panic Attacks and Panic Disorder

Individuals who have had panic attacks describe them as the most frightening experiences of their lives. Without reason or warning, their hearts race wildly. They may become light-headed or dizzy. Because they can't catch their breath, they may start breathing rapidly and hyperventilate. Parts of their bodies, such as their fingers or toes, may tingle or feel numb. Worst of all is the terrible sense that something horrible is about to happen—that they will die, lose their minds, or have a heart attack.

Most attacks reach peak intensity within 10 minutes. Afterward, individuals live in dread of another one. In the course of a lifetime, your risk of having a single panic attack is 7 percent.

✓**check-in** Have you ever had a panic attack?

Panic disorder develops when attacks recur or apprehension about them becomes so intense that individuals cannot function normally. Full-blown panic disorder occurs in about 2 percent of all adults in the course of a lifetime and usually develops before age 30. Women are more than twice as likely as men to experience panic attacks, although no one knows why. Parents, siblings, and children of individuals with panic disorders are also more likely to develop them than are others.

The two primary treatments for panic disorder are cognitive-behavioral therapy (CBT), which teaches specific strategies for coping with symptoms such as rapid breathing, and medication. Treatment helps as many as 90 percent of those with panic disorder either improve significantly or recover completely, usually within 6 to 8 weeks.

Generalized Anxiety Disorder

About 10 million adults in the United States suffer from a **generalized anxiety disorder (GAD)**, excessive or unrealistic apprehension that causes physical symptoms, such as restlessness, fatigue, and muscle tension that lasts for 6 months or longer. It usually starts when people are in their 20s. Unlike fear, which helps us recognize and avoid real danger, GAD is an irrational or unwarranted response to harmless objects or situations of exaggerated danger.

The most common symptoms are:

- Increased heart rate.
- Sweating.
- Increased blood pressure.
- Muscle aches.
- Intestinal pains.
- Irritability.

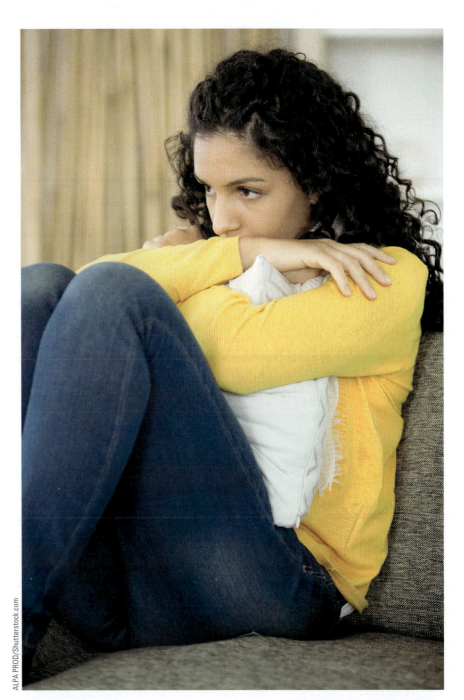

ALPA PROD./Shutterstock.com

- Sleep problems.
- Difficulty concentrating.

Undergraduates with generalized anxiety may find it especially difficult to deal with physical discomfort, uncertainty, negative emotions, ambiguity, and frustration.[103] Chronically anxious individuals worry—not just some of the time, and not just about the stresses and strains of ordinary life—but constantly, about almost everything: their health, families, finances, marriages, and potential dangers. Treatment for GAD may consist of a combination of psychotherapy, behavioral therapy, and antianxiety drugs.

Worry is a normal part of daily life, but individuals with generalized anxiety disorder worry constantly about everything that might go wrong.

panic disorder An anxiety disorder in which the apprehension or experience of recurring panic attacks is so intense that normal functioning is impaired.

generalized anxiety disorder (GAD) An anxiety disorder characterized as chronic distress.

Other Common Disorders

Obsessive–Compulsive Disorder

An estimated 1.9 to 3.3 percent of Americans have an **obsessive–compulsive disorder (OCD)**.[104] Some of these individuals suffer only from an *obsession*, a recurring idea, thought, or image that they realize, at least initially, is senseless.

The most common obsessions are:

- Repetitive thoughts that usually involve harm and danger.
- Contamination (e.g., becoming infected by shaking hands).
- Doubt (e.g., wondering whether one has performed some act, such as having hurt someone in a traffic accident).

Most people with OCD also suffer from a *compulsion*, a repetitive behavior performed according to certain rules or in a stereotyped fashion. The most common compulsions include:

- Handwashing.
- Cleaning.
- Repeating words silently.
- Counting.
- Checking (e.g., making sure dozens of times that a door is locked).

Individuals with OCD realize that their thoughts or behaviors are bizarre, but they cannot resist or control them. Eventually, the obsessions or compulsions consume a great deal of time and significantly interfere with normal routines, job functioning, or usual social activities or relationships with others. A young woman who must follow a very rigid dressing routine may always be late for class, for example; a student who must count each letter of the alphabet as he types may not be able to complete a term paper.

Treatment may consist of cognitive therapy to correct irrational assumptions, behavioral techniques such as progressively limiting the amount of time someone obsessed with cleanliness can spend washing and scrubbing, and medication. Deep brain stimulation, which is used to treat Parkinson's, has helped patients with severe OCD. Other related disorders include excoriation (skin-picking), hoarding (persistent difficulty discarding or parting with possessions), body dysmorphic disorder (preoccupation with perceived physical defects or flaws), and trichotillomania (hair-pulling).

Attention-Deficit/Hyperactivity Disorder

Attention-deficit/hyperactivity disorder (ADHD) is the most common mental disorder in childhood, affecting an estimated 6 to 7 percent of children and teenagers (and 5 percent of adults).[105] The characteristic symptoms of ADHD are:

- Inattention—wandering off task, difficulty sustaining focus, being disorganized, lacking persistence.
- Hyperactivity—excessive movements, such as fidgeting or tapping.
- Impulsivity—hasty actions done without forethought and with high potential for harm.

For many youngsters, ADHD persists into adolescence and adulthood. About one in three young adults diagnosed with childhood ADHD still had the disorder at an average age of 27. About twice as many had at least one other mental health issue, such as alcohol abuse, depression, or chronic anxiety.

ADHD on Campus In the ACHA survey, 6 percent of students report that they have been diagnosed with ADHD.[106] The normal challenges of college—navigating the complexities of scheduling, planning courses, and honing study skills—may be especially daunting for these students, who may find it hard to concentrate, read, make decisions, complete complex projects, and meet deadlines. Undergraduates with ADHD report significantly lower GPAs[107] and greater anxiety[108] and are at higher risk of becoming smokers, abusing alcohol and drugs, and having automobile accidents.

Relationships with peers can also become more challenging. Young people with ADHD may become frustrated easily, have a short fuse, and erupt into angry outbursts. Some become more argumentative, negative, and defiant than most other teens. Male students with ADHD typically begin dating at a later age, have fewer romantic relationships, and experience more rejection than undergraduate men without ADHD. Female undergraduates with ADHD report more difficulties regulating their emotions, more stress, more conflict, and lower satisfaction in their romantic relationships than other female students.[109]

Sleep problems, including sleeping much more or less than normal, are common. The likelihood of developing other emotional problems, including

obsessive–compulsive disorder (OCD) An anxiety disorder characterized by obsessions and/or compulsions that impair one's ability to function and form relationships.

attention-deficit/hyperactivity disorder (ADHD) A spectrum of difficulties in controlling motion and sustaining attention, including hyperactivity, impulsivity, and distractibility.

depression and anxiety disorders, is higher. As many as 20 percent of those diagnosed with depression, anxiety, or substance abuse also have ADHD. The risk of substance use disorders for individuals with ADHD is twice that of the general population.[110]

Treating ADHD

The medications used for this disorder include stimulants (such as Ritalin), which improve behavior and cognition for about 70 percent of adolescents with ADHD. Extended-release preparations (including a skin patch) are longer acting, so individuals do not have to take these medications as often as in the past.

As discussed in Chapter 12, an estimated 17 percent of college students misuse stimulant medications.[111] Some may be self-medicating themselves for attention problems, but it's not clear whether they suffer from true ADHD. Emergency department visits involving abuse of ADHD drugs have doubled in the past decade.

An alternative nonstimulant treatment is Strattera (atomoxetine), which treats ADHD and coexisting problems such as depression and anxiety but does not seem to have any known potential for abuse. Adverse effects include drowsiness, loss of appetite, nausea, vomiting, and headaches. Its long-term effects are not known.

✓**check-in** If you have an attention disorder, how do you cope with it?

Many students with ADHD benefit from strategies such as sitting in the front row to avoid distraction, recording lectures if they have difficulty listening and taking notes at the same time, being allowed extended time for tests, and taking oral rather than written exams. Some students have tried to feign ADHD to qualify for such special treatment or to obtain prescriptions for stimulants. However, a thorough examination by an experienced therapist can usually determine whether a student actually suffers from ADHD.

Autism Spectrum Disorder

Autism, a complex neurodevelopmental disability that causes social and communication impairments, is a "spectrum" disorder that affects individuals to varying degrees. Found in all racial, ethnic, and socioeconomic groups, this disorder can affect every aspect of an individual's life. As many as 70 percent of autistic individuals may also have another mental disorder requiring treatment.

According to recent estimates from the CDC, about 1 in 68 children has **autism spectrum disorder (ASD)**.[112] Boys are four to five times more likely to be diagnosed with ASD than girls,

perhaps because of genetic vulnerability. Among the possible factors that may increase the risk of ASD are genetic factors, maternal illness or trauma during pregnancy, abnormalities in brain circuitry, low birth weight, and parental age.

There is no scientific evidence that any part of a vaccine or combination of vaccines causes autism, nor is there proof that any material used to produce the vaccine, such as thimerosal, a mercury-containing preservative, plays a role in causing autism. Although past research fraudulently linked vaccines to autism, further investigations have refuted those findings and found no link, even in youngsters with siblings with autism.[113]

ASD symptoms, which include repetitive patterns of thoughts and behavior and deficits in communication and social interactions, usually start before age 2 and can create delays or problems in many different skills that develop from infancy to adulthood. The earlier interventions begin, the more effective they have proved to be.[114]

ASD on Campus

About a third of adolescents and young adults diagnosed with ASD—an estimated 2 percent of all undergraduates with disabilities—are entering colleges and universities. Although many have the cognitive ability to succeed academically, a high percentage of ASD-diagnosed undergraduates do not complete their postsecondary programs. One reason may be social exclusion, often based on misconceptions about autism.[115] Specific interventions, such as online training, have been shown to increase undergraduates' understanding and acceptance of their peers with autism.[116]

✓**check-in** How would you describe your knowledge of autism spectrum disorder and your attitude toward individuals with this disorder?

Adults with autism have significantly increased rates of all major psychiatric disorders, including depression, anxiety, bipolar disorder, obsessive–compulsive disorder, schizophrenia, and suicide attempts, as well as physical illnesses such as immune conditions, digestive and sleep disorders, seizures, obesity, hypertension, and diabetes.[117]

Schizophrenia

Schizophrenia, one of the most debilitating mental disorders, profoundly impairs an individual's sense of reality. As the National Institute of Mental Health (NIMH) puts it, schizophrenia, which is characterized by abnormalities in brain

autism spectrum disorder (ASD) A neurodevelopmental disorder that causes social and communication impairments.

schizophrenia A general term for a group of mental disorders with characteristic psychotic symptoms, such as delusions, hallucinations, and disordered thought patterns during the active phase of the illness, and a duration of at least six months.

structure and chemistry, destroys "the inner unity of the mind" and weakens "the will and drive that constitute our essential character." This disorder, which is diagnosed in about 1 percent of people worldwide, affects every aspect of psychological functioning, including the ways in which people think, feel, view themselves, and relate to others.

The symptoms of schizophrenia include:

- Hallucinations.
- Delusions.
- Disorganized thinking.
- Talking in rambling or incoherent ways.
- Making odd or purposeless movements or not moving at all.
- Repeating others' words or mimicking their gestures.
- Showing few, if any, feelings; responding with inappropriate emotions.
- Lacking will or motivation to complete a task or accomplish something.
- Functioning at a much lower level than in the past at work, in interpersonal relations, or in taking care of themselves.

Schizophrenia, which affects 0.3 to 0.7 percent of the world's population, is one of the leading causes of disability among young adults. Schizophrenia usually develops in the early to mid-20s in men and the late 20s in women. Although symptoms do not occur until then, they almost certainly result from failure in brain development that occurs very early in life, probably before birth. Schizophrenia has a strong genetic basis and is not the result of upbringing, social conditions, or traumatic experiences.

For the vast majority of individuals with schizophrenia, antipsychotic drugs are the foundation of treatment. Newer agents are more effective in making most people with schizophrenia feel more comfortable and in control of themselves, helping organize chaotic thinking, and reducing or eliminating delusions or hallucinations, allowing fuller participation in normal activities. Aerobic exercise has also proven beneficial.[118]

Self-Injury and Suicide

Deliberately harming oneself may take any form of damage to the body: cutting, burning, stabbing, hitting, and excessive rubbing. The intent is not to take one's life but to obtain relief from painful feelings or thoughts, to resolve an interpersonal difficulty, or to induce positive feelings, such as relief. Self-injury most often starts in the early teens and can continue for many years. Admission to hospitals for self-inflicted injuries peaks between the ages of 20 and 29 and then declines. In the ACHA survey, 7.8 percent of college students—4.8 percent of men and 8.4 percent of women—reported intentionally cutting, burning, bruising, or otherwise injuring themselves.[119]

Suicide is the second leading cause of death among 15- to 24-year-olds in the United States.[120] The most common methods are guns, hanging, and poisoning. Suicide, often the tragic consequence of emotional and psychological problems, affects millions of lives every year:

- An estimated 8.5 million American adults (3.8 percent) report having had serious thoughts of suicide in the past year.
- 1.1 million (0.5 percent) attempt suicide.
- Some 38,000 Americans—among them many young people who seem to have "everything to live for"—commit suicide.
- An average of 105 suicides occur in the United States every day.
- An estimated 811,000 people attempt to take their own lives per year.
- There may be 4.5 million suicide "survivors" in the United States.
- The suicide rate for African American and Caucasian men peaks between ages 20 and 40 and rises again after age 65 among white men and after age 75 among blacks.
- In general, whites are at highest risk for suicide, followed by American Indians, African Americans, Hispanic Americans, and Asian Americans.

Long considered a threat to younger and older Americans, suicide has increased significantly among middle-aged men and women. Although the reasons are unknown, researchers speculate that baby boomers, who also had high suicide rates in adolescence, may be particularly vulnerable to self-inflicted harm. They also tend to choose the most lethal suicide methods, such as guns and hanging. At all ages, men *commit* suicide three to four times more frequently than women, but women *attempt* suicide much more often than men (see Table 2.1).

Suicide on Campus

More than 1,100 college students take their own lives every year; many more—an estimated 1.2 percent of undergraduates—attempt to do so. However, rates of suicidal thoughts and behaviors for college students are significantly lower than those of their same-age peers who are not in college.[121]

About 8 percent of undergraduates report having seriously considered suicide in the last 12 months; 1.2 percent attempt suicide.[122] College students who are serving or have served in the military do not have higher rates of depression and are not more likely to plan or attempt suicide than other undergraduates.[123]

Suicide rarely stems from a single cause. Researchers have identified several common ones for college students, including:

- Depression and depressive symptoms.
- Family history of mental illness.
- Personality traits such as hopelessness, helplessness, impulsivity, and aggression.
- Alcohol use and binge drinking. (Among college students, binge drinkers are significantly more likely to contemplate suicide, to have attempted suicide in the past, and to believe they would make a future suicide attempt than non-binge drinkers.)
- Interpersonal difficulties with a romantic partner, family, or friends, which may reflect what researchers call "thwarted belongingness" or a lack of connectedness with peers, loved ones, and the school community.[124]
- Ineffective problem solving and coping skills.
- Recent sexual or physical victimization; being in an emotionally or physically abusive relationship.
- Family problems.
- Exposure to trauma or stress.
- Feelings of loneliness or social isolation.
- Harassment because of sexual orientation.
- Disturbed sleep and insomnia.[125]

Although many schools offer counseling and crisis services, students often don't know where to turn when they feel hopeless or are thinking about suicide.

Risk Factors

The most important risk factors for suicide appear to be impulsivity, high levels of arousal and aggression, and past suicidal behavior (see Table 2.2). Others are as follows:

- **Suicidal behavior disorder**. Individuals who have tried to take their own lives are at higher risk for further attempts and for death in the 2 years following a failed attempt. About 25 to 30 percent of persons who try to kill themselves attempt to do so again.

- **Mental disorders**. More than 95 percent of those who commit suicide have a mental disorder, such as depression.
- **Substance abuse**. Alcoholics and drug abusers who attempt suicide often have other risk factors, including major depression, poor social support, serious medical illness, and unemployment.
- **Hopelessness**. When hope dies, individuals view every experience in negative terms and come to expect the worst possible outcomes for their problems. Given this way of thinking, suicide often seems a reasonable response to a life seen as not worth living.

TABLE 2.1 Suicide Risk

	Who Attempts Suicide?	Who Commits Suicide?
Sex	Female	Male
Age	Under 35	Under 20 or over 60
Means	Less deadly, such as a wrist slashing	More deadly, such as a gun
Circumstances	High chance of rescue	Low chance of rescue

TABLE 2.2 Risk Factors for Suicide

Biopsychosocial Risk Factors

- Mental disorders, particularly depressive disorders, schizophrenia, and anxiety disorders
- Alcohol and other substance use disorders
- Hopelessness
- Impulsive and/or aggressive tendencies
- History of trauma or abuse
- Some major physical illness
- Previous suicide attempt
- Family history of suicide

Environmental Risk Factors

- Job or financial loss
- Relational or social loss
- Easy access to lethal means
- Local clusters of suicide that have a contagious influence

Sociocultural Risk Factors

- Lack of social support and sense of isolation
- Stigma associated with help-seeking behavior
- Barriers to accessing health care, especially mental health and substance abuse treatment
- Certain cultural and religious beliefs (for instance, the belief that suicide is a noble resolution of a personal dilemma)
- Exposure to suicide, including through the media, and the influence of others who have died by suicide

Source: Suicide Prevention Resource Center: www.sprc.org/.

Steps to Prevent Suicide

If you worry that someone you know may be contemplating suicide, express your concern. Here are some specific guidelines:

- **Ask concerned questions.** Listen attentively. Show that you take the person's feelings seriously and truly care.

- **Don't offer trite reassurances.** Don't list reasons to go on living, try to analyze the person's motives, or try to shock or challenge him or her.

- **Suggest solutions or alternatives to problems.** Make plans. Encourage positive action, such as getting away for a while to gain a better perspective on a problem.

- **Don't be afraid to ask whether your friend has considered suicide.** The opportunity to talk about thoughts of suicide may be an enormous relief and—contrary to a longstanding myth—will not fix the idea of suicide more firmly in a person's mind.

- **Don't think that people who talk about killing themselves never carry out their threat.** Most individuals who commit suicide give definite indications of their intent to die.

- **Watch out for behavioral clues.** If your friend begins to behave unpredictably or suddenly emerges from a severe depression into a calm, settled state of mind, these could signal increased danger of suicide. Don't leave your friend alone. Call a suicide hotline, or get in touch with a mental health professional.

- **If a friend expresses suicidal thoughts on Facebook, report the post to its "Report Suicidal Content" link.** The person who posted the suicidal content will receive an email or call from the National Suicide Prevention Lifeline (1-800-273-TALK).

If you are thinking about suicide . . .

- **Talk to a mental health professional.** If you have a therapist, call immediately. If not, call a suicide hotline.

- **Find someone you can trust and talk honestly about what you're feeling.** If you suffer from depression or another mental disorder, educate trusted friends or relatives about your condition so they are prepared if called upon to help.

- **Write down your more uplifting thoughts.** Even if you are despondent, you can help yourself by taking the time to retrieve some more positive thoughts or memories. A simple record of your hopes for the future and the people you value in your life can remind you of why your own life is worth continuing.

- **Avoid drugs and alcohol.** Most suicides are the results of sudden, uncontrolled impulses, and drugs and alcohol can make it harder to resist these destructive urges.

- **Go to the hospital.** Hospitalization can sometimes be the best way to protect your health and safety.

- **Combat stress**. Conditions that may increase a veteran's risk of suicide include depression, PTSD, traumatic brain injury, and lack of social support. The Veterans Administration has set up a Suicide Prevention Hotline number at 1-800-274-TALK.

- **Family history**. One of every four people who attempt suicide has a family member who also tried to commit suicide. "Poor parental attachment" may increase the risk of suicide in college students during their transition to adulthood.[126]

- **Physical illness**. People who commit suicide are likely to be ill or to believe that they are. While suicide may seem to be a decision rationally arrived at in persons with serious or fatal illness, depression, not uncommon in such instances, can warp judgment.

- **Brain chemistry**. Investigators have found abnormalities in the brain chemistry of individuals who complete suicide, especially low levels of a metabolite of the neurotransmitter serotonin.

- **Access to guns**. Unlike other methods of suicide, guns almost always kill. Although only 5 percent of suicide attempts involve firearms, more than 90 percent of these attempts are fatal.

- **Other factors**. Individuals who kill themselves have often gone through more major life crises—job changes, births, financial reversals, divorce, and retirement—in the previous 6 months, compared with others.

✓**check-in** Do you know anyone who attempted or committed suicide?

Overcoming Problems of the Mind

At any given time, about 25 percent of men, women, and children meet the criteria for a mental disorder, yet 75 percent of those in need of psychological help never receive the treatment they need. As discussed earlier in this chapter, college students are especially likely to delay getting help for a psychological problem.

Without treatment, mental disorders take a toll on every aspect of life, including academics, relationships, careers, and risk-taking. Symptoms or episodes of a disorder typically become more frequent or severe. Individuals with one mental disorder are at high risk of having a second one; this is called *comorbidity*.

Self-Care Strategies

Self-care, defined as "providing adequate attention to one's own physical and psychological wellness," can contribute enormously to both physical and psychological health.[127]

Eating Right Both body and mind require good nutrition to run efficiently. Poor eating habits—skipping meals, wolfing them down, munching on junk foods—can make people psychologically uneasy and unable to concentrate on tasks at hand, relax, or enjoy being with others. A healthful, balanced diet is essential to a feeling of well-being.

People who are depressed need to be especially watchful because they may lose their appetite, eat less, lose weight, and be at risk for nutritional deficiencies. Although various nutritional "cures" for depression have been touted over the years, none has been scientifically validated.

Excessive caffeine (discussed in Chapters 5 and 12) can cause many symptoms associated with anxiety or panic. Anyone troubled by an anxiety disorder should avoid caffeinated beverages.

Many people increase the amount of alcohol they drink when under stress. Depressed individuals may try to drown their sorrows; those who are anxious may drink to calm their "nerves." However, drinking only makes these problems worse. As discussed in Chapter 13, alcohol, a central nervous system depressant, can intensify a depressed mood or exacerbate anxiety.

Exercise In addition to its head-to-toe physical benefits, as discussed in Chapter 6, exercise may be, as one therapist puts it, the single most effective way to lift a person's spirits and to restore feelings of potency about all aspects of life (see Health on a Budget). People who exercise regularly report a more cheerful mood, higher self-esteem, and less stress. Their sleep and appetite also tend to improve. In clinical studies, exercise has proved effective as a treatment for depression and anxiety disorders. But remember: Although exercise can help prevent and ease problems for many people, it's no substitute for professional treatment of serious psychiatric disorders.

Books and Websites A wealth of informational and motivational material is available online and in books. Research has shown that such "low-intensity interventions," which do not require the expense and time of a professional therapist, can help individuals with disorders that range from mild to more severe.

Virtual Support Increasingly, mental health professionals are utilizing "e-health" or "m-health" (the delivery of health care by electronic means via the Internet using phones, watches, apps, and other devices). Such technology makes psychological support available 24 hours a day, 7 days a week—a boon for many patients.

Peer Support Support groups have long been a staple of treatment for individuals who have a chronic illness; are wrestling with a substance use disorder; have experienced common traumatic experiences, such as child abuse; or are dealing with similar challenges, such as widowhood. Often these groups do not have a professional leader or formal structure. Their primary goal is to provide support and encouragement, overcome a sense of isolation, and share information. Some schools have begun offering online peer support forums to decrease isolation and boost problem solving skills for students with problems such as symptoms of depression.

With an estimated half million veterans, active-duty personnel, reservists, and National Guardsmen attending college, more peer support groups for fellow service members or veterans are appearing on campus. Compared with their civilian counterparts, they focus on issues such as the challenge of adjusting from military service to student life, tobacco- and

$ HEALTH ON A BUDGET

The Exercise Prescription

Imagine a drug so powerful it can alter brain chemistry, so versatile it can help prevent or treat many common mental disorders, so safe that moderate doses cause few, if any, side effects, and so inexpensive that anyone can afford it. This wonder drug, proved in years of research, is exercise.

Chapter 6 provides detailed information on improving your fitness. To make a difference in the way you look and feel, follow these simple guidelines:

- **Work in short bouts.** Three 10-minute intervals of exercise can be just as effective as exercising for 30 minutes straight.

- **Mix it up.** Combine moderate and vigorous intensity exercises to meet the guidelines. For instance, you can walk briskly two days a week and jog at a faster pace on the other days.

- **Set aside exercise times.** Schedule exercise in advance so you can plan your day around it.

- **Find exercise buddies.** Recruit roommates, friends, family, coworkers. You'll have more fun on your way to getting fit.

alcohol-related risky behaviors, psychological symptoms, and suicide risk.

Where to Turn for Help

✓**check-in** Should you seek professional help? Consider therapy if you:

- Feel an overwhelming and prolonged sense of helplessness and sadness, which does not lift despite your efforts and help from family and friends.
- Find it difficult to carry out everyday activities such as homework, and your academic performance is suffering.
- Worry excessively, expect the worst, or are constantly on edge.
- Are finding it hard to resist or are engaging in behaviors that are harmful to you or others, such as drinking too much alcohol, abusing drugs, or becoming aggressive or violent.

About 10 percent of students seek care from a mental health counseling center on campus. Your health education instructor can tell you about general and mental health counseling available on campus, school-based support groups, community-based programs, and special emergency services. On campus, you can also turn to the student health services or the office of the dean of student services or student affairs.

Within the community, you may be able to get help through the city or county health department and neighborhood health centers. Local hospitals often have special clinics and services, and there are usually local branches of national service organizations, such as United Way or Alcoholics Anonymous, other 12-Step programs, and various support groups. You can call the psychiatric or psychological association in your city or state for the names of licensed professionals. (Check the telephone directory for listings.) Your primary physician may also be able to help. Search the Internet for special programs, found either by the nature of the service, by the name of the neighborhood or city, or by the name of the sponsoring group.

In addition to suicide-prevention programs, look for crisis intervention, violence prevention, and child-abuse prevention programs; drug treatment information; shelters for battered women; senior citizen centers; and self-help and counseling services. Many services have special hotlines for coping with emergencies. Others provide information as well as support over the phone, or by email or texts.

Types of Therapy

The term **psychotherapy** refers to any type of counseling based on the exchange of words in the context of the unique relationship that develops between a mental health professional and a person seeking help. The process of talking and listening can lead to new insight, relief from distressing psychological symptoms, changes in unhealthy or maladaptive behaviors, and more effective ways of dealing with the world. Psychotherapy does not just benefit the mind but actually changes the brain. In studies comparing psychotherapy and psychiatric medications as treatments for depression, both proved about equally effective.

Most mental health professionals today are trained in a variety of psychotherapeutic techniques and tailor their approach to the problem, personality, and needs of each person seeking their help. Because skilled therapists may combine different techniques in the course of therapy, the lines between the various approaches often blur.

Psychodynamic Psychotherapy For the most part, today's mental health professionals base their assessment of individuals on a **psychodynamic** understanding that takes into account the role of early experiences and unconscious influences in *actively* shaping behavior. (This is the *dynamic* in psychodynamic.) Psychodynamic treatments work toward the goal of providing greater insight into problems and bringing about behavioral change. Therapy may be brief, intermittent, or long term, continuing for several years.[128]

Cognitive-behavioral therapy (CBT) focuses on inappropriate or inaccurate thoughts or beliefs to help individuals break out of a distorted, maladaptive way of thinking. The techniques of **cognitive therapy** include identification of an individual's beliefs and attitudes, recognition of negative thought patterns, and education in alternative ways of thinking. Individuals with major depression or anxiety disorders are most likely to benefit, usually in 15 to 25 sessions. In a recent study, telephone CBT proved as effective as face-to-face therapy.[129]

The goal of **behavioral therapy** is to substitute healthier ways of behaving for maladaptive patterns used in the past. Some therapists believe that changing behavior also changes how people think and feel. As they put it, "Change the behavior, and the feelings will follow." Behavioral therapies work best for disorders characterized by specific, abnormal patterns of acting—such as alcohol and

psychotherapy Treatment designed to produce a response by psychological rather than physical means, such as suggestion, persuasion, reassurance, and support.

psychodynamic Interpreting behaviors in terms of early experiences and unconscious influences.

cognitive therapy A technique used to identify an individual's beliefs and attitudes, recognize negative thought patterns, and educate in alternative ways of thinking.

behavioral therapy A technique that emphasizes application of the principles of learning to substitute desirable responses and behavior patterns for undesirable ones.

drug abuse, anxiety disorders, and phobias—and for individuals who want to change habits.

Interpersonal Therapy

Originally developed for research into the treatment of major depression, **interpersonal therapy (IPT)** does not deal with the psychological origins of symptoms but, rather, concentrates on current problems of getting along with others. The emphasis is on the here-and-now and on interpersonal—rather than intrapsychic—issues. Individuals with major depression, chronic difficulties developing relationships, and chronic mild depression are most likely to benefit.

Other Treatment Options

Psychiatric Drugs

Thanks to the development of more precise and effective **psychiatric drugs**, success rates for treating many common and disabling disorders—depression, panic disorder, schizophrenia, and others—have soared. Often used in conjunction with psychotherapy, these medications have revolutionized mental health care.

At some point in their lives, about half of all Americans will take a psychiatric drug. The reason may be depression, anxiety, a sleep difficulty, an eating disorder, alcohol or drug dependence, impaired memory, or another disorder that disrupts the intricate chemistry of the brain.

✓**check-in** Have you ever taken a psychiatric drug?

Psychiatric medications, among the most commonly prescribed drugs in the United States, account for almost 12 percent of drug prescriptions.[130] Sedatives and hypnotics are the most widely prescribed, followed by antidepressants. Adverse reactions to psychiatric medications, including antidepressants, lead to about 90,000 visits to emergency departments every year. Selective serotonin reuptake inhibitors (SSRIs), the

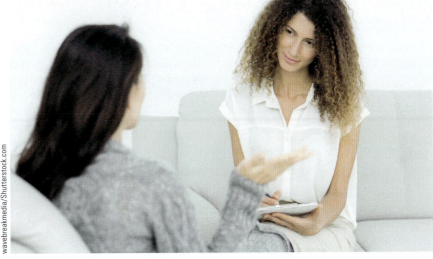
wavebreakmedia/Shutterstock.com

drugs of choice in treating depression, are also effective in treating obsessive–compulsive disorder, panic disorder, social phobia, posttraumatic stress disorder, premenstrual dysphoric disorder, and generalized anxiety disorder. In patients who don't respond, psychiatrists may add another drug to boost the efficacy of the treatment.

Alternative Mind—Mood Products

Some "natural" products, such as herbs and enzymes, claim to have psychological effects. However, they have not undergone rigorous scientific testing. The most well-known product is St. John's wort, which has been used to treat anxiety and depression in Europe for many years. In 10 carefully controlled studies in the United States, the herb did not prove more effective than a placebo. Side effects include dizziness, abdominal pain and bloating, constipation, nausea, fatigue, and dry mouth. St. John's wort should not be taken in combination with other prescription antidepressants. An added precaution: It can lower the efficacy of oral contraceptives and increase the risk of unwanted pregnancy.

When choosing a therapist, always consider professional qualifications, such as education, as well as personal qualities, such as compassion.

interpersonal therapy (IPT) A technique used to develop communication skills and relationships.

psychiatric drugs Medications that regulate a person's mental, emotional, and physical functions to facilitate normal functioning.

WHAT DID YOU DECIDE?

- How does the brain affect our thoughts and behavior?
- What are common mental disorders on college campuses?
- How do depression and anxiety affect individuals?
- Why do college students commit suicide?

Reflection

As this chapter makes clear, everyone experiences psychological and emotional difficulties. How has what you've learned about mental health helped you understand yourself or someone close to you?

TAKING CHARGE OF YOUR HEALTH
Caring for Your Mind

Like physical health, psychological well-being is not a fixed state of being but a process. The way you live every day affects how you feel about yourself and the world. Here are some basic guidelines that you can rely on to make the most of the process of living. Check those that you commit to making part of your mental and psychological self-care:

_____ **Accept yourself.** As a human being, you are, by definition, imperfect. Come to terms with the fact that you are a worthwhile person despite your mistakes.

_____ **Respect yourself.** Recognize your abilities and talents. Acknowledge your competence and achievements and take pride in them.

_____ **Trust yourself.** Learn to listen to the voice within you and let your intuition be your guide.

_____ **Love yourself.** Be happy to spend time by yourself. Learn to appreciate your own company and to be glad you're you.

_____ **Stretch yourself.** Be willing to change and grow, to try something new and dare to be vulnerable.

_____ **Look at challenges as opportunities for personal growth.** "Every problem brings the possibility of a widening of consciousness," psychologist Carl Jung once noted. Put his words to the test.

_____ **When your internal critic—the negative inner voice we all have—starts putting you down, force yourself to think of a situation that you handled well.**

_____ **Set a limit on self-pity.** Tell yourself, "I'm going to feel sorry for myself this morning, but this afternoon, I've got to get on with my life."

SELF-SURVEY

The Satisfaction with Life Scale

Below are five statements that you may agree or disagree with. Using the 1–7 scale below, indicate your agreement with each item by placing the appropriate number on the line preceding that item. Please be open and honest in your responding. Once you have completed filling in your agreement with each item, add up your total score to determine your satisfaction with life by matching it to the scores below.

7 - Strongly agree
6 - Agree
5 - Slightly agree
4 - Neither agree nor disagree
3 - Slightly disagree
2 - Disagree
1 - Strongly disagree

_____ In most ways my life is close to my ideal.
_____ The conditions of my life are excellent.
_____ I am satisfied with my life.
_____ So far I have gotten the important things I want in life.
_____ If I could live my life over, I would change almost nothing.

31 - 35 Extremely satisfied
26 - 30 Satisfied
21 - 25 Slightly satisfied
20 Neutral
15 - 19 Slightly dissatisfied
10 - 14 Dissatisfied
5 - 9 Extremely dissatisfied

30–35 Very high score; highly satisfied

Respondents who score in this range love their lives and feel that things are going very well. Their lives are not perfect, but they feel that things are about as good as lives get. Furthermore, just because the person is satisfied does not mean she or he is complacent. In fact, growth and challenge might be part of the reason the respondent is satisfied. For most people in this high-scoring range, life is enjoyable, and the major domains of life are going well—work or school, family, friends, leisure, and personal development.

25–29 High score

Individuals who score in this range like their lives and feel that things are going well. Of course their lives are not perfect, but they feel that things are mostly good. Furthermore, just because the person is satisfied does not mean she or he is complacent. In fact, growth and challenge might be part of the reason the respondent is satisfied. For most people in this high-scoring range, life is enjoyable, and the major domains of life are going well—work or school, family, friends, leisure, and personal development. The person may draw motivation from the areas of dissatisfaction.

20–24 Average score

The average of life satisfaction in economically developed nations is in this range—the majority of people are generally satisfied, but have some areas where they very much would like some improvement. Some individuals score in this range because they are mostly satisfied with most areas of their lives but see the need for some improvement in each area. Other respondents score in this range because they are satisfied with most domains of their lives, but have one or two areas where they would like to see large improvements. A person scoring in this range is normal in that they have areas of their lives that need improvement. However, an individual in this range would usually like to move to a higher level by making some life changes.

15–19 Slightly below average in life satisfaction

People who score in this range usually have small but significant problems in several areas of their lives, or have many areas that are doing fine but one area that represents a substantial problem for them. If a person has moved temporarily into this level of life satisfaction from a higher level because of some recent event, things will usually improve over time and satisfaction will generally move back up. On the other hand, if a person is chronically slightly dissatisfied with many areas of life, some changes might be in order. Sometimes the person is simply expecting too much, and sometimes life changes are needed. Thus, although temporary dissatisfaction is common and normal, a chronic level of dissatisfaction across a number of areas of life calls for reflection. Some people can gain motivation from a small level of dissatisfaction, but often dissatisfaction across a number of life domains is a distraction, and unpleasant as well.

10–14 Dissatisfied

Furthermore, a person with low life satisfaction in this range is sometimes not functioning well because their unhappiness serves as a distraction. Talking to a friend, member of the clergy, counselor, or other specialist can often help the person get moving in the right direction, although positive change will be up to the person.

5–9 Extremely Dissatisfied

Individuals who score in this range are usually extremely unhappy with their current life. In some cases this is in reaction to some recent bad event such as widowhood or unemployment. In other cases, it is a response to a chronic problem such as alcoholism or addiction. In yet other cases the extreme dissatisfaction is a reaction due to something bad in life such as recently having lost a loved one. However, dissatisfaction at this level is often due to dissatisfaction in multiple areas of life. Whatever the reason for the low level of life satisfaction, it may be that the help of others is needed—a friend or family member, counseling with a member of the clergy, or help from a psychologist or other counselor. If the dissatisfaction is chronic, the person needs to change, and often others can help.

Common to each category

To understand life satisfaction scores, it is helpful to understand some of the components that go into most people's experience of satisfaction. One of the most important influences on happiness is social relationships. People who score high on life satisfaction tend to have close and supportive family and friends, whereas those who do not have close friends and family are more likely to be dissatisfied. Of course the loss of a close friend or family member can cause dissatisfaction with life, and it may take some time for the person to bounce back from the loss.

Another factor that influences the life satisfaction of most people is work or school, or performance in an important role such as homemaker or grandparent. When the person enjoys his or her work, whether it is paid or unpaid, and feels that it is meaningful and important, this contributes to life satisfaction. When work is going poorly because of bad circumstances or a poor fit with the person's strengths, this can lower life satisfaction. When a person has important goals, and is failing to make adequate progress toward them, this too can lead to life dissatisfaction.

A third factor that influences the life satisfaction of most people is personal satisfaction with the self, religious or spiritual life, learning and growth, and leisure. For many people these are sources of satisfaction. However, when these sources of personal worth are frustrated, they can be powerful sources of dissatisfaction. Of course there are additional sources of satisfaction and dissatisfaction—some that are common to most people such as health, and others that are unique to each individual. Most people know the factors that lead to their satisfaction or dissatisfaction, although a person's temperament—a general tendency to be happy or unhappy—can color their responses.

There is no one key to life satisfaction, but rather a recipe that includes a number of ingredients. With time and persistent work, people's life satisfaction usually goes up when they are dissatisfied. People who have had a loss recover over time. People who have a dissatisfying relationship or work often make changes over time that will increase their satisfaction. One key ingredient to happiness, as mentioned above, is social relationships, and another key ingredient is to have important goals that derive from one's values, and to make progress toward those goals. For many people it is important to feel a connection to something larger than oneself. When a person tends to be chronically dissatisfied, they should look within themselves and ask whether they need to develop more positive attitudes to life and the world.

Source: Ed Diener, Robert A. Emmons, Randy J. Larsen and Sharon Griffin. "The Satisfaction with Life Scale," *Journal of Personality Assessment*, 1985, vol. 49, issue 1, 71–75. http://labs.psychology.illinois.edu/~ediener/Documents/Diener -Emmons-Larsen-Griffin_1985.pdf

REVIEW QUESTIONS

(LO 2.1) 1. _____ health describes our ability to perceive reality as it is, to respond to its challenges, and to develop rational strategies for living.
   a. Emotional
   b. Spiritual
   c. Physical
   d. Mental

(LO 2.2) 2. The highest level of the "Maslow pyramid" of human needs is _____.
   a. safety
   b. esteem
   c. belonging
   d. self-actualization

(LO 2.2) 3. Which of the following approaches to practicing positive psychology requires a person to expect positive experiences from life?
   a. Boosting one's emotional intelligence
   b. Managing moods
   c. Becoming optimistic
   d. Ignoring the criticisms of others

(LO 2.2) 4. What is the first step in the process of values clarification?
   a. Publicly affirm your values by sharing them with others.
   b. Act out your values.
   c. Choose freely from among all available options.
   d. Carefully consider the consequences of each choice.

(LO 2.2) 5. When you forgive, _____.
   a. you lose your values
   b. you free yourself from anger, resentments, and reliving hurts over and over again
   c. you are not being kind to yourself
   d. you become powerless over your emotions

(LO 2.3) 6. According to the Centers for Disease Control and Prevention, which of the following statements is true of sleep-related problems among Americans?
   a. Normal sleep times range from 10 to 20 hours.
   b. Women are more likely than men to report not getting enough sleep.
   c. Poor-quality sleepers report drinking less alcohol than good sleepers.
   d. Asian Americans report getting less sleep as compared with all other ethnic groups.

(LO 2.3) 7. The most widely publicized dietary supplement for relieving insomnia contains _____.
   a. chamomile
   b. antihistamines
   c. an antipyretic
   d. melatonin

(LO 2.4) 8. Which of the following is a factor that increases vulnerability to a mental disorder among undergraduates?
   a. Regular exercise
   b. Long-term relationship
   c. Financial pressures
   d. Belonging to a fraternity or sorority

(LO 2.4) 9. Which of the following is a characteristic symptom of major depression?
   a. Racing thoughts
   b. Relationship problems
   c. Difficulty concentrating
   d. Increased sensory sensitivity

(LO 2.4) 10. Which of the following is a characteristic symptom of bipolar disorder?
   a. Lack of energy
   b. Persistent thoughts of death
   c. Mood swings
   d. Eating more or less than usual

(LO 2.5) 11. Which of the following anxiety disorders is treated with a process called systematic desensitization?
   a. Panic attack
   b. Phobia
   c. Generalized anxiety disorder
   d. Obsessive–compulsive disorder

(LO 2.5) 12. Panic attacks _____.
   a. occur more frequently among men than among women
   b. usually require hospitalization
   c. occur more frequently among family members with the disorder
   d. are resistant to treatment by therapy and medication

(LO 2.7) 13. Which of the following strategies will benefit students with attention-deficit/hyperactivity disorder (ADHD)?
   a. Stand in the last row rather than sitting in the front row.
   b. Draw images rather than writing notes.
   c. Take written exams rather than oral exams.
   d. Record lectures rather than taking notes.

(LO 2.6) 14. Which of the following is true of suicide?
  a. Individuals with a high level of serotonin may have a greater risk of committing suicide than those with lower levels.
  b. White Americans are at the lowest risk for suicide.
  c. Women attempt suicide much more often than men.
  d. Suicide usually stems from a single cause.

(LO 2.7) 15. _____ takes into account the role of early experiences and unconscious influences in *actively* shaping behavior.
  a. Interpersonal therapy
  b. Family-focused therapy
  c. Cognitive-behavioral therapy
  d. Psychodynamic psychotherapy

Answers to these questions can be found on page 531.

Sean Locke Photography/Shutterstock.com

LEARNING OBJECTIVES

After reading this chapter, you should be able to:

3.1 Outline the types of stress and the effects of stress on people.

3.2 Identify stressors commonly reported by different groups across the United States.

3.3 Summarize the incidence, symptoms, and treatment of the stress disorders associated with traumatic life events.

3.4 Outline the ways in which the body responds to stress.

3.5 Describe how stress can affect a person's heart, immune system, gastrointestinal system, and susceptibility to cancer.

3.6 Explain psychological responses to stress.

3.7 Discuss practical techniques of stress management.

3.8 Summarize how time management can help prevent stress and money management can lessen personal stress.

WHAT DO YOU THINK?

- Is stress always harmful?
- What stressors do college students typically encounter?
- How does the body respond to stress?
- What are some effective ways of managing stress?

3

Stress Management

Getting laid off felt like a punch in the stomach. Chayla had heard rumors that all part-time positions would be eliminated. But her boss always said she was the best assistant they had ever hired. And now she was without a job—with tuition, rent, and insurance bills all due in a month. And so in between writing papers and preparing for finals, Chayla would have to look for another job. Just thinking about all she had to do made her head throb.

Like Chayla, you live with stress every day, whether you're studying for exams, meeting people, facing new experiences, or figuring out how to live on a budget. You're not alone. College students rank stress as the number-one barrier to academic achievement, according to the American College Health Association (ACHA) National College Health Assessment survey. About 58 percent report "more than average" or "tremendous" stress.[1]

Freshmen, female, minority, and first-generation students register the most stress, but no one is immune. However old you are, wherever you come from, whatever your goals, stress is and always will be part of your life.

Yet stress in itself isn't necessarily bad. What matters most is not a stressful situation but an individual's response to it. This chapter helps you learn to anticipate stressful events, manage day-to-day hassles, prevent stress overload, and find alternatives to running endlessly on a treadmill of alarm, panic, and exhaustion. <

What Is Stress?

The word **stress** comes from the Latin *stringere*, which means "to draw tight." Many people use the word loosely to refer to an external force that causes someone to become tense or upset, to the internal state of arousal, and to the physical response of the body when it must adapt, cope, or adjust to a challenge.

Hans Selye, a pioneer in studying physiological responses to challenge, defined *stress* as "the nonspecific response of the body to any demand made upon it." Through years of research, he noted that laboratory animals and people responded in the same way to a **stressor** (anything that triggers a state of arousal), regardless of whether it was positive or negative.

You experience stress when you confront what you perceive as a potential challenge or a threat that you don't think you can handle. This thought stimulates feelings, such as fear and

stress The nonspecific response of the body to any demands made upon it; may be characterized by muscle tension and acute anxiety, or may be a positive force for action.

stressor A specific or nonspecific agent or situation that causes the stress response in a body.

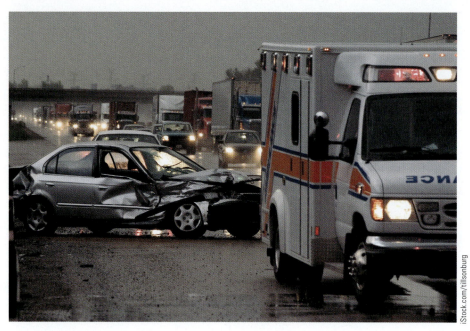
iStock.com/tillsonburg

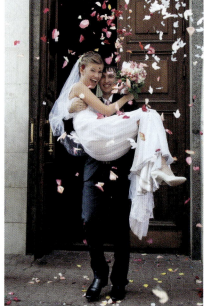
chaos/Shutterstock.com

An automobile accident is an acute negative stressor. A wedding is an example of a positive stressor that triggers both joy and anxiety. Watching television coverage of a mass shooting can provoke neustress.

iStock.com/Zoranm

anxiety, which lead to unconscious physiological responses as well as to conscious, deliberate behaviors.

Eustress, Distress, and Neustress

Not all stressors are negative. Some of life's happiest moments—births, reunions, weddings—are enormously stressful. We weep with the stress of frustration or loss; we weep, too, with the stress of love and joy.

Selye coined the term **eustress** for positive stress in our lives (*eu-* is a Greek prefix meaning

"good"). Eustress challenges us to grow, adapt, and find creative solutions in our lives. However, too much eustress can also be problematic. A wedding, for instance, is a joyful event, but planning, organizing, and pinning down details can create anxiety and take up so much time that they interfere with other commitments and cause anxiety.

Distress, the negative stress caused by trauma, loss, and other upsetting occurrences, breeds overreaction, confusion, poor concentration, and performance anxiety. We cannot function at our best; we feel off, distracted, or edgy. We're also likely to develop physical symptoms and ailments. For students, distress can be paralyzing, leading to increased frustration and a sense of hopelessness. Instead of seeking support, they may withdraw from people who could provide perspective, which leads to greater isolation.[2]

Some experts have introduced another category: **"neustress"** for neutral stressors that do not affect us immediately or directly but that may trigger anxiety, sadness, fear, and other stressful feelings. For example, an airplane crash or a mass shooting reported in the media may deeply upset you. You experience emotions commonly related to stress, such as anxiety, but your response is briefer and less severe than if you or a loved one had been in danger.

✓**check-in** How can you tell when you're stressed?

Read through this list of warning signs and check any that apply to you:

_____ You are experiencing physical symptoms, including chronic fatigue,

eustress Positive stress, which stimulates a person to function properly.

distress A negative stress that may result in illness.

neustress Neutral stressors that do not affect us immediately or directly but may trigger stressful feelings.

headaches, indigestion, diarrhea, and sleep problems.

_____ You are having frequent illness or worrying about illness.

_____ You are self-medicating, including using nonprescription drugs.

_____ You are having problems concentrating on studies or work.

_____ You are feeling irritable, anxious, or apathetic.

_____ You are working or studying longer and harder than usual.

_____ You are exaggerating, to yourself and others, the importance of what you do.

_____ You are becoming accident-prone.

_____ You are breaking rules, whether it's a curfew at the dorm or a speed limit on the highway.

_____ You are going to extremes, such as drinking too much, overspending, or gambling.

No checks? Congratulations! Continue to build the strengths that make stress manageable. Ask yourself: What is working? What's not working? If you checked one or more of these red flags, pay closer attention to both the number and the intensity of stressors in your life as you read through this chapter.

Stress and the Dimensions of Health

From a **holistic** perspective, which looks at health and an individual as a whole rather than part by part, stress can have an impact on every dimension of well-being.

Physical Stress, whether physical or psychological, triggers molecular changes within your body that affect your heart, muscles, immune system, bones, blood vessels, skin, lungs, gastrointestinal (digestive) tract, and reproductive organs.

Psychological Chronic stress affects thoughts and feelings, impairing your ability to learn and to remember and contributing to anxiety and depression. However, positive emotions and attitudes,

such as compassion and gratitude, can buffer the ill effects of stress and enhance satisfaction and genuine happiness.

Spiritual Stress can sidetrack our quest to identify our basic purpose in life and to experience the fulfillment of achieving our full potential. But your spirit, when nurtured, can help you both resist and recover from stress.

Social Your relationships with your family, friends, coworkers, and loved ones affect and are affected by the stress in your life—and in challenging times, social support can buffer the negative effects of stress.[3]

Intellectual Even mild stressors can interfere with your brain's functioning by impairing sleep, dampening creativity, disrupting concentration and memory, and undermining your ability to make good choices and decisions.

Occupational Most undergraduates—about 70 percent—are employed, with 20 percent working full time year-round. They are more likely to feel overwhelmed and report greater anxiety and stress than students without jobs.[4]

Environmental External forces such as pollution, noise, natural disasters, exposure to toxic chemicals, and threats to your safety can cause or intensify the stress in your life. These days, you also have to cope with a by-product of our 24/7, nonstop digital world: technostress, created by an unending barrage of texts, tweets, emails, notifications, pins, pokes, and other digital distractions.

✓**check-in** How does stress affect the various dimensions of your health?

Types of Stressors

Stressors come in all varieties: big, small, brief, long, intense, mild, trivial, and terrible. Here are some of the most common stressors:

- **Acute time-limited stressors** include anxiety-provoking situations such as having to give a talk in public or work out a math problem, such as calculating a tip or dividing a bill, under pressure. Even small daily hassles like misplacing your keys or cell phone can add to your stress.

- **Brief stressors** are more serious challenges such as taking the SAT or meeting a deadline for a big project.

holistic A perspective that looks at health and an individual as a whole rather than part by part.

acute time-limited stressor A temporary anxiety-provoking situation.

brief stressor A more serious and extended challenge.

- **Life-change events** include planned and predictable occurrences, such as graduation or marriage, as well as unexpected ones, such as the loss of a home in a fire or flood. Stress experts Thomas Holmes and Richard Rahe first documented an association between stressful life events and the onset of disease. Their Schedule of Recent Experiences (SRE) evaluates individual levels of stress and potential for coping on the basis of life-change units, determined by the degree of readjustment necessary to adapt successfully to an event. The death of a partner or parent ranks high on the list, but even positive events, such as a vacation trip, involve some degree of stress. Life changes do not in themselves cause diseases, however. Their actual impact depends on your response and coping skills.

- **Chronic stressors** are ongoing demands caused by life-changing circumstances, such as permanent disability following an accident or caregiving for a parent with dementia, that do not have any clear endpoint.

- **Distant stressors** are traumatic experiences that occurred long ago, such as child abuse or combat, yet continue to have an emotional and psychological impact.

✓**check-in** Which types of stressors have you encountered?

Stress in America

Every year the American Psychological Association (APA) asks men and women across the country to rank their stress level on a scale of 1 (little or no stress) to 10 (a great deal of stress). The 2018 *Stress in America* survey showed that the youngest American adults—Millennials (ages 22–37) and Generation Z (ages 15–21)—reported the highest levels of stress. The causes include immigration policy and status, sexual harassment and assault, issues in the news (including mass shootings, climate change, and the rise in suicide rates) and the current political climate. More personal sources of stress included personal debt, housing instability, and hunger or getting enough to eat.[5]

Here are the other key findings:

- Eight in ten Americans—but more than nine in ten of younger adults—reported at least one physical or emotional stress symptom in the previous month, including headache, feeling overwhelmed, feeling nervous or anxious, or feeling depressed or sad.

- Millennials report the highest stress levels of all generations (5.7 on a scale of 1 to 10) followed by Generation Xers (5.3). The average stress level for all adults is 4.9.[6]

- One in three Americans said personal safety is a very or somewhat significant source of stress.

- Americans are increasingly stressed about their country, with more than a third identifying the nation's future as a major stressor. Nearly a quarter of Americans identify discrimination as a significant source of stress, the highest percentage the APA has ever reported.[7]

- Women consistently report higher stress levels than men and feel more stressed about money, family responsibilities, and acts of terrorism.

- Women reported managing stress by exercise or walking, spending time with friends or family, reading, and praying. Men's top stress management approaches were exercise, watching TV, going online, or reading.

- Younger Americans report higher stress levels than older ones. Americans with household incomes less than $50,000 have higher stress levels than those earning more.

- Despite the many stressors in their lives, four in ten Americans say they are doing significantly or somewhat better at managing stress than they did a decade ago.

✓**check-in** What's your stress level?
Rank your current state of stress on a scale from 1 (low) to 10 (extreme). How does it compare with the national average of 4.9?

Stress on Campus

Being a student—full time or part time, in your late teens, early 20s, or later in life—can be extremely stressful. You may feel pressure to perform well to qualify for a good job or graduate school. To meet steep tuition payments, you may have to juggle part-time work and coursework. You may feel stressed about choosing a major, getting along with a difficult roommate, passing

life-change event An occurrence, planned or unplanned, that requires some degree of re-adjustment.

chronic stressor Unrelenting demands and pressures that go on for an extended time.

distant stressor Traumatic experience that occured long ago yet continue to have an emotional or psychological impact.

Stressed-Out Students

Within the past 12 months, students' ratings of the overall level of stress experienced:

This table summarizes the levels of stress reported by college students in the previous 12 months. How does your stress level compare?

	Percent (%)		
	Male	**Female**	**Average**
No stress	3.5	0.8	1.6
Less than average stress	11.7	4.4	6.5
Average stress	37.9	33.3	34.3
More than average stress	37.7	47.9	44.9
Tremendous stress	9.2	13.7	12.7

Source: American College Health Association. American College Health Association-National College Health Assessment II: Reference Group Executive Summary Spring 2018. Silver Spring, MD: American College Health Association, 2018.

a particularly hard course, or living up to your parents' and teachers' expectations. If you're an older student, you may have children, jobs, housework, and homework to balance. Your days may seem so busy and your life so full that you worry about coming apart at the seams. Multiple stressors—pychological, academic, physical, social, financial—can come together into what psychiatrists have called "a perfect storm" that can put any student at risk.[8]

The costs of health care and uncertainty about health insurance causes stress for many Americans, regardless of their age, income, racial background, or geographic location. Adults without health insurance reported a higher overall stress level than those who are insured. In the American College Health Association-National College Health Assessment (ACHA-NCHA) survey, about 87 percent—78 percent of men and 91 percent of women—reported feeling overwhelmed by all they had to do at some point in the past 12 months.[9] (See Snapshot: On Campus Now.) Perceived stress levels affect student grades and performance on tests.[10]

Stressors reported by students around the world include test pressures, financial problems, frustrations such as delays in reaching goals, problems in friendships and dating relationships, and daily hassles. Student athletes may experience the added stresses of anxiety about performing well, perfectionism, injuries, fitting in with their teammates, and balancing academics and sports.[11] The transition from military service to campus life may add to the stress of veterans as they adjust to new challenges and a new lifestyle.[12]

✓**check-in** Would you rate your stress as "average," "less than average," "more than average," or "tremendous"?

Stress and Student Health

Students may react to stress in various ways:

- Physiologically—by sweating, stuttering, trembling, or developing physical symptoms
- Emotionally—by becoming anxious, fearful, angry, guilty, or depressed
- Behaviorally—by crying, eating, smoking, or being irritable or abusive
- Cognitively—by thinking about and analyzing stressful situations and strategies that might be useful in dealing with them.

Students under stress may engage in behaviors that can harm their health, including smoking, excessive drinking, and substance abuse.[13] Students may experience both short- and long-term mental and physical consequences, including the worsening of chronic health conditions and increased risk of developing high blood pressure and heart and kidney disorders.[14]

The undergraduates who report higher stress levels differ from their classmates in various ways. They are:

- Less likely to exercise regularly.
- Less likely to consume fruits and vegetables.

- More likely to consume junk food and soft drinks.
- Shown to report more symptoms of depression and anxiety.[15]

In addition to its impact on health, stress can affect students physically, emotionally, academically, and socially.[16] Among its documented effects are:

- Difficulty paying attention and concentrating.
- Poor or inadequate sleep.
- Lack of exercise.
- Increased consumption of junk food.
- Greater risk of anxiety and depression.
- Lessened life satisfaction.

To get a sense of your personal stress level, complete the Self-Survey: Student Stress Scale in this chapter, modified to include college-specific stressors such as a failing grade or a change in major. If you score high, think about the reasons your life may be in turmoil. Of course, some events, such as your parents' divorce or a meningitis outbreak, are beyond your control. Even so, you can respond with coping techniques that will protect your long-term well-being.

✓**check-in** What is your greatest source of stress?

Gender Differences If you're a woman, you're more likely than your male classmates to be stressed about finances, social relationships, and daily hassles. In the ACHA-NCHA survey, more female than male students reported feeling hopeless, overwhelmed, or exhausted (but not from physical activity). Women also scored higher than men in feeling stressed about having too many things to do at once, being separated from people they care about, financial burdens, and important decisions about their education. Women react more intensely to stressful challenges, such as speaking before a group or singing in public.[17]

Neither gender necessarily handles stress better. College men are more likely to "disengage" by using alcohol. College women report more emotion-focused strategies, such as expressing feelings, seeking emotional support, and positive reframing. They're also more prone to acting impulsively and not dealing with a problem directly, sometimes by spending more time online.

Students under Age 25 Those of you between the ages of 18 and 25 are in the life stage termed "emerging adulthood." During this potentially risky transition period, young men and women of every racial and ethnic group are more likely to engage in behaviors that can increase stress and imperil health, such as eating more junk food, smoking, not exercising, and taking risks.

As neuroimaging research has revealed, the brain continues to develop throughout the first quarter-century of life, and this affects cognitive and problem solving skills. In dealing with daily stressors, for instance, a teenage or 20-something brain relies more on the amygdala, a small almond-shaped region in the medial and temporal lobes that processes emotions and memories. This is one reason any stressor—a poor grade or a friend's snub, for instance—feels as intensely upsetting as a major crisis. As individuals age, the frontal cortex, which governs reason and forethought, plays a greater role and helps put challenges into perspective.

✓**check-in** If you are under 25:
- Be aware that your brain may not always grasp the long-term consequences of your actions.
- Set realistic priorities.
- Restrain potentially harmful impulses.
- Learn to center yourself with breathing and relaxation techniques (described in section on "Routes to Relaxation").

Students over Age 25 The number of older undergraduates is skyrocketing. Many of these students, often parents with full- or part-time jobs, find themselves playing multiple roles and facing multiple stressors, including pressure to perform well to qualify for a better job or graduate school. Veterans may be processing their experiences in distant and dangerous lands. Finances are a huge source of stress, and many worry about the costs of housing and childcare and fear incurring additional debt.

Family typically emerges as the greatest source of both stress and support for women returning to school. On the one hand, women feel stressed about not earning money, missing special occasions like their children's track meets or dance recitals, and keeping up with endless household chores. On the other, they feel that short-term sacrifices will pay off in greater long-term security for their families. Single mothers face the most acute stressors, such as not being able to complete an assignment on time because they have to care for a sick child.

Minority Students *Minority stress* refers to negative experiences in the campus environment that students perceive to be linked to the social, physical, or cultural attributes characteristic of their racial or ethnic group.[18] Among its forms are the following:

- **University social climate stress**, which arises from perceptions of the campus environment as unwelcoming to members of the student's group.

- **Intergroup stress**, based on perceptions of negative relations among students from different racial and ethnic groups, primarily white students.

- **Discrimination stress**, which reflects concerns related to personal experiences of prejudice and discrimination. As research has confirmed, discrimination can cause chronic stress and take a significant toll on emotional and physical well-being.[19] Racial discrimination, which may be experienced more intensely than other forms of bias, has been linked to increased distress, depression, anxiety, and psychiatric symptoms in African Americans.[20]

- **Within-group stress**, which stems from perceived pressure to conform to the norms of the student's group regarding language, behaviors, and ways of thinking.

- **Achievement stress**, which reflects students' concerns about the relative inadequacy of their academic preparation and ability. For instance, Asian Americans between ages 15 and 24, who feel the stress of high expectations as the "model minority," have significantly higher suicidal rates than other racial/ethnic groups in the same age range.[21]

- **Acculturative stress**, the tension and anxiety that accompany efforts to adapt to the orientation and values of a dominant culture. In studies of minority freshmen, Asian American, Filipino, African American, and Native American students all felt more sensitive and vulnerable to the college social climate, to interpersonal tensions between themselves and nonminority students and faculty, to experiences of actual or perceived racism, and to discrimination. Minority students, despite scoring above the national average on the SAT, may not feel accepted as legitimate undergraduates and may sense that others view them as unworthy beneficiaries of affirmative action initiatives. These experiences can influence their confidence and career aspirations as well as their mental health.[22]

- While many minority students say that overt racism is rare and relatively easy to deal with, subtle racial expressions—sometimes termed **microaggressions**—may undermine their academic confidence and their ability to bond with the university. Researchers have identified three common types:

  - **Microassaults**. These are conscious and intentional actions or slurs, such as using racial epithets, displaying swastikas, or deliberately responding to a white customer before a person of color in a restaurant or store.

  - **Microinsults**. These verbal and nonverbal communications subtly convey rudeness and insensitivity and demean a person's racial heritage or identity. An example is a student implying that a classmate won admission to a university on the basis of race rather than merit.

  - **Microinvalidations**. These communications subtly exclude, negate, or nullify the thoughts, feelings, or experiential reality of a person of color—for instance, asking Asian Americans where they were born, which conveys the message that they are perpetual foreigners in their own land.

....
✓**check-in** Have you ever encountered
....
microaggressions on your campus?
....

Entering Freshmen The first year of college is the most stressful for all undergraduates, even when they begin with positive expectations and attitudes. One intervention that has proven helpful is mindfulness (discussed later in this chapter), an approach that focuses attention on the present rather than regrets about the past or worries about the future.[23]

First-generation college students—those whose parents never experienced at least a full year of college—may feel greater stress because their family and friends may not be able to relate to and understand college-related stressors. They are more likely to be female, Hispanic, older, to come from lower economic status, and to have children of their own.[24] As a result, they have no experience, even vicarious, to draw from as they negotiate the transition to university life. Some first-generation students see themselves taking on the challenging roles of being trailblazers and role models in addition to the usual academic and personal demands.

Students whose parents and perhaps grandparents attended college may have several

microaggressions Subtle racial expressions.

microassaults Conscious and intentional actions and slurs.

microinsults Verbal and nonverbal communications that subtly convey rudeness and insensitivity.

microinvalidations Communications that subtly exclude, negate, or nullify the thoughts, feelings, or experiential reality of a person of color.

How to Handle Test Stress

- **Plan ahead.** A month before finals, map out a study schedule for each course. Set aside a small amount of time every day or every other day to review the course materials.

- **Be positive.** Picture yourself taking your final exam. Imagine yourself walking into the exam room feeling confident, opening up the test booklet, and seeing questions for which you know the answers.

- **Take regular breaks.** Get up from your desk, breathe deeply, stretch, and visualize a pleasant scene. You'll feel more refreshed than you would if you chugged another cup of coffee.

- **Practice.** Some teachers are willing to give practice finals to prepare students for test situations, or you and your friends can test each other.

- **Talk to other students.** Chances are that many of them share your fears about test taking and may have discovered some helpful techniques of their own. Sometimes talking to your adviser or a counselor can also help.

- **Be satisfied with doing your best.** You can't expect to ace every test; all you can and should expect is your best effort. Once you've completed the exam, allow yourself the sweet pleasure of relief that it's over.

advantages, including more knowledge of college life, greater social support, more preparation for college in high school, a greater focus on college activities, and more financial resources. However, some report increased stress because of the high expectations of their college-educated parents.

✓**check-in** Did your parents attend college?

Test Stress How many tests have you taken in your life? Hundreds? Thousands? After so much experience, you'd think that tests would be no big deal. And they're not—unless you have developed a thought pattern that sets you up to stress out. For some students, test anxiety provokes a marked elevation in blood pressure, a potential threat to their cardiovascular health. Even if you react this intensely, you can take steps to ease your stressful feelings.

Students feel stressed by tests because they are afraid of a negative outcome, whether it's failing or just not getting an excellent grade. Sometimes they become so preoccupied with the possibility of failing that they can't concentrate on studying. Bright students may freeze up during tests and be unable to comprehend multiple-choice questions or write essay answers, even if they know the material.

Locus of control, discussed in Chapter 1, is crucial. If you see external forces as determining how well you do on tests, you give away your power, and your sense of helplessness creates disabling symptoms of anxiety. The students most susceptible to exam stress are those who believe they'll do poorly and who see tests as extremely threatening.

Unfortunately, negative thoughts often become a self-fulfilling prophecy. As they study, these students keep wondering, "What good will studying do? I never do well on tests." As their fear increases, they try harder. Fueled by caffeine and sugary snacks, they become edgy and find it harder to concentrate. By the time of the test, they're nervous wrecks, scarcely able to sit still and focus on the exam.

You can overcome test stress by knowing—even mastering—the subject and by controlling the way you think about and talk to yourself about tests. Rather than waste energy worrying about the test, shift your attention to studying and the pleasure of learning. Rather than remind yourself of tests you blew in the past, train yourself to ace tests in the future.

Relaxation training also helps. Students who learn relaxation techniques—such as controlled breathing, meditation, progressive relaxation, and guided imagery (visualization)—before finals tend to have higher levels of immune cells during the exam period and feel in better control during their tests.

✓**check-in** How would you rate your test anxiety?

Other Stressors

At every stage of life, you will encounter challenges and stressors. Among the most common are those related to money, anger, work, and illness. (See Health on a Budget.)

Financial Stress

Money ranks second only to academics as a source of stress for college students. In the National Student Financial Wellness Study of almost 19,000 undergraduates at 52 colleges and universities, 7 in 10 undergraduates felt stressed about their personal finances. Nearly 6 in 10 worry about having enough money to pay for school; half are concerned about paying their monthly expenses.[25] Students stressed out by financial pressure are more likely to reduce their

Frugal Living

When you were living with—and off—your parents, you may never have thought twice about your daily take-out cappuccino or the price of tickets for a weekend concert. That was then; this is now. You have to make choices and set priorities. If money was tight in your family, you may have already mastered ways to stretch your dollars. If you've never had to worry about money before, frugal living may be one of most useful skills you acquire in college.

Here are some tips to get started:

- If you drink a lot of coffee, buy an inexpensive coffee maker, brew your own, pour it into an insulated mug, and carry it with you rather than buying a pricey coffee drink.

- Explore thrift stores when you need furniture, sports equipment, or clothing.

- Even if it's allowed, don't bring a car to campus. You can take a campus shuttle, walk, or bike to class.

- Before you make a purchase, find out if there's a student discount for it. (Search online for "student discount" and the item you want.) You can save money on everything from movie tickets to a new computer.

- If you have access to a microwave or stove and a refrigerator, prepare simple meals on your own.

- Take advantage of free or inexpensive leisure activities: hike, play sports, go to campus-sponsored lectures and performances.

- Use apps to check prices in a store against online retailers. Read reviews before making a significant purchase. Search for online coupons and promotions.

- Know your triggers. Do you buy more than you need just because it's a "Buy two, get one free" sale? Are you a sucker for end-of-season markdowns?

- Avoid late fees on anything—library books, DVD rentals, parking tickets. They add up faster than you expect.

- Don't blow bonus money. If your grandparents send a check for your birthday, resist the temptation to splurge. Put most of it into a backup fund for unexpected expenses or new money goals.

---

courseload, withdraw from college to get full-time jobs, and take longer to graduate.[26] (See Managing Your Money section on page 82.)

✓**check-in** Do you think you would be less stressed if you had more money?

Occupational Stress

About half of undergraduates have jobs, which helps make ends meet but can create other difficulties. Those working more than 10 hours a week are more likely to report academic difficulties. In the workforce, employees with dead-end jobs with little or no control or status are especially vulnerable to stress-related problems such as hypertension. The workplace itself can contribute to stress if it's noisy, crowded, poorly lit and ventilated, or tolerant of insensitive jokes and comments. Yet as pressured as a job may be, losing one can be even more stressful. In various studies, unemployment has emerged as a major stressor that causes significant anxiety, depression, and health complaints.

High job strain—defined as high psychological demands combined with low control or decision-making ability over one's job—may increase blood pressure, particularly among men. People who become obsessed by their work and careers can turn into workaholics, so

caught up in racing toward the top that they forget what they're racing toward and why. In some cases, they throw themselves into their work to mask or avoid painful feelings or difficulties in their own lives.

✓**check-in** If you work, what aspects of your job do you find most stressful?

Burnout

You don't need a job to experience **burnout**, a state of physical, emotional, and mental exhaustion brought on by constant or repeated emotional pressure. Many people, especially those caring for others at work or at home, get to a point where there's an imbalance between their own feelings and dealing with difficult, stressful issues on a day-to-day basis. If they don't recognize what's going on and make some changes, their health and the quality of their work suffer.

The risk of burnout may depend on your perception of anxiety, a low-intensity fear triggered by apprehension about ongoing or future challenges. Individuals who perceive anxiety as motivational may be energized and channel this energy into productive effort so they outperform under stress, while those who experience anxiety as debilitating or unpleasant may not perform to their full potential in stressful circumstances.[27]

burnout A state of physical, emotional, and mental exhaustion resulting from constant or repeated emotional pressure.

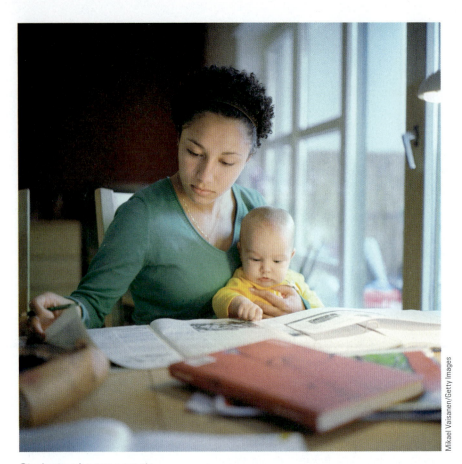
Mikael Vaisanen/Getty Images

Students who are parents must deal with the stress of juggling multiple tasks and responsibilities— often at the same time.

The early signs of burnout overlap with the symptoms of stress: exhaustion, sleep problems or nightmares, increased anxiety or nervousness, muscular tension (headaches, backaches, etc.), increased use of alcohol or medication, digestive problems (nausea, vomiting, diarrhea), loss of interest in sex, frequent body aches or pain, quarrels with family or friends, negative feelings about everything, problems concentrating, mistakes and accidents on the job, and feelings of depression, hopelessness, or helplessness.

Illness and Disability

Just as the mind can have profound effects on the body, the body can have an enormous impact on our emotions. Whenever we come down with the flu or pull a muscle, we feel under par. When we face a more serious or persistent problem— a chronic disease such as diabetes, for instance, or a lifelong hearing impairment—the emotional stress of constantly coping with it is even greater.

A common source of stress for college students is learning disabilities, which may affect 1 of every 10 Americans. Most people with learning disabilities have average or above-average intelligence, but they rarely live up to their ability in school. Some have only one area of difficulty, such as reading or math. Others have problems

trauma The experience of a direct or perceived uncontrollable threat to the safety of individuals, their loved ones or their community.

with attention, writing, communicating, reasoning, coordination, and social skills.

✓**check-in** Have you ever experienced stress because of an illness or a disability?

Traumatic Life Events

Bad things happen. Cars crash. Close friends and relatives die. Floods, tornadoes, and earthquakes wreak havoc on communities. Armed students shoot senselessly at classmates and professors. Bombs explode in peaceful public places. Mental health professionals define **trauma** as the experience of a direct or perceived uncontrollable threat to the safety of individuals, their loved ones or their community.

According to epidemiological studies, about 90 percent of individuals will experience at least one potentially traumatic event—natural or human caused, large scale or small—during the course of their lives.[28] Nine in 10 college women report having directly experienced at least one traumatic event, usually involving a threat to their own lives or to others. The most frequently reported trauma was a motor vehicle accident.

Students who have experienced a potentially traumatic event generally have more difficulty fitting in than those who have not being alone, feeling tired, hungry, or overwhelmed, and dealing with new schedules and demands are common experiences for students—but also common elements of traumatic events that can trigger emotional responses in traumasurvivors.[29] Students who've experienced adverse or traumatic experiences during childhood are often more vulnerable to stressors in college.[30]

✓**check-in** Have you ever experienced a traumatic event?

As profoundly disturbing as such experiences can be, current research has shown that after a trauma, the vast majority of people, including children, cope well, continue to meet the demands of their daily lives, and recover fully. However, some people suffer from a mental disorder as a result of the trauma, in the form of acute stress disorder and posttraumatic stress disorder.

Acute Stress Disorder

In acute stress disorder, disabling symptoms occur within 3 days to a month after exposure to a traumatic event, such as threatened or actual personal or sexual assault, mugging, violence, physical or sexual abuse, kidnapping, being taken hostage, a terrorist attack, a natural disaster, an airplane crash, or a severe industrial or automobile accident.

Symptoms of acute stress disorder may include:

- Recurrent, involuntary, and intrusive distressing memories of the trauma.

- Recurrent distressing dreams related to the trauma.

- Dissociative reactions, such as flashbacks, in which an individual feels that the traumatic event is recurring.

- Persistent inability to experience happiness, satisfaction, or other positive emotions.

- Altered sense of the reality of one's surroundings or oneself, such as time slowing down.

- Inability to remember an important aspect of the traumatic event.

- Efforts to avoid distressing memories, thoughts, or feelings related to the trauma.

- Efforts to avoid reminders, such as certain people, places, activities, objects, or situations, that arouse distressing feelings or thoughts.

- Sleep disturbances, including difficulty falling or staying asleep and restless sleep.

- Irritable behavior and angry outbursts.

- Hypervigilance.

- Problems with concentration.

- Intensified startle response.

Acute stress disorder causes significant distress and interferes with a person's ability to work, study, relate to others, and maintain usual routine and social activities. People with acute stress disorder initially need protection, consolation, assurance of safety, and assistance with decisions and plans. Self-compassion, discussed in Chapter 2, can help survivors of traumatic events reach out for social support, engage in less self-blame and self-criticism, and view the memory as an emotionally difficult event rather than an experience that defines or changes them.[31]

Posttraumatic Stress Disorder

In the past, **posttraumatic stress disorder (PTSD)** was viewed as a psychological response to out-of-the-ordinary stressors, such as captivity or combat. However, other experiences can also forever change the way people view themselves and their world. Individuals with PTSD directly

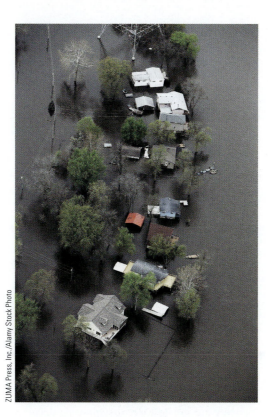

ZUMA Press, Inc./Alamy Stock Photo

Natural disasters such a hurricanes or tornadoes can be traumatic for an entire community.

experience or witness a trauma, learn of an actual or threatened act of violence toward a family member or friend, or experience repeated or extreme exposure to the traumatic events (as happens with soldiers in combat and first responders).

An estimated 9 percent of all college students suffer from PTSD. In the general population, an estimated 8 to 10 percent of women and 4 to 5 percent of men develop PTSD in their lifetime. Childhood traumas occur equally in both sexes. Adult men encounter more traumas—accidents, violence, combat, terrorism, disasters, injuries—than adult women. Women experience more sexual assaults and abuse.

Symptoms of PTSD, which usually begin within the first 3 months after a trauma, include:

- Recurrent, involuntary, and intrusive distressing memories of the traumatic event.

- Recurrent distressing dreams related to the trauma.

- Persistent avoidance of external reminders and distressing memories of the trauma.

- Persistent feelings of guilt, shame, anger, horror, fear, or other negative emotions.

- Hypervigilance and other changes in arousal and alertness.

Some individuals reexperience their terror and helplessness again and again in their dreams or intrusive thoughts. Some engage in aggressive, reckless, or self-destructive behavior. Others

posttraumatic stress disorder (PTSD) The repeated reliving of a trauma through nightmares or recollection.

enter a state of emotional numbness and can no longer respond to people and experiences the way they once did, especially when it comes to showing tenderness or affection.

Individuals with PTSD may require different types of help at different stages. During the first days after a trauma, protection, reassurance of safety, help making decisions and plans, and the support of those closest to them can be most significant in easing their distress. Some approaches, such as immediate "debriefing" to release emotions or treatment with anxiety-reducing medications, may not help and may even hinder long-term recovery. Behavioral, cognitive, and psychodynamic therapy, sometimes along with psychiatric medication, can help individuals suffering with PTSD. Mind–body practices, such as exercise, mindfulness, meditation, and deep breathing (described later in this chapter), have also proven effective.

Without recognition and treatment, PTSD can last for decades, with symptoms intensifying during periods of stress. When identified and treated, more than half of affected persons achieve complete recovery. The odds of recovery are greatest when symptoms develop soon after the trauma, when the individual had previously been in good psychological condition, when there are strong social supports,

and when there are no other mental or medical disorders. In time, individuals with PTSD can learn to increase their control over anguishing memories and feelings and come to accept what happened, however horrible, as a tragic reality of the past that does not have to shape their future.

Mental health professionals have found that no single approach to treatment works for all trauma victims. Some approaches, such as immediate "debriefing" to release emotions or treatment with anxiety-reducing medications, may not help and may even hinder long-term recovery. Behavioral, cognitive, and psychodynamic therapy, sometimes along with psychiatric medication (described in Chapter 3), can also help individuals suffering from PTSD. Mind–body practices—such as exercise, mindfulness, meditation, and deep breathing—along with family support have proven effective in treating PTSD.[32]

Inside Stress

The **stress response** refers to a cascade of internal changes that mobilize the body's resources for action. Various models explain this process from different perspectives.

General Adaptation Syndrome

In his general adaptation syndrome (GAS) model of the stress response, Hans Selye postulated that our bodies continually strive to maintain a stable and consistent physiological state, called **homeostasis** (Figure 3.1). When a stressor disrupts this state, it triggers a nonspecific physiological response, consisting of three distinct stages:

1. *Alarm.* As it becomes aware of a stressor, the body mobilizes various systems for action. Levels of certain hormones rise; blood pressure and flow to the muscles increase; the digestive and immune systems slow down.

2. *Resistance.* If the stress continues, the body draws on its internal resources to try to sustain homeostasis, but this requires greater and greater effort.

3. *Exhaustion.* If stress continues long enough, normal functioning becomes impossible. Even a small amount of additional stress at this point can lead to a breakdown. In animal experiments, Selye

stress response The cascade of internal changes that mobilize the body's resources for action.

homeostasis The body's natural state of balance or stability.

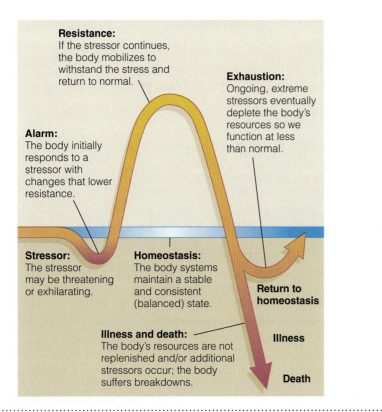

Resistance:
If the stressor continues, the body mobilizes to withstand the stress and return to normal.

Exhaustion:
Ongoing, extreme stressors eventually deplete the body's resources so we function at less than normal.

Alarm:
The body initially responds to a stressor with changes that lower resistance.

Stressor:
The stressor may be threatening or exhilarating.

Homeostasis:
The body systems maintain a stable and consistent (balanced) state.

Return to homeostasis

Illness and death:
The body's resources are not replenished and/or additional stressors occur; the body suffers breakdowns.

Illness

Death

FIGURE 3.1 General Adaptation Syndrome (GAS)
The three stages of Selye's GAS are alarm, resistance, and exhaustion.

found that persistent stress caused illnesses similar to those seen in humans, such as heart attack, stroke, kidney disease, and rheumatoid arthritis.

Scientists have argued that Selye's theory is too abstract and general and have challenged his assertions that any type of stressor triggers the same kind of response in the body and that positive stress (eustress) produces the same physiological changes as negative stress (distress). Selye's GAS model also does not take into account variations among individuals and differences between minor and major stresses, but it remains fundamental to our understanding of the impact of stress on the body.

Fight or Flight

Physiologist Walter Cannon, another pioneer in stress research, dubbed the complex, near-instantaneous sequence of internal changes that kicks in when you confront any potential danger the **"fight-or-flight" response**. When your brain perceives a threat, it sounds the body's alarm and sends signals for production of natural stimulants that speed up thinking, heart rate, breathing, immunity, metabolism, and blood flow.

Your heart beats harder to pump blood to your large muscles. You breathe faster to take in more oxygen. Your body mobilizes energy and delivers it to the brain, heart, and lungs; shuts off nonessential functions such as digestion and the sex drive; and ramps up the immune system to prepare for quick healing in case of injury. This classic threat response primes you to run for your life or go on the offense and fight back.

In interpersonal situations, individuals "fight" by arguing, opposing, demanding, criticizing, accusing, insisting, or refusing. Alternatively, they may take flight—literally by physically removing themselves or by withdrawing, not talking, dissociating, changing the topic, or otherwise "checking out."

Freezing

More recently, scientists have identified an acute stress response that may precede fight or flight: freezing, a survival mechanism that stems from some of the oldest circuits within the brain. Animals, such as a deer suddenly caught in the headlights of car, often stop as soon as they become aware of a danger. Freezing makes them less likely to be detected by a predator some distance away and may delay an attack if a predator is nearby.

Freezing may last for seconds or minutes—although it may feel longer. As evolutionary scientists explain, early humans may also have frozen in place at the sight or sound of a potential hazard, using this time to stop, look, listen, and assess what was happening. During this time, their bodies mobilized action. If, for instance, they spotted a predator at some distance, they would turn and flee. If the predator was already charging at them, they braced for a fight.

Submission

If unable to flee from or fight off a predator, animals may become immobile in the hope that their attacker will lose interest. In humans, this sort of reaction is called *dissociation*. Their minds go blank. Too overwhelmed to say a word or move a muscle, they submit, forfeit, yield, give up or give in, lower their expectations, settle, agree with others, or surrender their aspirations.

Submission occurs when no other option seems possible. Hostages held by armed gunmen, for instance, comply with their orders because they fear for their lives. In a less dramatic situation, you might discover that a friend's romantic partner is cheating, but you may not say anything because you fear that the emotional fallout would be devastating for everyone.

Challenge Response Model

Imagine that you are an athlete preparing for an Olympics final or a paramedic racing to an accident scene. Just as in the fight-or-flight response, your body mobilizes—not to save your life but to perform at your peak. Your heart pumps more blood through your body. You breathe more deeply to take in more oxygen. Your pupils take in more light. Your hearing sharpens. Your brain focuses. You are ready to give your all.

Unlike a threat response, which rewires the brain to heighten a sense of danger, a **challenge response** strengthens connections between the parts of the brain that suppress fear and enhance learning and positive motivation. In various studies of people in high-stakes situations, the challenge response consistently predicted better performance under pressure than fight or flight or than the absence of any stress response. Students scored higher on exams. Athletes ran faster, jumped higher, or scored more points for their team.

What determines if you react with a threat or a challenge response? The most important factor is how you perceive your ability to handle it. As you size up a stressor, you consciously or

"fight-or-flight" response The body's automatic physiological response that prepares the individual to take action upon facing a perceived threat or danger.

challenge response A physiological response that strengthens connections between the parts of the brain that suppress fear and enhance learning and positive motivation so as to prepare and enable a person to face a stressor directly.

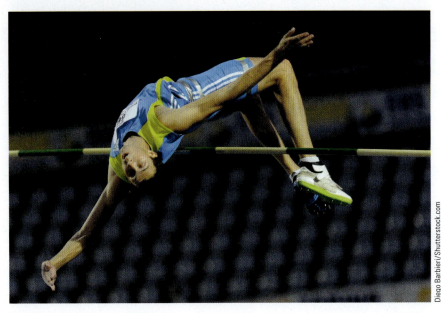

The challenge of competition can push athletes to perform at their peak.

unconsciously ask yourself: How tough is this going to be? Do I have the skills or resources I need to handle it? Where can I turn for help? Just as in the cognitive reappraisal model of stress (see upcoming discussion), you respond differently if you believe that the challenge exceeds your resources or if you believe you can cope with it successfully.

Individuals who consistently respond to stress as if it were a challenge rather than a threat are more likely to:

- Focus on their resources.
- Acknowledge their personal strengths.
- Think about how they prepared for a particular challenge in the past.
- Remember how they overcame previous challenges.
- Imagine the support of their loved ones.
- Pray or know that others are praying for them.

tend-and-befriend model A behavioral response to stress characterized by increased feelings of trust.

transactional or cognitive-relational model A framework for evaluating the process of coping with a stressful event in four stages (primary appraisal, secondary appraisal, coping, and reevaluation); based on the theory that the level of stress that people experience depends on their assessment of a stressor and on the resources available to deal with it.

✓**check-in** Tune into your stress signals. As soon as you notice early stress signals, think of how they are preparing you to meet a challenge. Pounding heart? Tell yourself that you are getting more-energizing blood throughout your body. Sweaty palms? They signal anticipation and excitement. Butterflies in your stomach? The nerve cells in your digestive tract are telling you that something significant is happening. Take a deep breath to sense your inner energy. Ask: What step should I take now to make the most of this moment?

Tend-and-Befriend Model

The classic threat response that prepares us for fight or flight can make people angry, defensive, aggressive, or withdrawn. But some individuals respond differently under pressure and become more caring, compassionate, and cooperative. The reason, according to the **tend-and-befriend model**, is that an urge to forge social connections under stress may be, like fight or flight, an essential survival instinct, especially for the females of a species.

Rather than the "stand-and-defend" reaction of the men in a prehistoric tribe or clan, the women may have responded by "tending" to offspring in harm's way and "befriending" those who would threaten them. Women may not be as innately driven as men to opt for fight or flight because of estrogen. Other female hormones as well as social support may moderate the effects of the powerful stress hormones.[33]

In times of crisis, both sexes may become more trusting, generous, and willing to risk their own well-being to protect others. The tend-and-befriend response creates what some call the "biology of courage," a physiological state that reduces fear and induces hope. The very acts of connecting and caring for others enable individuals to overcome feelings of powerlessness and hopelessness by inducing increases in several key brain chemicals, including:

- Oxytocin, which regulates the social caregiving system so you feel less fear and more empathy, connection, and trust.
- Dopamine, which boosts optimism about ability to cope and primes the brain for action so you don't freeze under pressure.
- Serotonin, which enhances your perception, intuition, and self-control so you can understand what is needed and take the most effective action.

Although the tend-and-befriend response may have evolved to protect children, it can emerge in response to any challenge you face. This is why nothing may help you more than helping others when you're feeling overwhelmed. When you reach out to tend and befriend someone in need, you benefit as well.

Transactional or Cognitive-Relational Model

The **transactional or cognitive-relational model**, developed by psychologist Richard Lazarus, is a framework for evaluating the processes of coping with stressful events. In his view, stress is "neither an environmental stimulus, a characteristic of the person, nor a response but a relationship between demands and the power to deal with them without unreasonable or destructive costs." The level of stress you experience depends on your appraisal of a stressor and on the social and cultural resources available to deal with it.[34]

According to this model, stress stems from an interaction or "transaction" between a person and a stress-inducing trigger. When individuals confront a stressor—whether it's a painful injury or an argument with a partner—they make immediate judgments about whether it poses a threat and whether they will be able to respond to it. Lazarus identified four stages in this process:

- The *primary appraisal* is the evaluation of the significance of the stressor or threatening event. You judge its severity based on previous experience, self-knowledge, and available information about the challenge. You determine whether or not it is threatening or thrilling, positive or negative, controllable or overwhelming, major or minor. If you do not perceive any danger, you do not experience a stress response because your well-being is not at stake.

- If you perceive the situation as threatening, you proceed to the *secondary appraisal* and assess whether you have the power and social, cultural, financial, and other resources to act. In essence, you ask yourself: What can I do about this? Can I control it? If you perceive that you can cope with the stressor, you experience positive stress. If you conclude that you may not be able to handle the stressor, you experience negative stress.

- In the *coping stage*, you may try a variety of efforts and processes with different outcomes. These include:
  - Problem-based coping, used when you feel you have control of the situation. For instance, you might deal with the stress of a failing grade by setting up a study schedule for upcoming exams.
  - Emotion-based coping, used when you feel you have little control over the situation. You might try avoidance (e.g., cutting class so you don't have to see the instructor), distancing yourself (e.g., telling yourself the bad grade doesn't really matter), venting your frustration in an argument with a friend, or numbing yourself with alcohol or drugs.

- In the fourth stage of *reappraisal* you evaluate the outcome in terms of your emotional well-being, ability to function, and health behaviors. Depending on whether the original stressor has been eliminated, you may need to try again or use a different approach. If, for instance, you realize you can't keep skipping class, so you make up any late assignments and focus on studying for future exams.

✓check-in Appraise your stress. When stressed, ask yourself: What is happening? Is it in any way dangerous or threatening? What can I do about it? Is this strategy working? If not, what else can I do?

Yerkes-Dodson Law

With too little stress, you might not be motivated enough to get out of bed in the morning and work toward your goals. With too much, you can't function at your best. But when your stress level is neither too high nor too low but just right, you are energized, effective, and efficient.

Psychology explains this phenomenon in terms of the Yerkes-Dodson law (named for the psychologists who first described it in 1908). In laboratory experiments, these researchers found that mild electrical shocks motivated rats to complete a maze, but when the shocks became too strong, the rats scurried around in random directions to escape. Their conclusion: Increasing stress can boost performance—but only to a certain point.

✓check-in How do you rate your current stress level: Too little? Too much? About right?

The Impact of Stress

In recent years, stress has been implicated as a culprit in a range of medical problems. While stress alone doesn't cause disease, it triggers molecular changes throughout the body that make us more susceptible to many illnesses (Figure 3.2).

Stress and the Heart

The links between stress, behavior, and the heart are complex. Scientists continue to explore the

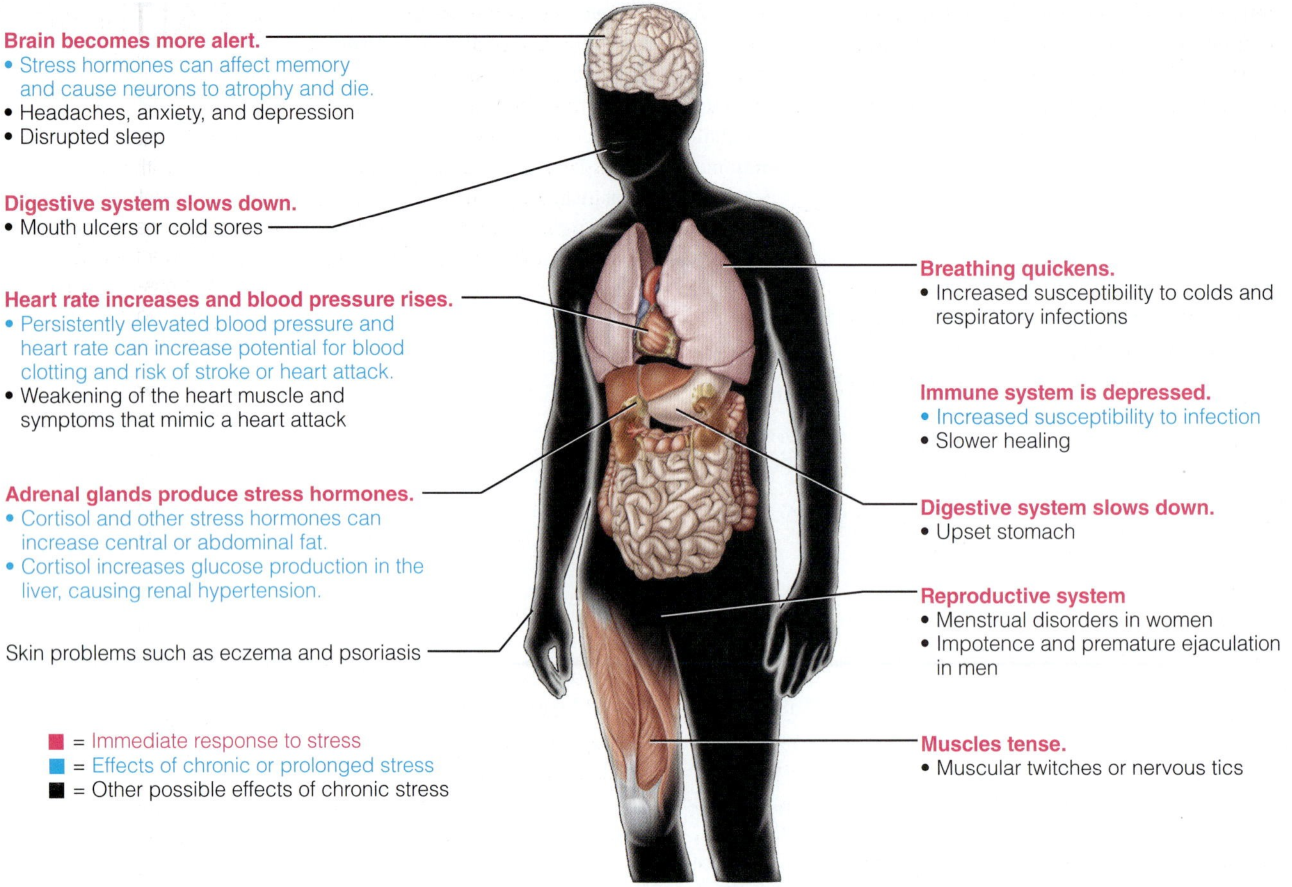

Brain becomes more alert.
- Stress hormones can affect memory and cause neurons to atrophy and die.
- Headaches, anxiety, and depression
- Disrupted sleep

Digestive system slows down.
- Mouth ulcers or cold sores

Heart rate increases and blood pressure rises.
- Persistently elevated blood pressure and heart rate can increase potential for blood clotting and risk of stroke or heart attack.
- Weakening of the heart muscle and symptoms that mimic a heart attack

Adrenal glands produce stress hormones.
- Cortisol and other stress hormones can increase central or abdominal fat.
- Cortisol increases glucose production in the liver, causing renal hypertension.

Skin problems such as eczema and psoriasis

■ = Immediate response to stress
■ = Effects of chronic or prolonged stress
■ = Other possible effects of chronic stress

Breathing quickens.
- Increased susceptibility to colds and respiratory infections

Immune system is depressed.
- Increased susceptibility to infection
- Slower healing

Digestive system slows down.
- Upset stomach

Reproductive system
- Menstrual disorders in women
- Impotence and premature ejaculation in men

Muscles tense.
- Muscular twitches or nervous tics

FIGURE 3.2 The Effects of Stress on the Body

impact of acute and chronic stress, gender, race, and socioeconomic status. One way in which stress increases the risk of heart attack and other cardiovascular problems is by pushing people toward bad habits. Men and women with high stress levels smoke and drink more and exercise less—and have higher rates of heart attack, stroke, and bypass surgeries.

Stress may be as great a threat for cardiovascular disease as smoking, hypertension, and other major risk factors (discussed in Chapter 10)—depending on how individuals respond to a stressor. According to a recent large-scale longitudinal study, men with low stress resilience in adolescence faced a greater danger of cardiovascular illness in middle age—perhaps because of unhealthy habits they acquired at an early age or because of inadequate coping skills.[35]

Chronic stress, whether because of finances, a demanding job, racial discrimination, or marital problems, can contribute to hypertension (discussed in depth in Chapter 10). Ruminating—mulling over stressful events or upsetting thoughts—may be the mechanism that elevates blood pressure even

hours or days after a stressful occurrence. The relaxation technique that has proven most effective in reducing blood pressure is meditation (discussed later in this chapter).

Stress and Immunity

The immune system is the network of organs, tissues, and white blood cells that defend against disease. Impaired immunity makes the body more susceptible to many diseases, including infections (from the common cold to tuberculosis) and disorders of the immune system itself. Acute time-limited stressors, the type that produce a fight-or-flight response, prompt the immune system to ready itself for the possibility of infections resulting from bites, punctures, or other wounds.[36]

However, long-term, or chronic, stress creates excessive wear and tear, and the system breaks down. Chronic stressors, so profound and persistent that they seem endless and beyond a person's control, suppress immune responses the most. The longer the stress, the more the immune system shifts from potentially adaptive changes to potentially harmful ones, first in cellular immunity and then in broader immune function. Traumatic stress, such as losing a loved one through death or divorce, can impair immunity for as long as a year.

Stress and the Gastrointestinal System

The "brain–gut axis," as gastroenterologists have called it, links the brain with the organs involved in digesting food as it enters your mouth, moves down the esophagus to the stomach, passes through the small and large intestines, and finally exits through your rectum and anus. During this journey, stress can:

- Decrease saliva so your mouth becomes dry (a frequent occurrence when under the stress of speaking in public).
- Cause contractions in the esophagus that interfere with swallowing.
- Increase the amount of hydrochloric acid in the stomach.
- Constrict blood vessels in the digestive tract.
- Alter the rhythmic movements of the small and large intestines necessary for the transport of food (leading to diarrhea if too fast or constipation if too slow).
- Contribute to or exacerbate gastroesophageal reflux disease (GERD).
- Lead to blockage of the bile and pancreatic ducts.
- Increase the risk of pancreatitis (inflammation of the pancreas), ulcerative colitis, and irritable bowel syndrome.

For many years stress alone was blamed for causing stomach ulcers, but scientists have discovered that a bacterium, *Helicobacter pylori*, infects the digestive system and sets the stage for ulcers. However, stress may increase susceptibility by reducing the protective gastric mucus that lines the stomach so ulcers develop more readily. With other chronic digestive diseases, such as irritable bowel syndrome, stress can be both a contributor and a consequence, causing or worsening symptoms that in turn intensify stress.

Stress directly affects what researchers call our "drive to eat." Under any type of stress, individuals eat more, binge more, and choose "palatable nonnutritious foods" (better known as junk foods) such as candy and cookies rather than healthier options. Foods high in sugar and fat may target pleasure centers in the brain and provide temporary comfort and relief. However, sweet treats can send blood sugar levels on a roller-coaster ride—up one moment and down the next.

Even if they don't consume more calories, some people, perhaps especially sensitive to cortisol, put on "belly," or visceral, fat (deposited deep within the central abdominal area of the body) when stressed. This type of fat poses a greater health threat than subcutaneous (under-the-skin) fat because it enters the bloodstream more readily, raises levels of harmful cholesterol, and heightens the risk of diseases such as diabetes, high blood pressure, and stroke.

Stress and Cancer

Among the latest findings from psychooncology, the field that combines medical and psychological approaches to cancer, are the following:

- Stress-related abnormalities in cortisol, inflammation, and the sympathetic nervous system can affect cancer growth.
- Stressful life experiences and depression are associated with poorer survival and greater mortality from various types of cancer, including breast, lung, and head and neck tumors.
- Psychosocial support and improved coping skills help even terminally ill patients to live better at the end of life—and in some cases to live longer as well.

Other Stress Symptoms

The first signs of stress include muscle tightness, tension headaches, backaches, upset stomach, and sleep disruptions (caused by stress-altered brain-wave activity). Some people feel fatigued, their hearts may race or beat faster than usual at rest, and they may feel tense all the time, easily frustrated, and often irritable. Others feel sad; lose their energy, appetite, or sex drive; and develop psychological problems, including depression, anxiety, and panic attacks.

Stress is also closely linked to skin conditions. If you break out the week before an exam, you know firsthand that skin can be extremely sensitive to stress. Skin conditions worsened by stress include acne, psoriasis, herpes, hives, and eczema. With acne, increased touching of the face, perhaps while cramming for a test, may be partly responsible. Other factors, such as temperature, humidity, and cosmetics and toiletries, may also play a role.[37]

Managing Stress

Although many students experience high levels of stress, relatively few seek counseling. Yet various approaches, including online stress management

HEALTH NOW!

Write It Out!

One of the most effective ways of coping with stress and other psychological challenges is by using a journal to monitor and express your feelings. Try the following stress-reducing exercises and record your responses and reflections in your online journal:

- **Assess your stress.** Take a strain inventory of your body every day to determine where things aren't feeling quite right. Ask yourself, "What's keeping me from feeling terrific today?" Focusing on problem spots such as stomach knots or neck tightness increases your sense of control over stress.

- **Reconstruct stressful situations.** Think about a recent episode of distress; then write down three ways it could have gone better and three ways it could have gone worse. This should help you see that the situation wasn't as disastrous as it might have been and help you find ways to cope better in the future.

- **Practice self-compassion.** As discussed in Chapter 2, treating yourself kindly in the face of stressful circumstances helps turn wisdom and awareness inward and provides a sense of perspective and connectedness.

- **Soothe yourself.** List some of the nice things you can do to soothe yourself, and include at least three of them in your daily routine. Make notes on how you feel after such experiences and which ones seem to have the most lasting impact.

and problem-solving interventions, have proven effective in reducing perceived stress and symptoms of anxiety and depression.[38] Apps for smartphones, watches, and other mobile devices are offering novel ways to monitor stressful situations and modify reactions to them.

✓check-in Complete this sentence: "When I'm stressed, I…." Eat a candy bar? Get a beer? Call Mom? Listen to music? Go for a run? Binge-watch? List all of the things you've done when stressed. Place a "+" next to those that helped, and a "–" next to those that didn't. Review your list, and add some new behaviors to try the next time you're in need of stress relief.

Journaling

One of the simplest yet most effective ways to work through stress is by putting your feelings into words that only you will read. The more honest and open you are as you write, the better (see Health Now!).

College students who wrote in their journals about traumatic events felt much better afterward than those who wrote about superficial topics. Focus on intense emotional experiences and "autopsy" them to try to understand why they affected you the way they did. Rereading and thinking about your notes may reveal the underlying reasons for your response.

✓check-in Have you ever tried journaling?

Exercise

Regular physical activity can relieve stress, boost energy, lift mood, and keep stress under control. Young adults who adopt and continue regular aerobic exercise show less intense cardiovascular responses to stress, which may protect them against coronary heart disease as they age. Strength training may have similar benefits (see Chapter 7).

There is a correlation between physical activity and stress in college students. Students who report higher levels of leisure-time exercise, along with a good social network and time management skills, generally enjoy better mental health, even when they report as much stress as less active undergraduates.

✓check-in Try an experiment with yourself: Keep track of the days when you work out in some way and those you don't. Rate your stress level every day, and see if exercise makes a difference for you.

Routes to Relaxation

Relaxation is the physical and mental state opposite that of stress. Rather than gear up for fight or flight, during relaxation our bodies and minds grow calmer and work more smoothly. We're less likely to become frazzled, and we're more capable of staying in control. A growing number of studies have confirmed the benefits of relaxation techniques. Although they differ in many ways, the various approaches may alter brain chemistry in fundamental ways, such as increasing the levels of pleasure-inducing chemicals in the brain.

When you practice **progressive relaxation**, you intentionally increase and then decrease tension in the muscles. While sitting or lying down in a quiet, comfortable setting, you tense and release various muscles, beginning with those of the hand, for instance, and then proceeding to the arms, shoulders, neck, face, scalp, chest, stomach, buttocks, genitals, and so on, down each leg to the toes. Relaxing the muscles can quiet the mind and restore internal balance.

Visualization or **guided imagery** involves creating mental pictures that calm you down and focus your mind. Some people use this technique to promote healing when they are ill. Visualization skills require practice and, in some cases, instruction by qualified health professionals.

Biofeedback is a method of obtaining feedback, or information, about some physiological activity occurring in the body. An electronic monitoring device attached to the body detects a change in an internal function and communicates it to the person through a tone, light, or meter. By paying attention to this feedback, most people can gain some control over functions previously thought to be beyond conscious control, such as body temperature, heart rate, muscle tension, and brain waves.

The goal of biofeedback for stress reduction is a state of tranquility, usually associated with the brain's production of alpha waves (which are slower and more regular than normal waking waves).

Meditation and Mindfulness

Meditation has been practiced in many forms over the ages, from the yogic techniques of the Far East to the Quaker silence of more modern times. Brain scans have shown that meditation activates the sections of the brain in charge of

progressive relaxation A method of reducing muscle tension by contracting, then relaxing, certain areas of the body.

visualization or **guided imagery** An approach to stress control, self-healing, or motivating life changes by means of seeing oneself in the state of calmness, wellness, or change.

biofeedback A technique of becoming aware, with the aid of external monitoring devices, of internal physiological activities in order to develop the capability of altering them.

meditation A group of approaches that use quiet sitting, breathing techniques, and/or chanting to relax, improve concentration, and become attuned to one's inner self.

the autonomic nervous system, which governs bodily functions, such as digestion and blood pressure, that we cannot consciously control. Research with a group of Tibetan monks and lay practitioners with extensive experience in meditation has demonstrated that meditation produces changes in various regions of the brain and can actually cause people to be more compassionate. The effects continue even after sessions of meditation.

Although many studies have documented the benefits of meditation for overall health, it may be particularly helpful for people dealing with stress-related medical conditions such as high blood pressure and heart problems, as well as for preventing stress-induced changes in the immune system (Figure 3.3).

Meditation helps a person reach a state of relaxation, with the goal of achieving inner peace and harmony. There is no one right way to meditate, and many people have discovered how to meditate on their own, without even knowing what it is they are doing.

Increasing numbers of college students are turning to meditation as a way of coping with stress. Most forms of meditation have common elements: sitting quietly for 15 to 20 minutes once or twice a day, concentrating on a word or an image, and breathing slowly and rhythmically. If you wish to try meditation, it often helps to have someone guide you through your first sessions. Or try tape-recording your own voice (with or without your favorite music in the background) and playing it back to yourself, freeing yourself to concentrate on the goal of turning the attention within.

Regular practice of transcendental meditation has reduced sleepiness in college students and improved their alertness and brain functioning. Undergraduates who began meditating during the first week of the term report being less tired and more resistant to the stress of finals than others.

Mindfulness is a modern form of an ancient Asian technique that involves maintaining awareness in the present moment. Some define it as an awareness that emerges by paying attention deliberately in the present to an experience as it happens moment by moment.

In mindful meditation, you tune in to each part of your body, scanning from head to toe, noting every sensation, however slight. You allow whatever you experience—an itch, an ache, or a feeling of warmth—to enter your awareness. Then you open yourself to focus on all the thoughts, sensations, sounds, and feelings that enter your awareness. Mindfulness keeps you in the here and now, thinking about *what is* rather than about *what if* or *if only*. For college students, mindfulness has

Meditation
- Reduces activation of the sympathetic nervous system—which, in turn, dilates the blood vessels and reduces levels of stress hormones, such as adrenaline, noradrenaline, and cortisol
- Reduces high blood pressure and use of hypertension medications
- Reduces atherosclerosis
- Reduces constriction of blood vessels
- Reduces thickening of coronary arteries
- Reduces mortality rates
- Slows aging
- Reduces hospitalization rates
- Decreases medical care utilization and hospitalization
- Increases creativity
- Improves memory
- Increases intelligence
- Decreases anxiety
- Reduces alcohol abuse
- Increases productivity

FIGURE 3.3 Many college students use meditation as a way of coping with stress. Have you tried it?

proven to enhance well-being and improve confidence in the ability to handle the complex challenges of adulthood.[39]

Mindfulness-based stress reduction, a group program that focuses on progressive acquisition of mindful awareness, has been used for patients with a wide variety of health problems as well as in healthy people coping with daily stress. Its proven psychological benefits include greater self-compassion and decreased absentmindedness, difficulty regulating emotions, fear of emotion, worry, and anger. Researchers have documented benefits for individuals suffering from chronic pain (including fibromyalgia), cancer, anxiety disorders[40] depression, and the stresses of the transition from high school to college.[41]

Yoga

An estimated 14.9 million Americans practice yoga, which has been defined as a union of mind, body, and spirit. In addition to easing conditions such as lower-back pain, migraine, asthma, and hypertension, yoga has proven to reduce anxiety and cortisol levels in those with moderate levels of stress.[42] Compared with other forms of exercise, yoga has a greater positive impact on mood and anxiety, possibly because it increases neurotransmitters (messenger chemicals) in the brain. "Expert" yoga practitioners, with 1 to 2 years of yoga practice, generally have lower levels of markers of

mindfulness A method of stress reduction that involves experiencing the physical and mental sensations of the present moment.

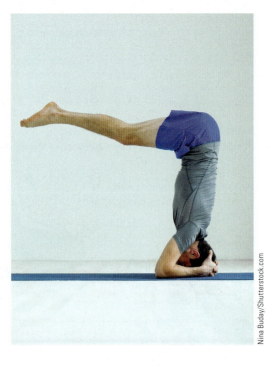

Yoga combines physical, mental, and spiritual practices to enhance fitness, increase flexibility, and reduce stress.

Nina Buday/Shutterstock.com

chronic inflammation than novices. Yoga may have another payoff for students: improved cognitive performance.[43]

Resilience

Adversity—whether in the form of a traumatic event or chronic stress—has different effects on individuals. Some people never recover and continue on a downward slide that may ultimately prove fatal. Others return, though at different rates, to their prior level of functioning. Life challenges, according to recent research, may increase mental toughness, build resilience, and help people cope with adversity.

Resilience can take many forms. A father whose child is kidnapped and killed may become a nationwide advocate for victims' rights. A student whose roommate dies in a car crash after a party may campaign for tougher laws against drunk driving. A couple whose premature baby spends weeks in a neonatal intensive care unit may find that their marriage has grown closer and stronger. Even though their experiences were painful, the individuals often look back at them as bringing positive changes into their lives.

Researchers have studied various factors that enable individuals to thrive in the face of adversity. These include the following:

- **An optimistic attitude**. Rather than react to a stressor simply as a threat, resilient men and women view it as a challenge—one they believe they can and will overcome. Researchers have documented that individuals facing various stressors, including serious illness and bereavement, are more likely to report experiencing growth if they have high levels of hope and optimism.

- **Self-efficacy**. A sense of being in control of one's life can boost health and lessen perceived stress and its impact on life satisfaction.[44]

- **Stress inoculation**. People who deal well with adversity often have had previous experiences with stress that toughened them in various ways, such as teaching them skills that enhanced their ability to cope and boosting their confidence in their ability to weather a rough patch.

- **Secure personal relationships**. Individuals who know they can count on the support of their loved ones are more likely to be resilient.

- **Spirituality or religiosity**. Religious coping may be particularly related to growth and resilience. In particular, two types seem most beneficial: spiritually-based religious coping (receiving emotional reassurance and guidance from God) and good-deeds coping (living a better, more spiritual life that includes altruistic acts).

Resilience sometimes means developing new skills simply because, in order to get through the stressful experience, people had to learn something they hadn't known how to do before—for instance, wrangling with insurance companies or other bureaucracies. By mastering such skills, they become more fit to deal with an unpredictable world and develop new flexibility in facing the unknown.

Individuals who engage in proactive coping, a concept based on the principles of positive psychology discussed in Chapter 2, perceive stressful situations as challenges instead of threats. Teaching such skills to incoming freshmen, recent research shows, builds their resilience and helps them deal better with the transition to college.

Along with new coping abilities comes the psychological sense of mastery. "I survived this," an individual may say, "so I'll be able to deal with other hard things in the future." Such confidence keeps people actively engaged in the effort to cope and is itself a predictor of eventual success. Stress can also make individuals more aware of the fulfilling aspects of life, and they may become more interested in spiritual pursuits. Certain kinds of stressful experiences also have social consequences. If a person experiencing a traumatic event finds that the significant others in his or her life can be counted on, the result can be a strengthening of their relationship.

Stress Prevention: Taking Control of Your Time

Although you may struggle to cram all that you need and want to do into your allotted 24 hours each day, you can take control of how you use the time you have. Becoming conscious of time and how you use it is crucial to reducing stressors and preventing stress overload.

✓**check-in** Are you running out of time? How can you tell if you've lost control of your time? The following are telltale symptoms of poor time management:

- Rushing.
- Chronic inability to make choices or decisions.
- Fatigue or listlessness.
- Constantly missed deadlines.
- Not enough time for rest or personal relationships.
- A sense of being overwhelmed by demands and details and having to do what you don't want to do most of the time.

One of the hard lessons of being on your own is that your choices and your actions have consequences. Stress is just one of them. But by thinking ahead, being realistic about your workload, and sticking to your plans, you can gain better control over your time and your stress levels.

Time Management

Time management involves skills that anyone can learn, but they require commitment and practice to make a difference in your life. It may help to know the techniques that other students have found most useful:

- **Schedule your time.** Use a calendar or planner. Beginning the first week of class, mark down deadlines for each assignment, paper, project, and test scheduled that semester. Develop a daily schedule, listing very

YOUR STRATEGIES FOR CHANGE

How to Cope with Distress after a Trauma

Senseless acts of violence or terrorism can trigger a variety of emotions, including shock, sorrow, fear, anger, and grief. You may have problems sleeping, concentrating, or going about simple chores. Because the world seems more dangerous, it may take a while for you to regain your sense of equilibrium. The following recommendations from the American Psychological Association can help.

- **Talk about it.** Ask for support from people who will listen to your concerns. It often helps to speak with others who have shared your experience so you do not feel so different or alone.

- **Strive for balance.** Remind yourself of people and events that are meaningful and comforting, even encouraging.

- **Take a break.** While you may want to keep informed, limit your exposure to news on television, the Internet, newspapers, or magazines. Schedule breaks to focus on something you enjoy.

- **Take care of yourself.** Engage in healthy behaviors, such as exercise, that will enhance your ability to cope. Avoid alcohol and drugs because they can suppress your feelings rather than help you to manage your distress.

- **Help others or do something productive.** Try volunteering at your school or within your community. Helping someone else often helps you feel better, too.

specifically what you will do the next day, along with the times. Block out times for working out, eating dinner, calling home, and talking with friends, as well as for studying.

- **Develop a game plan.** Allow at least two nights to study for any major exam. Set aside more time for researching and writing papers. Make sure to allow time to revise and print out a paper—and to deal with emergencies such as a computer breakdown. Set daily and weekly goals for every class. When working on a big project, don't neglect your other courses. When possible, try to work ahead in all your classes.

- **Identify time robbers.** For several days, keep a log of what you do and how much time you spend doing it. You may discover that disorganization is eating away at your time or that you have a problem getting started. (See the section, "Overcoming Procrastination.")

- **Make the most of classes.** Read the assignments before class rather than waiting until just before you have a test. By reading ahead of time, you'll make it easier to understand the lectures. Go to class yourself. Your own notes will be more helpful than a friend's or those from a note-taking service. Read your lecture notes at the end of each day or at least at the end of each week.

- **Develop an efficient study style.** Some experts recommend studying for 50 minutes and then breaking for 10 minutes. Small incentives, such as allowing yourself to call or visit a friend during those 10 minutes, can provide the motivation to keep you at the books longer. When you're reading, don't just highlight passages. Instead, write notes or questions to yourself in the margins, which will help you retain more information. Even if you're racing to start a paper, take a few extra minutes to prepare a workable outline. This will help you better structure your paper when you start writing.

- **Focus on the task at hand.** Rather than worry about how you did on yesterday's test or how you'll ever finish next week's project, focus intently on whatever you're doing at any given moment. If your mind starts to wander, use any distraction—the sound of the phone ringing or a noise from the hall—as a reminder to stay in the moment.

- **Turn elephants into hors d'oeuvres.** Cut a huge task into smaller chunks so it seems less enormous. For instance, break down your term paper into a series of steps, such as selecting a topic, identifying sources of research information, taking notes, developing an outline, and so on.

- **Keep your workspace in order.** Even if the rest of your room is in a shambles, try to keep your desk clear. Piles of papers are distracting, and you can end up wasting a lot of time searching piles for notes you misplaced or an article you have to read by morning. Try to spend the last 10 minutes of the day getting your desk in order so you get a fresh start on the next day.

Overcoming Procrastination

Putting off until tomorrow what should be done today creates a great deal of stress for many students. In various studies, 30 to 60 percent of undergraduates have reported postponing academic tasks, such as studying for exams, writing papers, and reading weekly assignments, so often that their performance and grades have suffered. Occasional delay becomes a more serious problem when it triggers internal discomfort, such as anxiety, irritation, regret, despair, and self-blame, as well as external consequences, such as poor performance and lost opportunities.

✔**check-in** Do you have a procrastination problem?

The three most common types of procrastination are putting off unpleasant things, difficult tasks, and tough decisions. Procrastinators are most likely to delay by wishing they didn't have to do what they must or by telling themselves they "just can't get started," which means they never do.

To get out of the procrastination trap, keep track of the tasks you're most likely to put off and try to figure out why you don't want to tackle them. Think of alternative ways to get tasks done. If you put off library readings, for instance, is the problem getting to the library or the reading itself? If it's the trip to the library, arrange to walk over with a friend whose company you enjoy.

Do what you like least first. Once you have that out of the way, you can concentrate on the tasks you enjoy. Build time into your schedule for interruptions, unforeseen problems, and unexpected events so you aren't constantly racing around. Establish ground rules for meeting your own needs (including getting enough sleep and making time for friends) before saying yes to any activity. Learn to live according to a three-word motto: Just do it!

Managing Your Money

✔ **Check-in:** You and your money.

How would you rate your financial management skills?

_____ Excellent

_____ Good

_____ Fair

_____ Poor

_____ Terrible

Money ranks second only to academics as a source of stress for college students.[45] However, money itself isn't a stressor. It's what you do—or don't do—with it that creates stress. Not having enough may be the most common complaint about money, but even with unlimited resources, you need to know how to manage money wisely and well.

College offers an ideal opportunity to learn how to handle everything from spare change to long-term loans. Once you know how to take control of your money, your money will not take control of you or your life. You will also be better prepared to pursue your goals—and have the financial resources to reach them.

College represents a huge investment for a family. If your parents are your primary source of support, talk with them about their expectations for how you handle your money. Do they expect you to get a job while taking classes? Do they expect you to work summers rather than backpacking through Costa Rica? Be very clear on which expenses are your responsibility and your spending limits.

About two thirds of students use loans to pay for college; more than 20 percent of loan recipients expect they will have a debt of $50,000 or more by the time they graduate. The average college student graduates with $24,000 in debt, according to the Project on Student Debt. With easy access to credit cards and so many things to spend money on, many students end up owing much more.

The information and exercises in the following section can boost both your financial understanding and your confidence in handling money now and in the future. We also recommend participating in the money management seminars that many schools offer. Or you can visit www.cashcourse.org, a free online resource specially designed for college students sponsored by the National Endowment for Education with plenty of practical information, but no ads or agenda.

Financial Homeostasis

As with any other aspect of stress management, homeostasis or balance is key. Your income, the amount of money available to you, must cover your expenses. If you spend more, you go into debt, which generates stress as well as other problems. As a first step, you need to organize your financial records and keep track of your monthly income and expenses (see Table 3.1).

Organizing Basics For bills and documents, buy a simple accordion file or a portable file. Make separate folders for documents from your school, bank, and service providers. As you put things away, add reminders of any deadlines and due dates to your phone. If you know you'll be more organized with virtual files, set up a system on your computer or on cloud storage. Save electronic files to specific folders, and scan or take pictures of paper documents and upload them. You may want also to back up your files on an external hard drive.

- Bills. Set alerts on your phone and computer, or circle days on your calendar to remind you of due dates so you pay bills on time.

TABLE 3.1 A College Student's Budget Template

Monthly income for the month of: _____	
Item	**Amount**
Estimated monthly income	
Financial awards	
Allowance from parents	
Other income	
Total	

Monthly expenses for the month of: _____	
Item	**Amount**
Rent	
Utilities	
Cell phone	
Groceries	
Car expenses	
Student loans	
Insurance	
Medical expenses	
Credit card debt	
Entertainment	
Laundry	
Miscellaneous	
Total	

Semester costs for the month of: _____	
Item	**Amount**
Tuition	
Books	
Lab fees	
Transportation	
Deposits	
Other	
Total	

How am I doing?	
Item	**Amount**
Monthly income	
Subtract monthly expenses	
Subtract semester expenses	
Difference	

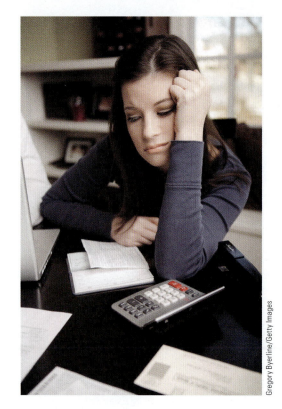

Gregory Byerline/Getty Images

Keeping up with paperwork and figuring out how to stay on a budget can add to a student's stress level.

- Insurance. File whatever policies you have, such as car or medical coverage.
- Loan and credit records. Keep loan agreements and payment records for car loans, credit card payments, and so on.
- Receipts and warranties. File the paperwork that comes with all major purchases, such as phones, tablets, and computers.
- Taxes. Include your tax returns, W2s, pay stubs, and so on.
- Keep records that are difficult to replace, such as your original birth certificate and Social Security card, in a bank deposit box or a fire-resistant safe.

- Checking account. Save your canceled checks and bank statements. If they are online, save them as a PDF and print them out. You should keep three to seven years' worth of bank statements in your records for tax purposes.
- Savings and investment. File all statements from your bank savings account and any other investments such as Certificates of Deposit (CDs) or mutual funds.
- College. Keep records of your tuition payments, receipts for textbooks and supplies, courses, grades, and credits.
- Financial aid. Save applications, award letters, student loan agreements, and notes about important telephone conversations.

Making a Budget Use your money for rent, bills, and groceries first. Then look ahead to upcoming expenses to see what you need to save for. This will give you a reality check on how much you have for going out or buying new clothes. Ideally, you should be able to save as well as spend. Financial planning starts with defining your financial goals, making plans for how to reach them, and taking action to make your goals a reality (see Table 3.2). If you write down your goals and incorporate them into your budget, you'll have a better chance of achieving them.

✓ **check-in** Do I Need This? Or Do I Just Want It?

You need to buy a bus pass or gas for your car. Do you need a morning latte? A cool phone cover?

Get in the habit of distinguishing between needs and wants. After a few months on campus, track your expenses, and put a plan into action.

TABLE 3.2 Your Money Goals

Goal	Amount Needed	By Date	How I'll Reach My Goal
Trip home	$300	Mom's birthday	Baby-sitting, tutoring
Car	$10,000	Next summer	Savings, bank loan, part-time job
New phone	$200	Within 3 months	Catering job, dog walking
Running shoes	$60	Two weeks	Not eating out, biking not driving
_____	_____	_____	_____
_____	_____	_____	_____
_____	_____	_____	_____

Personal Finances 101

Even the smartest students can end up making dumb money mistakes. The less students know about personal finances, the greater their credit card debt—and their financial stress.

Banking Basics

To decide which bank is best for you, compare what different ones offer. Here are some important questions to ask:

- How much money do I need to deposit to open an account?
- Is there a transaction fee for debit card transactions?
- Is there a charge for withdrawing money from an ATM machine?
- Does it offer a student or basic checking account with low or no monthly fees?
- Does it offer online banking, mobile deposits, text alerts, and 24-hour customer service?
- Can you set up automatic transfers or bill-pay services?
- Are there penalties for monthly account use? Falling below a minimum balance? Using an ATM not owned by the bank? Overdrafts?
- Will you receive statements via mail or electronically?

Banking rules allow consumers to choose whether or not they will be charged overdraft fees for debit card and ATM transactions. By opting in, you authorize your bank to allow your transactions to go through even if you are short money in your account. This will result in the financial institution charging you fees for the overdraft. If you opt-out, your transaction will be denied.

Here are some guidelines to avoid banking penalties and problems:

- Every time you write a check, enter the amount into your checkbook register and subtract it from your balance.
- Make sure to list ATM, debit card, credit card, and online transactions in your register as well.
- Don't assume your account balance at the ATM is correct. If you made purchases that haven't been processed by your bank yet, the ATM balance will be higher than the amount of money you really have. The same is true for your online bank balance.
- When the bank mails or posts your checking account statement each month, compare the bank's figures with your own and balance your checkbook. If you have questions, ask someone at the bank to help you.
- Keep your records safe. If you suspect someone else has gained access to your checking account, report it to your bank immediately. They can place a freeze on your account so it cannot be used.

Avoid Debit and Credit Card Stress

Using credit cards—as the majority of undergraduates do—is not only convenient but also a good way to start building credit. However, it's easy for students to amass a large amount of credit debt.

Here's how to avoid this common and serious source of stress:

- Keep one or, at most, two credit or debit cards (see Table 3.3). Resist the temptation to

TABLE 3.3 Credit Cards versus Debit Cards

Debit Card	Credit Card
Can get from bank	Can get from bank or other company
Might charge fees	Might charge fees
Can make purchases online	Can make purchases online
Money taken interest-free from checking account	Money borrowed interest-free from card provider, if paid back on time (charged interest, if paid back later)
Does not help build credit history	Helps build credit history
Free to withdraw cash from bank's ATM (charged fee if another bank's ATM)	Charged interest on cash advance from ATM or card
Does not offer rewards	Often offers rewards for use

sign up for more simply to get a mug, flash drive, or whatever else on-campus vendors are offering.

- Shop around for a card that has no annual fee, a lower interest rate, and a 20- to 30-day grace period (the amount of time you have to pay for new purchases before interest is charged). Avoid cards that charge a one-time processing fee and cards with low introductory interest rates that shoot up in a few months. You can shop for the best credit card deals on sites such as www.bankrate.com.

- Consider getting a credit card that's secured by a bank deposit, meaning that you have enough money in a savings account to equal the credit limit on the card. A secured credit card can help you get used to handling credit while building a good credit history.

- Don't charge anything you can't pay for right away. If you have a real emergency, allow yourself three months to repay the charge in full.

- Stick with the card you've chosen. The longer your credit history, the more your credit score will rise.

- Subtract your credit card purchases from your checking account so you'll have enough money to pay the bill in full each month.

- Do not use a cash advance from a credit card unless you have a serious emergency. You'll probably pay a fee for the money, and you'll be charged interest immediately.

- Avoid lending your cards to anyone, even close friends. Never leave your cards in plain sight, even in your room.

Each credit card has a different **APR (annual percentage rate)**, the amount of interest it charges each year on your balance. A **fixed interest rate** stays the same over time. A **variable interest rate** changes over time and can be raised at any time, or in response to your credit behavior. An **introductory interest rate** starts low—sometimes as low as 0 percent—but increases after a certain period of time. Many cards charge different interest rates for different types of purchases. For example, you might incur a lower interest rate on everyday purchases such as groceries and gas and a higher interest rate on a cash advance.

Digital Financial Management

Do you use Apple Pay at the bookstore? Venmo for your share of the rent or take-out bill? Affirm for a sweater on an online clothing retailer? As smartphones are replacing wallets, digital financial services are transforming consumer banking.

Thanks to electronic deposits, debits, and statements, you can make financial transactions from almost anywhere, often with a single swipe.

While digital solutions may make many routine transactions faster and simpler, they don't alter the fundamentals of financial responsibility. You still need to balance income and expenses, meet payment deadlines, and monitor where your money is going. Keep track of your spending, and download records of your daily transactions. Check the balance in your accounts frequently to avoid overdrafts or spot fraudulent transactions. It may be easier than ever to buy something on impulse, but that doesn't mean you can afford to do so.

When shopping or banking online:

- Shop only on secured sites (sites with a Web address that starts with https).

- Log out of any accounts before you shut down your computer (e.g., email, bank account, student account).

- Password-protect your phone and apps. Download software updates regularly. Take advantage of security technology such as fingerprint logins.

Protect Your Private Information

Identity thieves often prey on college students. Avoid checking your bank balance with a public computer. If you must use one, be sure to log out of your account completely and clear the cache on the web browser. Here are some other steps to take to prevent someone else from spending your money or using your credit cards:

- Don't give anyone your Social Security, credit card, or bank account numbers unless you know why the individual or organization is requesting them. If you are unsure, ask the person to send you a request by mail instead of asking for it over the telephone. Delete e-mails requesting personal information.

- Don't just throw away papers that list important account numbers or other financial numbers. Shred anything with your name, address, credit card information, or bank account numbers before putting it in the trash or recycle bin. This includes unused credit card offers.

- Don't send your credit card number over the Internet unless you are sure the website is secure and your computer is protected by a firewall and anti-virus, anti-spyware, and other security software. Keep your security software updated.

- Keep your credit card and ATM receipts in a safe place until you've paid the credit card bill

APR (annual percentage rate) The amount of interest a credit card company charges each year on the unpaid balance.

fixed interest rate An interest rate that stays the same over time.

variable interest rate A rate that changes over time and can be raised at any time, or in response to your credit behavior.

introductory interest rate A rate that starts low but increases after a certain period of time.

or balanced your checkbook. Then tear them up or shred them before throwing them away.

- Review your credit card statements and telephone bills for unauthorized use. If you suspect fraud, call the company immediately.
- Check your computer for malware (malicious software that affects your computer).
- If you're a victim of identity theft, report the crime to the police and your bank immediately.
- Opt out of pre-approval offers.
- Sign up for paperless billing.
- Avoid oversharing on social networks. Leave your full name, address, and birth date out of your profiles. Ignore friend requests from people you don't know.

If you suspect your identity has been stolen, act quickly. Most people who steal financial information use it within 48 hours. With a credit card, your maximum liability is $50. However, with a debit card you have to report fraud quickly to ensure you get your money back. If you report a lost or stolen debit card within 48 hours, your liability for unauthorized charges is $50. Between 49 hours and 60 days, your liability goes up to $500. After 60 days, you might be liable for all of the charges.

Alert the credit reporting agencies. Contact one of the credit reporting agencies (Equifax, TransUnion, or Experian). Ask the agency to place a fraud alert on your file to make it harder for someone to open new accounts in your name. A basic alert lasts 90 days, but you can extend it to 7 years.

Report the theft to the Federal Trade Commission (FTC). Complete its online complaint form, giving as many details as you can. Save and print out your FTC Identity Theft Affidavit. Report the theft to the police so you have an official record of the fraud. You'll need this, along with the FTC Affidavit, to prove to businesses that identity theft occurred. To remedy some of the damage, close any new accounts that have been opened in your name. Remove any unauthorized charges from your accounts. Correct any fraudulent entries on your credit report.

WHAT DID YOU DECIDE?

- Is stress always harmful?
- What stressors do college students typically encounter?
- How does the body respond to stress?
- What are some effective ways of managing stress?

Reflection
Based on what you've learned in this chapter, identify the major stressors in your life and the early signs of distress. Choose one stress management technique to incorporate immediately into your daily life.

TAKING CHARGE OF YOUR HEALTH
Strengthening Your Stress Muscles

If you decide to run a charity 5-kilometer race, you don't start training by heading for the gym or track and immediately going the full distance. You build up your muscles and your aerobic capacity by starting with a lap or two and gradually increasing your distance and pace. Similarly, with stress management, you need to acquire and enhance fundamental skills that lay the foundation for developing all kinds of new, more complex habits and skills. Check the strategies you might use to manage stress better in your daily life:

____ **Think back to times in the past week or so when you managed stress well.** Write down the practical skills you used. Go further into the past and think about other times you handled stress successfully. Also add these to your list of strengths.

____ **Review the times in the past when you did not handle stress well.** Write down why you think you handled stress badly in certain situations. Identify specific steps or skills that would have enabled you to handle the situations better.

____ **In assessing your strengths and weaknesses in handling stress, separate what you did, especially any mistakes you made, from who you are.** Instead of saying, "I'm so stupid," tell yourself, "That wasn't the smartest move I ever made, but I learned from it."

____ Pause but don't panic when confronting a stressor. Pay attention to what's happening around you and analyze the situation thoughtfully but refrain from getting caught up in gloom-and-doom thinking, which can lead to high levels of anxiety and poor decision making.

____ Avoid the tendency to overreact or to become passive.
____ Remain calm and stay focused.
____ If you find yourself turning more to escape routes such as drinking, gambling, or emotional eating, seek help from a campus counselor before the problem gets worse.

SELF-SURVEY

Student Stress Scale

The Student Stress Scale, an adaptation of Holmes and Rahe's Life Events Scale for college-age adults, provides a rough indication of stress levels and possible health consequences.

In the Student Stress Scale, each event, such as beginning or ending school, is given a score that represents the amount of readjustment a person has to make as a result of the change. In some studies, using similar scales, people with serious illnesses have been found to have high scores.

To determine your stress score, add up the number of points corresponding to the events you have experienced in the past 12 months.

1.	Death of a close family member	100
2.	Death of a close friend	73
3.	Divorce of parents	65
4.	Jail term	63
5.	Major personal injury or illness	63
6.	Marriage	58
7.	Getting fired from a job	50
8.	Failing an important course	47
9.	Change in the health of a family member	45
10.	Pregnancy	45
11.	Sex problems	44
12.	Serious argument with a close friend	40
13.	Change in financial status	39
14.	Change of academic major	39
15.	Trouble with parents	39
16.	New girlfriend or boyfriend	37
17.	Increase in workload at school	37
18.	Outstanding personal achievement	36
19.	First quarter/semester in college	36
20.	Change in living conditions	31
21.	Serious argument with an instructor	30
22.	Getting lower grades than expected	29
23.	Change in sleeping habits	29
24.	Change in social activities	29
25.	Change in eating habits	28
26.	Chronic car trouble	26
27.	Change in number of family get-togethers	26
28.	Too many missed classes	25
29.	Changing colleges	24
30.	Dropping more than one class	23
31.	Minor traffic violations	20
	Total Stress Score_____	

Scoring and Interpretation

Here's how to interpret your score: If your score is 300 or higher, you're at high risk for developing a health problem. If your score is between 150 and 300, you have a 50–50 chance of experiencing a serious health change within 2 years. If your score is below 150, you have a one in three chance of a serious health change.

Source: Mullen, Kathleen, and Gerald Costello. *Health Awareness Through Discovery*. Minneapolis: Burgess Publishing Company, 1981.

REVIEW QUESTIONS

(LO 3.1) 1. Stress is defined as _____.
   a. a negative emotional state related to fatigue and similar to depression
   b. a response to any event or situation that either upsets or excites us
   c. the end result of the general adaptation syndrome
   d. a motivational strategy for making life changes

(LO 3.1) 2. "Neustress" is a term that has been introduced to refer to _____stresses.
   a. novel
   b. neutral
   c. internal
   d. external

(LO 3.1) 3. Another term for looking at an individual's health as a whole rather than part by part is _____.
   a. comprehensive
   b. holistic
   c. unrealistic
   d. transcendental

(LO 3.2) 4. College students who report higher stress levels are more likely to _____.
   a. be male
   b. work hard
   c. consume junk food and soft drinks
   d. come from nontraditional backgrounds

(LO 3.2) 5. In a recent American Psychological Association survey of men and woman across the country, one in three Americans said _____ is/are a very or somewhat significant source of stress.
   a. parenting problems
   b. personal safety
   c. one's job
   d. relationship problems

(LO 3.2) 6. What kind of experiences that racial minorities have are referred to as *microaggressions*?
   a. Being insulted
   b. Academic challenges
   c. Limited opportunities
   d. Subtle negations of identity

(LO 3.3) 7. What is burnout?
   a. The aftermath of extreme anger triggered by stress
   b. A feeling of complete defeat
   c. The feeling that comes after a long evening of partying
   d. A state of exhaustion brought on by constant or repeated emotional pressure

(LO 3.3) 8. Traumatic events that may trigger acute stress disorder include which of the following?
   a. Loss of a friend in an accident
   b. Breakup of a relationship
   c. Personal or physical assault
   d. Failing a course

(LO 3.4) 9. Which of the following is true of posttraumatic stress disorder (PTSD)?
   a. Psychiatric medication has not proven effective for individuals with PTSD.
   b. Without recognition and treatment, PTSD can last for decades.
   c. The odds of recovering from PTSD are worst when symptoms develop soon after the trauma.
   d. Immediate "debriefing" to release emotions or treatment with anxiety-reducing medications is the best approach to treating PTSD.

(LO 3.4) 10. A person suffering from PTSD may experience which of the following symptoms?
   a. Procrastination
   b. Constant thirst
   c. Drowsiness
   d. Terror-filled dreams

(LO 3.4) 11. According to the general adaptation syndrome theory, how does the body typically respond to an acute stressor?
   a. The heart rate slows, blood pressure declines, and eye movement increases.
   b. The body enters a physical state called eustress and then moves into the physical state referred to as distress.
   c. If the stressor is viewed as a positive event, there are no physical changes.
   d. The body demonstrates three stages of change: alarm, resistance, and exhaustion.

(LO 3.4) 12. Which of the following is produced by the adrenal gland as a response to stress?
   a. Melanin
   b. Cortisol
   c. Epinephrine
   d. Oxytocin

(LO 3.4) 13. Which of the following statements is true of stress and the gastrointestinal system?
   a. Stress can constrict blood vessels in the digestive tract.
   b. Stress can increase saliva in the mouth.
   c. Stress can decrease the amount of hydrochloric acid in the stomach.
   d. Stress can dilate the esophagus.

(LO 3.5) 14. _____ produce a fight-or-flight response and prompt the immune system to ready itself for the possibility of infections resulting from bites, punctures, or other wounds.
a. Distant stressors
b. Acute time-limited stressors
c. Chronic stressors
d. Brief naturalistic stressors

(LO 3.6) 15. The transactional model views stress as _____.
a. based on the "fight-or-flight" response
b. an opportunity to strengthen relationships
c. being triggered primarily by physiological factors
d. a function both of stressors and a person's reaction to them

(LO 3.6) 16. The Yerkes-Dodson Law states that _____.
a. people are most motivated when they are stress-free
b. the lower the stress, the more energized people are
c. when your stress level is neither too high nor too low but just right, you are energized, effective, and efficient
d. the impact of stress has nothing to do with physical health

(LO 3.7) 17. Which of the following is a factor that enables individuals to thrive in the face of adversity?
a. Self-sacrifice
b. Self-schema
c. Selflessness
d. Self-efficacy

(LO 3.7) 18. A relaxed, peaceful state of being can be achieved with which of the following activities?
a. An aerobic exercise class
b. Playing a computer game
c. Meditating for 15 minutes
d. Attending a rap concert

(LO 3.8) 19. Which of the following techniques will help a student with time management?
a. Chunking smaller tasks together into larger tasks.
b. Focusing on past activities.
c. Providing small incentives at regular intervals.
d. Seeking a note-taking service.

Answers to these questions can be found on page 531.

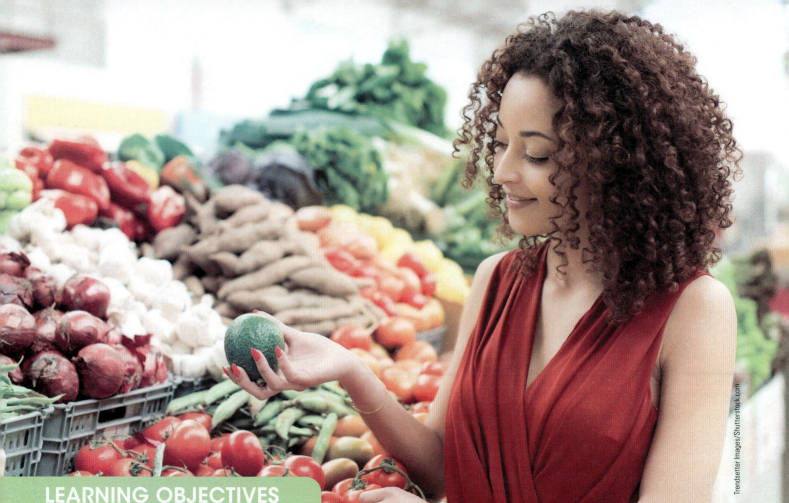

Trendsetter Images/Shutterstock.com

After reading this chapter, you should be able to:

4.1 Analyze the recommendations of the most recent *Dietary Guidelines for Americans.*

4.2 Identify the six categories of essential nutrients.

4.3 Differentiate between simple and complex carbohydrates.

4.4 Describe the forms of fat and their effects on health.

4.5 Review the components of various healthy eating patterns.

4.6 Assess the importance and accuracy of food labels.

4.7 Discuss the causes, effects, and prevention of foodborne infections.

4.8 Outline ways to identify nutrition quackery.

WHAT DO YOU THINK?

- What are the essential nutrients you need every day?

- What are some healthy eating patterns recommended by nutritionists?

- What steps can students take to eat a healthier diet?

- What are the healthiest beverages to drink?

4

Personal Nutrition

Jenna is a vegan. Ryan wolfs down a double cheeseburger with fries several times a week. Yuko counts calories but never checks labels for fat or sugar content. Max chugs energy drinks to stay alert during marathon study sessions. Shona avoids anything containing gluten. What about you? What are your food preferences and patterns?

College students, diverse in every way, vary greatly in the foods they choose. Those that are generally in good health pay little attention to the choices they make at every meal. But at every stage of life, **nutrition**—the connection between our bodies and the foods we eat—matters. Healthful eating enhances vitality, provides energy for daily tasks, and protects against many chronic illnesses.

About half of all American adults have one or more preventable diseases related to poor eating patterns and physical inactivity. These include cardiovascular disease, high blood pressure, type 2 diabetes, certain types of cancer, and poor bone health. As nutritional experts and health officials have realized, there is no one prescription or formula for a healthy eating pattern.

Sixty percent of adults in the United States report following some type of special diet–to avoid allergens, such as nuts or lactose, limit sodium or fat intake, or avoid food intolerances, such as gluten.[1] By customizing general evidence-based guidelines, individuals can enjoy foods that meet their personal, cultural, and traditional preferences.

This chapter can help you create a healthy eating pattern, regardless of your financial or time constraints. It translates the latest scientific research and government dietary guidelines into specific advice designed to promote and preserve good health. By learning more about nutrients, food groups, eating patterns, nutrition labels, and safety practices, you can nourish your body with foods that not only taste good but are also good for you. <

✓**check-in** How would you rate your knowledge of nutrition?

_____ Excellent

_____ Good

_____ Average

_____ Poor

Ask yourself the same question at the end of this course.

Dietary Guidelines for Americans

The *Dietary Guidelines for Americans*, revised every 5 years by a team of experts assembled by the Departments of Agriculture and Health

nutrition The science devoted to the study of dietary needs for food and the effects of food on organisms.

93

and Human Services, provide "science-based advice for healthy people ages 2 years and older to assist them in their efforts to make food and physical activity choices that promote health and prevent the risk of disease." Every revision generates some controversy among nutritionists and health professionals.[2] However, following the guidelines, particularly by increasing vegetable, fruit, and dietary fiber intake, has proved to lower the risk of dying of cancer or cardiovascular disease.[3]

The five official *Dietary Guidelines* are as follows:

1. **Follow a healthy eating pattern across the lifespan.** Choose a healthy eating pattern at an appropriate calorie level to help achieve and maintain a healthy body weight, support nutrient adequacy, and reduce the risk of chronic disease.

2. **Focus on variety, nutrient density, and amount.** To meet nutrient needs within calorie limits, choose a variety of nutrient-dense foods across and within all food groups in recommended amounts.

3. **Limit calories from added sugars and saturated fats and reduce sodium intake.** Cut back on foods and beverages higher in these components to amounts that fit within a healthy eating pattern.

4. **Shift to healthier food and beverage choices.** Choose nutrient-dense foods and beverages across and within all food groups in place of less healthy choices. Consider cultural and personal preferences to make these shifts easier to accomplish and maintain.

5. **Support healthy eating patterns for all.** Everyone has a role in helping to create and support healthy eating patterns in multiple settings nationwide, from home to school to work to communities.[4]

The current *Guidelines* recommend a healthy eating pattern that includes:

- A variety of vegetables from all of the subgroups—dark green, red and orange, legumes (beans and peas), starchy, and others.

- Fruits, especially whole fruits—fresh, canned, dried, or frozen.

- Grains, at least half of which are whole grains.

- Fat-free or low-fat dairy, including milk, yogurt, cheese, and/or fortified soy beverages.

- A variety of protein foods, including seafood, lean meats, poultry, eggs, legumes, nuts, seeds, and soy products.

- Oils, such as canola, corn, olive, peanut, safflower, soybean, and sunflower.

Additional recommendations set specific limits on nutrients:

- **Consume less than 10 percent of calories per day from added sugars.** For example, added sugar should be limited to 50 grams (about 12 teaspoons) on a 2,000-calorie diet. Added sugars include brown sugar, corn sweetener, corn syrup, dextrose, fructose, glucose, high-fructose corn syrup, honey, invert sugar, malt syrup, molasses, raw sugar, and turbinado sugar. Naturally occurring sugars, such as those found in fruits or milk, are not added sugars.

- **Consume less than 10 percent of calories per day from saturated fats.** Replacing saturated fats with unsaturated fats—but not with carbohydrates—can reduce the risk of cardiovascular disease.

- **Limit the intake of *trans* fats, such as partially hydrogenated oils, to as low as possible.**

- **Consume less than 2,300 milligrams of sodium per day.** Adults with prehypertension and hypertension are encouraged to cut sodium to 1,500 milligrams per day.[5]

The Building Blocks of Good Nutrition

The digestive system (Figure 4.1) breaks down food into **macronutrients**, the nutrients required by the human body in the greatest amounts. We also need vitamins and minerals, the so-called **micronutrients**, but in only very small amounts (see Tables 4.1 and 4.2).

Every day your body needs certain **essential nutrients** that provide energy, build and repair body tissues, and regulate body functions. The six classes of essential nutrients are water,

macronutrients Nutrients required by the human body in the greatest amounts, including water, carbohydrates, proteins, and fats.

micronutrients Vitamins and minerals needed by the body in very small amounts.

essential nutrients Nutrients that the body cannot manufacture for itself and must obtain from food.

Organs That Aid Digestion

Salivary Glands
Produce a starch-digesting enzyme
Produce a trace of fat-digesting enzyme (important to infants)

Liver
Manufactures bile, a detergent-like substance that facilitates digestion of fats

Gallbladder
Stores bile until needed

Bile Duct
Conducts bile to small intestine

Pancreatic Duct
Conducts pancreatic juice into small intestine

Pancreas
Manufactures enzymes to digest all energy-yielding nutrients
Releases bicarbonate to neutralize stomach acid that enters small intestine

Digestive Tract Organs That Contain the Food

Mouth
Chews and mixes food with saliva

Esophagus
Passes food to stomach

Stomach
Adds acid, enzymes, and fluid
Churns, mixes, and grinds food to a liquid mass

Small Intestine
Secretes enzymes that digest carbohydrate, fat, and protein
Cells lining intestine absorb nutrients into blood and lymph fluids

Large Intestine (Colon)
Reabsorbs water and minerals
Passes waste (fiber, bacteria, any unabsorbed nutrients) and some water to rectum

Rectum
Stores waste prior to elimination

Anus
Holds rectum closed
Opens to allow elimination

FIGURE 4.1 The Digestive System
The organs of the digestive system break down food into nutrients that the body can use.

protein, carbohydrates, fats, vitamins, and minerals (Figure 4.2).

Water

Essential for health and survival, water makes up 85 percent of blood, 70 percent of muscles, and about 75 percent of the brain and performs many essential functions, including carrying nutrients, maintaining temperature, lubricating joints, aiding digestion, ridding the body of waste through urine, and contributing to the production of sweat, which evaporates from the skin to cool the body.

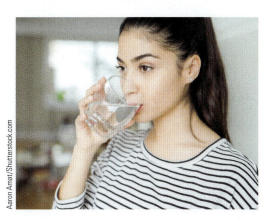

Aaron Amat/Shutterstock.com

Water is crucial to well-being at every age.

The Building Blocks of Good Nutrition

TABLE 4.1 Recommended Dietary Allowances (RDA) and Adequate Intakes (AI) for Vitamins

Age (yr)	Thiamin RDA (mg/day)	Riboflavin RDA (mg/day)	Niacin RDA (mg/day)[a]	Biotin AI (µg/day)	Pantothenic Acid AI (mg/day)	Vitamin B$_6$ RDA (mg/day)	Folate RDA (µg/day)[b]
Infants							
0–0.5	0.2	0.3	2	5	1.7	0.1	65
0.5–1	0.3	0.4	4	6	1.8	0.3	80
Children							
1–3	0.5	0.5	6	8	2	0.5	150
4–8	0.6	0.6	8	12	3	0.6	200
Males							
9–13	0.9	0.9	12	20	4	1.0	300
14–18	1.2	1.3	16	25	5	1.3	400
19–30	1.2	1.3	16	30	5	1.3	400
31–50	1.2	1.3	16	30	5	1.3	400
51–70	1.2	1.3	16	30	5	1.7	400
>70	1.2	1.3	16	30	5	1.7	400
Females							
9–13	0.9	0.9	12	20	4	1.0	300
14–18	1.0	1.0	14	25	5	1.2	400
19–30	1.1	1.1	14	30	5	1.3	400
31–50	1.1	1.1	14	30	5	1.3	400
51–70	1.1	1.1	14	30	5	1.5	400
>70	1.1	1.1	14	30	5	1.5	400
Pregnancy							
≤18	1.4	1.4	18	30	6	1.9	600
19–30	1.4	1.4	18	30	6	1.9	600
31–50	1.4	1.4	18	30	6	1.9	600
Lactation							
≤18	1.4	1.6	17	35	7	2.0	500
19–30	1.4	1.6	17	35	7	2.0	500
31–50	1.4	1.6	17	35	7	2.0	500

NOTE: For all nutrients, values for infants are AI.

[a] Niacin recommendations are expressed as niacin equivalents (NE), except for recommendations for infants younger than 6 months, which are expressed as preformed niacin.

[b] Folate recommendations are expressed as dietary folate equivalents (DFE).

[c] Vitamin A recommendations are expressed as retinol activity equivalents (RAE).

[d] Vitamin D recommendations are expressed as cholecalciferol and assume an absence of adequate exposure to sunlight. Pregnant or lactating girls ages 14–18 also need 15 micrograms vitamin D per day.

[e] Vitamin E recommendations are expressed as ∞-tocopherol.

Vitamin B$_{12}$ RDA (µg/day)	Choline AI (mg/day)	Vitamin C RDA (mg/day)	Vitamin A RDA (µg/day)[33]	Vitamin D RDA (IU/day)[44]	Vitamin E RDA (mg/day)[55]	Vitamin K AI (µg/day)
0.4	125	40	400	400 (10 µg)	4	2.0
0.5	150	50	500	400 (10 µg)	5	2.5
0.9	200	15	300	600 (15 µg)	6	30
1.2	250	25	400	600 (15 µg)	7	55
1.8	375	45	600	600 (15 µg)	11	60
2.4	550	75	900	600 (15 µg)	15	75
2.4	550	90	900	600 (15 µg)	15	120
2.4	550	90	900	600 (15 µg)	15	120
2.4	550	90	900	600 (15 µg)	15	120
2.4	550	90	900	800 (20 µµg)	15	120
1.8	375	45	600	600 (15 µg)	11	60
2.4	400	65	700	600 (15 µg)	15	75
2.4	425	75	700	600 (15 µg)	15	90
2.4	425	75	700	600 (15 µg)	15	90
2.4	425	75	700	600 (15 µg)	15	90
2.4	425	75	700	800 (20 µg)	15	90
2.6	450	80	750	600 (15 µg)	15	75
2.6	450	85	770	600 (15 µg)	15	90
2.6	450	85	770	600 (15 µg)	15	90
2.8	550	115	1200	600 (15 µg)	19	75
2.8	550	120	1300	600 (15 µg)	19	90
2.8	550	120	1300	600 (15 µg)	19	90

TABLE 4.2 Recommended Dietary Allowances (RDA) and Adequate Intakes (AI) for Minerals

Age (yr)	Sodium AI (mg/day)	Chloride AI (mg/day)	Potassium AI (mg/day)	Calcium RDA (mg/day)	Phosphorus RDA (mg/day)	Magnesium RDA (mg/day)	Iron RDA (mg/day)
Infants							
0–0.5	120	180	400	200	100	30	0.27
0.5–1	370	570	700	260	275	75	11
Children							
1–3	1000	1500	3000	700	460	80	7
4–8	1200	1900	3800	1000	500	130	10
Males							
9–13	1500	2300	4500	1300	1250	240	8
14–18	1500	2300	4700	1300	1250	410	11
19–30	1500	2300	4700	1000	700	400	8
31–50	1500	2300	4700	1000	700	420	8
51–70	1300	2000	4700	1000	700	420	8
>70	1200	1800	4700	1200	700	420	8
Females							
9–13	1500	2300	4500	1300	1250	240	8
14–18	1500	2300	4700	1300	1250	360	15
19–30	1500	2300	4700	1000	700	310	18
31–50	1500	2300	4700	1000	700	320	18
51–70	1300	2000	4700	1200	700	320	8
>70	1200	1800	4700	1200	700	320	8
Pregnancy							
≤18	1500	2300	4700	1300	1250	400	27
19–30	1500	2300	4700	1000	700	350	27
31–50	1500	2300	4700	1000	700	360	27
Lactation							
≤18	1500	2300	5100	1300	1250	360	10
19–30	1500	2300	5100	1000	700	310	9
31–50	1500	2300	5100	1000	700	320	9

NOTE: For all nutrients, values for infants are AI.

Zinc RDA (mg/day)	Iodine RDA (µg/day)	Selenium RDA (µg/day)	Copper RDA (µg/day)	Manganese AI (mg/day)	Fluoride AI (mg/day)	Chromium AI (µg/day)	Molybdenum RDA (µg/day)
2	110	15	200	0.003	0.01	0.2	2
3	130	20	220	0.6	0.5	5.5	3
3	90	20	340	1.2	0.7	11	17
5	90	30	440	1.5	1.0	15	22
8	120	40	700	1.9	2	25	34
11	150	55	890	2.2	3	35	43
11	150	55	900	2.3	4	35	45
11	150	55	900	2.3	4	35	45
11	150	55	900	2.3	4	30	45
11	150	55	900	2.3	4	30	45
8	120	40	700	1.6	2	21	34
9	150	55	890	1.6	3	24	43
8	150	55	900	1.8	3	25	45
8	150	55	900	1.8	3	25	45
8	150	55	900	1.8	3	20	45
8	150	55	900	1.8	3	20	45
12	220	60	1000	2.0	3	29	50
11	220	60	1000	2.0	3	30	50
11	220	60	1000	2.0	3	30	50
13	290	70	1300	2.6	3	44	50
12	290	70	1300	2.6	3	45	50
12	290	70	1300	2.6	3	45	50

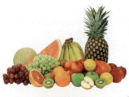

1. CARBOHYDRATES are substances in food that each consist of a single sugar molecule, or of multiple sugar molecules in various forms. They provide the body with energy.

Simple sugars are the most basic type of carbohydrates. Examples include glucose (blood sugar), sucrose (table sugar), and lactose (milk sugar). **Starches** are complex carbohydrates consisting primarily of long, interlocking chains of glucose units. **Dietary fiber** consists of complex carbohydrates found principally in plant cell walls. Dietary fiber cannot be broken down by human digestive enzymes.

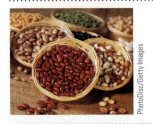

2. PROTEINS are substances in food that are composed of amino acids. Amino acids are specific chemical substances from which proteins are made. Of the 20 amino acids, 9 are "essential," or a required part of our diet.

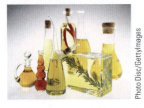

3. FATS are substances in food that are soluble in fat, not water.

Saturated fats are found primarily in animal products, such as meat, butter, and cheese, and in palm and coconut oils. Diets high in saturated fat may elevate blood cholesterol levels. **Unsaturated fats** are found primarily in plant products, such as vegetable oil, nuts, and seeds, as well as in fish. Unsaturated fats tend to lower blood cholesterol levels. **Essential fatty acids** are two specific types of unsaturated fats that are required in the diet. *Trans* fats are a type of unsaturated fat present in hydrogenated oil, margarine, shortening, pastries, and some cooking oils that increase the risk of heart disease. **Cholesterol** is a fat-soluble, colorless liquid primarily found in animals. It can be manufactured by the liver.

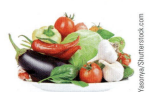

4. VITAMINS are chemical substances found in food that perform specific functions in the body. Humans require 13 different vitamins in their diet.

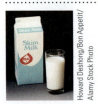

5. MINERALS are chemical substances that make up the "ash" that remains when food is completely burned. Humans require 15 different minerals in their diet.

6. WATER is essential for life. Most adults need about 11–15 cups of water each day from food and fluids.

FIGURE 4.2 Six Categories of Nutrients

You lose about 64 to 80 ounces of water a day—the equivalent of eight to ten 8-ounce glasses—through perspiration, urination, bowel movements, and normal exhalation. You lose water more rapidly if you exercise, live in a dry climate or at a high altitude, drink a lot of caffeine or alcohol (which increases urination), skip a meal, or become ill. To ensure adequate water intake, nutritionists advise drinking enough so that your urine is not dark in color. Healthy individuals can get adequate hydration from beverages other than plain water, including juice.

✓**check-in** How much water do you drink every day?

Protein

Every living cell in the body contains protein. Critical for growth and repair, **proteins** form the basic framework for our muscles, bones, blood, hair, and fingernails.

Twenty different **amino acids** join together to make all types of protein. Our bodies cannot make nine of these amino acids. These are known as *essential* amino acids that we must get from our diets. Dietary protein sources are categorized according to how many of the essential amino acids they provide:

- A **complete protein**, or high-quality protein, source provides all the essential amino acids. Animal-based foods such as meat, poultry, fish, milk, eggs, and cheese are considered complete protein sources.

- An **incomplete protein** source is low in one or more of the essential amino acids.

- **Complementary proteins** are two or more incomplete protein sources that together provide adequate amounts of all the essential amino acids. Two good examples are rice and dry beans, which together can provide adequate amounts of all the essential amino acids the body needs.

You need to eat protein every day because your body doesn't store it the way it stores fats or carbohydrates. The average person needs 50 to 65 grams of protein daily. This is the amount in 4 ounces of meat plus 1 cup of cottage cheese.

Protein-rich foods help people feel full sooner by releasing a hormone that regulates feelings of satiety, or fullness, so they may eat less—an advantage if they are trying to lose weight.[6] Higher protein intake may also help promote healthy aging by preventing the loss of muscle mass and strength that makes older adults more vulnerable to frailty, disability, and loss of independence.[7] Eating two protein-rich meals a day may provide the greatest benefit in maintaining lean body mass and muscle strength.[8]

Protein Sources

Protein is found in the following foods:

- Meats, poultry, and fish
- Legumes (dry beans and peas)
- Tofu
- Eggs
- Nuts and seeds
- Milk and milk products
- Grains, some vegetables, and some fruits (only small amounts relative to other sources)

Protein contributes to calorie intake, so if you eat too much, your overall calorie intake could be greater than your calorie needs, and you could gain weight. Animal proteins also are sources of saturated fat, which has been linked to elevated low-density lipoprotein (LDL) cholesterol, a risk factor for cardiovascular disease. Red meat in particular may increase the risk of death from cancer and heart disease—and the more of it that men and women eat, the greater the risk. Processed meats, such as bologna and hot dogs, also contain high amounts of sodium, unhealthy saturated fats, and nitrates, preservatives that have been linked to cancer.

✓check-in How often do you eat meat in a week?

Because it is rich in omega-3 fatty acids, seafood, another good protein source, has been linked with fewer cardiac deaths among individuals with or without cardiovascular disease. The American Heart Association recommends two servings of fish a week, although even a single fish meal a month may have a positive effect. These benefits outweigh the risks associated with methyl mercury, a heavy metal found in varying levels in different types of seafood. The types of seafood that are generally lower in mercury include salmon, anchovies, herring, sardines, Pacific oysters, trout, and Atlantic and Pacific mackerel (but not king mackerel, which is high in mercury).

Beyond protein, dairy products provide many nutrients, including calcium, vitamin D, and potassium, and may improve bone health, lower blood pressure, and reduce the risk of cardiovascular disease and type 2 diabetes. Health officials recommend 3 cups a day or the equivalent for adults—ideally from nonfat or low-fat dairy products. Soy beverages fortified with calcium and vitamins A and D are considered part of the dairy product food group.

Vegetarians who avoid eating all (or most) animal foods must rely on plant-based sources to meet their protein needs. Even for meat-eaters, substituting vegetable protein for animal protein confers health benefits, including lowering the risk of type 2 diabetes in both men and women.[9] Among the best options are certain nuts—peanuts, walnuts, almonds, and pistachios—that reduce risk factors for cardiovascular disease. In a study of more than 200,000 people, those who ate more nuts, including peanuts and peanut butter, had lower rates of premature death from heart disease and other causes. The recommended daily amount: about 2 tablespoons of shelled peanuts.[10]

Carbohydrates

Carbohydrates are organic compounds that provide our brains and bodies with *glucose*, their basic fuel. The major sources of carbohydrates are plants—including grains, vegetables, fruits, and beans—and milk. There are two types: *simple carbohydrates* (sugars) and *complex carbohydrates* (starches and fiber). All carbohydrates provide 4 calories per gram. Both adults and children should consume at least 130 grams of carbohydrates each day, the minimum needed to produce enough glucose for the brain to function.[11]

Simple carbohydrates include *natural sugars*, such as the lactose in milk and the fructose in fruit, and *added sugars* that are found in candy, soft drinks, fruit drinks, pastries, and other sweets.

On average, Americans consume more than 20 teaspoons of sweet calories a day. Some come from the teaspoons of sucrose (simple sugar) you add to coffee or tea. Those whose diets are higher in added sugars typically have lower intakes of other essential nutrients. The risk of cardiovascular disease and death increases once added sugar intake exceeds 15 percent of daily calories.[12]

✓check-in How much sugar do you consciously add to your diet every day?

A common hidden source of simple carbohydrates is high-fructose corn syrup, a sweetener and preservative made by changing the sugar glucose in cornstarch to fructose. Because it extends the shelf life of processed foods and is cheaper than sugar, high-fructose corn syrup has become a popular ingredient in many sodas, fruit-flavored drinks, and other processed foods. Although not intrinsically less healthy than sugar, high-fructose corn syrup might stimulate the pancreas to produce more insulin. It also makes beverages very sweet, which may increase consumption and contribute to obesity and other health problems.[13]

proteins Organic compounds composed of amino acids; one of the essential nutrients.

amino acids Organic compounds containing nitrogen, carbon, hydrogen, and oxygen; the essential building blocks of proteins.

complete protein Proteins that contain all the amino acids needed by the body for growth and maintenance.

incomplete protein Proteins that lack one or more of the amino acids essential for protein synthesis.

complementary proteins Incomplete proteins that, when combined, provide all the amino acids essential for protein synthesis.

carbohydrates Organic compounds, such as starches, sugars, and glycogen, that are composed of carbon, hydrogen, and oxygen and are sources of bodily energy.

simple carbohydrates Sugars; like all other carbohydrates, they provide the body with glucose.

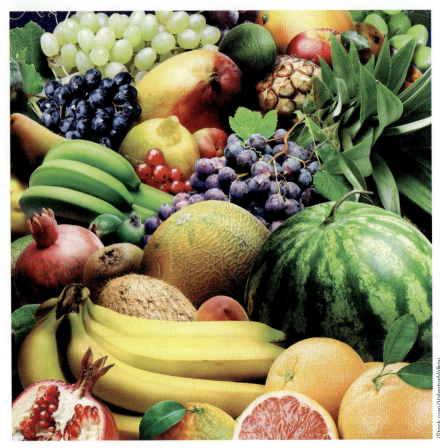

Fresh fruits offer variety, flavor, and essential nutrients to your daily diet.

nutritionists contend that the amount of added sugars even in nutrient-rich, recommended foods such as yogurt and whole grains may make this goal difficult to achieve[15] (Figure 4.3).

✓**check-in** Do you think foods high in added sugars should be taxed or restricted to reduce their consumption?

Complex carbohydrates include grains, cereals, vegetables, beans, and nuts. Americans get most of their complex carbohydrates from refined grains, which have been stripped of fiber and many nutrients, in breads and desserts. Far more nutritious are whole grains, which consist of all components of a grain, including:

- The *bran*—the fiber-rich outer layer.
- The middle layer, called the *endosperm*.
- The *germ*—the nutrient-packed inner layer.

Whole grains should make up at least half of all the grains you consume. Their health benefits include improved digestion, a lower mortality rate,[16] and reduced risk of cardiovascular disease, diabetes, and some cancers.[17]

Fiber **Dietary fiber** is the nondigestible form of complex carbohydrates that occurs naturally in plant foods, such as leaves, stems, skins, seeds, and hulls. **Functional fiber** consists of isolated, nondigestible carbohydrates that may be added to foods and that provide beneficial effects in humans. Total fiber is the sum of both.

Inadequate fiber intake may increase the risk of weight gain and obesity, chronic disease, and premature aging and mortality. The health benefits of adequate fiber intake include:

- Helping to maintain a healthy body weight by slowing the eating process, decreasing appetite, and increasing feelings of satiety.
- Enhancing movement of digested food through the intestines and colon.
- Lowering blood lipids (fats) and blood pressure and improving cardiometabolic health.
- Increasing insulin sensitivity and lowering systemic inflammation to reduce the risk of diabetes.
- Lowering the risk of strokes.
- Lowering the risk of colorectal cancer.
- Promoting healthy aging by preventing or delaying the onset of chronic diseases and helping to preserve good physical and cognitive functioning.[18]

✓**check-in** Are you getting enough fiber in your daily diet?

Sugar consumption, especially added sugar, has been implicated as a major cause of several chronic diseases, including obesity, heart disease, diabetes, and dental cavities.[14] Americans have cut back on sugar over recent years, but health authorities are calling for greater reductions to as low as 5 percent of total calories. However, some

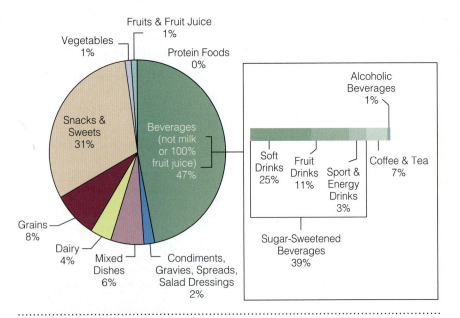

FIGURE 4.3 Sources of Added Sugars in the U.S. Diet

The National Academy of Medicine has set recommendations for daily intake levels of total fiber (dietary plus functional fiber): 38 grams of total fiber for men; 25 grams for women; for both men and women over 50 years of age, who consume less food, 30 and 21 grams, respectively.

Good fiber sources include wheat and corn bran (the outer layer); leafy greens; the skins of fruits and root vegetables; oats, beans, and barley; and the pulp, skin, and seeds of many vegetables and fruits, such as apples and strawberries (see Table 4.3). Because sudden increases in fiber can cause symptoms like bloating and gas, experts recommend gradually adding more fiber to your diet, with an additional serving or two of vegetables, fruit, or whole-wheat bread.

✓check-in Should you avoid gluten?

Gluten The number of consumers who say they are trying to avoid gluten has doubled in the past decade.[19] However, more than 85 percent of those claiming gluten intolerance actually have no symptom changes with a gluten-free diet.[20] The estimated 1 percent of Americans—some 3 million adults and children—with celiac disease are the only ones who clearly need to avoid gluten. In this autoimmune disorder, immune cells attack the lining of the small intestine, through which nutrients are absorbed. For genetically susceptible people, gluten—a protein in wheat, barley, rye, and other grains—can trigger symptoms such as abdominal pain, bloating, diarrhea, headache, and fatigue. If you don't have celiac disease or a sensitivity to gluten, doctors caution that a gluten-free diet can do more harm than good because it may not provide necessary vitamins, minerals, and fiber.

Glycemic Index and Glycemic Load

The glycemic index is a ranking of carbohydrates, gram for gram, based on their immediate effect on blood glucose (sugar) levels. Carbohydrates that break down quickly during digestion and trigger a fast, high glucose response have the highest glycemic index rating. Those that break down slowly, releasing glucose gradually into the bloodstream, have low glycemic index ratings. Potatoes, which raise blood sugar higher and faster than apples, for instance, earn a higher glycemic index rating than apples. The glycemic index does not account for the amount of food you typically eat in a serving.

complex carbohydrates Starches, including cereals, fruits, and vegetables.

dietary fiber The nondigestible form of carbohydrates found in plant foods, such as leaves, stems, skins, seeds, and hulls.

functional fiber Isolated, nondigestible carbohydrates that have beneficial effects in humans.

TABLE 4.3 Fiber Sources

Grains

Whole-grain products provide about 1 to 2 grams (or more) of fiber per serving:
- 1 slice whole-wheat, pumpernickel, rye bread
- 1 oz ready-to-eat cereal (100% bran cereals contain 10 grams or more)
- ½ cup cooked barley, bulgur, grits, oatmeal, brown rice, quinoa

Vegetables

Most vegetables contain about 2 to 3 grams of fiber per serving:
- 1 cup raw bean sprouts
- ½ cup cooked broccoli, brussels sprouts, cabbage, carrots, cauliflower, collards, corn, eggplant, green beans, green peas, kale, mushrooms, okra, parsnips, potatoes, pumpkin, spinach, sweet potatoes, swiss chard, winter squash
- ½ cup chopped raw carrots, peppers

Fruits

Fresh, frozen, and dried fruits have about 2 grams of fiber per serving:
- 1 medium apple, banana, kiwi, nectarine, orange, pear
- ½ cup applesauce, blackberries, blueberries, raspberries, strawberries

Fruit juices contain very little fiber.

Legumes

Many legumes provide about 6 to 8 grams of fiber per serving:
- ½ cup cooked baked beans, black beans, black-eyed peas, kidney beans, navy beans, pinto beans

Some legumes provide about 5 grams of fiber per serving:
- ½ cup cooked garbanzo beans, great northern beans, lentils, lima beans, split peas

Elena Schweitzer/Shutterstock.com

monticello/Shutterstock.com

art nick/Shutterstock.com

PhotoDisc/Getty Images

Glycemic load is a measure of how much a typical serving size of a particular food raises blood glucose. For example, the glycemic index of table sugar is high, but you use so little to sweeten your coffee or tea that its glycemic load is low.

Low-Carb Foods

You can get low-carb versions of everything from beer to bread. However, the Food and Drug Administration (FDA), which regulates health claims on food labels in the United States, hasn't defined what "low-carb" means. Words like "low-carb," "carb-wise," or "carb-free" are marketing terms created by manufacturers to sell their products.

Although many people may buy low-carb foods because they believe that they're healthier, that isn't necessarily the case. A low-carb nutrition bar, for instance, may be high in saturated fat and calories. Some low-carb food products cause digestive symptoms because food companies often replace the carbohydrates in a cookie or cracker with substances such as the sweetener sorbitol, which can cause diarrhea or stomach cramps.

Dieters often buy low-carb products to lose weight. According to proponents of low-carb diets, if carbohydrates raise blood sugar and insulin levels and cause weight gain, a decrease in carbs should result in lower blood sugar and insulin levels—and weight loss. With limited carbohydrates in the diet, the body would break down fat to provide needed energy.

Some people do lose weight when they switch to low-carb foods, but the reasons are probably that they consume fewer calories, lose water weight, and have decreased appetite because of a buildup of ketones (a by-product of fat metabolism) in the blood. As discussed in Chapter 6, a low-carb diet can lead to fairly rapid weight loss but is no easier to maintain over the long run than any other diet.[21]

Refined Grains

The refining of whole grains removes vitamins, minerals, and fiber. Although most refined grains are enriched with iron, thiamin, riboflavin, niacin, and folic acid before being used as food ingredients, not all of the vitamins and minerals and none of the dietary fiber are routinely added back. Many refined grain products, such as cookies and cake, also are high in solid fats and added sugars. On average, the recommended amount is no more than 3 ounce-equivalents.

Fats

Fats carry the fat-soluble vitamins A, D, E, and K; aid in absorption in the intestine; protect organs from injury; regulate body temperature; and play an important role in growth and development. They provide 9 calories per gram—more than twice the amount in carbohydrates or proteins.

Both high- and low-fat diets can be unhealthy. When people eat very low levels of fat and very high levels of carbohydrates, their levels of high-density lipoprotein, the so-called good cholesterol, decline. On the other hand, high-fat diets can lead to obesity and its related health dangers.

Solid fats make up an average of 19 percent of the total calories in the average daily diet, but contribute few essential nutrients and no dietary fiber. Reducing solid fats, most commonly consumed in grain-based desserts, pizza, regular cheese, processed meat products, and fried potatoes, can reduce extra calories, saturated fats, *trans*-fatty acids, and cholesterol.

Saturated fats and *unsaturated fats* are distinguished by the type of fatty acids in their chemical structures. All dietary fats are a mix of saturated and unsaturated fats but are predominantly one or the other. **Saturated fats** have long been considered a major threat to cardiovascular health, although current research has raised some questions about their impact.[22] However, there is ample evidence that lowering saturated fats to the recommended 10 percent of all calories—or lower—can significantly reduce the risk of cardiovascular disease. The American Heart Association recommends that people restrict saturated fats to as little as 5 percent of daily calories—roughly 2 tablespoons of butter or 2 ounces of cheddar cheese if you are consuming 2,000 calories a day.

To reduce your saturated fat intake:

- **Cut back on the major sources of saturated fats in your diet:** regular (full-fat) cheese, pizza, grain-based desserts (cakes, cookies, pies, sweet rolls, pastries, doughnuts, etc.), dairy-based desserts (ice cream, frozen yogurt, milkshakes, pudding, etc.), sausages, franks, bacon, and ribs.

- **Switch to nonfat or low-fat milk and dairy products.** When preparing or ordering fish, **choose grilled**, **baked**, **broiled, or poached fish**, not fried. Fried fish at fast-food restaurants is often low in omega-3 fatty acids and high in *trans* and saturated fats.

- **Trim all visible fat from meat.**

- **Use oils that are rich in monounsaturated fatty acids,** such as canola, olive, and safflower oils, or polyunsaturated fatty acids, such as soybean, corn, and cottonseed oils.

Unsaturated fats can be divided into monounsaturated and polyunsaturated, again depending on their chemical structure. Unsaturated fats,

saturated fats A chemical term indicating that a fat molecule contains as many hydrogen atoms as its carbon skeleton can hold. These fats are normally solid at room temperature.

like oils, are likely to be liquid at room temperature; and saturated fats, like butter, are likely to be solid. In general, vegetable and fish oils are unsaturated, and animal fats are saturated.

Olive, soybean, canola, cottonseed, corn, and other vegetable oils are unsaturated fats. Olive oil is considered a good fat and one of the best vegetable oils for salads and cooking. Used for thousands of years, this staple of the Mediterranean diet (discussed later in this chapter) has been correlated with a lower incidence of heart disease, including strokes and heart attacks.[23]

Omega-3 and omega-6 are polyunsaturated fatty acids with slightly different chemical compositions. Regular consumption of omega-3 fatty acids, found in fatty fish such as salmon and sardines, flaxseed, and walnuts, helps prevent blood clots, protect against irregular heartbeats, and lower blood pressure, especially among people with high blood pressure or atherosclerosis. Omega-6 fatty acids are found in vegetable oils, nuts, seeds, meat, poultry, and eggs. There is controversy over the benefits of increasing omega-6 fatty acids, and nutritionists do not recommend replacing oils made from vegetables with those made from saturated fats or fish oil supplements. For years, fish oil supplements were touted for their health benefits. However, large-scale studies have concluded that fish oil does not reduce the incidence of strokes or the overall risk of cardiovascular disease.[24]

The body makes more cholesterol than it uses, and people do not need additional amounts. The main sources of cholesterol, which is found only in animal foods, include eggs, chicken, and beef. *Trans*-fatty acids or **trans fats**, found naturally in some foods and formed during food processing, are not essential in the diet.

In response to consumer and health professionals' demand for less saturated fat in the food supply, many manufacturers switched to partially hydrogenated oils. The process of hydrogenation creates *trans* fats, which are found in some margarine products and most foods made with partially hydrogenated oils, such as baked goods and fried foods.

Even though *trans* fats are unsaturated, they have an even more harmful effect on cholesterol than saturated fats because they increase harmful LDL and, in large amounts, decrease helpful HDL (blood fats are discussed in Chapter 12). Some food manufacturers have reduced or eliminated *trans* fats in snacks and other products. Cities and communities across the country have banned *trans* fats in restaurants. Some campuses also have stopped using *trans* fats in their dining halls and food outlets.

Vitamins

Americans generally get adequate amounts of most micronutrients. However, intakes of several nutrients are low enough to be of concern:

- **For adults:** vitamins A, C, and E; calcium; magnesium; potassium; fiber
- **For children:** vitamin E, calcium, magnesium, potassium, fiber

Among the groups at highest risk of nutritional deficiencies are:

- **Teenage girls**
- **Women of childbearing age:** iron, folic acid
- **People over age 50:** vitamin B_{12}
- **Older adults, people with dark skin, and those who do not get adequate exposure to sunshine:** vitamin D

✓**check-in** Are you getting the recommended amounts of vitamins and minerals?

Vitamins, which help put proteins, fats, and carbohydrates to use, are essential to regulating growth, maintaining tissue, and releasing energy from foods. Together with the enzymes in the body, they help produce the right chemical reactions at the right times.

The body produces some vitamins, such as vitamin D, which is manufactured in the skin after exposure to sunlight. Other vitamins must be ingested. Vitamins A, D, E, and K are fat soluble; they are absorbed through the

trans fats Fat formed when liquid vegetable oils are processed to make table spreads or cooking fats; also found in dairy and beef products; considered to be especially dangerous dietary fats.

vitamins Organic substances that the body needs in very small amounts and that carry out a variety of functions in metabolism and nutrition.

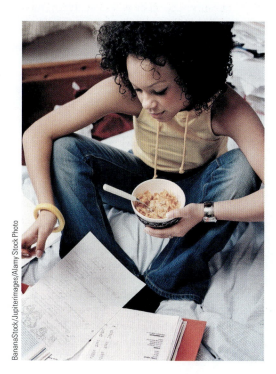

BananaStock/Jupiterimages/Alamy Stock Photo

A whole-grain cereal with low- or no-fat milk can sustain your energy while studying for a big test.

intestinal membranes and stored in the body. The B vitamins and vitamin C are water soluble; they are absorbed directly into the blood and then used up or washed out of the body in urine and sweat. They must be replaced daily. Nutritionists generally recommend nutritious foods as the best sources of vitamins and minerals. However, about two-thirds of American adults consume take nutritional supplements on a daily basis.[25]

Antioxidants prevent the harmful effects caused by oxidation within the body. They include vitamins C and E and beta-carotene (a form of vitamin A), as well as compounds like carotenoids and flavonoids. They all share a common target: renegade oxygen cells called free radicals released by normal metabolism as well as by pollution, smoking, radiation, and stress.

Diets high in antioxidant-rich fruits and vegetables have been linked with lower rates of esophageal, lung, colon, and stomach cancer. Nevertheless, scientific studies have not proved conclusively that any specific antioxidant, particularly in supplement form, can prevent cancer.

Folic Acid **Folic acid** or folate, a B vitamin, reduces the risk of neural tube defects in children. Women planning to become pregnant are advised to take a daily supplement of folic acid starting 1 month before conception. Another potential benefit, based on a study of more than 85,710 new mothers, may be a lower risk of the most severe form of autism in children.[26] However, folic acid supplementation does not substantially decrease—or increase—the incidence of cancer overall or of specific types, such as cancer of the breast, lung, prostate, or large intestine.[27]

Vitamin D This vitamin, essential for bone health, cognitive function, pain control, and many other processes within the body, comes in two forms:

- Vitamin D_2, from plants (that have been exposed to sunlight) and foods fortified with vitamin D, such as milk, cheese, bread, and juice.
- Vitamin D_3, formed in the skin after exposure to the sun's ultraviolet rays and ingested from animal sources, including some fish.

The benefits of vitamin D include better absorption of calcium, formation and maintenance of strong bones, and enhanced immunity. Studies of the relationship of vitamin D with specific conditions and illnesses have yielded mixed results.

It is not clear whether low vitamin D causes disease or simply reflects behaviors that contribute to poor health, such as a sedentary lifestyle,

smoking, and a diet high in processed and otherwise unhealthy foods. Low levels of vitamin D have been associated with a wide range of medical problems, including diabetes, depression, high blood pressure, cancer, and heart disease.[28] To avoid these problems, millions of Americans take vitamin D supplements. However, large-scale studies have concluded that high doses of vitamin D do not lower cancer rates in healthy adults, nor do they reduce the risk of heart attacks, strokes, and deaths from cardiovascular disease.[29]

Vitamin D supplements have shown no benefit in preventing or slowing cognitive impairment or dementia.[30] Either alone or with calcium, vitamin D does not reduce the incident of fractures among adults without a known deficiency, osteoporosis, or prior fracture, and it has been associated with an increase in the incidence of kidney stones.[31]

✓**check-in** Have you ever taken a vitamin D supplement?

Minerals

Carbon, oxygen, hydrogen, and nitrogen make up 96 percent of our body weight. The other 4 percent consists of **minerals** that help build bones and teeth, aid in muscle function, and help our nervous systems transmit messages. Every day we need the following:

- About one-tenth of a gram (100 milligrams) or more of the major minerals: sodium, potassium chloride, calcium, phosphorus, magnesium, and sulfur.
- About one-hundredth of a gram (10 milligrams) or less of each of the trace minerals: iron (although young women need more, particularly if they are physically active), zinc, selenium, molybdenum, iodine, copper, manganese, fluoride, and chromium.

Calcium Calcium, the most abundant mineral in the body, builds strong bone tissue throughout life and plays a vital role in blood clotting and muscle and nerve functioning. Nursing women need more calcium to meet the additional needs of their babies' bodies. Calcium may also help control high blood pressure, prevent colon cancer in adults, and promote weight loss. Adequate calcium and vitamin D intake during childhood, adolescence, and young adulthood is crucial to prevent osteoporosis, a bone-weakening disease that strikes one of every four women over the age of 60.

The safest way to ensure adequate calcium and vitamin D is by adding foods rich in these

antioxidants Substances that prevent the damaging effects of oxidation in cells.

folic acid A form of folate used in vitamin supplements and fortified foods.

minerals Naturally occurring inorganic substances, small amounts of some being essential in metabolism and nutrition.

nutrients to your diet. The recommended daily intake amounts are: for women ages 19 to 50 and men ages 19 to 70—1,000 milligrams; for women older than age 50 and men over age 70—1,200 milligrams. Amounts greater than 2,000 milligrams can cause constipation and kidney stones and may put individuals at risk for calcification within their blood vessels and other serious health threats.

In both men and women, bone mass peaks between the ages of 25 and 35. Over the next 10 to 15 years, bone mass remains fairly stable. At about age 40, bone loss equivalent to 0.3 to 0.5 percent per year begins in both men and women. Women may experience greater bone loss, at a rate of 3 to 5 percent, at the time of menopause. This decline continues for approximately 5 to 7 years and is the primary factor leading to postmenopausal osteoporosis.

The higher a young adult's peak bone mass, the longer it takes for age- and menopause-related bone loss to increase the risk of fractures. Osteoporosis is less common in groups with higher peak bone mass—men versus women, blacks versus whites. More than 60 percent of middle-aged and older women regularly take calcium supplements, but their benefits have not been proven, and they may pose potential risks, including kidney stones and high death rates from cardiovascular disease and other causes.[32]

✓**check-in** Are you taking steps to strengthen your bones?

Sodium Sodium helps maintain proper fluid balance, regulates blood pressure, transmits muscle impulses, and relaxes muscles. However, excess sodium contributes to high blood pressure, a leading cause of heart disease, kidney disorders, and stroke; it can also directly harm the blood vessels, heart, kidneys, and brain.[33] African Americans, who have higher rates of high blood pressure and diseases related to hypertension, such as stroke and kidney failure, tend to be more sensitive to salt.

Nine in 10 Americans consume more sodium (primarily in the form of salt) than they need. The average intake for Americans over age 2 is about 3,266 milligrams per day—much higher than the 1,500 milligrams that the Institute of Medicine has set as the "adequate intake" for individuals ages 9 to 50 and its "tolerable upper limit" of 2,300 milligrams for adolescents over age 14 and all adults. African Americans; individuals with hypertension, diabetes, or chronic kidney disease; and those older than age 51 should cut back to 1,500 milligrams per day.

Salt added at the table and in cooking provides only a small proportion of the sodium Americans consume. The most common sources are commercially packaged and restaurant foods.[34] Although Americans have significantly cut back on some high-sodium products, such as breads and salty snacks, the sodium levels in their total food and beverage purchases continue to exceed the recommended upper limit of 2,300 milligrams of sodium per 2,000 calories. The main sources are prepared meals/mixed dishes, processed meat, and cheese.[35]

✓**check-in** Are you consuming too much sodium?

Here is what you can do to lower your sodium intake:

- **Look for labels that say "low sodium."** They contain 140 milligrams or less of sodium per serving.
- **Learn to use spices and herbs** rather than salt to enhance the flavor of food.
- **Go easy on condiments** such as soy sauce, pickles, olives, ketchup, and mustard, which can add a lot of salt to your food.
- **Always check the amount of sodium in processed foods,** such as frozen dinners, packaged mixes, cereals, salad dressings, and sauces. The amount in different types and brands can vary widely.

Calories

Calories are the measure of the amount of energy that can be derived from food. How many calories you need depends on your gender, age, body-frame size, weight, percentage of body fat, and your **basal metabolic rate (BMR)**—the number of calories needed to sustain your body at rest. Your activity level also affects your calorie requirements (Table 4.4). Regardless of whether you consume fat, protein, or carbohydrates, if you take in more calories than required to maintain your size and don't work them off in some sort of physical activity, your body will convert the excess to fat (see Chapter 6).

Calorie balance refers to the relationship between calories consumed from foods and beverages and calories expended in normal body functions and through physical activity. You cannot control the calories your body burns to maintain temperature and other basic processes. However, you can control what you eat and drink and how many calories you use in physical activity. To maintain a healthy weight, you must expend as much energy (calories) as you take in.

calories The amount of energy required to raise the temperature of 1 gram of water by 1 degree Celsius. In everyday usage related to the energy content of foods and the energy expended in activities, a calorie is actually the equivalent of a thousand such calories, or a kilocalorie.

basal metabolic rate (BMR) The number of calories required to sustain the body at rest.

calorie balance The relationship between calories consumed from foods and beverages and calories expended in normal body functions and through physical activity. If the calories consumed equal calories expended, you will have calorie balance.

TABLE 4.4 Estimated Calorie Needs

• Most women, some older adults, children age 2–6:	1,600
• Average adult:	2,000
• Most men, active women, teenage girls, older children:	2,200
• Active men, teenage boys:	2,800

Source: U.S. Department of Health and Human Services and U.S. Department of Agriculture. *2015–2020 Dietary Guidelines for Americans.* 8th Edition. Appendix 2. Estimated Calorie Needs per Day, by Age, Sex, and Physical Activity Level. December 2015. Available at https://health.gov /dietaryguidelines/2015/guidelines/.

Among the best ways to balance this energy equation are:

- Limiting portion sizes (discussed later in this chapter).
- Substituting nutrient-dense foods (such as raw vegetables or low-fat soups) for nutrient-poor foods (such as candy and cake).
- Limiting added sugars, solid fats, and alcoholic beverages.
- Increasing physical activity. As discussed in Chapter 7, adults may need up to 60 minutes of moderate to vigorous physical activity—the equivalent of 150 to 200 calories, depending on body size—daily to prevent unhealthy weight gain. Men and women who have lost weight may need 60 to 90 minutes to keep off excess pounds.

✓**check-in** How do you balance the calories you consume with the calories you use?

YOUR STRATEGIES FOR CHANGE

Creating a Healthy Eating Pattern

- **Limit calorie intake to the amount needed** to attain or maintain a healthy weight.
- **Consume foods from all food groups** in nutrient-dense forms and in recommended amounts.
- **Reduce intake of solid fats.**
- **Replace solid fats with oils.**
- **Reduce intake of added sugars.**
- **Reduce intake of refined grains** and replace some refined grains with whole grains.
- **Reduce intake of sodium.**
- If consumed, **limit alcohol intake to moderate levels**.
- **Increase intake of vegetables and fruits.**
- **Increase intake of whole grains.**
- **Increase intake of milk and milk products** and replace whole milk and full-fat milk products with nonfat or low-fat choices to reduce solid fat intake.
- **Increase seafood intake** by replacing some meat or poultry with seafood.

Alcohol

As discussed in Chapter 12, about half of Americans regularly drink alcohol. Depending on the amount consumed, age, and other factors, alcohol can have harmful or beneficial effects. However, there is no nutritional need for alcohol. The *Dietary Guidelines* note that no one should begin drinking or drink more frequently on the basis of potential health benefits because moderate alcohol consumption, though associated with a lower risk of cardiovascular disease, also is linked with increased risks of breast cancer, violence, drowning, and injuries from falls and motor vehicle crashes.

Healthy Eating Patterns

There is no one "right" way to eat. A healthy eating pattern is not a rigid prescription but an array of options that can accommodate cultural, ethnic, traditional, and personal preferences as well as food costs and availability.

Although healthy eating patterns vary around the world, most:

- Are abundant in vegetables and fruits
- Emphasize whole grains
- Suggest moderate portions
- Emphasize a variety of foods high in protein (seafood, beans and peas, nuts, seeds, soy products, meat, poultry, and eggs)
- Include only limited amounts of food high in added sugars
- May include more oils than solid fats
- Are generally low in full-fat dairy products, although some include substantial amounts of low-fat milk and milk products

Compared to typical American diets, these patterns tend to have a high unsaturated to saturated fat ratio and a high dietary fiber and potassium content. Some are also relatively low in sodium compared to current American intake.

✓**check-in** How does your diet compare with this healthy eating pattern?

Among the research-based healthy eating patterns are the U.S. Department of Agriculture's (USDA's) MyPlate and Food Patterns, the Dietary Approaches to Stop Hypertension (DASH) plan, the Mediterranean diet, and vegetarian diets.

MyPlate

The USDA's MyPlate icon (Figure 4.4) serves as a visual reminder for healthy eating based on the following principles:

- Enjoy your food but eat less.
- Avoid oversized portions.
- Make half your plate fruits and vegetables.
- Make at least half your grains whole grains.
- Switch to nonfat or low-fat (1%) milk.
- Compare sodium in foods such as soup, bread, and frozen meals and choose those with lower numbers.
- Drink water instead of sugary drinks.

The USDA Food Patterns

These approaches identify daily amounts of foods to eat from five major food groups and subgroups: vegetables, fruits and juices, grains, milk and milk products, and protein foods. They also include an allowance for oils and limits on the maximum number of calories that should be consumed from solid fats and added sugars. Amounts and limits are given at different calorie levels, ranging from 1,000 to 3,200. All the USDA Food Patterns emphasize selection of a variety of foods in nutrient-dense forms—that is, with little or no solid fats and added sugars—from each food group.

The USDA Food Patterns include a vegan pattern, which consists of only plant foods and substitutes calcium-fortified beverages and foods for dairy products, and a lacto-ovo-vegetarian pattern, which includes milk, milk products, and eggs.

The DASH Eating Plan

DASH emphasizes vegetables, fruits, and low-fat milk and milk products; includes whole grains, poultry, seafood, and nuts; and is lower in sodium, red and processed meats, sweets, and sugar-containing beverages than typical intakes in the United States (Table 4.5). In research studies, DASH approaches have proven to lower blood pressure, improve blood lipids, and reduce the risk of cardiovascular disease.

The Mediterranean Diet

Many cultures and agricultural patterns exist in the countries that border the Mediterranean Sea. The "Mediterranean diet" is not the cuisine of a particular nation but an eating pattern that emphasizes vegetables, fruits and nuts, olive oil, and grains (often whole grains), with only small

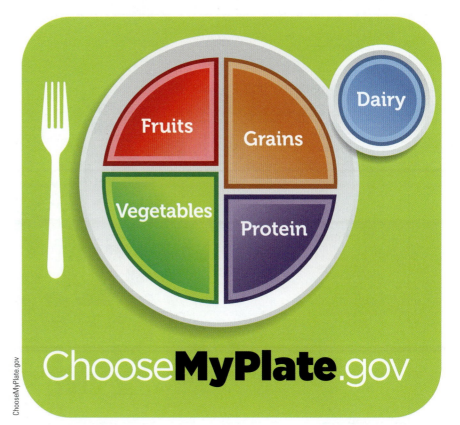

ChooseMyPlate.gov

FIGURE 4.4 The MyPlate System

The most recent food pattern from the USDA reminds Americans to balance calories, increase foods such as fruits and vegetables, and drink fat-free or low-fat milk.

TABLE 4.5 The DASH Eating Plan

USDA/DASH recommendations for a 2,000-calorie daily diet include
• Fruit Group—2–2.5 cups (4–5 servings) of fresh, frozen, canned, or dried fruit, with only limited juice
• Vegetable Group—2–2.5 cups (4–5 servings)
• Dark greens, such as broccoli and leafy greens—3 cups per week
• Orange vegetables, such as carrots and sweet potatoes—2 cups per week
• Legumes, such as pinto or kidney beans, split peas, or lentils—3 cups per week
• Starchy vegetables—3 cups per week
• Other vegetables—6.5 cups per week
• Grain Group—6–8 ounce-equivalents of cereal, bread, crackers, rice, or pasta, with at least 50% whole grain
• Meat and Beans Group—5.5–6 ounce-equivalents of baked, broiled, or grilled lean meat, poultry, or fish, eggs, nuts, seeds, beans, peas, or tofu
• Milk Group—2–3 cups low-fat/fat-free milk, yogurt, or cheese, or lactose-free, calcium-fortified products
• Oils—2–6 teaspoons
• Discretionary—267 calories; for example, solid fats (saturated fat such as butter, margarine, shortening, or lard) or added sugar

www.usda.gov

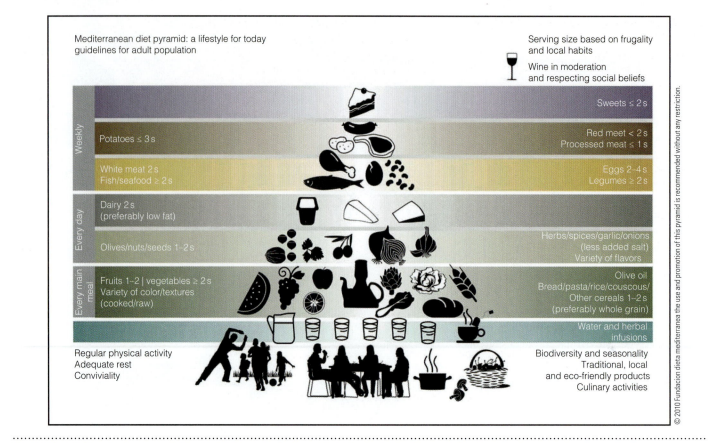

Mediterranean diet pyramid: a lifestyle for today
guidelines for adult population

Serving size based on frugality
and local habits

Wine in moderation
and respecting social beliefs

Weekly

Sweets ≤ 2 s

Potatoes ≤ 3 s

Red meet < 2 s
Processed meat ≤ 1 s

White meat 2 s
Fish/seafood ≥ 2 s

Eggs 2–4 s
Legumes ≥ 2 s

Every day

Dairy 2 s
(preferably low fat)

Olives/nuts/seeds 1–2 s

Herbs/spices/garlic/onions
(less added salt)
Variety of flavors

Every main meal

Fruits 1–2 | vegetables ≥ 2 s
Variety of color/textures
(cooked/raw)

Olive oil
Bread/pasta/rice/couscous/
Other cereals 1–2 s
(preferably whole grain)

Water and herbal
infusions

Regular physical activity
Adequate rest
Conviviality

Biodiversity and seasonality
Traditional, local
and eco-friendly products
Culinary activities

© 2010 Fundacion dieta mediterranea the use and promotion of this pyramid is recommended without any restriction.

FIGURE 4.5 The Traditional Healthy Mediterranean Diet Pyramid

amounts of meats and full-fat milk and milk products. It is also a cultural model involving the way foods are selected, produced, processed, and distributed.[36]

Scientists have identified antioxidants in red wine and olive oil that may account for the beneficial effects on the heart of the Mediterranean diet, which features lots of fruits and vegetables, legumes, nuts, and grains (Figure 4.5). The proven health benefits of the Mediterranean diet include:

- Reducing rates of carrdiovascular disease and deaths.

- Reducing rates of cancer, including breast, colorectal, and lung cancers.

- Lowering risk of mild age-related cognitive impairment and of its progression to Alzheimer's disease.

- Ameliorating the symptoms of rheumatoid arthritis.

- Protecting against respiratory diseases, including asthma.[37]

Strict adherence to the Mediterranean diet has proven so beneficial that many physicians recommend its use for the general population, regardless of gender, age, family history of heart disease, diabetes, smoking status, hypertension, or fitness.

Vegetables and Fruits

Nutritionists and health officials consistently recommend eating more vegetables and fruits. Why? They:

- Provide many nutrients that many Americans lack.

- Lower the risk of many chronic illnesses, including type 2 diabetes, cardiovascular disease (including heart attack and stroke), and certain cancers.

- Help individuals reach and maintain a healthy weight.

- Lessen the risk of dying. In a recent study, individuals who ate seven or more portions of fresh fruits and vegetables a day had a 42 percent lower risk of death at any age than those who ate less than one portion a day. Even those who ate just one portion had lower death rates.[38]

Fewer than one-third of American adults eat the recommended amounts of fruits and vegetables. College-age young adults between ages 18 and 24 eat the fewest vegetables. Nearly four-fifths of this group don't put vegetables on their plates—or scrape them to the side if they do. About one in four teenagers eats fruit less than once a day.

✓check-in Which is better for you: fruit or fruit juice?

As long as you drink 100 percent juice, you can choose either—or, better yet, both. According to a nutritional analysis, a combination of whole fruit and 100 percent juice boosts potassium and vitamin C without significantly increasing total calories. Not only does 100 percent fruit juice deliver essential nutrients and phytonutrients, but it also provides year-round access to a variety of fruits and is a cost-effective way to help people meet fruit recommendations.[39]

Phytochemicals, compounds that exist naturally in plants, serve many functions, including helping a plant protect itself from bacteria and disease, giving tomatoes their red color, and putting "fire" into hot peppers. In the body, they act as antioxidants, mimic hormones, and reduce the risk of various illnesses, including cancer and heart disease. Good sources include broccoli, tomatoes, and soybeans.

Phytochemicals give tomatoes their red color and hot peppers their "fire." In the body, they act as antioxidants, mimic hormones, and reduce the risk of various illnesses, including cancer and heart disease. Broccoli may contain as many as 10,000 different phytochemicals, each capable of influencing some action or organ in the body. Tomatoes provide lycopene, a powerful antioxidant that seems to offer protection against cancers of the esophagus, lungs, prostate, and stomach. Soybeans, a rich source of an array of phytochemicals, appear to slow the growth of breast and prostate cancer.

Vegetarian Diets

Among the followers of vegetarian diets are:

- Lacto-ovo-pesco-vegetarians, who eat dairy products, eggs, and fish but not red meat.

- Lacto-vegetarians, who eat dairy products as well as grains, fruits, and vegetables.

- Ovo-lacto-vegetarians, who also eat eggs.

- Vegans, or pure vegetarians, who eat only plant foods. They may take vitamin supplements because that vitamin is normally found only in animal products.

The key to getting sufficient protein from a vegetarian diet is understanding the concept of complementary proteins. Recall that meat, poultry, fish, eggs, and dairy products are complete proteins that provide the nine essential amino acids—substances that the human body cannot produce itself. Incomplete proteins, such as legumes or nuts, may have relatively low levels of one or two essential amino acids but fairly high levels of others.

By combining complementary protein sources, vegetarians can make sure their bodies make the most of the nonanimal proteins they eat. Many cultures rely heavily on complementary foods for protein. In Middle Eastern cooking, sesame seeds and chickpeas are a popular combination; in Latin American dishes, beans and rice, or beans and tortillas; in Chinese cuisine, soy and rice.

Vegetarians can best meet their nutrient needs by paying special attention to protein, iron, vitamins, calcium, and vitamin D. Instead of a 6-ounce serving of meat, they can substitute one egg, 1.5 ounces of nuts, or 2/3 cup of legumes. Those who avoid milk because of its lactose content may obtain all the nutrients of milk by using lactose-reduced milk or eating other calcium-rich foods, such as broccoli, calcium-fortified orange juice, and fortified soy milk.

Vegetarian diets have proven health benefits, including:

- Lower cholesterol levels.

- Healthier weight.

- Decreased risk of heart disease.

- Lower incidences of breast, colon, and prostate cancer; high blood pressure; and osteoporosis.

- Weight reduction.[40]

Even people who are not strict vegetarians but who eat more plant foods (whole grains, beans, vegetables, fruits, and nuts) than animal products lower their risk of dying from heart disease or a stroke.

✓check-in Are you a vegetarian? If so, which type? How do you ensure an adequate amount of protein in your diet?

Ethnic Cuisines

Whatever your cultural heritage, you have probably sampled Chinese, Mexican, Indian, Italian, and Japanese foods. If you belong to any of these ethnic groups, you may eat these cuisines regularly. Each type of ethnic cooking has its own nutritional benefits and potential drawbacks (Table 4.6).

phytochemicals Chemicals such as indoles, coumarins, and capsaicin, which exist naturally in plants and have disease-fighting properties.

TABLE 4.6 Ethnic Food Choices

	Grains	Vegetables	Fruits	Meats and Legumes	Milk
Asian	Rice, noodles, millet	Amaranth, baby corn, bamboo shoots, chayote, bok choy, mung bean sprouts, sugar peas, straw mushrooms, water chestnuts, kelp	Carambola, guava, kumquat, lychee, persimmon, melons, mandarin orange	Soybeans and soy products such as soy milk and tofu, squid, duck eggs, pork, poultry, fish and other seafood, peanuts, cashews	Usually excluded
Mediterranean	Pita pocket bread, pastas, rice, couscous, polenta, bulgur, focaccia, Italian bread	Eggplant, tomatoes, peppers, cucumbers, grape leaves	Olives, grapes, figs	Fish and other seafood, gyros, lamb, chicken, beef, pork, sausage, lentils, fava beans	Ricotta, provolone, parmesan, feta, mozzarella, and goat cheeses; yogurt
Mexican	Tortillas (corn or flour), taco shells, rice	Chayote, corn, jicama, tomato salsa, cactus, cassava, tomatoes, yams, chilies	Guava, mango, papaya, avocado, plantain, bananas, oranges	Refried beans, fish, chicken, chorizo, beef, eggs	Cheese, custard

topnatthapon/Shutter-stock.com

Photodisc/Getty Images

Mitch Hrdlicka/Photodisc/Getty Images

The cuisine served in Mexico features rice, corn, and beans, which are low in fat and high in nutrients. However, the dishes Americans think of as Mexican are far less healthful. Burritos, especially when topped with cheese and sour cream, are very high in fat. Although guacamole has a high fat content, it contains mostly monounsaturated fatty acids, a better form of fat.

African American cuisine traces some of its roots to food preferences from western Africa (e.g., peanuts, okra, and black-eyed peas), as well as to traditional American foods, such as fish, game, greens, and sweet potatoes. It uses many nutritious vegetables, such as collard greens and sweet potatoes, as well as legumes. However, some dishes include high-fat food products such as peanuts and pecans or involve frying, sometimes in saturated fat.

The mainland Chinese diet, which is plant-based, high in carbohydrates, and low in fats and animal protein, is considered one of the most healthful in the world. However, Chinese restaurants in the United States serve more meat and sauces than are generally eaten in China. According to laboratory tests of typical take-out dishes from Chinese restaurants, many have more fats and cholesterol than hamburger or egg dishes from fast-food outlets.

Traditional French cuisine, which includes rich, high-fat sauces and dishes, has never been considered healthful. Yet, nutritionists have been stumped to explain the so-called French paradox. Despite a diet high in saturated fats, the French have had one of the lowest rates of coronary artery disease in the world. The French diet increasingly resembles the American diet, but French portions tend to be one-third to one-half the size of American portions.

Many Indian dishes highlight healthful ingredients such as vegetables and legumes (beans and peas). However, many also use *ghee* (a form of butter), which is rich in harmful saturated fats. The best advice in an Indian restaurant is to ask how each dish is prepared. Good choices include *daal* or *dal* (lentils), *karbi* or *karni* (chickpea soup), and *chapati* (tortilla-like bread).

The traditional Japanese diet is very low in fat, which may account for the low incidence of heart disease in Japan. Dietary staples include soybean products, fish, vegetables, noodles, and rice. A variety of fruits and vegetables are also included in many dishes. However, Japanese cuisine is high in salted, smoked, and pickled foods. Watch out for deep-fried dishes such as tempura and salty soups and sauces.

Campus Cuisine: How College Students Eat

Often on their own for the first time, college students typically change their usual eating patterns. When they are making meal choices, the top two influences on students are price and convenience, with nutrition coming in third.

A growing problem on many campuses is "food insecurity," defined as limited or uncertain availability of healthful foods and limited or uncertain ability to acquire healthful foods.[41]

Many factors may be contributing to the increase in food insecurity, including rising costs for tuition, room, and board; parents' more limited resources; greater competition for work–study jobs; and lack of food stamps or other safety-net services.[42]

Even when cost is not an issue, college students don't necessarily get all the nutrients they need. The proportion of 18- to 24-year-olds who eat the recommended amounts of fruits and vegetables is generally lower than in the population as a whole. College men eat fewer fruits and vegetables than women do; Caucasian and Asian students eat more than African American undergraduates. Both African American and Hispanic students consume less than multiracial or other racial/ethnic groups.[43]

Nutrition Knowledge

Undergraduates vary greatly in their awareness and understanding of basic nutrition. Students often believe that they need fewer vegetables and fruits and more milk servings than recommended. Those in health or nutrition courses are significantly more likely to meet dietary recommendations than those who hadn't taken such courses. Those who've been living on their own for more than a year rate their food skills higher than those who left home more recently.[44] In general, male undergraduates do not consume high-calorie foods and beverages under stress as often as women, but few students of either sex are aware of age- and gender-specific recommendations.[45]

Nutrition majors make different—and better—choices than other majors, including eating breakfast, choosing healthier, nutrient-dense foods for their meals and snacks, following more of the *Dietary Guidelines*, monitoring portion size, reading food labels, and exercising regularly (for an hour at least three times a week). Perhaps as a result of these smart choices, nutrition majors have lower body mass indexes (BMIs; discussed in Chapter 6) than other majors.[46]

✓**check-in** Are nutritious food choices easily available at your school?

Fast Food: Eating on the Run

Young adults (ages 20–29) consume approximately 40 percent of their daily calories away from home and eat at fast-food restaurants an average of two to three times a week. Those who frequently eat at burger-and-fries restaurants have a higher intake of sugar-sweetened beverages, total calories, and total fat and saturated fats; a lower intake of healthful foods and key ingredients; and a greater risk of being overweight or obese.

Although fast-food chains have increased the total number of menu offerings, the average calorie count has not changed much. The average lunch or dinner entrée has 453 calories; the average side dish has 263 calories (see Figure 4.6 for more information about choices at fast-food eateries).

Even a single junk-food meal can damage arteries. A recent study compared the effects on blood vessels of a Mediterranean-style meal of salmon, almonds, and vegetables cooked in olive oil and a meal of a sausage, cheese, and egg sandwich with hash browns. Within hours, the junk-food meal constricted blood flow through the arteries; the Mediterranean-style meal did not. Individuals who eat fast food also have higher blood levels of potentially harmful plastic-related compounds, which may leach into foods during processing, packaging, or preparation, than others.[47]

✓**check-in** How many fast-food meals do you eat in a week?

You Are What You Drink

Water—tap or bottled, sparkling or still, chilled or room temperature—is the medical experts' beverage of choice. But don't think that "fortified" or "enriched" water is better. There is no evidence that nutrients added to water confer any health benefits. Consumers who assume that they're getting vitamins in their drinks may think they don't need to eat healthful foods and could end up shortchanging themselves of vital nutrients.

Soft Drinks According to the most recent government data, two thirds of children and half of adults drink at least one sugar-sweetened soda or other beverage daily.[48] Although soda consumption has decreased among young adults, one in five still qualifies as a heavy user. One 12-ounce can of regular soda contains 9 teaspoons of sugar (about 140 calories)—enough to put individuals into a higher-risk category for heart disease if they drink soda daily. Drinkers of sugar-sweetened beverages tend to consume more calories, exercise less, smoke more, and eat less nutriously.[49]

HEALTH NOW!

More Healthful Fast-Food Choices

Fast-food restaurants may be the cheapest option, but unfortunately, they are not usually the most healthful one. Eating just one fast-food meal can pack enough calories, sodium, and fat for an entire day:

- Just two or more high-fat fast-food meals a week have been linked to increased risk of diabetes.
- Seemingly healthful choices, such as a "Mac Snack Wrap," can be low in calories (330) but extremely high in fat (19 grams).

Steps to Take

- **Drink water instead of soda.** One 32-ounce Big Gulp with regular cola packs about 425 calories.
- **Eat your food naked.** Avoid calorie- and fat-packed spreads, cheese, sour cream, and so on. If you sample the salad bar, steer clear of mayonnaise, bacon bits, oily vegetable salads, and rich dressings.
- **Choose small portions.** Since an average fast-food meal can run as high as 1,000 calories or more, don't supersize anything. A single serving often provides enough for two meals. Take half home or divide with a friend.
- **Hold the salt.** Fast-food restaurant food tends to be very high in sodium, so don't add any more.
- **Savor each bite.** If you order fries, eat each one slowly and pay attention to its smell, texture, and taste. Ask yourself, "Do I really need to eat a whole container, or am I satisfied after a handful?"

Try these tips the next time you go to a fast-food restaurant, and describe your experience in your online journal.

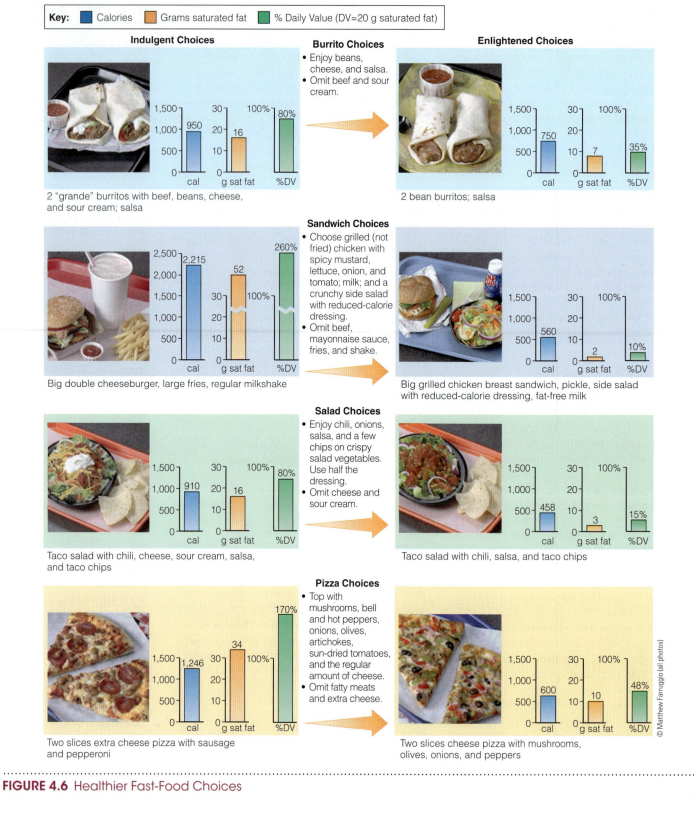

Key: ■ Calories ■ Grams saturated fat ■ % Daily Value (DV=20 g saturated fat)

Indulgent Choices

Burrito Choices
- Enjoy beans, cheese, and salsa.
- Omit beef and sour cream.

Enlightened Choices

2 "grande" burritos with beef, beans, cheese, and sour cream; salsa

950 cal, 16 g sat fat, 80% %DV

2 bean burritos; salsa

750 cal, 7 g sat fat, 35% %DV

Sandwich Choices
- Choose grilled (not fried) chicken with spicy mustard, lettuce, onion, and tomato; milk; and a crunchy side salad with reduced-calorie dressing.
- Omit beef, mayonnaise sauce, fries, and shake.

Big double cheeseburger, large fries, regular milkshake

2,215 cal, 52 g sat fat, 260% %DV

Big grilled chicken breast sandwich, pickle, side salad with reduced-calorie dressing, fat-free milk

560 cal, 2 g sat fat, 10% %DV

Salad Choices
- Enjoy chili, onions, salsa, and a few chips on crispy salad vegetables. Use half the dressing.
- Omit cheese and sour cream.

Taco salad with chili, cheese, sour cream, salsa, and taco chips

910 cal, 16 g sat fat, 80% %DV

Taco salad with chili, salsa, and taco chips

458 cal, 3 g sat fat, 15% %DV

Pizza Choices
- Top with mushrooms, bell and hot peppers, onions, olives, artichokes, sun-dried tomatoes, and the regular amount of cheese.
- Omit fatty meats and extra cheese.

Two slices extra cheese pizza with sausage and pepperoni

1,246 cal, 34 g sat fat, 170% %DV

Two slices cheese pizza with mushrooms, olives, onions, and peppers

600 cal, 10 g sat fat, 48% %DV

© Matthew Farruggio (all photos)

FIGURE 4.6 Healthier Fast-Food Choices

✓**check-in** Did you know that drinking a can of soda a day could increase your risk of dying of heart disease by one-third?

Among the health dangers associated with sweetened drinks are:

- Increased calorie intake, higher body weight, lower consumption of calcium and other nutrients, and greater risk of diabetes.

Frugal Food Choices

Many people feeling a budget squeeze opt for the cheapest foods they can find, even if they're high in fat and calories and low in nutrients. Such short-term choices can lead to long-term health problems. Here are some ways to eat healthfully for less:

- **Drink tap water.** It's cheaper than bottled and just as safe. Don't waste money on fortified drinks, which offer no proven additional nutritional value. Sugar-sweetened drinks add extra calories as well as extra costs.

- **Consider the cost of convenience.** Prepackaged grab-and-go items such as individual packets of baby carrots or crackers and cheese may be handy but cost more. Buy larger bags or boxes and create your own easy-carry single servings with small reusable containers.

- **Avoid fad fruits.** Pomegranates and other exotic fruits are indeed rich in antioxidants but so are much cheaper oranges and seasonal berries.

- **Freeze.** If you have access to a freezer, take advantage of grocery store sales and stock up on frozen fruits and vegetables, which—thanks to advances in preservation and freezing methods—provide plenty of nutrients.

- **Bulk up.** Join with your roommates or friends and check for low prices on large quantities at the local co-op as well as national mega-stores.

- **Eat seasonally.** Take advantage of the low prices on watermelon in summer or apples in autumn.

- **Look for an Asian grocery store**, if you're a vegan and eat a lot of ramen dishes. Ramen usually costs much less at such stores, but be sure to ask for vegetarian ramen.

- **Sign up for "loyalty" cards** that qualify you for discount or special offers at local grocery stores.

- **Compare unit prices** listed on shelves to get the best price.

- Possible greater risk of heart disease.
- Increased likelihood of metabolic syndrome, even with just a single daily soft drink, either diet or regular.
- Damage to tooth enamel from sweetened iced tea and many carbonated beverages.
- Thinning of hip bones in women who drink regular and diet cola.
- Greater risk of kidney disease.[50]

✓**check-in** Do you love sugary soda? Swapping just one soda a day for water or unsweetened coffee or tea could lower your risk of diabetes by up to 25 percent.[51]

Rather than satisfying a sweet tooth, soft drinks seem to do the opposite and either increase hunger or decrease feelings of satiety or fullness. Even diet drinks made with artificial sweeteners may "condition" people to eat more sweets and increase the risk of diabetes.

Energy Drinks Energy drinks have become the fastest-growing part of the beverage market in the United States. Americans consume more than 6 billion of these caffeinated beverages a year. The most frequent users include younger adults, males, Hispanics, blacks, unmarried individuals, adults with higher family incomes, those living in the South or West, and those who engage in some leisure-time physical activity.

About 8 in 10 students at 2-year and 4-year colleges, online universities, and technical schools report using energy drinks in the previous year. Although many students use caffeine-fueled concoctions for a physical or mental edge, there is little scientific evidence to indicate that they provide any benefit. Although student-athletes are less likely to consume energy drinks, those who do tend to be male and have lower overall knowledge of nutrition.[52] College students who frequently consume energy drinks are more likely to engage in binge drinking and abuse of prescription stimulants.[53]

✓**check-in** Do you consume energy drinks? If so, how often?

Espresso drinks from Starbucks and other vendors contain significantly more caffeine than regular coffee.[54] Some energy drinks contain 15 times the amount of caffeine in a 12-ounce serving of cola. Red Bull, for instance, contains nearly 80 milligrams of caffeine per can, about the same amount of caffeine as a cup of brewed coffee and twice the caffeine of a cup of tea. Other brands contain several times this amount.

Energy drink formulations vary widely. Some contain fruit juices, teas, and dietary supplements such as ginseng, glucuronolactone, and taurine, a substance that plays an important role in muscle contraction (especially in the heart) and the nervous system. We know very little about the effects of such ingredients, which may work synergistically with caffeine to boost its stimulant power. Frequent or heavy use can trigger physical and psychological complications, including:

- Disrupted sleep
- Exaggerated stress response
- Heart palpitations
- Increased risk of high blood pressure
- Panic attacks
- Irritability
- Tremors
- Anxiety
- Depression
- Substance abuse
- Digestive problems
- Cardiac arrhythmia

Toxic levels of caffeine can cause sudden death or life-threatening conditions, such as acute kidney damage, hepatitis, seizures, strokes, coronary artery spasms, and heart attack. Emergency department visits related to energy drinks have more than doubled in recent years.

Doctors recommend that all adults limit their caffeine intake to 500 milligrams a day, with a lesser amount for those who have heart problems, high blood pressure, or trouble sleeping or who are taking medications. The recommended maximum for adolescents is 100 milligrams of caffeine a day.

The practice of mixing energy drinks with alcohol (discussed in Chapter 16) is especially dangerous, leading to a state some call "wide-awake drunkenness," in which drinkers cannot fully assess their true level of impairment and are more likely to engage in risky behaviors, such as driving while intoxicated.

✓**check-in** How much caffeine do you consume every day?

Choosing Healthful Snacks

Snacking has become more widespread on campuses, as in other places. College students snack primarily "to satisfy hunger"; the second most common reason is "no time for meals." Other reasons for munching between meals: "for energy," "to be sociable," and "to relieve stress." One-third snack at 9:00 p.m. or later.

In response to consumer demands for smart snack choices, food manufacturers are offering "better-for-you" options that are lower in salt and sugar or free of *trans* fat and artificial colors. Some new snack items promoted as healthful options, such as sugar-free chocolate or organic potato chips, offer little nutritional value. Meat-based snacks, increasingly popular among young men, also can be high in fat and sodium. Read labels carefully and be sure to check total calories and fat.

A best-for-you option is fruit such as bananas, apples, or berries—rich in vitamins, low in calories, and packed with fiber. Other nutritious snacks include nuts, trail mix, granola bars, yogurt, sunflower seeds, soy nuts, and dried fruit (such as cranberries). If you enjoy fruit juice, buy 100-percent fruit juice without added sugar. Limit yourself to one serving of these calorie-rich beverages a day.

✓**check-in** What are your favorite snacks?

If you rely on snacks to keep you energized throughout the day, take time to plan in advance so you have choices other than the nearest vending machine. Try to prepare snacks from different food groups: low-fat or nonfat milk and a few graham crackers, for instance, or celery sticks with peanut butter and raisins. Save part of one meal—half of your breakfast bagel or lunch sandwich—to eat a few hours later. If you're trying to add fiber to your diet, eat high-fiber snacks, such as prunes, popcorn, or sunflower seeds.

Taking Charge of What You Eat

You can't control what you don't know. Because of the Nutrition Labeling and Education Act, food manufacturers must provide information about fat, calories, and ingredients in large type on packaged food labels, and they must show how a food item fits into a daily diet of 2,000 calories. The law also restricts nutritional claims for terms such as *healthy*, *low fat*, and *high fiber*.

A growing number of cities and states are mandating calorie-posting by fast-food restaurants. Some national health reform proposals would require restaurant chains to post the number of calories, grams of saturated fat, and milligrams of sodium next to menu items, although menu labeling has not proven to affect dietary choices. Often the problem is not a lack of information, health officials note, but a lack of self-control. You can find detailed nutritional information for restaurants of all price levels at www.healthydiningfinder.com.

In evaluating food labels and product claims, keep in mind that while individual foods vary in their nutritional value, what matters is your total diet. If you eat too much of any one food—regardless of what its label states—you may not be getting the variety and balance of nutrients that you need.

Portions and Servings

Consumers often are confused by what a *serving* actually is, especially since many American restaurants have supersized the amount of food they put on their customers' plates. The average bagel has doubled in size in the past 10 to 15 years. A standard fast-food serving of French fries is larger in the United States than in the United Kingdom.

A food-label *serving* is a specific amount of food that contains the quantity of nutrients described on the Nutrition Facts label. A *portion* is the amount of a specific food that an individual eats at one time. Portions can be bigger or smaller than the servings on food labels. According to nutritionists, "marketplace portions"—the actual amounts served to customers—are two to eight times larger than the standard serving sizes defined by the USDA. In fast-food chains, today's portions are two to five times larger than the original sizes. As studies have shown, people presented with larger portions eat 30 to 50 percent more than they otherwise would.

If you are trying to balance your diet or control your weight, it's important to keep track of the size of your portions so that you do not exceed recommended servings. For instance, a 3-ounce serving of meat is about the size of a pack of playing cards (see Figure 4.7). If you eat a larger amount, count it as more than one serving.

Nutrition Labels

Nutrition labels can influence consumers' purchases—if they are clear and comprehensible.[55]

To achieve this goal, nutrition labels have been revised to include:

- Information about the amount of "added sugars" or empty calories in a food product.

- Updated serving size requirements to reflect the amounts people actually eat, not what they "should" be eating.

- Calorie and nutrition information for both "per serving" and "per package" calorie for larger packages that could be consumed in one sitting or multiple sittings.

- Inclusion of potassium and vitamin D, nutrients that some in the U.S. population need more of. Vitamins A and C are no longer required on the label.

- Revised Daily Values (the total amount of a nutrient that the average adult should aim to get or not exceed on a daily basis) for a variety of nutrients such as sodium, dietary fiber, and vitamin D to help consumers understand the nutrition information in the context of a total daily diet.

✓**check-in** Do you read nutrition labels on the foods you buy?

Nutrition labels can influence purchasing decisions—but learning how to read them takes practice and motivation.[56]

What Is an "Organic" Food?

Consumers, including college students, say they prefer "organic" foods because they believe they are fresher, better tasting, more nutritious, and free of chemicals and pesticides. That's not

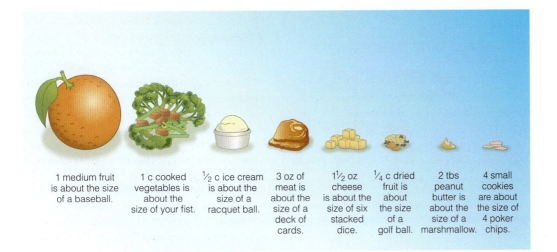

1 medium fruit is about the size of a baseball.

1 c cooked vegetables is about the size of your fist.

½ c ice cream is about the size of a racquet ball.

3 oz of meat is about the size of a deck of cards.

1½ oz cheese is about the size of six stacked dice.

¼ c dried fruit is about the size of a golf ball.

2 tbs peanut butter is about the size of a marshmallow.

4 small cookies are about the size of 4 poker chips.

FIGURE 4.7 Portion Sizes
Here are some quick estimates of portion sizes.

The U.S. Food and Drug Administration has finalized a new Nutrition Facts label for packaged foods that will make it easier for you to make informed food choices that support a healthy diet. The updated label has a fresh new design and reflects current scientific information, including the link between diet and chronic diseases.

1. Servings

The number of "servings per container" and the "Serving Size" declaration have increased and are now in larger and/or bolder type. Serving sizes have been updated to reflect what people actually eat and drink today. For example, the serving size for ice cream was previously 1/2 cup and now is 2/3 cup.

There are also new requirements for certain size packages, such as those that are between one and two servings or are larger than a single serving but could be consumed in one or multiple sittings.

2. Calories

"Calories" is now larger and bolder.

3. Fats

"Calories from Fat" has been removed because research shows the type of fat consumed is more important than the amount.

4. Added Sugars

"Added Sugars" in grams and as a percent Daily Value (%DV) is now required on the label. Added sugars includes sugars that are either added during the processing of foods, or are packaged as such (e.g., a bag of table sugar), and also includes sugars from syrups and honey, and

sugars from concentrated fruit or vegetable juices. Scientific data shows that it is difficult to meet nutrient needs while staying within calorie limits if you consume more than 10 percent of your total daily calories from added sugar.

5. Nutrients

The lists of nutrients that are required or permitted on the label have been updated. Vitamin D and potassium are now required on the label because Americans do not always get the recommended amounts. Vitamins A and C are no longer required since deficiencies of these vitamins are rare today. The actual amount (in milligrams or micrograms) in addition to the %DV must be listed for vitamin D, calcium, iron, and potassium.

The daily values for nutrients have also been updated based on newer scientific evidence. The daily values are reference amounts of nutrients to consume or not to exceed and are used to calculate the %DV.

6. Footnote

The footnote at the bottom of the label has been changed to better explain the meaning of %DV. The %DV helps you understand the nutrition information in the context of a total daily diet.

Current Label

Nutrition Facts

Serving Size 2/3 cup (55g)
Servings Per Container About 8

Amount Per Serving

Calories 230	Calories from Fat 72

	% Daily Value*
Total Fat 8g	12%
Saturated Fat 1g	5%
Trans Fat 0g	
Cholesterol 0mg	0%
Sodium 160mg	7%
Total Carbohydrate 37g	12%
Dietary Fiber 4g	16%
Sugars 12g	
Protein 3g	

Vitamin A	10%
Vitamin C	8%
Calcium	20%
Iron	45%

* Percent Daily Values are based on a 2,000 calorie diet. Your daily value may be higher or lower depending on your calorie needs.

	Calories:	2,000	2,500
Total Fat	Less than	65g	80g
Sat Fat	Less than	20g	25g
Cholesterol	Less than	300mg	300mg
Sodium	Less than	2,400mg	2,400mg
Total Carbohydrate		300g	375g
Dietary Fiber		25g	30g

New Label

Nutrition Facts

1 8 servings per container
Serving size 2/3 cup (55g)

2 **Amount per serving**
Calories **230**

	% Daily Value*
3 **Total Fat** 8g	10%
Saturated Fat 1g	5%
Trans Fat 0g	
Cholesterol 0mg	0%
Sodium 160mg	7%
Total Carbohydrate 37g	13%
Dietary Fiber 4g	14%
Total Sugars 12g	
4 Includes 10g Added Sugars	20%
Protein 3g	
5 Vitamin D 2mcg	10%
Calcium 200mg	15%
Iron 8mg	45%
Potassium 235mg	6%

6 * The % Daily Value (DV) tells you how much a nutrient in a serving of food contributes to a daily diet. 2,000 calories a day is used for general nutrition advice.

Transitioning to the New Label

Manufacturers still have time to begin using the new and improved Nutrition Facts label, so you will see both label versions for a while. However, the new label is already starting to appear on products nationwide.

FIGURE 4.8 The revised food label makes it easier to check calories and servings per container.

necessarily true of all the foods that claim to be natural and healthy. **Certified organic** foods must meet strict criteria set by the USDA, including the following:

- Processing or preservation only with substances approved by the USDA for organic foods.

- Processing without genetic modification or ionizing radiation.

- No use of most synthetic chemicals, such as pesticides, herbicides, or fertilizers.

- Fertilization without sewage sludge.

- Food-producing animals grown without medication such as antibiotics or hormones, provided with living conditions similar to their natural habitat, and fed organic feed.

Foods with some organic ingredients may use wholesome-sounding words such as "natural," "free-range," or "locally grown."

Are organic foods better for you? In a recent study of 70,000 adults, the most frequent consumers of organic food had significantly fewer cancers than those who never ate organic food.[57]

Some studies have shown higher levels of specific nutrients, such as flavonoids, in organic produce, but no one knows if this translates into specific health benefits. However, you can avoid exposure to pesticides and other chemicals by opting for certified organic foods.

Genetically Engineered Foods

Biotechnology, the science of manipulating organisms to modify their genetic makeup, has created a new generation of foods. Using recombinant DNA technology, scientists directly manipulate the genes of living things—removing some, adding others, changing gene positions—in order to influence how an organism grows and develops. This technology allows scientists to introduce desirable traits, such as resistance to disease or mold, and eliminate undesirable traits, such as an apple's tendency to turn brown after slicing.

Although you may not realize it, you've probably eaten genetically modified organisms (GMOs) produced by recombinant DNA engineering.

certified organic Foods that meet strict criteria set by the U.S. Department of Agriculture

Are You Eating Your Veggies?

College students who report:	Male	Female	Average	College students who report:	Male	Female	Average
Eating no servings of fruits and vegetables a day	10.2	7.5	8.4	Eating three to four servings	23.1	26.1	25.2
				Eating five or more servings	4.3	5.0	4.8
Eating one to two servings	62.5	61.4	61.6				

Source: American College Health Association. American College Health Association-National College Health Assessment II: Reference Group Executive Summary Spring 2018. Silver Spring, MD: American College Health Association, 2018.

✓check-in For a 3-day period (including one weekend day), keep track of your veggie intake. Put a star by those you like most. If you aren't getting at least five servings a day, add at least one of your favorites every day. Record your observations in your online journal.

Many food additives—such as high-fructose corn syrup, used in many processed foods—are made with GMOs. Other foods, such as the papayas sold in many markets, are themselves GMOs.

Some consumers worry about the safety of GMOs, and "certified organic" products do not contain them. The Food and Drug Administration, which evaluates the safety of genetically engineered foods, views them as safe unless they differ significantly from similar foods.

Dietary Supplements

✓check-in Do you take dietary supplements? If so, why do you use them?

More than half the adults in the United States consume dietary supplements.[58] Many supplements, including vitamins C, D, and E and fish oil, have failed to deliver on their promised benefits in rigorous, randomized controlled trials. Folic acid and other B vitamins, once believed to prevent heart disease and strokes, may increase cancer risk in high doses. Here are the most recent findings[59]:

- Treatment with beta-carotene, vitamin A, and vitamin E may increase mortality

- Vitamin B supplementation may protect against stroke but has no effect on cardiovascular disease or cancer.

- Omega-3 fatty acids and fish oil supplements have shown no protective effects on cardiovascular disease.

Years of research have found no clear evidence of a beneficial effect of supplements on all-cause mortality, cardiovascular disease, or cancer.

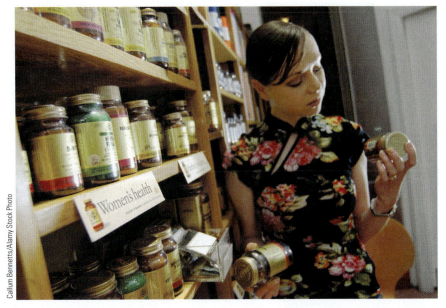

Callum Bennetts/Alamy Stock Photo

Be sure to read labels carefully before you start taking a dietary supplement.

Students take supplements primarily to promote general health, provide more energy, increase muscle strength, or enhance performance. Yet, researchers note, college students typically are not deficient in crucial nutrients, and there is little or no evidence that the supplements provide the desired benefits.[60]

Food Safety

Foodborne infections cause an estimated 76 million illnesses, 325,000 hospitalizations, and 5,000 deaths in the United States every year.

Three organisms—*Salmonella*, *Listeria*, and *Toxoplasma*—are responsible for more than 75 percent of these deaths. Although most foodborne infections cause mild illness, severe infections and serious complications—including death—do occur. College students are one of the most at-risk population groups due to risky food safety behaviors.

Scares about tainted food have led to massive recalls of such popular foods as peanut butter, jalapenos, lettuce, spinach, and tomatoes. As a result, consumer advocates, as well as manufacturers and trade associations, are calling for stricter regulations.

✓**check-in** What can you do to improve your food safety?

- Pay attention when you hear that a food or product is under suspicion.
- Make note of the brands, the production dates, and the manufacturer(s) involved.
- Check the labels of the foods in your pantry and refrigerator, and throw out any that may be contaminated.

Fight BAC!

"BAC" stands for food bacteria, an invisible threat to your health. To improve food safety awareness and practices, government and private agencies have developed the Fight BAC! campaign, which identifies four key culprits in foodborne illness: (see Figure 4.9)

- Improper cooling
- Improper handwashing
- Inadequate cooking
- Failure to avoid cross-contamination

Avoiding *E. coli* Infection

Eating unwashed produce, such as spinach or lettuce, or undercooked beef, especially hamburger, can increase your risk of infection with *Escherichia coli* (*E. coli*) bacteria. These bacteria, which live in the intestinal tract of healthy people and animals, are usually harmless. However, infection with the strain *E. coli* O157:H7 produces symptoms that can range from mild to life threatening. This strain has made its way into hamburger in fast-food chains and into packaged spinach. *E. coli* can cause severe bloody diarrhea, kidney failure, and even death. Symptoms usually develop within 2 to 10 days and can include severe stomach cramps, vomiting, mild fever, and bloody diarrhea. Most people recover within

Clean— keep hands, utensils, and surfaces clean.

Separate— keep raw foods separated from ready-to-eat foods.

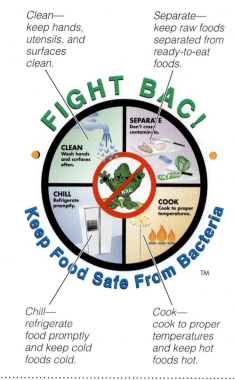

Chill— refrigerate food promptly and keep cold foods cold.

Cook— cook to proper temperatures and keep hot foods hot.

FIGURE 4.9 Fight BAC!

7 to 10 days. Others—especially older adults, children under the age of 5, and those with weakened immune systems—may develop complications that lead to kidney failure.

Food Poisoning

Salmonella is a bacterium that contaminates many foods, particularly undercooked chicken, eggs, and sometimes processed meat. Eating contaminated food can result in salmonella poisoning, which causes diarrhea and vomiting. The Centers for Disease Control and Prevention (CDC) estimates 40,000 reported cases of salmonella poisoning a year; the actual number of cases could be anywhere from 400,000 to 4 million. The FDA has warned consumers about the dangers of unpasteurized orange juice because of the risk of salmonella contamination.

Another bacterium, *Campylobacter jejuni*, may cause even more stomach infections than salmonella. Found in water, milk, and some foods, campylobacter poisoning causes severe diarrhea and has been implicated in the growth of stomach ulcers.

Bacteria can also cause illness by producing toxins in food. *Staphylococcus aureus* is the most common culprit. When cooked foods are cross-contaminated with the bacteria from raw foods and not stored properly, staph infections can result, causing nausea and abdominal pain anywhere from 30 minutes to 8 hours after ingestion.

An uncommon but sometimes fatal form of food poisoning is botulism, caused by the *Clostridium botulinum* organism. Improper home-canning procedures are the most common cause of this potentially fatal problem.

Even many healthful foods can pose dangers. The FDA has urged consumers to avoid eating raw sprouts because of the risk of getting sick. Sprouts, particularly alfalfa and clover, can be contaminated by *Salmonella* or *E. coli* bacteria. The FDA advises people to either cook sprouts before eating them or request that they be left off sandwiches and other food ordered in restaurants. Home-grown sprouts can also present a risk if they come from contaminated seeds.

There have been several outbreaks of listeriosis, caused by the bacterium *Listeria*, commonly found in deli meats, hot dogs, soft cheeses, raw meat, and unpasteurized milk. Although rare, listeriosis can be life threatening. At greatest risk are pregnant women, infants, and those with weakened immune systems. You can reduce your risk by cooking meats and leftovers thoroughly and by washing everything that may come into contact with raw meat.

Pesticides

Plants and animals naturally produce compounds that act as pesticides to aid in their survival. The vast majority of the pesticides we consume are therefore natural, not added by farmers or food processors. *Commercial pesticides* save billions of dollars of valuable crops from pests, but they also may endanger human health and life. Fearful of potential risks in pesticides, many consumers are purchasing organic foods.

Food Allergies

The National Institute of Allergy and Infectious Diseases defines a food allergy as "an adverse health effect arising from a specific immune response that occurs reproducibly on exposure to a given food." As many as 50 to 90 percent of presumed food allergies are not allergic reactions.

The symptoms that different foods provoke vary. One person might sneeze if exposed to an irritating food; another might vomit or develop diarrhea; others might suffer headaches, dizziness, hives, or a rapid heartbeat. Symptoms may not develop for up to 72 hours, making it hard to pinpoint which food was responsible.

✓**check-in** Do you have any food allergies? Have they been diagnosed by a physician?

YOUR STRATEGIES FOR PREVENTION

How to Protect Yourself from Food Poisoning

- **Always wash your hands with liquid or clean bar soap before handling food.** Rub your hands vigorously together for 10 to 15 seconds; the soap combined with the scrubbing action dislodges and removes germs.

- **When preparing fresh fruits and vegetables, discard outer leaves, wash under running water, and, when possible, scrub with a clean brush or hands.** Do not wash meat or poultry.

- **To avoid the spread of bacteria to other foods, utensils, or surfaces, do not allow liquids to touch or drip onto other items.** Wipe up all spills immediately.

- **Clean out your refrigerator regularly.** Throw out any leftovers stored for 3 or 4 days.

- **To kill bacteria and viruses, sterilize wet kitchen sponges by putting them in a microwave for 2 minutes.** Make sure they are completely wet to guard against the risk of fire.

If you suspect that you have a food allergy, see a physician with specialized training in allergy diagnosis. Medical opinion about the merits of many treatments for food allergies is divided. Once you've identified the culprit, the wisest and sometimes simplest course is to avoid it.

Nutritional Quackery

The Academy of Nutrition and Dietetics (AND) describes nutritional quackery as a growing problem for unsuspecting consumers. Because so much nutritional nonsense is garbed in scientific-sounding terms, it can be hard to recognize bad advice when you get it. One basic rule: If the promises of a nutritional claim sound too good to be true, they probably are.

Before you try any new nutritional approach, check with your doctor or a registered dietitian. Don't believe ads or advisers basing their nutritional recommendations on hair analysis, which is not accurate in detecting nutritional deficiencies. Question personal testimonies about the powers of some magical pill or powder, and be wary of "scientific articles" in journals that aren't reviewed by health professionals.

- What are the essential nutrients you need every day?

- What are some healthy eating patterns recommended by nutritionists?

- What steps can students take to eat a healthier diet?

- What are the healthiest beverages to drink?

Reflection

"You are what you eat," according to an old saying. Reflect on what your current way of eating—what you choose to eat, where and when you eat, how quickly or slowly you eat, how you feel after eating—says about you. Based on what you've learned in this chapter, imagine the difference changes in your food choices or eating habits might make. Give one dietary change a try in the coming week.

TAKING CHARGE OF YOUR HEALTH
Making Healthful Food Choices

As nutritional knowledge expands and evolves, it's easy to be confused by changing advice on which foods to avoid and which to eat. But even though research may challenge or change thinking on a specific food, some basic principles always apply. Start an online food diary in your journal. For 1 week, record which of the following healthful eating habits that you follow on most days. Identify at least one other behavior that you would like to adopt. Identify any barriers that are keeping you from implementing this change. Then consciously put it into practice for a week. Write a brief summary of how you did.

____ **Eat breakfast.** Easy-to-prepare breakfasts include cold cereal with fruit and low-fat milk, whole-wheat toast with peanut butter, yogurt with fruit, or whole-grain waffles.

____ **Don't eat too much of one thing.** Your body needs protein, carbohydrates, fat, and many different vitamins and minerals, such as vitamins C and A, iron, and calcium, from a variety of foods.

____ **Eat more grains, fruits, and vegetables.** These foods give you carbohydrates for energy, plus vitamins, minerals, and fiber. Try breads such as whole-wheat, bagels, and pita. Spaghetti and oatmeal are also in the grain group.

____ **Don't ban any food.** Fit in a higher-fat food, like pepperoni pizza, at dinner by choosing lower-fat foods at other meals.

And don't forget about moderation. If two pieces of pizza fill you up, don't eat a third.

____ **Make every calorie count.** Load up on nutrients, not on big portions. Choosing foods that are nutrient dense will help protect against disease and keep you healthy.

____ **Avoid high-fat fast foods.** Hot dogs, fried foods, packaged snack foods, and pastries are most likely to be laden with fat.

____ **Check the numbers.** When buying prepared foods, choose items that contain no more than 3 grams of fat per 100 calories.

____ **Think small.** A dinner-size serving of meat should be about the size of a deck of cards; half a cup is the size of a woman's fist; a pancake is the diameter of a CD.

____ **Read labels carefully.** Remember that "cholesterol free" doesn't necessarily mean fat free. Avoid products that contain saturated coconut oil, palm oil, lard, or hydrogenated fats.

____ **Switch to low-fat and nonfat dairy products.** Rather than buy whole-fat dairy products, choose skim milk, fat-free sour cream, and low- or nonfat yogurt.

____ **The brighter the better.** When selecting fruits and vegetables, choose the most intense color. A bright orange carrot has more beta-carotene than a pale one. Dark green lettuce leaves have more vitamins than lighter ones. Orange sweet potatoes pack more vitamin A than yellow ones.

SELF-SURVEY

How Healthful Is Your Diet?

STEP 1

Keep a food diary for a week, writing down everything you eat and drink for meals and snacks. Include the approximate amount eaten (for example, 1/2 cup, 1 large, 12-oz can, and so on).

	Mon.	Tues.	Wed.	Thurs.	Fri.	Sat.	Sun.
Grains							
Vegetables							
Fruits							
Milk, yogurt, cheese							
Meat, poultry, dry beans, eggs, nuts							
Fats, oil, sweets							

STEP 2   Are You Getting Enough Vegetables, Fruits, and Grains?

How often do you eat	Seldom/ Never	1–2 times a week	3–5 times a week	Almost daily
At least three servings of vegetables a day?				
Starchy vegetables like potatoes, corn, or peas?				
Foods made with dry beans, lentils, or peas?				
Dark green or deep yellow vegetables (broccoli, spinach, collards, carrots, sweet potatoes, squash)?				
At least two servings of fruit a day?				
Citrus fruits and 100% fruit juices (oranges, grapefruit, tangerines)? Whole fruit with skin or seeds (berries, apples, pears)?				
At least six servings of breads, cereals, pasta, or rice a day?				

The best answer for each is "almost daily." Use your food diary to see which foods you should be eating more often.

STEP 3   Are You Getting Too Much Fat?

How often do you eat	Seldom/ Never	1–2 times a week	3–5 times a week	Almost daily
Fried, deep-fat fried, or breaded food?				
Fatty meats, such as sausages, luncheon meat, fatty steaks or roasts? Whole milk, high-fat cheeses, ice cream?				
Pies, pastries, rich cakes?				
Rich cream sauces and gravies?				
Oily salad dressings or mayonnaise?				
Butter or margarine on vegetables, rolls, bread, or toast?				

Ideally, you should be eating these foods no more than one or two times a week. If your food diary indicates that you're eating them more frequently, your fat intake may well be too high.

STEP 4   Are You Getting Too Much Sodium?

How often do you eat	Seldom/ Never	1–2 times a week	3–5 times a week	Almost daily
Cured or processed meats, such as ham, sausage, frankfurters, or luncheon meats?				
Canned vegetables or frozen vegetables with sauce?				
Frozen TV dinners, entrées, or canned or dehydrated soups?				
Salted nuts, popcorn, pretzels, corn chips, or potato chips?				
Seasoning mixes or sauces containing salt?				
Processed cheese?				
Salt added to table foods before you taste them?				

Ideally, you should be eating these high-sodium items no more than one or two times a week. If your food diary indicates that you're eating them more frequently, your sodium intake may well be too high.

REVIEW QUESTIONS

(LO 4.1)   1. According to the most recent *Dietary Guidelines for Americans*, which of the following nutrients do most people need to cut back on?
   a. Iron
   b. Zinc
   c. Sodium
   d. Potassium

(LO 4.2)   2. _____ refers to the relationship between calories consumed from foods and beverages and calories expended in normal body functions and through physical activity.
   a. Calorimetry
   b. Bioenergetics
   c. Basal metabolic rate
   d. Calorie balance

(LO 4.2)   3. The classes of essential nutrients include which of the following?
   a. Amino acids, antioxidants, fiber, and cholesterol
   b. Proteins, calcium, calories, and folic acid
   c. Protein, carbohydrates, fats, minerals, vitamins, and water
   d. Iron, whole grains, fruits, and vegetables

(LO 4.3)   4. Which of the following is a simple carbohydrate?
   a. Fiber
   b. Grains

   c. Glucose
   d. Artificial sweetener

(LO 4.3)   5. Americans get most of their complex carbohydrates from _____.
   a. Fiber
   b. Refined grains
   c. Added sugars
   d. High fructose corn syrup

(LO 4.3)   6. Which of the following health dangers is associated with sweetened soft drinks?
   a. Damage to tooth enamel
   b. Exaggerated stress response
   c. Irritability
   d. Tremors

(LO 4.4)   7. Reducing intake of saturated fats can significantly reduce the risk of _____.
   a. cancer
   b. diabetes
   c. dental cavities
   d. cardiovascular disease

(LO 4.4)   8. Which of the following is an unsaturated fat?
   a. Milkfat
   b. Animal fat
   c. Cholesterol
   d. Vegetable oil

(LO 4.5) 9. The "Mediterranean diet" includes healthy, heart-beneficial foods that are rich in _____.
 a. antioxidants
 b. cholesterol
 c. vitamins
 d. protein

(LO 4.5) 10. "Food insecurity" on college campuses is defined as _____.
 a. lack of knowledge about nutrition
 b. limited availability of healthy foods
 c. contamination of food by pathogens
 d. students' concerns about their weight

(LO 4.5) 11. Which of the following information is now required by the FDA on Nutrition Facts labels?
 a. Portion size requirements to reflect the amounts people should be eating, not what they actually eat.
 b. Information about the amount of added sugars or empty calories in a food product.
 c. Inclusion of sodium and vitamin E, nutrients that some in the U.S. population lack.
 d. Calorie and nutrition information for "per serving" rather than "per package" for larger packages.

(LO 4.6) 12. Which of the following criteria must be met by foods that are certified as organic?
 a. Not using preservation techniques.
 b. Processing with genetic modification.
 c. Processing only with ionizing radiation.
 d. Not using pesticides or herbicides.

(LO 4.7) 13. _____ is a bacterium that contaminates many foods, particularly undercooked chicken, eggs, and sometimes processed meat.
 a. *Staphylococcus aureus*
 b. *Clostridium botulinum*
 c. *Salmonella*
 d. *Campylobacter*

(LO 4.8) 14. Nutritional quackery can be difficult to recognize because _____.
 a. determining which nutrients are essential is controversial
 b. it is often expressed in scientific-sounding terms
 c. the Academy of Nutrition and Dietetics does not define it
 d. people follow many different eating patterns

Answers to these questions can be found on page 531.

Terry J/Getty Images

LEARNING OBJECTIVES

After reading this chapter, you should be able to:

5.1   Summarize differences in weight among different populations in America.

5.2   Identify ways to assess body composition.

5.3   Explain the factors that have contributed to the obesity epidemic.

5.4   Discuss the impact of excess weight on health.

5.5   Review healthy approaches to gaining weight.

5.6   Assess ways of attaining and maintaining a healthy weight.

5.7   List the treatment options for extreme obesity.

5.8   Discuss the factors that lead to unhealthy eating on campus.

5.9   Recognize common forms of disordered eating and of eating disorders.

WHAT DO YOU THINK?

- How common is obesity in the United States?
- How does your weight affect your health?
- What are the best ways to lose excess pounds?
- What are the most common eating disorders on college campuses?

5

Weight Management and the Obesity Epidemic

Sarah's mother called it "baby fat." "You'll outgrow it soon enough," she said. Yet Sarah's cheeks grew chubbier and her waist wider every year. She went on her first diet in high school. For three days she ate nothing but carrot sticks, cottage cheese, and apples. Then she scarfed down two double cheeseburgers with fries and a chocolate shake. Her other attempts at dieting didn't last much longer. By graduation, Sarah was grateful to hide under the flowing black robe as she walked on stage to get her diploma.

When Sarah heard about the "freshman 15," the extra pounds many students acquire during their first year at college, she groaned at the prospect of putting on more weight. In her Personal Health class, Sarah set one primary goal: not to gain another pound. Rather than going on—and inevitably falling off—one diet after another, she developed a weight management plan that included healthful food choices and regular exercise. Armed with the information and tools provided in this chapter, Sarah, for the first time in her life, took charge of her weight.

You can do the same. This chapter explains why excess pounds are dangerous and what obesity is, describes current approaches to weight loss, discusses diets that work (and some that don't), offers practical guidelines for exercise and behavioral approaches to losing weight, and examines unhealthy eating patterns and eating disorders. If you're already at a healthy weight, this chapter can ensure that you remain so in the future. If, like two-thirds of Americans, you are overweight or obese, you will find help in these pages. Remember: You can lose excess weight. And you can start now. <

✓**check-in** Do you know your current weight?

Obesity in America

For the first time in history, more people worldwide—some 2.1 billion—are overweight or obese than underweight. Global obesity rates have risen to 11 percent among men and 15 percent among women. Overweight and obesity are the fifth leading cause of death, accounting for nearly 3.4 million deaths annually.[1]

More than a quarter of severely obese men and about a fifth of severely obese women live in the United States, where nearly 40 percent of adults are classified as obese.[2] The prevalence of obesity among children ranges from 14 percent for those ages 2 to 5; 18 percent for those

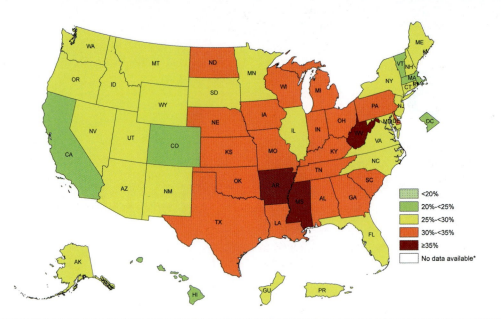

FIGURE 5.1 Adult Obesity in the United States.

Source: Behavorial Risk Factor Surveillance System, CDC.

ages 6 to 11; and 21 percent for 12- to 19-year-olds.[3] Despite efforts to educate Americans about healthy eating habits and food choices, excess weight continues to be a widespread problem (Figure 5.1):

- More than 2 in 3 adults are overweight or obese.
- About 2 in 5 adults are obese.
- More than 1 in 20 adults have extreme obesity.
- About one-third of children and adolescents age 6 to 19 are overweight or obese.[4] The key factors contributing to childhood obesity include more hours of screen time (including television viewing and use of computers and mobile devices) and diets high in saturated fat and sugar-sweetened beverages and low in protein.[4]
- About 1 in 20 teenagers are obese—and may face an increased risk of dying of heart disease or stroke by middle age. About 1 in 5 teenagers are obese--and may face an increased risk of dying of heart disease or stroke by middle age. An estimated 75 to 80 percent will become obese.[5]

The prevalence of obesity among women has remained relatively stable, at about 35 percent, since 2000, but the prevalence among men has increased from 27.5 percent to 35.5 percent.[6] Age and sex affect obesity rates. About 35 percent of men between ages 20 and 39 are obese, compared with 41 percent of those between ages 40 and 50. Among women ages 20–39, some 37 percent are obese, compared with 45 percent of those between ages 40 and 59.[7] Americans of all races carry excess pounds, but there are racial differences.

- Asian Americans have the lowest obesity rates (12.7 percent).
- The overall prevalence of obesity is higher among black and Hispanic adults than among white and Asian adults.[8]

✓**check-in** Are you between the ages of 18 and 35? If so, you are likely to put on weight more quickly than your parents.

Weight on Campus

Whether or not they are enrolled in college, young adults gain an average of 30 pounds between ages 18 and 35. In the last decade, the prevalence of overweight and obesity increased from 62.2 to 67.1 percent among young men and from 51.7 to 55.8 percent among young women age 20 to 39. More than a third of undergraduates report being overweight, obese, or severely or extremely obese.[9] A recent study found a significant association between **body mass index (BMI)** and academic performance, with students who gained weight over 4 years of college getting lower grades in junior/senior college level courses.[10]

Here are some specifics about weight issues on campus:

- Almost a quarter of undergraduates are overweight; another 16 percent are obese.[11]

body mass index (BMI)
A mathematical formula that correlates with body fat; the ratio of weight to height squared.

$ HEALTH ON A BUDGET

Hold the Line!

You can leave college a whole lot smarter but no heavier than when you entered—without spending extra money. Here are some suggestions:

- **Plan meals.** Most campus cafeterias post the week's menus in advance. Plan which items you will eat before you see or smell high-fat dishes.

- **Don't linger.** If you use the cafeteria as a social gathering place, you may end up eating with two or three different groups of people. Set a time limit to eat—then leave.

- **Develop alternative behavior.** People who eat when they are stressed or bored need to have substitute activities

ready when they need them. Make a list of things you can do—shower, phone a friend, take a hike—when stress strikes.

- **Eat at "home."** If the dormitory has a small kitchen, cook some healthful dishes and invite friends to join you.

- **Take advantage of physical activity programs.** Many college students become less active during their years in college. Aim to maintain or increase the amount of exercise you did in high school. Join a biking club, take a salsa class, learn yoga, or try tennis or racquetball.

- Students at 2-year colleges may be twice as likely to be obese as those at 4-year institutions.[12]

- Bisexual and lesbian female undergraduates are more likely to be obese than heterosexual women and may be at greater risk for unhealthy dietary, exercise, and weight control behaviors.[13]

- Obese and overweight students do not express greater concern about health or adapt different health-related behaviors than other undergraduates.[14]

- Excess weight is associated with symptoms of depression, significantly higher rates of lifetime trichotillomania (hair-pulling disorder) in

obese male undergraduates, and higher rates of panic disorder in overweight and obese college women.[15]

Many factors contribute to weight gain in college. Students in a hurry often opt for fast food and consume more fatty foods and sugared drinks, which increase their risks of obesity and other health problems. Limited finances are a common reason for students' unhealthy choices, but it is possible to hold the line on calories as well as costs. (See Health on a Budget.) According to researchers' analysis, the primary cause of weight gain among students is a decline in

📷 SNAPSHOT: ON CAMPUS NOW

The Weight of Student Bodies

BMI	Percent (%)		
	Male	Female	Average
<18.5, underweight	3.5	4.6	4.3
18.5–24.9, healthy weight	52.2	57.4	55.7
25–29.9, overweight	29.0	21.7	23.8
30–34.9, class I obesity	9.9	9.4	9.6
35–39.9, class II obesity	3.5	4.2	4.0
≥40, class III obesity	1.9	2.8	2.6

✓**check-in** Using Figure 5.1, determine your BMI. Which of the categories presented here do you fit in? Have you ever been overweight or obese? Are you now? Do you want to lose weight? Why or why not? Record your feelings on your weight today and in the past in your online journal.

Source: American College Health Association. American College Health Association-National College Health Assessment II: Reference Group Executive Summary Spring 2018. Silver Spring, MD: American College Health Association, 2018.

exercise frequency and, even more significantly, in exercise intensity[16] (see Chapter 7).

✓check-in Do you eat differently in college than you did before? Do you work out less?

Here are some of the ways weights change in college (see Snapshot: On Campus Now):

- Only about 5 percent of students gain the legendary "freshman 15," although most put on some weight, an average of about 11 pounds. The students who gain the most weight tend to be less physically active than their peers.
- Percentage of body fat, absolute body fat, and BMI tend to increase in the first semester at school. Normal-weight college women who try to restrict or lose weight are, ironically, most likely to gain body fat in their freshman year.[17]
- A certain percentage of incoming students—about a quarter to a third in different studies—lose weight during their first year.
- In male students, increased alcohol consumption and peer pressure to drink account for extra pounds.
- In college women, the strongest correlation of weight gain was with an increased workload, which may lead to more stress-related eating, greater snacking, or less exercise.[18]
- An estimated 10 to 13 percent of college students report using prescription stimulants to lose weight.

Health courses or university programs that promote healthy behaviors have proven effective in leading to better nutritional choices, lower weights, and increased exercise.[19]

✓check-in Have you gained or lost weight since starting college?

Body Composition

Rather than rely on a range of ideal weights for various heights, as they once did, medical experts use various methods to assess body composition and weight, including BMI, waist circumference, waist-to-hip ratio, and body fat.

Body Mass Index

Body mass index (BMI), a ratio between weight and height, is a mathematical formula that correlates with body fat. You can determine your BMI from Figure 5.2. Here is how to interpret the reading:

- A healthy BMI ranges from 18.5 to 24.9.
- A BMI of 25 or greater defines **overweight** and marks the point at which excess weight increases the risk of disease. If your BMI is between 25 (23.4 for Asians) and 29.9, your weight is undermining the quality of your life. You suffer more aches and pains. You find it harder to perform everyday tasks. You run a greater risk of serious health problems.
- A BMI of 30.0 or greater defines **obesity** and marks the point at which excess weight increases the risk of death. If your BMI is between 30.0 and 34.9 (class 1 obesity), you face all the preceding dangers plus one more: dying.
- A BMI between 35.0 and 39.9 (class 2 obesity) means increased risk of premature death.
- A BMI of 40 or higher indicates class 3 or severe obesity, a truly life-threatening condition.

✓check-in Do you know your BMI?

Experts debate which measure of body composition—BMI, waist circumference, or waist-to-hip ratio—is the best indicator of central or visceral obesity, which increases the risk of heart disease, metabolic syndrome, diabetes, and other illnesses. Among the limitations to the usefulness of BMI as an assessment tool are the following:

- Muscular individuals, including athletes and bodybuilders, may be miscategorized as overweight or obese because they have greater lean muscle mass.
- BMI does not reliably reflect body fat, an independent and possibly more accurate predictor of health risk.[20]
- BMI is not an accurate indicator of cardiometabolic health, which is more accurately reflected by blood pressure, lipids (fats), glucose, insulin resistance, and C-reactive protein[21] (discussed in Chapter 12).
- BMI is not useful for growing children, women who are pregnant or nursing, or older adults.
- BMI, which was developed in Western nations, may not accurately indicate the risk of obesity-related diseases in Asian men and women.

Waist Circumference

A widening waist, or "apple" shape, is a warning signal of increased risk of heart disease, lung problems, and cancer. Particularly combined with a high BMI, it can also be an indicator of premature death.[22]

overweight A condition of having a BMI between 25.0 and 29.9.

obesity The excessive accumulation of fat in the body; class 1 obesity is defined by a BMI between 30.0 and 34.9; class 2 obesity is a BMI between 35.0 and 39.9; class 3, or severe obesity, is a BMI of 40 or higher.

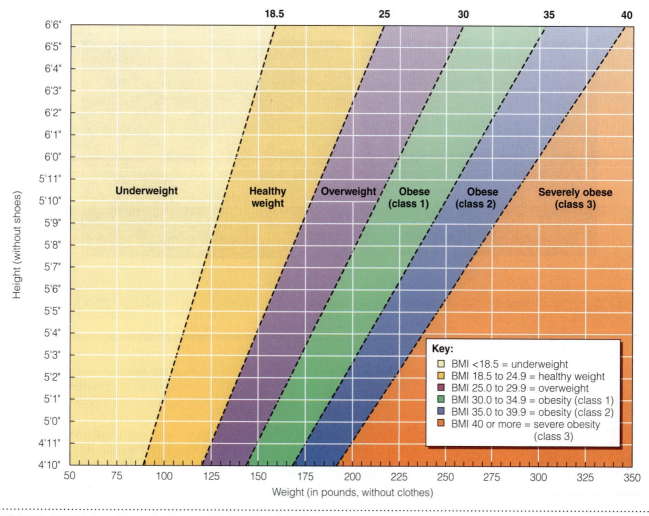

FIGURE 5.2 BMI Values Used to Assess Weight for Adults

✓**check-in** What is your waist measurement? Place a tape measure around your bare abdomen just above your hip bone. Be sure that the tape is snug but does not compress your skin. Relax, exhale, and measure.

When is a waist too wide? Various studies have produced different results, but the general guideline is that a waist measuring more than 35 inches in a woman or more than 40 inches in a man signals greater health risks. The larger the waist, the greater the risk of premature death.

Waist circumference indicates "central" obesity, which is characterized by fat deposited deep within the central abdominal area of the body. Such "visceral" fat is more dangerous than "subcutaneous" fat just below the skin because it moves more readily into the bloodstream and directly raises levels of harmful cholesterol.

Waist-to-Hip Ratio

Men of all ages are more prone to develop the "apple" shape characteristic of central obesity; women in their reproductive years are more likely to accumulate fat around the hips and thighs and acquire a pear shape (Figure 5.3). Another indicator of shape-related health risks is your **waist-to-hip ratio (WHR)**. In addition to measuring your waist, measure your hips at the widest part. Divide your waist measurement by your hip measurement.

✓**check-in** What is your WHR?

For women, a ratio of 0.80 or less is considered safe; for men, the recommended ratio is 0.90 or less. For both men and women, a 1.0 or higher is considered "at risk" or in the danger zone for undesirable health consequences, such as heart disease and other ailments associated with being overweight.

waist-to-hip ratio (WHR)
The proportion of one's waist circumference to one's hip circumference.

Body Composition   131

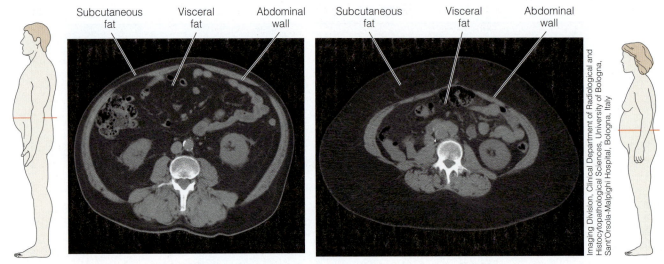

Subcutaneous fat   Visceral fat   Abdominal wall   Subcutaneous fat   Visceral fat   Abdominal wall

Male: BMI 29   Female: BMI 32

Imaging Division, Clinical Department of Radiological and Histocytopathological Sciences, University of Bologna, Sant'Orsola-Malpighi Hospital, Bologna, Italy

FIGURE 5.3 Central Obesity. In both men and women a larger waist circumference indicates more visceral fat and an increased risk of heart disease.

Measuring Body Fat

Ideal body fat percentages for men range from 7 to 25 percent and for women from 16 to 35 percent. Methods of assessing body composition include a variety of approaches.

Skinfold Measurement

Skinfold measurement is determined using a caliper to measure the amount of skinfold. The usual sites include the chest, abdomen, and thigh for men and the tricep, hip, and thigh for women. Various equations determine body fat percentage, including calculations that take into account age, sex, race, and other factors. This relatively simple and low-cost method requires considerable technical skill for an accurate reading.

Home Body Fat Analyzers

Handheld devices and stand-on monitors sold online and in specialty stores promise to make measuring your body fat percentage as easy as finding your weight. None has been extensively tested.

Laboratory Methods

- **Bioelectrical Impedance Analysis (BIA).** This noninvasive method is based on the principle that electrical current applied to the body meets greater resistance with different types of tissue. Lean tissue, which contains large amounts of water and electrolytes, is a good electrical conductor; fat, which does not, is a poor conductor. In theory, the easier the electrical conduction, the greater an individual's lean body mass.

- **Hydrostatic (underwater) weighing.** According to the Archimedes' principle, a body immersed in a fluid is buoyed by a force equal to the weight of the displaced fluid. Since muscle has a higher density than water and fat has a lower density, fat people tend to displace less water than lean people.

- **Dual-energy X-ray absorptiometry (DXA).** X-rays are used to quantify the skeletal and soft tissue components of body mass. The test requires just 10 to 20 minutes, and radiation dosage is low (800 to 2,000 times lower than a typical chest X-ray). Some researchers believe that DXA will supplant hydrostatic testing as the standard for body composition assessment.

- **The Bod Pod®.** This large, egg-shaped fiberglass chamber uses an approach based on air displacement plethysmography—that is, the calculation of the relationship between pressure and volume—to derive body volume.

✓**check-in** Do you know your body fat percentage?

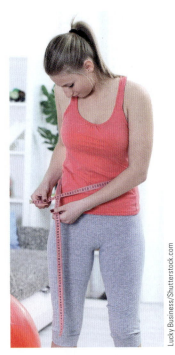

Your waist-to-hip ratio can indicate if you are at risk for undesirable health conditions.

Lucky Business/Shutterstock.com

Understanding Weight Problems

Ultimately, all weight problems result from a prolonged energy imbalance caused by consuming too many calories and burning too few in daily activities. How many calories you need depends on your sex, age, body-frame size, weight, percentage of body fat, activity level, and *basal metabolic rate (BMR)*—the number of calories needed to sustain your body at rest.

How Did So Many Get So Fat?

A variety of factors, ranging from behavior to environment to genetics, played a role in the increase in overweight and obesity in the United States. They include the following:

- **Bigger portions.** The size of many popular restaurant and packaged foods has increased two to five times during the past 20 years. According to studies of appetite and satiety, people presented with larger portions eat up to 30 percent more than they otherwise would (see Table 5.1).

- **Consuming more calories than we burn.** American adults have been eating steadily fewer calories for almost a decade, but may still not be getting enough exercise to burn the calories they do consume.

- **Fast food.** Young adults who eat frequently at fast-food restaurants gain more weight and develop metabolic abnormalities that increase their risk of diabetes in early middle age.

- **Sugar-sweetened beverages.** More than half of adults in the United States consume at least one or more sugar-sweetened beverage per day, which researchers calculate could lead to a pound of weight gain every 20 days.[23]

- **Physical inactivity.** The heaviest individuals tend to move the least. Obese men and women are much more sedentary and log more hours sitting or reclining than others.[24]

- **Screen Time.** Watching television, playing video games, and using computers and mobile devices may contribute to lower fitness and higher weights.

✓**check-in** How much television do you watch every day? Every week?

- **Emotional eating.** College students who are prone to boredom and have difficulty coping with negative emotions are likely to eat when they have nothing else to do or are feeling upset.[25]

- **Genetics.** Scientists have identified a particular variation in a gene associated with fat mass and obesity, called *FTO*, that increases the risk of excess weight by 20 to 30 percent. However, physical activity can counteract its effect.

TABLE 5.1 Supersized Portions

Food/Beverage	Original Size (year introduced)	Today (largest available)
Soda (Coca-Cola)	6.5 oz (1916)	34 oz
French fries (Burger King)	2.6 oz (1954)	6.9 oz
Hamburger (McDonald's; beef only)	1.6 oz (1965)	8 oz
Nestlé Crunch	1.6 oz (1938)	5 oz
Budweiser (bottle)	7 oz (1976)	40 oz

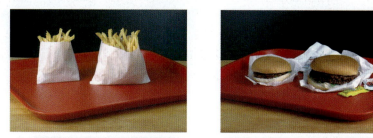

Source: "Are Growing Portion Sizes Leading to Expanding Waistlines?" *Academy of Nutrition and Dietetics,* www.eatright.org.

- **Social networks.** Researchers are not sure if overweight people seek out other overweight people or whether normal-weight individuals become heavier as a result of their relationships with heavier partners.

- **Marriage.** Although marriage confers many health benefits, it also puts on pounds—particularly among the happily married. The reason may be that, having found a mate, spouses no longer try to stay slim to attract a partner.

- **Perceived discrimination.** Among African Americans, perceived everyday discrimination may contribute to a higher BMI, larger waist circumference, and greater risk of obesity.[26]

Health Dangers of Excess Weight

If you have put on weight, you may be most concerned about looking fat or not fitting into your clothes. But the younger individuals are when they gain weight, the more health risks they may face over their lifetimes, including:

- A 70 percent chance of becoming overweight or obese throughout life.

- Greater likelihood of high total cholesterol levels and other cardiovascular disease risk factors such as elevated blood pressure.

- Higher prevalence of type 2 diabetes and cardiometabolic disorders.[27]

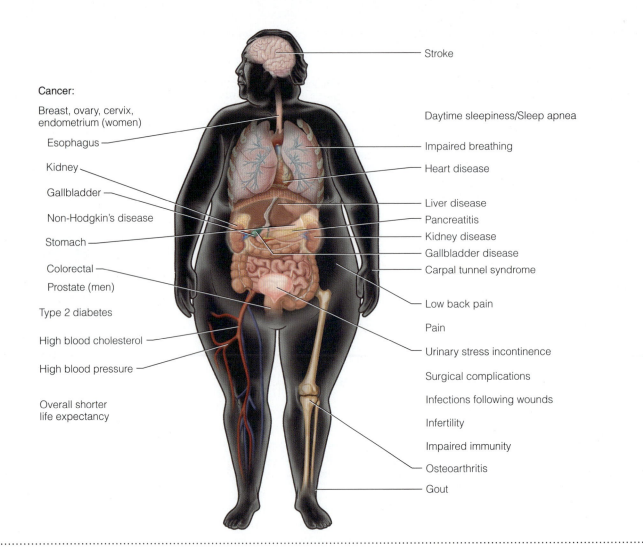

Cancer:

Breast, ovary, cervix, endometrium (women)

Esophagus

Kidney

Gallbladder

Non-Hodgkin's disease

Stomach

Colorectal

Prostate (men)

Type 2 diabetes

High blood cholesterol

High blood pressure

Overall shorter life expectancy

Stroke

Daytime sleepiness/Sleep apnea

Impaired breathing

Heart disease

Liver disease

Pancreatitis

Kidney disease

Gallbladder disease

Carpal tunnel syndrome

Low back pain

Pain

Urinary stress incontinence

Surgical complications

Infections following wounds

Infertility

Impaired immunity

Osteoarthritis

Gout

FIGURE 5.4 Health Dangers of Excess Weight

- Increased risk of premature death. Obesity, smoking, and high blood sugar levels significantly increase the risk of dying before age 55.

- Physiological changes that are the equivalent to 20 years of aging, including increased risk of cardiovascular disease, diabetes, cancer, rheumatoid arthritis, sleep apnea, gout, and liver disease (Figure 5.4), as well as difficulties in walking, balance, and rising from a chair.

The Impact on the Body

Major diseases linked to obesity include the following:

- **Type 2 diabetes.** More than 80 percent of people with type 2 diabetes are overweight. According to the International Diabetes Foundation, the rise in obesity may lead to a "catastrophic" epidemic of diabetes, affecting as many as 642 million people around the world

by 2040.[28] Although the reasons are not known, being overweight may make cells less efficient at using sugar from the blood. This then puts stress on the cells that produce insulin (a hormone that carries sugar from the blood to cells) and makes them gradually fail. Those with BMIs of 35 or more are approximately 20 times more likely to develop diabetes. Excess weight also increases the risk of premature death among people with type 2 diabetes.

- **Cardiovascular disease and heart attacks.** People who are overweight are more likely to suffer from high blood pressure, high levels of triglycerides (blood fats), harmful low-density lipoprotein (LDL) cholesterol, and low levels of beneficial high-density lipoprotein (HDL) cholesterol.[29] Even relatively small amounts of excess fat—as little as 5 pounds—can add to the dangers in those already at risk for hypertension. People with more body fat have higher blood levels of substances that cause inflammation, which may raise heart disease risk. Obesity is implicated in 40 percent of severe heart attacks, which are striking younger, fatter Americans.[30]

- **Strokes.** Obesity increases the danger of a particular type of stroke in women who take oral contraceptives, although the absolute risk is low.[31]

- **Cancer.** Obesity contributes to more than 100,000 cases of cancer—among them cancers of the endometrium, esophagus, pancreas, gallbladder, kidney, breast, ovaries, and colon—in the United States every year. Excess weight may account for 14 percent of all cancer deaths in men and 20 percent of those in women. Obesity quadruples the risk of prostate cancer in black men.[32] Women who were overweight as children or teens may have a greater risk of colon cancer as adults.[33] Losing weight, researchers estimate, could prevent as many as one in every six cancer deaths.[34]

Other Health Problems Overweight men and women are also more likely to develop:

- Knee injuries that require surgery to repair.
- Spinal disc degeneration, a common cause of lower back pain.
- Alterations in various measures of immune function.
- Greater risk of gallstones, kidney stones, and kidney disease.
- Liver disease.
- Less responsiveness to flu vaccination.
- Cognitive problems and dementia.
- Worsened symptoms of fibromyalgia, a musculoskeletal disorder.
- Poor sleep, which could add to the risk of medical problems.

Premature Death Obese American adults die an average of almost 4 years earlier than those with normal weight, and middle-aged obese adults face the highest risk of early death. According to recent research, obesity is associated with at least a 20 percent increased risk of death from all causes or from heart disease.

✓**check-in** What do you see as the greatest health risk of excess weight and obesity?

The Emotional and Social Toll

In our calorie-conscious and thinness-obsessed society, obesity also affects quality of life, including emotional and physical pain.

Many see excess weight as a psychological burden, a sign of failure, laziness, or inadequate willpower. Overweight men and women often blame themselves for becoming heavy and feel guilty and depressed as a result. In fact, the psychological problems once considered the cause of obesity may be its consequence. Obesity is associated with a higher prevalence of suicide risk in women, but not necessarily in men.[35]

Obesity also has social consequences. Heavy women are less likely to marry, earn less, and have lower rates of college graduation. Obese individuals of both sexes often experience unfair treatment, which can contribute to binge eating, irregular mealtimes, and greater consumption of convenience foods, because of their body weight.[36]

✓**check-in** Do you think that there is a bias against obese people?

If You're Too Thin: How to Gain Weight

Being underweight is not an uncommon problem, particularly among adolescent and young adult men as well as among those who diet excessively or suffer from eating disorders (discussed later in this chapter).

If you lose weight suddenly and don't know the reason, talk to a doctor. Rapid weight loss can be an early symptom of a health problem.

If you're trying to put on pounds, you need to do the opposite of dieters—that is, consume more calories than you burn. But as with losing weight, you should try to gain weight in healthy ways. Here are some suggestions:

- **Eat more of a variety of foods** rather than more high-fat, high-calorie foods. Get no more than 30 percent of your daily calories from fat. A higher percentage poses a threat to your heart and your health.

- **If your appetite is small, eat more frequently.** Try for five or six smaller meals rather than a big lunch and dinner.

- **Choose some calorie-rich foods,** such as dried fruits rather than fresh ones. Add nuts and cheese to salads and main dishes.

- **Drink juice** rather than regular or diet soda.

- **Try adding a commercial liquid meal** replacement as a snack.

- **Exercise regularly** to build up both appetite and muscle.

Thinking Thinner

Do you ease onto your scale, hoping for a certain number to appear—maybe what you weighed when you graduated from high school? If so, you may be setting yourself up for disappointment. Rather than focus on just one number, consider other ways to think about weight:

- **"If-only weight"**: A weight you would choose if you could weigh whatever you wanted— just like the height or eye color you'd have chosen if you could.

- **"Happy weight"**: A weight that is not the one you'd choose as your ideal but that you'd be happy with.

- **"Acceptable weight"**: A weight that would not make you particularly happy but that you could be satisfied with.

- **"Disappointed weight"**: A weight that would not be acceptable.

- **"Never-again weight"**: The all-time high you never want to hit again.

In your online journal, jot down your if-only weight, happy weight, acceptable weight, disappointed weight, and never-again weight. Then write down your actual weight, as of today. How many pounds is your real weight from your acceptable weight?

Assuming that you can lose a pound a week, how many weeks would it take to get to that weight? How do you envision yourself feeling and behaving once you reach your acceptable weight? Do you have any plans once you reach your acceptable weight, such as buying clothes or taking a weekend trip? How will your life be different?

A Practical Guide to a Healthy Weight

More than half of college women and about one-third of college men intend to lose weight. (See "Health Now!"). However, individuals vary in their readiness to change their diets, increase their physical activity, and seek professional counseling. Take the self-survey that accompanies this chapter in MindTap to determine your readiness to lose weight.

There are only two effective strategies for losing weight: eating less and exercising more. Unfortunately, most people search for easier alternatives that almost invariably turn into dietary dead-ends or unexpected dangers. Among young people, the most successful strategies for attaining and maintaining a healthy weight include[37]:

- Drinking less soda.
- Eating less junk food.
- Drinking more water.
- Increasing physical activity.
- Weighing themselves regularly.
- Adding more protein to their diets.
- Watching less television.
- Adding more fiber to their diets.

✓**check-in** Have you tried any of these strategies to lose weight?

Preventing Weight Gain

✓**check-in** What do you do when you notice that you've gained a few pounds?

As with other medical problems, the best approach to excess weight and obesity is prevention. "Self-regulation" by eating less and exercising more can prevent weight gain. However, losing excess pounds and keeping them off may take more. In a study of about 600 people (average age, 28), big changes, such as cutting back 500 to 1,000 calories a day and engaging in moderate exercise 250 minutes a week (more than the standard recommendation of 150 minutes), produced a much greater weight loss compared with smaller changes, such as eating about 100 calories less a day and exercising a little more. The "big changers" were more likely to maintain their weight loss during 3 years of follow-up.[38]

Weight Loss Diets

Every year, sometimes every season, seems to bring a breakthrough diet that promises to take off pounds, reshape your body, and recharge your life. You can "shred" 4 inches in 6 weeks, fast your way to a lower weight and longer life, or follow the dictates of Doctor Oz, Phil, or Ornish. Or you can try diets with roots in the Paleolithic Age, South Beach, Beverly Hills, or Park Avenue.

Some popular diets are high in protein; others are low in complex carbohydrates. Some allow no fat; others ban sugar or gluten. Which ones work? As long as you are burning more calories than you consume, they all do.[39] But not all diets are practical, inexpensive, easy to stay on, or good for your overall nutrition and health. (You can find an authoritative analysis of the latest diets at www.webmd.com/diet/evaluate-latest-diets.)

Relatively few weight loss approaches reach the national standards developed by the American Heart Association, the American College of Cardiology, and the Obesity Society:

- High-intensity interventions of at least 14 sessions over a 6-month period.
- An evidence-based diet.
- Physical activity guidelines.
- Self-monitoring tools such as food tracking.
- No endorsement of nutritional supplements.[40]

High-Protein Diets Many popular diets emphasize more protein and fewer carbohydrates. The Institute of Medicine considers a range of 10 to 35 percent of calories from protein as acceptable for adults, and some diets advise even higher levels. Protein is more satiating than carbohydrates and fat, so dieters complain less of hunger. However, severe restriction of carbohydrates can induce ketosis, which is caused by an incomplete breakdown of fats that can lead to nausea, fatigue, and light-headedness and can worsen kidney disease and other medical problems.

Recent studies have shown that high-protein diets are effective in controlling appetite, reducing body fat, maintaining lean body mass, and improving blood pressure and other health biomarkers. Ongoing studies are weighing their long-term impact on weight and well-being.[41]

Low-Carbohydrate, Low-Fat Diets Some popular diets are based on the premise that the correct proportions of various nutrients, particularly carbohydrates, fats, and proteins, lead to hormonal balance, weight loss, and greater vitality. They also promise additional health benefits, including lower blood pressure and cholesterol.

While dieters may eat just as much or even more food, they ingest fewer calories and much less fat. In research studies, dieters have burned more calories by cutting back on carbohydrates.[42] However, many people cannot stay on these diets for a sustained period.

Low-Carbohydrate, High-Fat Diets This approach remains controversial, in part because they have variable effects on blood cholesterol in different people. However, a diet low in carbohydrates and high in fats can have positive effects on other cardiovascular risk factors, possibly because it reduces hunger so dieters consume fewer calories. A recent review concluded that this dietary pattern, while "not suitable for everyone," is a "safe and efficacious dietary option" for others.[43]

The Bottom Line Researchers have identified the key components of a successful diet:

- Daily caloric intake of about 500 calories less than usual (or a recommended 1,200 calories for women and 1,500 for men).
- Relatively high in protein.
- Moderately low in calories.
- Low glycemic index (discussed in Chapter 4).

In a 12-month weight loss diet study, there was no significant difference in weight change between a healthy low-fat diet and a healthy low-carbohydrate diet. Dieters who cut back on added sugars, refined grains, and highly processed foods, while eating more vegetables and whole grains, without limiting calories or portion sizes, lost the most significant amounts of weight.[44] The behavioral strategies that lead to the greatest weight loss focus on dietary impulse control, weight-loss planning and monitoring, motivational support, information seeking, and self-monitoring.[45]

Not all diets are safe or effective. To spot a dubious approach to weight loss, see the Consumer Alert feature.

Although people lose weight on any diet that helps them eat less, most dieters lose only about 5 percent of their initial weight and gain some of that back. However, even such a modest weight loss can lower cardiovascular risk factors, such as elevated blood pressure, total cholesterol, and blood glucose.[46]

Do Weight Loss Programs Work?

✓**check-in** Would you turn to a commercial weight loss program to help you shed excess pounds? Before you answer, read the following section.

ⓘ CONSUMER ALERT

Dubious Diets

Facts to Know
The National Council Against Health Fraud cautions dieters to watch for these warnings of dangerous or fraudulent programs:

- Promises of very rapid weight loss.
- Claims that the diet can eliminate "cellulite" (a term used to describe dimply fatty tissue on the arms and legs).
- "Counselors" who are really salespersons pushing a product or program.
- No mention of any risks associated with the diet.
- Unproven gimmicks, such as body wraps, starch blockers, hormones, diuretics, or "unique" pills or potions.
- No maintenance program.

Steps to Take
If you hear about a new diet that promises to melt away fat, don't try it until you get answers to the following questions:

- Does it include a wide variety of nutritious foods?
- Does it provide at least 1,200 calories a day?
- Is it designed to reduce your weight by 0.5 to 2 pounds per week?
- Does it emphasize moderate portions?
- Does it use foods that are easy to find and prepare?
- Can you follow it wherever you eat—at home, work, restaurants, or parties?
- Is its cost reasonable?

If the answer to any of these questions is no, don't try the diet; then ask yourself one more question: Is losing weight worth losing your well-being?

Americans spend $2.5 billion a year on programs and products to help them lose weight and keep it off. Yet there has been little scientific evidence to show whether or not these plans lead to successful long-term weight loss. A recent study analyzed published studies on

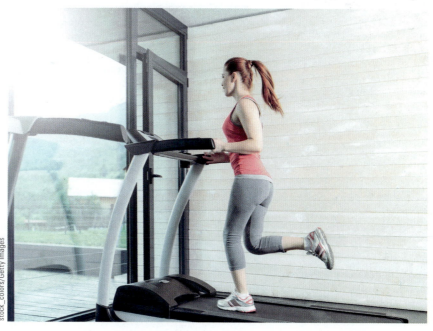

Regular exercise provides many health benefits while also helping to control weight.

stock_colors/Getty Images

some of the most popular programs. Here are the findings:

- **Counseling plus calorie control** (Weight Watchers and Jenny Craig). These are the only two programs backed by scientific evidence showing that their clients maintained weight loss for at least a year. Nutrisystem clients also lost weight but were followed for only 3 months.

- **Very-low-calorie and low-calorie meal replacement programs** (Medifast, Optifast, and Health Management Resources). Consumers using these products initially reported greater weight loss than those given counseling alone, but attrition was high and the difference was not statistically significant by 9 months. The very-low-calorie methods increased the risk of gallstones.

- **Self-directed** (Atkins and Slimfast). Individuals following the Atkins diet reported greater weight loss than those in education-counseling programs at 6 and 12 months. Adherence was not reported; the most common complication was constipation. Slimfast users lost more weight than a control group but had results similar to those who received counseling alone.

- **Internet-based programs** (The Biggest Loser Club, eDiets, and Lose it!). Results varied, with Biggest Loser Club members showing greater weight loss than a control group at 3 months but no difference between eDiets and LoseIt! participants and controls.

Because so little solid research is available, the researchers' conclusion was inconclusive: "We still don't know whether a lot of these programs work."[47] For years individuals have tried to lose or control weight by smoking; more recently, some have tried electronic cigarettes (discussed in depth in Chapter 17). Among those most likely to try "vaping" are overweight individuals who restrict calories, have poor impulse controls, and prefer coffee or vanilla flavors.[48]

Physical Activity and Exercise

Unplanned daily activity, such as fidgeting or pacing, can make a difference in preventing weight gain. Scientists use the acronym **NEAT (nonexercise activity thermogenesis)** to describe such "nonvolitional" movement, which may be an effective way of burning calories. In research on self-confessed couch potatoes, the thinner ones sat an average of 2 hours less and moved and stood more often than the heavier individuals.

Although physical activity and exercise can prevent weight gain and improve health, they typically burn up just 200 calories a day and do not lead to significant weight loss.[49] However, when combined with a low-fat diet, exercise helps preserve lean body mass, helps keep off excess pounds, and promotes greater cardiovascular fitness.[50] Moderate exercise, such as 30 to 60 minutes of daily physical activity, reduces the risk of heart disease and other health threats. More exercise—a minimum of 200 to 300 minutes weekly of moderately intense activity—is necessary to maintain weight loss.

Among its other benefits (discussed in Chapter 7), exercise contributes to a healthy weight by:

- Increasing energy expenditure.
- Building up muscle tissue.
- Burning off fat stores.
- Stimulating the immune system.
- Possibly reprogramming metabolism so that more calories are burned during and after a workout.

An exercise program designed for both health benefits and weight loss should include both aerobic activity and resistance training. People who start and stick with an exercise program during or after a weight loss program are consistently more successful in keeping off most of the pounds they've shed.

Complementary and Alternative Medicine for Obesity

Complementary and alternative medicine (CAM) is defined as "varied medical and health-care systems, practices, and products that are not considered to be part of any Western health-care system" (see Chapter 14). These include the following:[51]

- **Herbal supplements.** Although widely advertised, the researchers concluded that "the evidence in support of their effectiveness is either nonexistent or points to a negligible effect."

- **Acupuncture.** In randomized trials, acupuncture was more effective than lifestyle modification and placebo in reducing BMI and weight. However, scientists have criticized the design and validity of the studies.

- **Mindfulness.** Weight loss programs that incorporate mindfulness (discussed in Chapter 2) along with diet and exercise have proven effective in helping participants shed pounds, but the impact of mindfulness alone is not clear.[52]

NEAT (nonexercise activity thermogenesis) Nonvolitional movement that can be an effective way of burning calories.

✓**check-in:** Want to eat less? Keep food out of sight. Leaving food in plain sight increases the likelihood of consuming it—and gaining weight. Seeing food can trigger thoughts about eating and increase stress about resisting the temptation to do so.

Common Diet Traps

A multimillion-dollar industry thrives on marketing various diet aids, most of dubious value. Here is what you should know about some of the most widespread:

- **Over-the-counter diet pills.** An estimated 15 percent of adults—21 percent of women and 10 percent of men—have used weight loss supplements. The weight loss prescription drug Orlistat (Xenical) is available as an over-the-counter weight loss pill called Alli. The drug, which blocks about one-quarter of the fat consumed, works best with a low-fat diet. If dieters eat a meal made up of more than 15 grams of fat, they can suffer nasty side effects, including flatulence, an urgent need to defecate, oily stools, and diarrhea.

- **Diet foods.** Diet products, including diet sodas and low-fat foods, are a very big business. Many people rely on meal replacements, usually shakes or snack bars, to lose or keep off weight. If used appropriately—as actual replacements rather than supplements to regular meals and snacks—they can be a useful strategy for weight loss. Yet people who use these products often gain weight because they think that they can afford to add high-calorie treats to their diets.

- **Artificial sweeteners and fake fats.** Nutritionists caution to use these products in moderation and not as substitutes for basic foods, such as grains, fruits, and vegetables. A recent review of studies of "non-sugar sweeteners" found no conclusive evidence of either benefit or harm.[53]

  Foods made with fat substitutes may have fewer grams of fat, but they don't necessarily have significantly fewer calories. Many people who consume reduced-fat, fat-free, or sugar-free sodas, cookies, chips, and other snacks often cut back on more nutritious foods, such as fruits and vegetables. They also tend to eat more of the low- or no-fat foods so that their daily calorie intake either stays the same or actually increases.

YOUR STRATEGIES FOR PREVENTION

Keeping the Pounds Off

Once you've reached your weight goal, try the following suggestions for long-term success:

- **Set a danger zone.** Once you've reached your desired weight, don't let your weight climb more than 3 or 4 pounds higher. Take into account normal fluctuations but watch out for an upward trend. Once you hit your upper weight limit, take action immediately rather than wait until you gain 10 pounds.

- **Be patient.** Think of weight loss as a road trip. If you're going across town, you expect to get there in 20 minutes. If your destination is 400 miles away, you know it'll take longer. Give yourself the time you need to lose weight safely and steadily.

- **Try, try again.** Dieters don't usually keep weight off on their first attempt. The people who eventually succeed don't give up. Through trial and error, they find a plan that works for them.

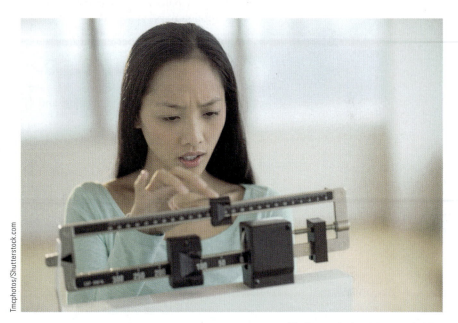

Tmcphotos/Shutterstock.com

Vigilance helps keep weight off. If the number on the scale creeps upward, take action immediately.

Maintaining Weight Loss

Surveys of people who lost significant amounts of weight and kept it off for several years show that most did so on their own—without medication, meal substitutes, or membership in an organized weight loss group. "Weight loss maintainers" are more active, have fewer TVs in their homes, and don't keep high-fat foods in their pantries. (See Your Strategies for Prevention.)

Rather than focus on why dieters fail, the creators of the National Weight Control Registry study the habits and lifestyles of those who've maintained a weight loss of at least 30 pounds for at least a year. The nearly 6,000 people in the registry have maintained their weight loss for almost 6 years.

No one diet or commercial weight loss program helped all these formerly overweight individuals. Many, through years of trial and error, eventually came up with a permanent exercise and eating program that worked for them. Despite the immense variety, their customized approaches share certain characteristics:

- **Personal responsibility for change.** Weight loss winners develop an internal locus of control. Rather than blame others for their weight problem or rely on a doctor or trainer to fix it, they believe that the keys to a healthy weight lie within themselves.

- **Exercise.** Registry members report an hour of moderate physical activity almost every day. Their favorite exercise? Three in four say walking, followed by cycling, weightlifting, aerobics, running, and stair climbing. On average, they burn about 2,545 calories per week through physical activity.

- **Monitoring.** About 44 percent of registry members count calories, and almost all keep track of their food intake in some way, written or not. New technology-based apps have proven easier to use, more motivating, and more accurate in tracking food intake.[54]

- **Vigilance.** Rather than avoid the scale or tell themselves their jeans shrank in the wash, successful losers keep tabs on their weight and size. About one-third check the scale every week. If the scale notches upward or their waistbands start to pinch, they take action.

- **Frequent eating.** Individuals who manage to maintain a significant weight loss typically eat more frequently (an average of three meals and two snacks a day) than those who eat less often.

....
✓**check-in** What steps do you take to
....
maintain a healthy weight?
....

Treating Severe Obesity

The biggest Americans are getting bigger, as the following statistics indicate:

- The prevalence of severe, or "morbid," obesity is increasing faster than obesity itself.

- The number of extremely obese adults—those at least 100 pounds overweight with BMIs over 40—has quadrupled in the past two

decades from 1 in 200 to about 1 in every 50 men and women.

- The number with BMIs greater than 50 has jumped from 1 in 2,000 in the 1980s to 1 in 400.

Extreme obesity poses extreme risks to health and survival and undermines quality of life. The options for treating this dangerous condition include medication and surgery.

Obesity Medications

Millions of Americans, including some who are not overweight, take over-the-counter pills, powders, herbs, and other supplements to shed extra pounds. However, they have not been extensively tested and may not be either safe or effective.

For individuals with a BMI higher than 30 (or 27 for those with heart disease or its risk factors), the Food and Drug Administration (FDA) has approved several medications. Although they can lead to temporary weight loss, lifestyle changes are still needed to maintain a healthy weight.

Obesity Surgery

Obesity, or bariatric, surgery is becoming the most popular weight loss approach for the estimated 15 million men and women who qualify as "morbidly obese" (100 or more pounds overweight) because of their increased health risks. It has proven effective in promoting weight loss among teenagers as well as older adults.[55]

Bariatric surgery has proven more effective in inducing weight loss and remission of type 2 diabetes and metabolic syndrome than other approaches.[56] The individuals most likely to benefit from obesity surgery generally:

- Have a BMI over 40.

- Have a BMI over 35 and a serious obesity-related problem, such as type 2 diabetes or severe sleep apnea (when breathing stops for brief periods during sleep).

- Have made repeated unsuccessful attempts to lose weight.

- Do not have any significant or untreated psychological problems.

- Are well-informed about the risks of the surgery.

- Recognize the need for lifestyle changes and daily vitamin and mineral supplements.

According to the Agency for Healthcare Research and Quality, three of four bariatric surgery patients lose 50 to 75 percent of their excess weight within 2 years and keep it off. Among its other potential benefits are the following:

- Improvement in or elimination of diabetes in some people, including teenagers.[57]
- Alleviation of high cholesterol, hypertension, and sleep apnea.
- Reduction of odds of dying by nearly half.
- Reduction of cardiovascular disorder, such as heart attack or stroke, and heart-related deaths.[58]
- Lower risk of gestational (pregnancy) diabetes.[59]

The types of procedures are as follows:

- **Gastric bypass.** Surgeons create an egg-sized pouch with staples and reroute food around part of the upper intestine to block absorption of calories and nutrients. About 75 percent of bypass patients lose 50 to 75 percent of their excess weight within 2 years.[60]
- **Banding.** In this newer, less risky procedure, surgeons slip an inflatable silicon band around the stomach; it can be tightened or loosened at a doctor's office without the need for further surgery. Patients lose about 40 to 55 percent of excess weight but may be more likely to regain lost pounds. The band also may slip or erode.
- **Endoscopic sleeve gastroplasty.** This new alternative for people who are mildly to moderately obese involves using an endoscope, a flexible tube inserted through the mouth.[61] When the endoscope reaches the stomach, the surgeon places sutures in the stomach, making it smaller and changing its shape. In a small study, the procedure resulted in a loss of about 50 percent of excess weight.[62]
- **Duodenal switch.** Duodenal switch or biliopancreatic diversion, a more extensive operation that removes a portion of the stomach and bypasses a large portion of the small intestine, may lead to greater long-term weight loss but carries a risk of more complications.

Long-term dangers—both physical and psychological—are unknown. Middle-aged and even older people may gain a boost in survival from gastric bypass surgery, but researchers have found no survival benefit for obese individuals under age 35 and also an increase in "externally caused deaths," including accident injuries, assaults, and suicides.[63] For obese teenagers, who generally do not respond well to dietary restrictions or medical treatments, bariatric surgery leads to a dramatic weight loss, but nearly three in four develop long-term nutritional deficiencies.[64]

Unhealthy Eating on Campus

Unhealthy eating behavior takes many forms, ranging from not eating enough to eating too much too quickly. Its roots are complex. In addition to media and external pressures, family history can play a role. Researchers have linked specific genes to some cases of anorexia nervosa and binge eating, but most believe that a variety of factors, including stress and culture, combine to cause disordered eating.

College students—particularly women, including varsity athletes—are at risk for unhealthy eating behaviors. Researchers estimate that only about one-third of college women maintain healthy eating patterns. Some college women have full-blown eating disorders; others develop "partial syndromes" and experience symptoms that are not severe or numerous enough for a diagnosis of anorexia nervosa or bulimia nervosa. Distress about body image increases the risk of all forms of disordered eating.

✓**check-in** Do you think unhealthy eating is common on your campus?

Body Image

Women have long been bombarded by idealized images in the media of female bodies that bear little resemblance to the way most women look. Increasingly, more advertisements and men's magazines are featuring idealized male bodies that bear little resemblance to the bodies most men have. As the gap between reality and ideal grows, both sexes struggle with issues related to body image, although men and women report different concerns as follows:

- Women express greater worry about thinness and more dissatisfaction with their lower rather than their upper bodies.
- College women are more likely to overestimate their weight, while men tend to underestimate their actual weight.
- The greater the discrepancy between a woman's current view of her body shape and the ideal she considers most attractive to men, the more likely she is to worry about how others will view her and to doubt her ability to make a desirable impression.
- "Social physique anxiety" occurs often in women who feel they do not measure up to

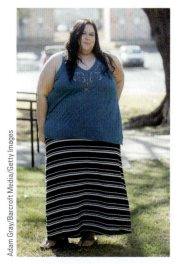

An estimated 15 million men and women are "morbidly obese" (100 or more pounds overweight).

Adam Gray/Barcroft Media/Getty Images

what they or others consider most desirable in terms of weight or appearance. Those reporting the greatest distress because of body image are at highest risk for eating disorders (discussed later in this chapter).

- Women compare their appearance to that of celebrities and models as well as peers more frequently than men and worry more that others will think negatively about their looks. Yet appearance matters just as much to men, who are as likely as women to engage in efforts to improve their bodies.

- Men often want either to lose or gain weight or to add muscle and bulk.

- College men in the United States overwhelmingly associate greater muscularity with feeling sexier, more confident, and more attractive to women. Pursuit of this idealized body type can lead to a dangerous obsession called muscle dysmorphia or reverse anorexia. Men with this disorder are at higher risk for depression and anxiety, abuse of substances such as anabolic steroids, and suicide.

College students of different ethnic and racial backgrounds express as much concern about their body shape and weight as whites—and sometimes more. In a study of university students, black and white men were similar in their ideals for body size and in their perceptions of their own shapes. Both black and white women perceive themselves as smaller than they actually are and desire an even smaller body size. However, black women are more accepting of larger size.

✓**check-in** Would more realistic media images affect how you feel about your body?

Disordered Eating

In a survey at a large, public, rural university in the mid-Atlantic states, 17 percent of the women were struggling with disordered eating. Younger students (ages 18–21) were more likely than older students to have an eating disorder. In this study, eating disorders equally affected women of different races (Caucasian, Asian, African American, Native American, and Hispanic), religions, athletic involvement, and living arrangements (on or off campus; with roommates, boyfriends, or family).

Although the students viewed eating disorders as both mental and physical problems and felt that individual therapy would be most helpful, all said that they would first turn to a friend for help. Women in sororities are at slightly increased risk of an eating disorder compared with those in dormitories. Loneliness has also emerged as a risk factor for eating disorders in college women.

Brief interventions, such as 4-hour Healthy Weight programs, have proven effective in preventing the onset of various forms of disordered eating.

Extreme Dieting

Extreme dieters go beyond cutting back on calories or increasing physical activity. They become preoccupied with what they eat and weigh. Although their weight never falls below 85 percent of normal, their weight loss is severe enough to cause uncomfortable physical consequences, such as weakness and sensitivity to cold. Technically, these dieters do not have anorexia nervosa (discussed later in this chapter), but they are at increased risk for it.

Extreme dieters may think they know a great deal about nutrition, yet many of their beliefs about food and weight are misconceptions or myths. For instance, they may eat only protein because they believe complex carbohydrates, including fruits and whole-grain breads, are fattening. Nutritional education alone can sometimes help change these eating patterns, but many extreme dieters who deny that they have a problem with food may need counseling to change their potentially dangerous eating behavior.[65]

✓**check-in** Have you ever tried an extreme diet?

Compulsive Overeating

People who eat compulsively cannot stop putting food in their mouth. They eat fast, and they eat a lot. They eat even when they're full. They may eat around the clock rather than at set mealtimes, often in private because they are embarrassed about how much they consume.

Some mental health professionals describe compulsive eating as a food addiction that is much more likely to develop in women. According to Overeaters Anonymous (OA), an international 12-step program, many women who eat compulsively view food as a source of comfort against feelings of inner emptiness, low self-esteem, and fear of abandonment.

The following behaviors may signal a potential problem with compulsive overeating:

- **Turning to food** when depressed or lonely, when feeling rejected, or as a reward.

- **A history of failed diets** and anxiety when dieting.

- **Thinking about food** throughout the day.

- **Eating quickly** and without pleasure.

- **Continuing to eat** even when no longer hungry.

- **Frequently talking about food or refusing to talk about food.**

- **Fear of not being able to stop** eating after starting.

Recovery from compulsive eating can be challenging because people with this problem cannot give up the substance they abuse entirely. Like everyone else, they must eat. However, they can learn new eating habits and ways of dealing with underlying emotional problems.

✓**check-in** Have you ever felt a compulsion to eat even when you weren't hungry?

Binge Eating

Binge eating—the rapid consumption of an abnormally large amount of food in a relatively short time—often occurs in compulsive eaters. The 25 million Americans with a binge-eating disorder typically eat a larger-than-ordinary amount of food during a relatively brief period, feel a lack of control over eating, and binge at least once a week for at least a 3-month period. During most of these episodes, binge eaters experience at least three of the following:

- **Eating much more rapidly** than usual.

- **Eating until they feel uncomfortably full.**

- **Eating large amounts of food** when not feeling physically hungry.

- **Eating large amounts of food** throughout the day with no planned mealtimes.

- **Eating alone** because they are embarrassed by how much they eat and by their eating habits.

The most commonly reported by those with binge-eating disorders is "stuffing oneself with food"; the least common, eating or drinking in secrecy.[66]

Binge eaters may spend up to several hours eating and consume 2,000 or more calories in a single binge—more than many people eat in a day. After such binges, they usually do not do anything to control weight but simply get fatter. As their weight climbs, they become depressed, anxious, or troubled by other psychological symptoms to a much greater extent than others of comparable weight.

Binge eating is probably the most common eating disorder. An estimated 8 to 19 percent of obese patients in weight loss programs are binge eaters.

✓**check-in** Have you ever gone on an eating binge?

If you occasionally go on eating binges, use the behavioral technique called *habit reversal* and replace your bingeing with a competing behavior. For example, every time you're tempted to binge, immediately do something—text-message a friend, play solitaire, check your email—that keeps food out of your mouth.

If you binge once a week or more for at least a 3-month period, you may have **binge-eating disorder**, a recently recognized psychiatric disorder that can require professional help.[67] Short-term talk treatment, such as cognitive-behavioral therapy, either individually or in a group setting, has proven most effective for binge eating.

Eating Disorders

Eating disorders affect an estimated 5 to 10 million women and 1 million men. Despite evidence that 5 to 10 percent of those with eating disorders are male, many college students believe mainly young white women develop eating disorders. More people—and more types of people—are developing full-blown or "partial syndrome" eating disorders, including young children, boys and men, people of color, and individuals with lower socioeconomic backgrounds.[68] Yet fewer of these individuals seek help than those with other mental disorders.[69]

The most common eating disorders are binge-eating disorder, anorexia nervosa, and bulimia nervosa. Among the factors that increase the risk are[70]:

- Genetic predisposition.

- Preoccupation with a thin body.

- Body dissatisfaction.

- Dieting.

- Overeating.

- Social pressure.

- Perfectionism and excessive cautiousness, which can reflect an obsessive-compulsive personality.

- Life transitions, such as puberty and the transition from adolescence to adulthood.

Female college students who spend a lot of time on Facebook, keeping track of "likes" and comparing their photos to others, could be at increased risk for an eating disorder. Male and

binge eating The rapid consumption of an abnormally large amount of food in a relatively short time.

binge-eating disorder Chronic or repeated episodes of uncontrollable binge eating.

eating disorders Unusual, often dangerous patterns of food consumption, including anorexia nervosa and bulimia nervosa.

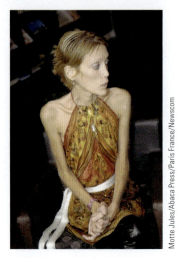

Individuals with eating disorders often have a distorted view of their weight. How do you decide what your ideal body size is?

anorexia nervosa A psychological disorder in which refusal to eat and/or an extreme loss of appetite leads to malnutrition, severe weight loss, and possibly death.

bulimia nervosa Episodic binge eating, often followed by forced vomiting or laxative abuse, and accompanied by a persistent preoccupation with body shape and weight.

female performers, dancers, and models are also at risk of developing eating disorders, as are athletes in sports involving pressure either to maintain ideal body weight or to achieve a weight that might enhance their performance, such as gymnastics, distance running, diving, figure skating, wrestling, and cycling.

Eating disorders affect ethnic minorities as much as whites, and there are more overlapping risk factors shared among various ethnic groups than differences.[71] In the few studies of eating disorders in minority college students that have been completed, African American female undergraduates had a slightly lower prevalence of eating disorders than did whites. Asian Americans reported fewer symptoms of eating disorders but more body dissatisfaction, concerns about shape, and more intense efforts to lose weight. Adolescents and adults with binge-eating disorder may be at higher risk of suicidal thoughts, plans, and attempts.[72]

The American Psychiatric Association has developed practice guidelines for the treatment of patients with eating disorders, which include medical, psychological, and behavioral approaches. One of the most scientifically supported is cognitive-behavioral therapy (discussed in Chapter 3). Mindfulness, discussed in Chapter 3, also has shown promise in helping individuals with or at risk for eating disorders.[73]

Anorexia Nervosa

Although *anorexia* means "loss of appetite," most individuals with **anorexia nervosa** are, in fact, hungry all the time. For them, food is an enemy—a threat to their sense of self, identity, and autonomy. In the distorted mirror of their mind's eye, they see themselves as fat or flabby even at a normal or below-normal body weight. Some simply feel fat; others think that they are thin in some places and too fat in others, such as the abdomen, buttocks, or thighs.

Anorexia, which affects about 0.4 percent of girls and young women per year, is 10 times more common in females than in males. Its key characteristics include the following:

- Restriction of food intake, leading to a significantly low body weight for their age, health, and sex.
- Intense fear of gaining weight or of becoming fat.
- Disturbance in the way individuals experience their body weight or shape.

The incidence of anorexia nervosa has increased in the past three decades in most developed countries. The peak ages for its onset are 14.5 to 18 years. Cases are increasing among males, minorities, women of all ages, and possibly preteens.

There are two recognizable forms of anorexia:

- In the *restricting type*, individuals lose weight by avoiding any fatty foods and by dieting, fasting, and exercising. Some start smoking as a way of controlling their weight. Some college women may numb their pain by drinking alcohol, a problem the media have dubbed "drunkorexia."
- In the *binge-eating/purging type*, individuals engage in binge eating, purging (through self-induced vomiting, laxatives, diuretics, or enemas), or both. Obsessed with an intense fear of fatness, they may weigh themselves several times a day, measure various parts of their body, check mirrors to see if they look fat, and try on different items of clothing to see if they feel tight.

Bulimia Nervosa

Individuals with **bulimia nervosa** go on repeated eating binges and rapidly consume large amounts of food, usually sweets, stopping only because of severe abdominal pain or sleep, or because they are interrupted. Those with purging bulimia induce vomiting or take large doses of laxatives to relieve guilt and control their weight. In nonpurging bulimia, individuals use other means, such as fasting or excessive exercise, to compensate for binges.

The characteristics of bulimia nervosa include:

- Repeated binge eating.
- A feeling of lack of control over eating behavior.
- Regular reliance on self-induced vomiting, laxatives, or diuretics.
- Strict dieting or fasting, or vigorous exercise, to prevent weight gain.
- A minimum average of one bingeing episode a week for at least 3 months.
- A preoccupation with body shape and weight.

An estimated 1 to 2 percent of adolescent and young American women develop bulimia. Some experiment with bingeing and purging for a few months and then stop when they change their social or living situation. Others develop longer-term bulimia. Among males, this disorder is about one-tenth as common. The average age for developing bulimia is 18.

- How common is obesity in the United States?
- How does your weight affect your health?
- What are the best ways to lose excess pounds?
- What are the most common eating disorders on college campuses?

Reflection

Has weight ever been an issue in your life? If so, think back to the first time you became concerned about your weight. How old were you? What was your life like at the time? How have your concerns about weight changed since then? Consider your answers as you reflect on what you learned in this chapter.

TAKING CHARGE OF YOUR HEALTH

Managing Your Weight

No diet—high-protein, low-fat, or high-carbohydrate—can produce permanent weight loss. Successful weight management, the Academy of Nutrition and Dietetics has concluded, "requires a lifelong commitment to healthful lifestyle behaviors emphasizing sustainable and enjoyable eating practices and daily physical activity." Studies have shown that successful dieters are highly motivated, monitor their food intake, increase their activity, set realistic goals, and receive social support from others. Another key to long-term success is tailoring any weight loss program to an individual's sex, lifestyle, and cultural, racial, and ethnic values.

Are you following these practical guidelines?

_____ **Be realistic.** Trying to shrink to an impossibly low weight dooms you to defeat. Start off slowly and make steady progress. If your weight creeps up 5 pounds, go back to the basics of your program.

_____ **Recognize that there are no quick fixes.** Ultimately, quick-loss diets are very damaging physically and psychologically because when you stop dieting and put the pounds back on, you feel like a failure.

_____ **Note your progress.** Make a graph, with your initial weight as the base, to indicate your progress. View plateaus or occasional gains as temporary setbacks rather than disasters.

_____ **Adopt the 90 percent rule.** If you practice good eating habits 90 percent of the time, a few indiscretions won't make a difference. In effect, you should allow for occasional cheating, so that you don't have to feel guilty about it.

_____ **Look for joy and meaning beyond your food life.** Make your personal goals and your relationships your priorities, and treat food as the fuel that allows you to bring your best to both.

_____ **Try again and again.** Remember, dieters usually don't keep weight off on their first attempt. The people who eventually succeed try various methods until they find the plan that works for them.

SELF-SURVEY

Are You Ready to Lose Weight?

As discussed in Chapter 1, people change the way they behave stage by stage and step by step. The same is true for changing behaviors related to weight. If you need to lose excess pounds, knowing your stage of readiness for change is a crucial first step. Here is a guide to identifying where you are right now.

If you are still in the *precontemplation* stage, you don't think of yourself as having a weight problem, even though others may. If you can't fit into some of your clothes, you blame the dry cleaners. Or you look around and think, "I'm no bigger than anyone else in this class." Unconsciously, you may feel helpless to do anything about your weight, so you deny or dismiss its importance.

In the *contemplation* stage, you would prefer not to have to change, but you can't avoid reality. Your coach or doctor may comment on your weight. You wince at the vacation photos of you in a swimsuit. You look in the mirror, try to suck in your stomach, and say, "I've got to do something about my weight."

In the *preparation* stage, you're gearing up by taking small but necessary steps. You may buy athletic shoes or check out several diet books from the library. Maybe you experiment with some minor changes, such as having fruit instead of cookies for an afternoon snack. Internally, you are getting accustomed to the idea of change.

In the *action* stage of change, you are deliberately working to lose weight. You no longer snack all evening long. You stick to a specific diet and track calories, carbs, or points. You hop on a treadmill or stationary bike for 30 minutes a day. Your resolve is strong, and you know you're on your way to a thinner, healthier you.

In the *maintenance* stage, you strengthen, enhance, and extend the changes you've made. Whether or not you have lost all the weight you want, you've made significant progress. As you continue to watch what you eat and to be physically active, you lock in healthy new habits.

Where are you right now? Read each of the following statements and decide which best applies to you.

1. I never think about my weight.   Precontemplation Stage

2. I'm trying to zip up a pair of jeans and wondering when was the last time they fit.   Contemplation Stage

3. I'm downloading a food diary to keep track of what I eat.   Preparation Stage

4. I have been following a diet for 3 weeks and have started working out. Action Stage

5. I have been sticking to a diet and engaging in regular physical activity for at least 6 months.   Maintenance Stage

REVIEW QUESTIONS

(LO 5.1) 1. _____ people have the lowest obesity rates.
   a. American Indian
   b. Asian American
   c. Pacific Islander
   d. Native Hawaiian

(LO 5.2) 2. Which of the following statements is true of BMI?
   a. A BMI between 35 and 39.9 means increased risk of premature death.
   b. A healthy BMI ranges from 11.5 to 21.
   c. A BMI of 30 or greater defines overweight.
   d. A BMI that ranges from 20 to 25 defines obesity.

(LO 5.2) 3. Which of the following statements is true about the waist-to-hip ratio?
   a. Women in their reproductive years are more likely to accumulate fat around the hips and thighs.
   b. A ratio of 1.0 or less is considered safe for women.
   c. A ratio of 1.5 or less is considered safe for men.
   d. Men of all ages are less prone to accumulate fat around the belly.

(LO 5.3) 4. _____ refers to the number of calories needed to sustain the human body at rest.
   a. Active metabolic rate
   b. Anaerobic metabolic rate
   c. Aerobic metabolic rate
   d. Basal metabolic rate

(LO 5.3) 5. Which of the following factors has resulted in an increase in overweight and obese people in the United States?
   a. Physical inactivity
   b. Excessive dieting
   c. Active work culture
   d. Excessive protein intake

(LO 5.4) 6. People who are overweight are at increased risk of suffering from _____.
   a. jaundice
   b. tuberculosis
   c. type 1 diabetes
   d. cancer

(LO 5.4) 7. Which of the following statements is true about the social consequences of obesity?
   a. Heavy women are less likely to marry.
   b. Heavy men are more likely to be well settled and earn more.
   c. Heavy women are more likely to be highly qualified.
   d. Obese individuals are likely to diet.

(LO 5.5) 8. Which of the following suggestions should be adopted in order to gain weight in healthy ways?
   a. Drink regular or diet soda rather than juice.
   b. Opt for a big lunch or dinner rather than five or six smaller meals.
   c. Eat more of a variety of foods rather than more high-fat, high-calorie foods.
   d. Choose fresh fruits rather than dried ones.

(LO 5.5) 9. If you lose weight suddenly without knowing why, you should _____.
   a. see a doctor
   b. try to exercise more
   c. increase your daily calorie intake
   d. maintain your current lifestyle

(LO 5.6)   10. Which of the following is a proven successful strategy for attaining and maintaining a healthy weight?
    a. Drinking less water.
    b. Weighing yourself regularly.
    c. Eating more carbohydrates.
    d. Cutting back on fiber and protein.

(LO 5.6)   11. Which of the following statements is true about weight-loss diets?
    a. Diets with strict proportions of fat, carbohydrates, and proteins are always more effective than diets that cut back on total calories.
    b. Many popular diets emphasize more carbohydrates and fewer proteins.
    c. To be successful, they should limit women to 1,600 calories and men to 2,000 calories.
    d. Most dieters lose only about 5 percent of their initial weight and gain some of that back.

(LO 5.7)   12. Individuals most likely to benefit from obesity surgery _____.
    a. are unaware of the risks of surgery
    b. have failed to recognize the need for lifestyle changes
    c. have a BMI over 40
    d. do not have any significant symptoms of sleep apnea

(LO 5.8)   13. Which of the following is a common concern of men about their body image?
    a. Men often want either to lose or gain weight or to add muscle and bulk.
    b. College men are most likely to overestimate their weight.

    c. Men express greater worry about thinness.
    d. Men express more dissatisfaction with their lower rather than their upper bodies.

(LO 5.8)   14. Which of the following is a common concern of women about their body image?
    a. Women express more dissatisfaction with their upper bodies rather than their lower bodies.
    b. College women are more likely to underestimate their weight.
    c. Women express greater worry about thinness.
    d. Women are at a higher risk of suffering from muscle dysmorphia.

(LO 5.9)   15. Which of the following behaviors may signal a potential problem with compulsive overeating?
    a. Relishing every bite and deriving pleasure from food.
    b. Frequently talking about food or refusing to talk about food.
    c. Eating only proteins due to a belief that carbohydrates are fattening.
    d. Being diagnosed with anorexia nervosa.

(LO 5.9)   16. For individuals with _____, food is a threat to their sense of self, identity, and autonomy.
    a. compulsive-eating disorder
    b. binge-eating disorder
    c. bulimia nervosa
    d. anorexia nervosa

Answers to these questions can be found on page 531.

wavebreakmedia/Shutterstock.com

LEARNING OBJECTIVES

After reading this chapter, you should be able to:

6.1 Explain the relationship between the dimensions of health and physical fitness.

6.2 Summarize the health risks of inactivity and the need for physical exercise.

6.3 Outline current physical activity recommendations.

6.4 Discuss the overload, FITT, and reversibility principles of exercise.

6.5 Specify methods to improve cardiovascular fitness.

6.6 Explain the significance of muscular fitness.

6.7 Compare static and dynamic flexibility.

6.8 Summarize the benefits of mind-body approaches to physical fitness and wellness.

6.9 Identify the causes and treatment of low back pain.

6.10 Discuss the nutritional requirements of athletes.

6.11 Specify precautions for preventing exercise-related problems.

WHAT DO YOU THINK?

• What are the dangers of physical inactivity?

• What are the health benefits of physical activity and exercise?

• What would be an ideal workout?

• How can you protect yourself from exercise injuries?

6

Physical Activity and Fitness

As a boy, Trevon never thought about doing anything special to stay physically fit. He could sprint faster, jump higher, and hit a ball harder than any of his friends. In high school, Trevon's life revolved around practices and games. Early in his first year in college, an injury sidelined Trevon. Frustrated that he had to sit out the season, he gave up his rigorous training routine.

Immersed in academics and other activities, Trevon stopped going to the gym or working out on his own. Yet he continued to think of himself as an athlete in excellent physical condition. When Trevon went home for spring break, he joined his younger brothers on a neighborhood basketball court. While he wasn't surprised that his long shots were off, Trevon was amazed by how quickly he got winded. In 15 minutes, he was panting for breath. "Getting old," one of his brothers joked. "Getting soft," the other teased.

Often the college years represent a turning point in physical fitness. Like Trevon, many other students, busy with classes and other commitments, devote less time to physical activity. This pattern often continues throughout life. An estimated 80 percent of adults and adolescents in the United States do not engage in the minimum amount of physical activity recommended for good health.[1] Excess sitting and inactivity have emerged as major threats to health around the world.

Ultimately, you decide how active to be. As you'll see in this chapter, exercise yields immediate rewards: It boosts energy, improves mood, soothes stress, improves sleep, and makes you look and feel better. In the long term, physical activity slows many of the changes associated with chronological aging, lowers the risk of serious chronic illnesses, and extends the lifespan. This chapter can help you reap these rewards. It presents the latest activity recommendations, documents the benefits of exercise, describes types of exercise, and provides guidelines for getting into shape and exercising safely. <

✓**check-in** How active are you:

____ Very

____ Moderately

____ Not very

____ Not at all

The Dangers of Inactivity

One in four adults on the planet is not active enough. According to the World Health Organization (WHO), physical inactivity has become the fourth leading risk factor for global mortality, accounting for about 3.2 million deaths annually.[2] The American College of Sports Medicine calls inactivity "the greatest public health problem of the twenty-first century."

"Sedentary" behavior includes sitting or reclining at work, at home, in school, getting to and from places, travelling in a car or bus, reading, playing cards, talking with friends, watching television, or using a computer or mobile device. "Screen time," whether involving a smartphone, computer, tablet, or television, has contributed to the sedentary lifestyle of many college students, who report from four to more than eight hours of screen time each day.[3]

New research on "the physiology of inactivity" has identified serious risks from "high-volume sitting" (sitting seven or more hours a day) and "prolonged uninterrupted sitting" (sitting for 30 minutes or longer at a time).[4] These include obesity, cardiovascular disease, diabetes, and certain cancers, as well as "all-cause mortality" (dying of any natural cause).[5]

Older adolescents, male adults, men and women over age 60, and people who are overweight or obese spend the most hours per day sitting. Individuals who both sit for long periods and are not physically active—an estimated one in ten Americans—are at highest risk of serious health complications.[6]

✓**check-in** Are you a couch potato? Over the next 3 days, keep track of the number of hours you spend sitting. Make note of periods of more than 30 minutes that you sit without interruption. If you sit for four hours or more a day, especially for prolonged periods without interruption, you qualify as a couch potato—and are at risk for the health complications of a sedentary lifestyle.

The best antidote to excessive sitting: Move! Health professionals suggest five minutes of activity for every 30 minutes of sitting: get up and stretch, walk around, jog in place, climb a flight of stairs. Pace when you're on the phone. Download an app or use an activity tracker to remind you to move. Check out online sites for sharing and getting supportive feedback.

Although brief bursts of activity are beneficial, to counter all the harmful effects of excessive sitting, you need more intense physical activity. The more movement that you build into your schedule, the more you can reduce the risks of a sedentary lifestyle.[7]

Physical Activity and Fitness

Physical activity refers to any movement produced by the muscles that results in expenditure of energy (measured in calories). Short stretches of physical activity, such as taking the stairs or walking several blocks, during the day can be as effective as structured exercise in preventing hypertension and other cardiovascular risk factors and in reducing the risk of premature death.

Fitness is the ability to respond to routine physical demands, with enough reserve energy to cope with a sudden challenge.

You can consider yourself physically fit if you:

- Meet your daily energy needs.
- Can handle unexpected extra demands.
- Are protecting yourself against potential health problems, such as heart disease.

The health-related components of physical fitness are as follows:

- **Cardiorespiratory fitness**, the ability of the heart to pump blood through the body efficiently. It is achieved through aerobic exercise—any activity, such as brisk walking or swimming, in which sufficient or excess oxygen is continually supplied to the body. In other words, aerobic exercise involves working out strenuously without pushing to the point of breathlessness. Cardiovascular fitness in school-aged children and adolescents is a key indicator of both current and future health.[8] In college women, aerobic fitness has proven to be the strongest predictor of healthy body composition.[9]

- **Metabolic fitness**, the optimal functioning of bodily systems, which reduces the risk for diabetes and cardiovascular disease. It can be achieved through a moderate-intensity exercise program, even with little or no improvement in cardiorespiratory fitness.

- **Muscular strength**, the force within muscles, measured by the absolute maximum weight that you can lift, push, or press in one effort. Strong

Making exercise a priority can boost your health and fitness during college and beyond.

Howard Sandler/Shutterstock.com

physical activity Any movement produced by the muscles that results in expenditure of energy.

fitness The ability to respond to routine physical demands, with enough reserve energy to cope with a sudden challenge.

muscles help keep the skeleton in proper alignment, improve posture, prevent back and leg aches, help in everyday lifting, and enhance athletic performance. Muscle mass increases along with strength, which makes for a healthier body composition and a higher metabolic rate.

- **Muscular endurance**, the ability to perform repeated muscular effort, measured by the number of times you can lift, push, or press a given weight. Important for posture, muscular endurance helps in everyday work as well as in athletics and sports.

- **Flexibility**, the range of motion around specific joints—for example, the stretching you do to touch your toes or twist your torso. Flexibility depends on many factors: your age, sex, and posture; how muscular you are; and how much body fat you have.

- **Body composition**, which refers to the relative amounts of fat and lean tissue (bone, muscle, organs, and water) in the body. A high proportion of body fat has serious health implications, including increased incidence of heart disease, high blood pressure, diabetes, stroke, gallbladder problems, back and joint problems, and some forms of cancer.

- **Functional fitness**, which refers to the performance of activities of daily living. Exercises that mimic job tasks or everyday movements can improve balance, coordination, strength, and endurance.

Fitness and the Dimensions of Health

The concept of fitness is evolving. Rather than focusing only on aerobic or strength training, instructors, coaches, and consumers are pursuing a broader vision of total fitness that encompasses every dimension of health:

- **Physical:** Becoming fit reduces your risk of major diseases, increases energy and stamina, and may prolong your life.

- **Emotional:** Fitness lowers tension and anxiety, lifts depression, relieves stress, improves mood, and promotes a positive self-image.

- **Social:** Physical activities provide opportunities to meet new people and to work out with friends or family.

- **Intellectual:** Fit individuals report greater alertness, better concentration, more creativity, and improved personal health habits.

- **Occupational:** Fit employees miss fewer days of work, are more productive, and incur fewer medical costs.

- **Spiritual:** Fitness fosters appreciation for the relationship between body and mind and may lead to greater realization of your potential.

- **Environmental:** Fit individuals often become more aware of their need for healthy air and food and develop a deeper appreciation of the physical world.

✓**check-in** How has your fitness affected the various dimensions of your health?

Working Out on Campus

Here is what we know about students' physical activity and fitness:

- Fewer than half of undergraduates meet the current recommendations for moderate or vigorous exercise (discussed later in this chapter).[10]

- College men are generally more active and more likely to meet recommended physical activity guidelines than women.[11]

- Students who identify as African or African American are equally likely to exercise, although they vary in how often and how intensely they work out.[12]

- Full-time students and those without jobs exercise more than part-time or employed students.

- Undergraduates living on campus are more active than those living off campus.

- Students living in fraternity or sorority housing engage in more exercise than those living in a house or an apartment.

- Single students report more days of vigorous workouts than married, divorced, or separated ones.

✓**check-in** Do you exercise more or less than when you first entered college?

As students progress from their first to fourth year of studies, they exercise less. The most drastic drop in physical activity occurs in the freshman year. As various studies have documented, fitness often declines, and levels of total cholesterol, harmful LDL (low-density lipoprotein) cholesterol, and fasting glucose (blood sugar) levels increase. A drop in exercise frequency and intensity has been identified as a major contributor to unhealthy changes in body composition and fitness.[13]

Various psychosocial factors can influence students' exercise behaviors[14]: Peer pressure to exercise (for men more than women), an exercise partner, a flexible class schedule, access to fitness facilities, stress, even a negative reaction

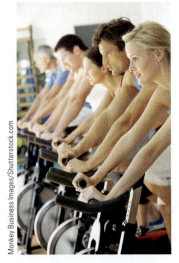

Regular exercise benefits every dimension of health, including physical well-being, self-image, stress level, and social relationships.

cardiorespiratory fitness The ability of the heart and blood vessels to circulate blood through the body efficiently.

metabolic fitness The reduction in risk for diabetes and cardiovascular disease, which can be achieved through a moderate-intensity exercise program.

muscular strength Physical power; the maximum weight one can lift, push, or press in one effort.

muscular endurance The ability to withstand the stress of continued physical exertion.

flexibility The range of motion allowed by one's joints; determined by the length of muscles, tendons, and ligaments attached to the joints.

body composition The relative amounts of fat and lean tissue (bone, muscle, organs, and water) in the body.

functional fitness The ability to perform real-life activities, such as lifting a heavy suitcase.

HEALTH NOW!

Eliminate Exercise Excuses

In your online journal, write down as many reasons as you can think of not to exercise. Then come up with quick excuse busters. Here are some ideas:

I can't afford a gym.

- Who needs a gym? You can get all the exercise you need on your own.
- Check out campus or community facilities.
- Walk or jog outdoors.
- Invest in inexpensive hand weights.

The school gym is always crowded.

- Always? Have you tried Sunday mornings, Friday evening at 7:00, Tuesdays at 3:00 p.m.? Ask the staff what times are quietest.
- If there are lines for the weight machines, use hand weights. If the treadmills are occupied, go to the outdoor track.
- Sign up for small-group training or classes to guarantee yourself a spot.

It's finals week.

- Break up study sessions with mini-workouts.
- Burn off tension with a jog.
- Unwind after studying with stretches, yoga, or Pilates.

I go to my dorm and just don't feel like leaving.

- Arrange to meet friends at the gym. If you know they're waiting, you'll go out even if it's rainy and cold.
- Sign up for a gym class during the day so that you don't have to make an extra trip.
- Recruit an exercise buddy so that the two of you can motivate each other to get moving.

📷 SNAPSHOT: ON CAMPUS NOW

Student Bodies in Motion

College students reported the following behaviors within the past 7 days:

- Do moderate-intensity cardio or aerobic exercise for at least 30 minutes:

	Percent (%)		
	Male	Female	Average
0 days	21.4	21.5	21.7
1–4 days	55.9	59.8	58.6
5–7 days	22.7	18.6	19.8

- Do vigorous-intensity cardio or aerobic exercise for at least 20 minutes:

	Percent (%)		
	Male	Female	Average
0 days	36.1	43.3	41.5
1–2 days	32.0	30.9	31.1
3–7 days	31.9	25.8	27.4

✓**check-in** Did you engage in moderate-intensity aerobic exercise for at least 30 minutes in the past seven days? Or did you exercise vigorously for at least 20 minutes? How often do you exercise? Are you in better shape now than you were a year ago? Would you like to improve your fitness? Record your feelings on your fitness today and in the past in your online journal.

Source: American College Health Association. American College Health Association-National College Health Assessment II: Reference Group Executive Summary Spring 2018. Silver Spring, MD: American College Health Association, 2018.

to Facebook posts all increase physical activity.[15] "Screen" time—whether with a mobile device, computer, or television—also has an impact on activity. Researchers describe college students who use smart phones from four to eight hours a day but also engage in some physical exertion as "active couch potatoes."[16]

✓**check-in** Did you know that trading 2 minutes of sitting for 2 minutes of walking every hour can cut your risk of premature death by one-third? Short bursts of activity—walking, going up and down stairs, doing household chores—can boost the longevity of sedentary individuals, according to researchers.[17]

Physical Activity and Exercise

Exercise refers to physical activity that requires planned, structured, and repetitive bodily movement with the intent of improving one or more components of physical fitness. If exercise could be packed into a pill, it would be the single most widely prescribed and beneficial medicine in the nation. Why? Because nothing can do more to help your body function at its best.

As hundreds of studies over the past few decades have documented, exercise is a powerful medicine.[18]

✓**check-in** What can exercise do for you?

- Cut your risk of dying of breast cancer by about 50 percent.
- Lower your risk of colon cancer by 60 percent.
- Reduce your risk of Alzheimer's by about 40 percent.
- Decrease your risk of heart disease and high blood pressure by about 40 percent
- Lower your risk of stroke by 27 percent.
- Reduce the likelihood of gestational diabetes in pregnant women.[19]

The Benefits of Exercise

The benefits of exercise start *now*—with both immediate and long-term effects. Physical fitness early in life lowers your risk of cardiovascular disease, diabetes, and psychiatric and neurological disorders, including depression and dementia, as you grow older.[20]

Regular physical activity can reduce the risk of more than 25 chronic medical conditions by 20 to 30 percent.[21] The reason may be that people who exercise, compared to those who don't, have different proteins moving through their bloodstreams and working together. Their activity may explain the complex process by which workouts lead to wellness.[22] As Figure 6.1 illustrates, exercise provides head-to-toe benefits, including the following:

- You may remain healthier, avoid chronic diseases, and live longer.
- Your heart muscles become stronger and pump blood more efficiently.
- Your heart rate and resting pulse slow down.
- Your blood pressure may drop slightly from its normal level.
- Your risk of a heart attack and of dying of heart disease declines.
- Your bones become denser, and the loss of calcium that normally occurs with age slows.

Longer and Healthier Life
In various studies, physical activity increased life expectancy by 1.3 to 5.5 years.[23] Aerobic activities, such as jogging, may make us biologically younger by extending telomeres, the tiny tips of our chromosomes that protect our DNA from damage but that tend to shorten and fray as cells age.[24]

The number of years you may be able to add to your life depends on your sex, age, and activity level. If you are a white, active or somewhat active 20-year-old man, your estimated life expectancy would be about 2.4 years longer than that of your inactive peers. If you are a black, active or somewhat active 20-year-old woman, you could gain an extra 5.5 years.

You can also improve the quality of life as you get older. According to a systematic review of recent studies, aerobic training improves cardiovascular, metabolic, and cognitive well-being. Exercise may also help reduce falls and slow the cognitive decline of older adults with Alzheimer's disease or other forms of dementia.[25]

✓**check-in** Did you know that for each hour you work out, you gain extra hours of life?

Even minutes count. A mere 10 minutes of daily physical activity may increase lifespans in adults by almost 2 years—even in those who are overweight.

Healthier Heart and Blood Vessels
Sedentary people are about twice as likely to die of a heart attack as people who are physically active. Although rigorous exercise somewhat increases the risk of sudden cardiac death for men, regular physical activity lowers the overall danger, especially in women.

Aerobic exercise lowers levels of the indicators of increased risk of heart disease, such as high cholesterol. Exercise itself, even without weight loss, may reduce dangerous blood fats in obese individuals. It also reduces the risk of developing the prediabetic condition called metabolic syndrome, which, if untreated, can lead to type 2 diabetes and increase the risk of heart disease. Two sessions of resistance training, for a total of an hour a week, can lower the risk of heart attacks, strokes, and death by about 50 percent.[26] Combining aerobic and resistance workouts has proven even more beneficial than either type of exercise alone.[27]

Healthier Lungs
In addition to its effects on the heart, exercise makes the lungs more efficient. The lungs take in more oxygen, and their vital capacity (the maximum amount of air volume the lungs can take in and expel) increases, providing more energy for you to use.

Cardiorespiratory fitness declines more rapidly after age 45, but exercising regularly, maintaining a healthy weight, and not smoking can help maintain cardiorespiratory health throughout life.

exercise A type of physical activity that requires planned, structured, and repetitive bodily movement with the intent of improving one or more components of physical fitness.

Health Benefits Associated with Regular Physical Activity

- Lower risk of all-cause mortality
- Lower risk of cardiovascular disease mortality
- Lower risk of heart disease and stroke
- Lower risk of hypertension
- Lower risk of type 2 diabetes
- Lower risk of adverse blood lipids (fats) profile
- Lower risk of cancer of the bladder, breast, colon, endometrium, esophagus, kidney, lung, and stomach
- Improved cognition
- Reduced risk of dementia, including Alzheimer's disease
- Improved quality of life
- Reduced anxiety
- Reduced risk of depression
- Improved sleep
- Slowed or reduced weight gain
- Weight loss, particularly when combined with reduced calorie intake
- Prevention of weight regain after initial weight loss
- Improved bone health
- Improved physical function
- Lower risk of falls and fall-related injuries (older adults)

New Evidence

- Reduced risk of cancer at additional sites
- Brain health benefits, including improved cognitive function, reduced anxiety and depression risk, improved sleep, and quality of life
- For pregnant women, reduced risk of excessive weight gain, gestational diabetes, and postpartum depression
- For people with various chronic conditions, reduced risk of dying, enhanced function, and improved quality of life

Source: U.S. Department of Health and Human Services, *Physical Activity Guidelines for Americans,* https://www.hhs.gov/fitness/be-active/physical-activity-guidelines-for-americans/index.html.

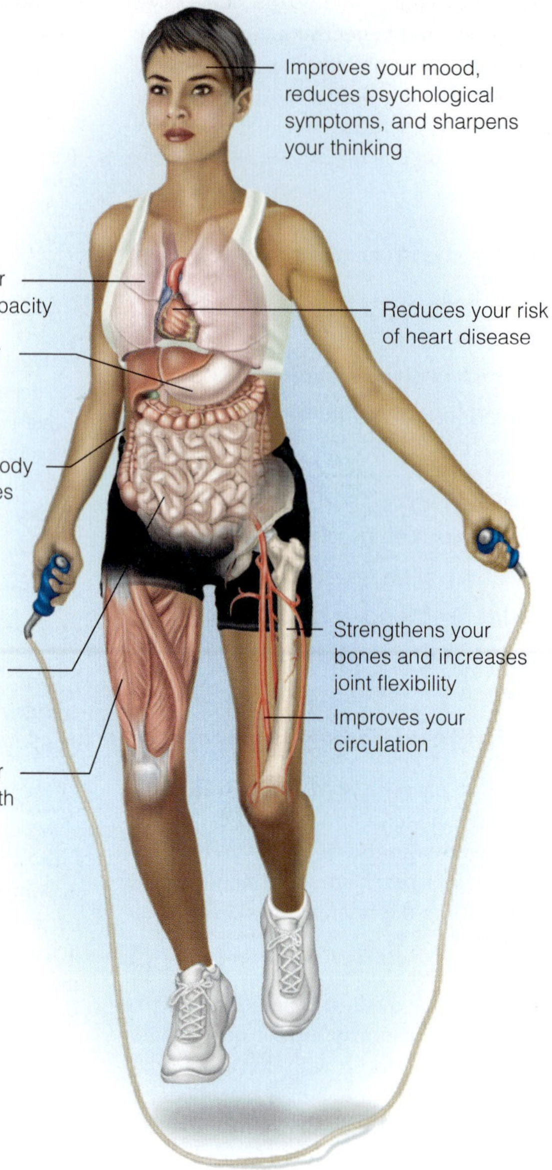

Improves your mood, reduces psychological symptoms, and sharpens your thinking

Increases your respiratory capacity

Reduces your risk of heart disease

Improves your digestion and your fat metabolism

Lowers your body fat and reduces your weight

Strengthens your bones and increases joint flexibility

Improves your circulation

Reduces the risk of several cancers

Increases your muscle strength and tone

FIGURE 6.1 The Benefits of Exercise

Regular physical activity enhances your overall physical and mental health and helps prevent disease.

Even individuals with a genetic predisposition to cardiovascular disease can improve their cardiorespiratory fitness.

Protection against Cancer Physical activity may reduce the risk of several cancers, including breast, colon, endometrial, prostate, and possibly pancreatic as well as non-Hodgkin's lymphoma.[28] In addition to helping maintain a healthy body weight, exercise may help prevent cancer by regulating sex hormones, insulin, and prostaglandins and by enhancing the immune system.

According to the American Institute for Cancer Research, physical activity may lower the risk of colon cancer by 40 to 50 percent; the risk of breast, endometrial, and lung cancers by 30 to 40 percent; and the risk of prostate cancer by 10 to 30 percent. The combination of excess weight and physical inactivity may account for one-quarter to one-third of all breast cancer cases. Regular, lifelong exercise may lower a woman's breast cancer risk by 20 percent, possibly by reducing weight and body mass and preventing metabolic syndrome and chronic inflammation (discussed in Chapter 12). Men who regularly get moderate exercise may have a lower risk of prostate cancer; those who do get the disease are less likely to have aggressive, fast-growing tumors.

Better Bones

You may think that weak, brittle bones are a problem only for older adults. However, 2 percent of college-age women have osteoporosis; another 15 percent have already sustained significant losses in bone density and are at high risk for osteoporosis.

The college women at greatest risk often are extremely skinny and maintain their low weights by dieting (often not eating calcium-rich dairy products) and by avoiding exercise so as not to increase their muscle mass. Depo-Provera, a method of birth control that consists of hormone injections every 3 months, is also associated with low bone density, especially with long-term use.

✓**check-in** Do you know the best exercises to boost bone density?

According to a study of college women, high-impact aerobics, such as Zumba, may offer the quickest route to building bone. Resistance exercises such as squats, leg presses, and calf presses were found to strengthen leg muscles but to have no effect on bone density. The American College of Sports Medicine (ACSM) recommends moderate- to high-intensity weight-bearing activities to maintain bone mass in adults.

Lower Weight

According to the ACSM's statement on "appropriate physical activity intervention strategies for weight loss and prevention of weight regain," long-term weight loss requires 150 or more minutes (2 hours and 30 minutes) of moderately intense physical activity per week. Less exercise can prevent a gain greater than 3 percent of current weight but provides what the ACSM describes as "only modest" weight loss. In addition to aerobic workouts, the ACSM recommends resistance training to increase lean tissue and decrease fat.

For individuals on a diet, exercise provides extra benefits: Dieters who work out lose more fat than lean muscle tissue, which improves their body composition. Exercise may also help to control weight by suppressing appetite.

Better Mental Health and Functioning

Exercise is an effective—but underused—treatment for mild to moderate depression and may help in treating other mental disorders. Regular, moderate exercise—such as walking, running, or lifting weights—three times a week has proved as effective as medication in improving mood and beneficial for depression and anxiety

disorders, including panic attacks.[29] Exercise also helps prevent relapse.

Exercise, particularly long-duration aerobic workouts, may improve certain cognitive skills, such as multitasking and concentration.[30] Lifelong fitness also may preserve brain health as we age. According to numerous long-term studies, physically fit adults perform better on cognitive tests than their less fit peers. Exercise may protect the aging brain by means of increased blood flow, improved development and survival of neurons, and decreased risk of heart and blood vessel diseases.[31] The combination of physical fitness and a healthy body mass index (BMI) may lower the risk of stroke.[32]

Benefits for Students

Unlike middle-aged and older individuals, traditional-age college students cite improved fitness as the number one advantage that exercise offers, followed by improved appearance and muscle tone. Your brain may also benefit. Strong cardiorespiratory fitness in young adulthood is associated with higher intelligence, better grades, and greater success in life. The reasons may be improved blood flow to the brain, diminished anxiety, enhanced mood, and less fatigue.

Taking this course may in itself change your attitude toward fitness and healthy behaviors. In a recent study, students enrolled in a health and fitness course, who were already active and fit, did not necessarily increase their workouts.[33] However, their attitudes shifted from extrinsic motivators (such as looking good) to internal ones (enjoyment).

✓**check-in** Has this course affected your attitude toward exercise? If so, how?

Brighter Mood and Less Stress

As a multinational study recently demonstrated, physical activity produces an unexpected positive psychological benefit: happiness. Compared to sedentary individuals, active people report higher levels of happiness—from 20 to 52 percent higher, depending on the exercise "dose." For men, vigorous exercise yielded the greatest happiness dividends; for women, moderate-intensity activities such as walking were most likely to boost their moods.[34]

Exercise makes people feel good from the inside out in various ways, including:

- Boosting mood.
- Elevating self-esteem.
- Increasing energy.
- Reducing tension.
- Relieving stress.
- Improving concentration and alertness.

During long workouts, some people experience what is called "runner's high," which may be the result of increased levels of mood-elevating brain chemicals called endorphins. Psychological improvements occur even after a 20-minute bout of exercise, regardless of how intensely you work out. Exercise also may be beneficial as an adjunctive treatment for substance use disorders.[35] In a study of healthy young adults ages 18 to 29 years, aerobic fitness boosted both cardiovascular and neurocognitive functions, enhancing their cognitive abilities.[36]

✓check-in Don't worry: Get active—and happy! Tune into your mood before and after you engage in different activities. Do you feel happier after a bicycle ride or a run? A swim or a stretch class? Men and women of various ages in different countries report different responses, but around the world, moving makes people happier than staying still.

A More Active and Healthy Old Age

Exercise slows the changes that are associated with advancing age: loss of lean muscle tissue, increase in body fat, and decrease in work capacity. In addition to lowering the risk of heart disease and stroke, exercise helps older men and women retain the strength and mobility needed to live independently. Studies that followed competitive runners, cyclists, and swimmers for four decades found little evidence of deterioration in their musculature.

In a longitudinal study of mainly white, highly educated adults, those who were physically fit in middle age showed a lower risk of dementia later in life. Other research has shown that remaining physically active as you age may help protect parts of the brain related to memory and thinking from shrinking. Exercise increases the size of brain regions involved in balance and coordination, which in the long term could reduce the risk of falls in older individuals, including those with dementia.[37]

Enhanced Sexuality

By improving physical endurance, muscle tone, blood flow, and body composition, exercise improves sexual functioning. Simply burning 200 extra calories a day can significantly lower the risk of erectile dysfunction in sedentary men. Exercise may also increase sexual drive, activity, and sexual satisfaction in people of all ages.

More exercise may mean better sex—at least for men. In a recent study, men who engaged in the equivalent of 2 hours of strenuous exercise, 3.5 hours of moderate exercise, or 6 hours of light exercise a week reported enhanced sexual function, including the ability to have erections and orgasms and the quality and frequency of erections.[38]

Exercise Risks

Despite its many benefits, exercise can pose risks—and not just for those over age 40. According to the "extreme exercise hypothesis," high-volume and/or high-intensity exercise may trigger harmful cardiovascular events in individuals with underlying and unrecognized coronary artery disease.[39] Even young college athletes who seem in perfect health have collapsed and died while running and while playing sports such as football and basketball.

The most common cause is hypertrophic cardiomyopathy (HCM), a genetic disease that results in thickening or enlargement of the heart that affects up to 1 in 500 people. HCM accounts for 40 percent of all deaths on athletic fields in the United States. An average of 66 athletes younger than age 40 die each year from cardiac arrest in the United States. HCM can be detected and treated.[40] Medical experts are urging colleges to consider screening for all student athletes as well as to develop a protocol for emergency resuscitation in case of cardiac arrest.

College students who play contact sports such as football may be at risk of a condition called chronic traumatic encephalopathy (CTE), the result of multiple mild head injuries. Initial symptoms include headache and impaired concentration. As the condition worsens, sufferers may face depression, outbursts of anger, short-term memory loss, and difficulty thinking and making decisions. The most severe forms can cause dementia, aggression, and difficulty finding words.[41]

✓check-in If you are a college athlete, what steps are you taking to protect your long-term health?

Physical Activity Guidelines for Americans

The U.S. Department of Health and Human Services' *Physical Activity Guidelines for Americans*, based on the most significant research findings on the health benefits of physical activity, recognize that some activity is better than none. However, the most recent Guidelines emphasize that more activity—consisting of both aerobic (endurance) and muscle-strengthening (resistance) physical activity—is more beneficial.[42] It's never too soon to start. The most recent *Guidelines* encourage children ages 3 to 5 to engage in active play—about three hours—every day.[43] Exercise may also help to reduce falls and slow the cognitive decline of older adults with Alzheimer's disease or other forms of dementia.[44]

The Guidelines recommend various types of exercise, including:

- **Moderate-intensity physical activity,** such as brisk walking, swimming, or bicycling, increases a person's heart rate and breathing to some extent. Relative to a person's capacity, moderate-intensity activity would be 5 or 6 on a 0-to-10 scale of working to capacity.

- **Vigorous-intensity physical activity** greatly increases a person's heart rate and breathing, usually a 7 or 8 on a 0-to-10 scale. Examples include jogging, singles tennis, swimming continuous laps, and biking uphill.

- **Muscle-strengthening activity,** such as strength training, resistance training, and muscular strength and endurance exercises, increase skeletal muscle strength, power, endurance, and mass.

- **Bone-strengthening or weight-bearing activity,** such as running, jumping rope, and lifting weights, exerts a force on the bones, which promotes bone growth or strength.

- **Balance activities** improve the ability to resist forces within or outside the body that could cause falls while a person is stationary or moving. Strengthening muscles of the back, abdomen, and legs also improves balance.

- **Multicomponent physical activity** includes more than one type of physical activity, such as aerobic, muscle-strengthening, and balance training. Examples include some dancing and sports.

Here are the government's key recommendations:[45]

- Move more and sit less throughout the day. Some physical activity is better than none. Adults who do any amount of moderate-to-vigorous physical activity gain some health benefits.

- For substantial health benefits, **adults should do at least 150 minutes (2 hours and 30 minutes) a week of moderate-intensity or 75 minutes (1 hour and 15 minutes) a week of vigorous-intensity aerobic physical activity** or an equivalent combination of moderate- and vigorous-intensity aerobic activity. The ACSM recommends episodes lasting at least 10 minutes. However, new studies have found that physical activity for periods

TABLE 6.1 Exercise Options

Vigorous activities take more effort than moderate ones. Here are just a few moderate and vigorous aerobic physical activities. Do these for 10 minutes or more at a time.

Moderate Activities	Vigorous Activities
(I can talk while I do them, but I can't sing.)	(I can only say a few words without stopping to catch my breath.)
• Ballroom and line dancing	• Aerobic dance
• Biking on level ground or with few hills	• Biking faster than 10 miles per hour
• Canoeing	• Fast dancing
• General gardening (raking and trimming shrubs)	• Heavy gardening (digging and hoeing)
• Sports where you catch and throw (baseball, softball and volleyball)	• Hiking uphill
• Tennis (doubles)	• Jumping rope
• Using your manual wheelchair	• Martial arts (such as karate)
• Using hand cyclers—also called ergometers	• Race walking, jogging, or running
• Walking briskly	• Sports with a lot of running (basketball and soccer)
• Water aerobics	• Swimming fast or swimming laps
	• Tennis (singles)
	• Zumba

Sean Nel/Shutterstock.com

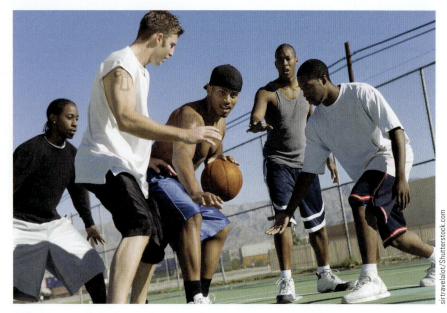

Group sports provide a fun alternative way to exercise, but an occasional game is no substitute for regular physical activity.

even briefer than 10 minutes may influence cardiometabolic risk.

- For additional and more extensive health benefits, **adults should increase their aerobic physical activity to 300 minutes (5 hours)** a week of moderate-intensity or 150 minutes a week of vigorous-intensity aerobic physical activity or an equivalent combination of moderate- and vigorous-intensity activity. Additional health benefits are gained by engaging in physical activity beyond this amount.

- Adults should also do **muscle-strengthening activities** that are moderate or high intensity and involve all major muscle groups **on 2 or more days a week,** as these activities provide additional health benefits.

Other health organizations recommend the following guidelines for average adults to improve health and reduce the risk of chronic disease:

- Moderately intense cardiorespiratory exercise 30 minutes a day, 5 days a week

or

- Vigorously intense cardiorespiratory exercise 20 minutes a day, 3 days a week

and

- 8 to 10 strength-training exercises, with 8 to 12 repetitions of each exercise, twice a week.

Although official guidelines call for a minimum of 150 minutes of moderate-to-vigorous-intensity physical activity per week, working at less than 50 percent of the recommended levels can lead to health benefits—particularly for sedentary individuals and/or those with a chronic medical condition.[45]

✓**check-in** Do you exercise often and intensely enough to meet these guidelines?

Your Exercise Prescription

For years, exercise has had what some call a "Goldilocks problem," with endless debate over how much is too much, too little, or just about the right amount. A large-scale, 14-year study of more than 661,000 people[46] produced some answers, including the following:

- Individuals who didn't exercise at all were at greatest risk of many diseases as well as of early death. Even a little exercise helped lower the likelihood of premature death.

- Individuals who got the recommended minimum of 150 minutes of moderate exercise per week significantly reduced their risk of dying (by 31 percent over a 14-year period) compared to those who didn't exercise.

- Individuals who tripled the recommended level of exercise, working out moderately (generally by walking) for 450 minutes per week (a little more than an hour per day), were even less likely to die prematurely.

- Those who engaged in 10 or more times the recommended amount of exercise did not gain any greater health benefits—but they also did not increase their risk of dying young.

The Principles of Exercise

Your body is literally what you make of it. Superbly designed for multiple uses, it adjusts to meet physical demands. If you need to sprint for a bus, your heart will speed up and pump more blood. Beyond such immediate, short-term adaptations, physical training can produce long-term changes in heart rate, oxygen consumption, and muscle strength and endurance. Although there are limits on the maximum levels of physical fitness and performance that any individual can achieve, regular exercise can produce improvements in everyone's baseline wellness and fitness.

The following principles of exercise are fundamental to any physical activity plan: the overload principle, frequency, intensity, time and type (FITT), and the reversibility principle.

Overload Principle

The **overload principle** requires a person exercising to provide a greater stress or demand on the body than it's usually accustomed to handling. For any muscle, including the heart, to get stronger, it must work against a greater-than-normal resistance or challenge. To continue to improve, you need further increases in the demands—but not too much too quickly. **Progressive overloading**—gradually increasing physical challenges—provides the benefits of exercise without the risk of injuries (Figure 6.2).

Overloading is specific to each body part and to each component of fitness. Leg exercises develop only the lower limbs; arm exercises, only the upper limbs. This is why you need a comprehensive fitness plan that includes a variety of exercises to develop different parts of the body. If you play a particular sport, you also need training to develop sports-specific skills, such as a strong, efficient stroke in swimming.

✓**check-in** Does your fitness program include exercises for different parts of the body?

FITT

Although low-intensity activity can enhance basic health, you need to work harder—that is, at a greater intensity—to improve fitness. Whatever exercise you do, there is a level, or threshold, at which fitness begins to improve; a target zone, where you can achieve maximum benefits; and an upper limit, at which potential risks outweigh any further benefits. The acronym FITT sums up the four dimensions of progressive overload: *frequency* (how often you exercise), *intensity* (how hard), *time* (how long), and *type* (specific activity).

Frequency   To attain and maintain physical fitness, you need to exercise regularly, but the recommended frequency varies with different types of exercise and with an individual's fitness goals. Health officials urge Americans to engage in moderate-intensity aerobic activity most days and in resistance and flexibility training 2 or 3 days a week. Recent research suggests that the health benefits of exercising one or two days a week are similar to those of working out three or more days a week. Even a single exercise session can make a difference, temporarily lowering blood pressure and improving blood fat levels and insulin sensitivity.[47]

Intensity   Exercise intensity varies with the type of exercise and with personal goals. To improve cardiorespiratory fitness, you need at a minimum to increase your heart rate to a target zone (the level that produces benefits). To develop muscular strength and endurance, you need to increase the amount of weight you lift or the resistance you work against and/or the number of repetitions. For enhanced flexibility, you need to stretch muscles beyond their normal length.

Time (Duration)   The amount of time, or duration, of your workouts is also important, particularly for cardiorespiratory exercise. The ACSM recommends 30 to 45 minutes of aerobic exercise, preceded by 5 to 10 minutes of warm-up and followed by 5 to 10 minutes of stretching. However, experts have found similar health benefits from a single 30-minute session of moderate exercise as from several shorter sessions throughout the day. Duration and intensity are interlinked. If you're exercising at high intensity (biking or running at a brisk pace, for instance), you don't need to exercise as long as when you're working at lower intensity (walking or swimming at a moderate pace). For muscular strength and endurance and for flexibility, duration is defined by the number of sets or repetitions rather than total time.

Type (Specificity)   The specificity principle refers to the body's adaptation to a particular type of activity or amount of stress placed on it.

overload principle The idea that for the body to get stronger, you must provide a greater stress or demand on the body than it is normally accustomed to handling.

progressive overloading Gradually increasing physical challenges once the body adapts to the stress placed upon it to produce maximum benefits.

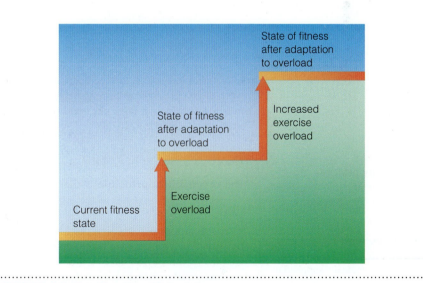

FIGURE 6.2 The Overload Principle

By increasing frequency, intensity, or duration, you will improve your level of fitness. Once your body adapts to (becomes comfortable with) the demands, you can again apply the overload principle to achieve a higher level of fitness.

Fitness Monitors

Millions of people have embraced the latest fitness fad: "wearable" mobile devices, including activity trackers, heart rate monitors, and apps for smartwatches and smartphones. Their features range from simple step-counting to sophisticated measures of speed, distance, and heart rate that analyze, track, and transmit data to a smartphone, laptop, or computer.

Do you need any of these to get or stay in shape? No, you can still rely on low-tech or no-tech approaches such as the exertion scale (page 159). But if you are intrigued by the new generation of exercise aids, here are some things to consider.

Facts to Know

The advantages of mobile trackers include:

- Increased awareness of habits, such as how sedentary or active you are.
- Immediate access to feedback, such as calories burned.
- Greater motivation to reach fitness goals, such as 10,000 steps a day.

Disadvantages include:

- Cost (most require a smartphone and a sufficient Wi-Fi data plan).
- Technical problems and malfunctions.
- Inaccurate results because of sweat, rain, or cold.

- Skin reactions, such as a red, itchy rash.
- Lack of rigorous scientific evidence demonstrating the value of self-monitoring over time.
- A high dropout rate, with as many as one-third to one-half of exercisers abandoning their mobile devices within months.

Steps to Take

- Choose a tracking device based on your individual needs. If you're simply counting steps, you don't need to pay for fancier features. If you want to monitor your sleep as well as your daytime activities, make sure the device is comfortable enough to wear 24/7.
- Don't substitute a mobile health (mHealth) device for a consultation with a health professional. It's easy to misinterpret data as a sign either that something is wrong when it isn't or that something is normal when it's not.
- Beware of becoming so focused on the data that you lose sight of the bigger picture. It's not worth dashing up and down the stairs late at night to reach your daily steps goal if the workout makes it harder for you to fall asleep.

Improving Cardiorespiratory Fitness

Cardiorespiratory endurance refers to the ability of the heart, lungs, and circulatory system to deliver oxygen to muscles working rhythmically over an extended period of time. Unlike muscular endurance (discussed later in this chapter), which is specific to individual muscles, cardiorespiratory endurance involves the entire body and can be aerobic or anaerobic.

- **Aerobic exercise**, which improves cardiorespiratory endurance, can take many forms, but all involve working strenuously without pushing to the point of breathlessness. A person who builds up good aerobic capacity can maintain long periods of physical activity without great fatigue.

- In **anaerobic exercise**, the amount of oxygen taken in by the body cannot meet the demands of the activity. This quickly creates an oxygen deficit that must be made up later. Anaerobic activities are high in intensity but short in duration, usually lasting only about 10 seconds to 2 minutes. An example is sprinting the quarter-mile, which leaves even the best-trained athletes gasping for air. In *nonaerobic exercise*, such as bowling, softball, or doubles tennis, there is frequent rest between activities. Because the body can take in all the oxygen it needs, the heart and lungs don't get much of a workout.

---

reversibility principle The idea that the physical benefits of exercise are lost through disuse or inactivity.

aerobic exercise Physical activity in which sufficient or excess oxygen is continually supplied to the body.

anaerobic exercise Physical activity in which the body develops an oxygen deficit.

Jogging, for instance, trains the heart and lungs to work more efficiently and strengthens certain leg muscles. However, it does not build upper-body strength or enhance flexibility.

Reversibility Principle

The **reversibility principle** is the opposite of the overload principle. Just as the body adapts to greater physical demands, it also adjusts to lower levels. If you stop exercising, you can lose as much as 50 percent of your fitness improvements within 2 months. If you have to curtail your usual exercise routine because of a busy schedule, you can best maintain your fitness by keeping the intensity constant and reducing frequency or duration. The principle of reversibility is aptly summed up by the phrase "Use it or lose it."

Monitoring Exercise Intensity

High-Tech Gadgets

Millions of people have bought fitness trackers and activity apps for smartphones and smartwatches. Despite the popularity of these devices, scientists have questioned their accuracy and usefulness.[48] In one recent study, various physical activity trackers either over- or underestimated energy expenditures during everyday activities such as housework as well as during workouts, although most proved to be as accurate as pedometers in counting steps.[49] (See the Consumer Alert feature in this chapter.)

In a study of college students, fitness trackers did not lead to a significant change in step count over 12 weeks. However, when utilized as part of a wellness course, there were some increases in knowledge and perception of wellness.[50]

✓check-in: **Have** you tried using a fitness tracker? If so, did it affect your exercise program?

Wearable activity monitors include the following:

- **Pedometers.** A pedometer, the classic in the field, uses a pendulum-based unit to count steps and translate them into miles. The new generation of advanced pedometers can calculate the number of calories burned, record several days of data, and download this information to your computer for analysis. The simplest, cheapest pedometers provide only estimates based on your average rather than actual step or stride.

- **Activity trackers.** Wearable trackers such as a Fitbit use an accelerometer, widely considered the most accurate and reliable step-counting mechanism. Most wristband models are so comfortable you can wear them around the clock to monitor your sleep as well as your waking activities. You can use waterproof models in the pool or shower. Many connect wirelessly to a smartphone or tablet and include a mobile app that tracks your progress toward your targets and allows you to share your data with others.

- **Smartwatches.** Available from Apple, Samsung, and other manufacturers, these offer sophisticated tracking of activity and exercise. Many provide a stopwatch, countdown timers, heart-rate monitoring, calorie consumption, and a training log. Most are sturdy and water-resistant. The top models are expensive, so compare the prices and features carefully before investing.

✓check-in Do you use an app or mobile tracker to monitor your daily activity?
If so, what do you like or dislike about it?
Has it had an impact on your behavior?

Nontech Methods

For a no-tech approach, you can use your pulse, or heart rate, as a guide. Here's how:

- Slightly tilt your head back and to one side.
- Use your middle finger or forefinger, or both, to feel for your pulse in the carotid artery in your neck. (Do not use your thumb; it has a beat of its own.)

- To determine your heart rate, count the number of pulses you feel for 10 seconds and multiply that number by 6, or count for 30 seconds and multiply that number by 2.

- Learn to recognize the pulsing of your heart when you're sitting or lying down. This is your resting heart rate.

Start taking your pulse during or immediately after exercise, when it's much more pronounced than when you're at rest. Three minutes after heavy exercise, take your pulse again. The closer that reading is to your resting heart rate, the better your condition. If it takes a long time for your pulse to recover and return to its resting level, your body's ability to handle physical stress is poor. As you continue working out, however, your pulse will return to normal much more quickly.

Target Heart Rate You don't want to push yourself to your maximum heart rate. The ACSM recommends working at 50 to 85 percent, depending on your level of fitness, of that maximum to get cardiorespiratory benefits from your training. This range is called your target heart rate. If you don't exercise intensely enough to raise your heart rate at least this high, your heart and lungs won't reap the most benefit from the workout. If you push too hard and exercise at or near your absolute maximum heart rate, you run the risk of placing too great a burden on your heart.

To find the best "zone" for your goals and activity, you must first know how to calculate your maximum heart rate. The following formula offers a rough baseline:

$$220 - \text{Age} = \text{Maximum heart rate (MHR)}$$

The ACSM recommends that for endurance training and general aerobic conditioning, you calculate 50 to 65 percent of your maximum heart rate if you're a beginner; 60 to 75 percent for intermediate-level exercisers; and 70 to 85 percent for established aerobic exercisers. For example, if you're a 45-year-old beginner with no known health issues, your maximum heart rate is approximately 175 beats a minute. Fifty to 65 percent of that maximum is 87 to 113 beats per minute.

Young men tend to have a lower resting heart rate and a higher peak heart rate than women. Men's heart rates also rise more dramatically during exercise and return to normal more quickly.

Your heart rate can also help you keep tabs on your progress: Measure your heart rate 15 to 60 minutes after exercising and compare these numbers over time as you get in better shape. The numbers decrease as your heart becomes stronger.

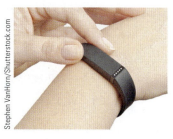

Stephen VanHorn/Shutterstock.com

A lightweight wrist monitor allows you to track your physical activity throughout the day.

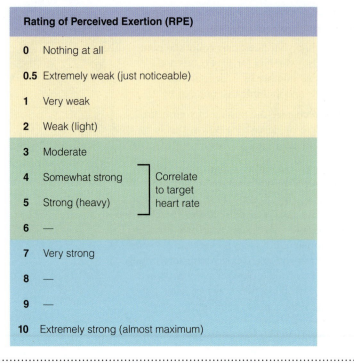

Rating of Perceived Exertion (RPE)	
0	Nothing at all
0.5	Extremely weak (just noticeable)
1	Very weak
2	Weak (light)
3	Moderate
4	Somewhat strong
5	Strong (heavy)
6	—
7	Very strong
8	—
9	—
10	Extremely strong (almost maximum)

4 Somewhat strong / 5 Strong (heavy) — Correlate to target heart rate

FIGURE 6.3 Revised Scale for Rating of Perceived Exertion (RPE)
You can learn to rate your exertion based on this scale.

Source: Original scale from Borg G, Psychophysical bases of perceived exertion. Medicine and Science in Sports and Exercise. 2003;14(5):377–81.

The Karvonen Formula The Karvonen formula is another mathematical formula for determining your target heart rate (HR) training zone. The formula uses maximum and resting heart rate with the desired training intensity to get a target heart rate.

Ideally, you should measure your resting and maximum heart rates for more accurate results. If the maximum heart rate cannot be measured directly, it can be estimated roughly using the traditional formula of 220 minus your age. You can also use an average value of 70 bpm (beats per minute) for your resting heart rate.

For example, if you are a 25-year-old male who has been exercising regularly, with a resting heart rate of 65, you would calculate your training heart rate for the intensity level of 70 percent, using the following formula:

$$220 - 25 \text{ (age)} = 195$$
$$195 - 65 \text{ (resting heart rate)} = 130$$
$$130 \times 0.70 \text{ (percent of maximum)} + 65 \text{ (resting}$$
$$\text{heart rate)} = 156 \text{ beats per minute}$$

Rating of Perceived Exertion Another option besides heart rate for monitoring your exercise intensity is the **rating of perceived exertion (RPE)**, a self-assessment scale that rates symptoms of breathlessness and fatigue.

rating of perceived exertion (RPE) A selfassessment cale that rates symptoms of breathlessness and fatigue.

You can use the RPE scale to describe your sensation of effort when exercising and gauge how hard you are working. The ACSM revised the original RPE scale to a range of 0 to 10 (Figure 6.3). Most exercisers should aim for a perceived exertion of "somewhat strong" or "strong," the equivalent of 4 or 5 on the RPE scale.

RPE is considered fairly reliable, but about 10 percent of the population tends to over- or underestimate their exertion. Your health or physical education instructor can help you learn to match what your body is feeling to the RPE scale. By paying attention to how you feel at different exercise intensities, you can learn to challenge yourself without risking your safety.

Designing an Aerobic Workout

Whatever activity you choose, your aerobic workout should consist of several stages: a warm-up, an aerobic activity, and a cooldown (Figure 6.4).

Warm-up Just as you don't get in your car and immediately gun your engine to 60 miles per hour, you shouldn't do the same with your body. You need to prepare your cardiorespiratory system for a workout, speed up the blood flow to your lungs, and increase the temperature and elasticity of your muscles and connective tissue to avoid injury. After reviewing more than 350 scientific studies, the ACSM concluded that preparing for sports or exercise should involve a variety of activities and not be limited to stretching alone. Researchers found little to no relationship between stretching and injuries or postexercise pain. A better option is a combination of warm up, strength training, and balance exercises.

✓**check-in** How do you warm up before exercising?

Aerobic Activity The two key components of this part of your workout are intensity and duration. As described in the previous section, you can use your target heart rate range to make sure you are working at the proper intensity. The current recommendation is to keep moving for 30 to 60 minutes, either in one session or several briefer sessions, each lasting at least 10 minutes.

Cooldown After you've pushed your heart rate up to its target level and kept it there for a while, the worst thing you can do is slam on the brakes. If you come to a sudden stop, you put your heart at risk. When you stand or sit immediately after vigorous exercise, blood can pool in

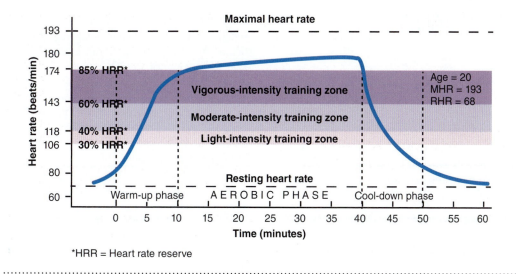

*HRR = Heart rate reserve

FIGURE 6.4 Recommended Cardiorespiratory or Aerobic Training Pattern

your legs. You need to keep moving at a slower pace to ensure an adequate supply of blood to your heart. Ideally, you should walk for 5 to 10 minutes at a comfortable pace before you end your workout session.

Your Long-Term Fitness Plan

One of the most common mistakes people make is to push too hard too fast. Often they end up injured or discouraged and quit entirely. If you are just starting an aerobic program, think of it as a series of phases: beginning, progression, and maintenance:

- **Beginning (4–6 weeks).** Start slow and low (in intensity). If you're walking, monitor your heart rate and aim for 55 percent of your maximum heart rate. Another good rule of thumb to make sure you're moving at the right pace: If you can sing as you walk, you're going too slow; if you can't talk, you're going too fast.

- **Progression (16–20 weeks).** Gradually increase the duration and/or intensity of your workouts. For instance, you might add 5 minutes every 2 weeks to your walking time. You can also gradually pick up your pace, using your target heart rate as your guide. Keep a log of your workouts so you can chart your progress until you reach your goal.

- **Maintenance (lifelong).** Once you've reached the stage of exercising for an hour every day, you may want to develop a repertoire of aerobic activities you enjoy. Combine or alternate activities (cross-training) to avoid monotony and keep up your enthusiasm.

Aerobic Options

You have lots of choices for aerobic exercise, so experiment. Focus on one for a few weeks; alternate different activities on different days; try something new every month.

Stepping Out: Walk the Walk   Walking may reduce the risk factors for cardiorespiratory disease, such as insulin resistance, as much as vigorous activity does. Walking briskly 3 hours a week has proven as effective as an hour and a half a week in more vigorous activities, such as aerobics or running, in protecting women's hearts. Women engaging in either form of exercise have a rate of heart attacks 30 to 40 percent lower than that of sedentary women.

Walking also protects men's hearts, whether they're healthy or have had heart problems. Men who regularly engage in light exercise, including walking, have a significantly lower risk of death than their sedentary counterparts.

✓**check-in** Do you track your steps with an app or monitor? If so, how many steps do you walk on an average day?

America on the Move   The typical adult averages about 5,310 steps; a child, from 11,000 to 13,000. According to the ACSM, college students who used a pedometer to count their daily steps took an average of 7,700 steps per day. This falls short of the 10,000 steps recommended as part of the national "America on the Move" program.

How far is 10,000 steps? The following statistics provide some guidance:

- The average person's stride length is approximately 2.5 feet.

YOUR STRATEGIES FOR CHANGE

The Right Way to Walk and Run

Here are some guidelines for putting your best foot forward, whether you are walking or running:

- Take time to warm up.

- Maintain good posture. Keep your back straight, your head up, and your eyes looking straight ahead. Hold your arms slightly away from your body—your elbows should be bent slightly so that your forearms are almost parallel to the ground.

- Use the heel-to-toe method. The heel of your leading foot should touch the ground before the ball or toes of that foot do. Push off the ball of your foot, and bend your knee as you raise your heel. You should be able to feel the action in your calf muscles.

- Pump your arms back and forth. This burns more calories and gives you an upper-body workout as well.

- Do not walk or run on the balls of your feet. This produces soreness in the calves because the muscles must contract for a longer time. Avoid running on hard surfaces and making sudden stops and turns.

- End your walk or run with a cooldown period. Let your pace become more leisurely for the last 5 minutes.

- This means it takes just over 2,000 steps to walk 1 mile, and 10,000 steps is close to 5 miles.

- Brisk walking, according to researchers' calculations, translates into an average of 118 steps—116 for men, 121 for women—per minute.

Why 10,000 steps? According to researchers' estimates, you take about 5,000 steps just to accomplish your daily tasks. Adding about 2,000 steps brings you to a level that can improve your health and wellness. Another 3,000 steps can help you lose excess pounds and prevent weight gain. People who walk at least 10,000 steps a day are more likely to have healthy weights. In addition, 10,000 steps generally translates into 30 minutes of activity, the minimum recommended by the U.S. surgeon general.

Treadmills are good alternatives to outdoor walks—and not just in bad weather. They keep you moving at a certain pace, and they allow you to exercise in a climate-controlled, pollution-free environment—a definite plus for many city dwellers. Holding onto the handrails while walking on a treadmill reduces both heart rate and oxygen consumption, so you burn fewer calories. Slow the pace if necessary so you can let go of the handrails while working out. Elliptical trainers are another aerobic option—with the additional benefit of being easier on the feet, knees, and other joints.

Jogging and Running If you have been sedentary, it's best to launch a walking program before attempting to jog or run indoors or out. Start by walking for 15 to 20 minutes three times a week at a comfortable pace. Continue at this same level until you no longer feel sore or unduly fatigued the day after exercising. Then increase your walking time to 20 to 25 minutes, speeding up your pace as well.

When you can handle a brisk 25-minute walk, alternate fast walking with slow jogging. Begin each session walking and gradually increase the amount of time you spend jogging. If you feel breathless while jogging, slow down and walk. Continue to alternate in this manner until you can jog for 10 minutes without stopping. If you gradually increase your jogging time by 1 or 2 minutes with each workout, you'll slowly build up to 20 or 25 minutes per session. For optimal fitness, you should jog at least three times a week.

The difference between jogging and running is speed. You should be able to carry on a conversation with someone on a long jog or run; if you're too breathless to talk, you're pushing too hard.

If your goal is to enhance aerobic fitness, then long, slow distance running is best. If you want to improve your speed, try *interval training*—repeated hard runs over a certain distance, with intervals of relaxed jogging in between. Depending on what suits you and what your training goals are, you can vary the distance, duration, and number of fast runs, as well as the time and activity between them.

High-Intensity Interval Training High-intensity interval training (HIIT) refers to an exercise session that includes short periods of strenuous aerobic exercise, usually alternating with moderate exercise. HIIT workouts, which may vary in length from 4 to 30 minutes, produce benefits similar to or sometimes greater than those of moderate aerobic exercise but in a much shorter period of time.[51] In various studies, periods of intense exercise divided into several bursts of 20 to 60 seconds within a longer total workout led to a significant improvement in markers of fitness and of cardiometabolic health.[52] An added bonus: Even though it's more physically demanding, individuals often find high-intensity workouts more enjoyable.[53]

HIIT usually consists of a warm-up; periods of intense, near-maximum exercise alternating with periods of moderate exercise; and a cooldown. This approach can be applied to any form of aerobic activity: jogging, running, biking, stair climbing, rowing, jumping, and so on.

✓**check-in** No time to exercise? Build HIIT into your daily routine by sprinting up stairs or running hard in place for 20 or 30 seconds.

Although HIIT has been shown to improve fitness,[54] glucose metabolism,[55] blood pressure, and blood vessel health,[56] it is not yet clear whether it is effective in lowering weight, altering blood fats, or strengthening muscles and bones.[57] The primary advantage of HIIT for busy college students may be its time efficiency.[58] For elite athletes, working at very high intensity for 10 to 15 percent of their workouts may produce optimum benefits.

Disadvantages of HIIT include keeping up motivation for the exhausting challenge of exercising near maximum capacity,[59] a lack of long-term studies, and safety concerns, particularly outside of a gym or controlled setting.[60]

✓**check-in** How do you know you're exercising intensely enough?

Here's a simple rule of thumb: You should be able to say a few words but not a complete sentence.

Other Aerobic Activities Because variety is the spice of an active life, many people prefer different forms of aerobic exercise. All can provide many health benefits. Among the popular options:

- **Swimming.** For aerobic conditioning, you have to swim laps using the freestyle, butterfly, breaststroke, or backstroke. (The sidestroke is too easy.) You must also be a good enough swimmer to keep churning through the water for at least 20 minutes. Your heart will beat more slowly in water than on land, so your heart rate while swimming is not an accurate guide to exercise intensity. Try to keep up a steady pace that's fast enough to make you feel pleasantly tired, but not completely exhausted, by the time you get out of the pool.

- **Cycling.** Bicycling, indoors and out, can be an excellent cardiovascular conditioner, as well as an effective way to control weight—provided you aren't just along for the ride. If you coast down too many hills, you'll have to ride longer up hills or on level ground to get a good workout. An 18-speed bike can make pedaling too easy unless you choose gears carefully. To gain aerobic benefits, mountain bikers have to work hard enough to raise their heart rates to their target zone and keep up that intensity for at least 20 minutes.

- **Spinning.** Spinning is a cardiovascular workout for the whole body that utilizes a special stationary bicycle. Led by an instructor, a group of bikers listens to music, and a participant modifies his or her individual bike's resistance and his or her own pace according to the rhythm. An average spinning class lasts 45 minutes.

- **Cardio kickboxing.** Also referred to as kickboxing or boxing aerobics, this hybrid of boxing, martial arts, and aerobics offers an intense total-body workout. An hour of kickboxing burns an average of 500 to 800 calories, compared to 300 to 400 calories in a typical step aerobics class.

- **Rowing.** Whether on water or a rowing machine, rowing provides excellent aerobic exercise as well as working the upper and lower body and toning the shoulders, back, arms, and legs. Correct rowing techniques are important to avoid back injury.

- **Skipping rope.** Essentially a form of stationary jogging with some extra arm action thrown in, skipping rope is excellent as both a heart conditioner and a way of losing weight. Always warm up before starting and cool down afterward.

- **Stair climbing.** You could run up the stairs in an office building or dormitory, but most people use stair-climbing machines available in home models and at gyms and health clubs.

- **Inline skating.** Inline skating can increase aerobic endurance and muscular strength and is less stressful on joints and bones than running or high-impact aerobics. Skaters can adjust the intensity of their workout by varying the terrain.

- **Tennis.** As with other sports, tennis can be an aerobic activity—depending on the number of players and their skill level. In general, a singles match requires more continuous exertion than playing doubles.

- **Zumba.** Zumba combines dance and aerobic elements with choreography that incorporates hip-hop, samba, salsa, merengue, mambo, martial arts, and belly dancing. Different types of classes target individuals of different ages and fitness levels. As many as 14 million people take weekly Zumba classes in more than 150 countries around the world.

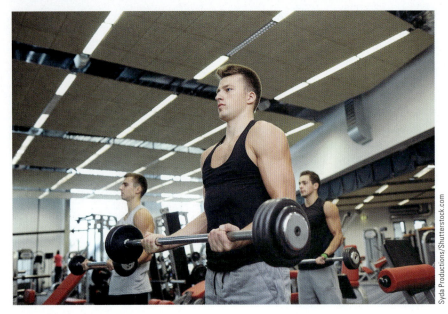

The use of free weights or strength-training machines can build muscle strength and endurance.

Building Muscular Fitness

Although aerobic workouts condition your internal organs (heart, blood vessels, and lungs), they don't exercise many of the muscles that shape your external form and provide power when you need it. Strength workouts are also important because they enable muscles to work more efficiently and reliably. Conditioned muscles function more smoothly and contract somewhat more vigorously and with less effort. With exercise, muscle tissue becomes firmer and can withstand much more strain—the result of toughening the sheath, protecting the muscle, and developing more connective tissue within it (Figure 6.5).

The two dimensions of muscular fitness are strength and endurance:

- *Muscular strength* is the maximal force that a muscle or group of muscles can generate for one movement.

- *Muscular endurance* is the capacity to sustain repeated muscle actions.

Both are important. You need strength to hoist a shovelful of snow and endurance so you can keep shoveling the entire driveway.

Regardless of your age, muscular fitness matters. Resistance training can lower the risk of heart attacks, strokes, and death by about 50 percent.[61] College students with high muscular fitness rate

higher in cardiometabolic health, with lower blood pressure, harmful blood fats, blood sugar, and waist measurements.[62] Resistance training also can improve mood and lessen symptoms of depression and anxiety.[63] In terms of longevity, maximizing and maintaining muscles may be as important as weight or body mass index.

The latest research on fat-burning shows that the best way to reduce your body fat is to add muscle-strengthening exercise to your workouts. Muscle tissue is your very best calorie-burning tissue, and the more you have, the more calories you burn, even when you are resting.

You don't have to become a serious bodybuilder. Using handheld weights (also called *free weights*) two or three times a week is enough.[64] Just be sure you learn how to use them properly because you can tear or strain muscles if you don't practice the proper weightlifting techniques. As more people have begun to lift weights, injuries have soared.

A balanced workout regimen of muscle building and aerobic exercise does more for you than just burn fat. It improves cardiovascular health and gives you more endurance by promoting better distribution of oxygen to your tissues and increasing the blood flow to your heart.[65]

Strength training has particular benefits for women: As numerous studies have documented, it makes their muscles stronger, their bodies leaner, and their bones more resistant to falls. In young women, it boosts self-esteem, body image, and emotional well-being. In middle-aged and older women, it enhances self-concept, boosts psychological health, and prevents weight gain.

Muscles at Work

Your muscles never stay the same. If you don't use them, they atrophy, weaken, or break down. If you use them rigorously and regularly, they grow stronger. The only way to develop muscles is by demanding more of them than you usually do. This is called **overloading**. (Remember the overload principle?)

The heart's right half pumps oxygen-poor blood to capillary beds in lungs. There, it diffuses into blood and diffuses out. The oxygenated blood flows into the heart's left half where it is then pumped to capillary beds throughout the body.

As you train, you have to gradually increase the number of repetitions or the amount of resistance and work the muscle to temporary fatigue. That's why it's important not to quit when your muscles start to tire. Progressive overload—steadily increasing the stress placed on the body—builds stronger muscles.

overloading A method of physical training that involves increasing the number of repetitions or the amount of resistance gradually to work the muscle to temporary fatigue.

Syda Productions/Shutterstock.com

Strength workouts increase circulation

The heart's right half pumps oxygen-poor blood to capillary beds in lungs. There, O_2 diffuses into blood and CO_2 diffuses out. The oxygenated blood flows into the heart's left half, where it is then pumped to capillary beds throughout the body.

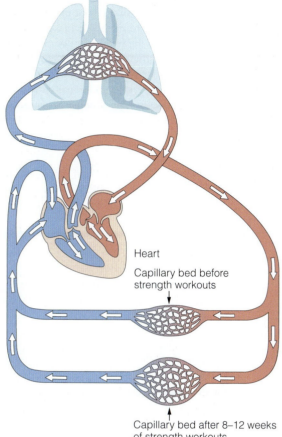

Heart

Capillary bed before strength workouts

Capillary bed after 8–12 weeks of strength workouts (extra capillaries develop, circulation increases)

Strength workouts build muscles

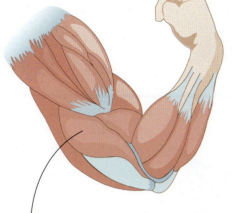

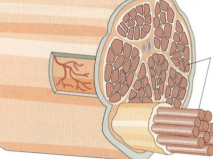

Outer sheath of connective tissue around muscle (toughened by strength workouts)

Bundles of muscle cells surrounded by connective tissue (more connective tissue develops from strength workouts)

FIGURE 6.5 Benefits of Strength Training on the Body

Strength training increases blood circulation to body tissues and promotes muscle development.

You need to exercise differently for strength than for endurance:

- *To develop strength*, do a few repetitions with heavy loads. As you increase the weight your muscles must move, you increase your strength.

- *To increase endurance*, do many more repetitions with lighter loads. If your muscles are weak and you need to gain strength in your upper body, you may have to work for weeks to do a half-dozen regular pushups. Then you can start building endurance by doing as many pushups as you can before collapsing in exhaustion.

Muscles can do only two things: contract and relax. As they do so, skeletal muscles either pull on bones or stop pulling on bones. All exercise involves muscles pulling on bones across a joint. The movement that takes place depends on the structure of the joint and the position of the muscle attachments involved.

In an **isometric** contraction, the muscle applies force while maintaining an equal length. The muscle contracts and tries to shorten but cannot overcome the resistance. An example is pushing against an immovable object, like a wall, or tightening an abdominal muscle while sitting. The muscle contracts, but there is no movement. Push or pull against the immovable object, with each muscle contraction held for 5 to 8 seconds; repeat 5 to 10 times daily.

An **isotonic** contraction involves movement, but the muscle tension remains the same. In an

isometric Of the same length; exercise in which muscles increase their tension without shortening in length, such as when pushing an immovable object.

isotonic Having the same tension or tone; exercise requiring the repetition of an action that creates tension, such as weight-lifting or calisthenics.

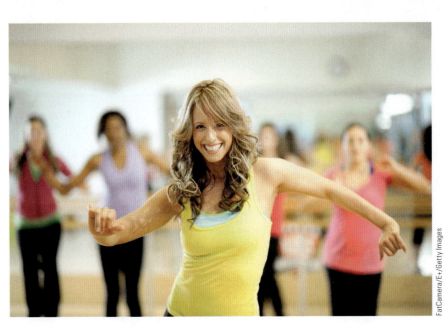

Bored with the typical aerobic exercises? Try a Zumba class or dance workout.

isotonic exercise, the muscle moves a moderate load several times, as in weightlifting or calisthenics. The best isotonic exercise for producing muscular strength involves high resistance and a low number of repetitions. On the other hand, you can develop the greatest flexibility, coordination, and endurance with isotonic exercises that incorporate lower resistance and frequent repetitions.

True **isokinetic** contraction is a constant-speed contraction. Isokinetic exercises require special machines that provide resistance to overload muscles throughout the entire range of motion.

Designing a Muscle Workout

A workout with weights should exercise your body's primary muscle groups (Figure 6.6):

- *Deltoids* (shoulders).
- *Pectorals* (chest).
- *Triceps* and *biceps* (back and front of upper arms).
- *Quadriceps* and *hamstrings* (front and back of thighs).
- *Gluteus maximus* (buttocks).
- *Trapezius* and *rhomboids* (back).
- *Abdomen*.

Various machines and free-weight routines focus on each muscle group, but the principle is always the same: Muscles contract as you raise and lower a weight, and you repeat the lift-and-lower routine until the muscle group is tired.

isokinetic Having the same force; exercise with specialized equipment that provides resistance equal to the force applied by the user throughout the entire range of motion.

reps (or repetitions) In weight training, multiple performances of a movement or an exercise.

sets In weight training, multiples of repetitions of the same movement or exercise.

A weight-training program is made up of:

- **Reps (or repetitions)**—Multiple performances of an exercise, such as lifting 50 pounds one time.

- **Sets**—A *set* number of repetitions of the same movement, such as a set of 20 push-ups. You should allow your breath to return to normal before moving on to each new set. Although the ideal number of sets in a resistance-training program remains controversial, recent evidence suggests that multiple sets lead to additional benefits in short- and long-term training in young and middle-aged adults.

Maintaining proper breathing during weight training is crucial. To breathe correctly, inhale when muscles are relaxed and exhale when you push or lift. Don't ever hold your breath because oxygen flow helps prevent muscle fatigue and injury.

Free Weights versus Machines No one type of equipment—free weight or machine—has a clear advantage in terms of building fat-free body mass, enhancing strength and endurance, or improving a sport-specific skill. Each type offers benefits but also has drawbacks.

Free weights offer great versatility for strength training. With dumbbells, for example, you can perform a variety of exercises to work specific muscle groups, such as the chest and shoulders. Machines, in contrast, are more limited; many allow only one exercise.

Strength-training machines have several advantages:

- They ensure correct movement for a lift, which helps protect against injury and prevent cheating when fatigue sets in.

- They isolate specific muscles, which is good for rehabilitating an injury or strengthening a specific body part.

- Because they offer high-tech options like varying resistance during the lifting motion, they can tax muscles in ways that a traditional barbell cannot.

Recovery

The ACSM recommends a minimum of 8 to 10 exercises involving the major muscle groups 2 to 3 days a week. Recent research has shown no greater improvement in strength from more frequent or intense workouts.[66]

Remember that your muscles need sufficient time to recover from a weight-training session. Never work a sore muscle because soreness may

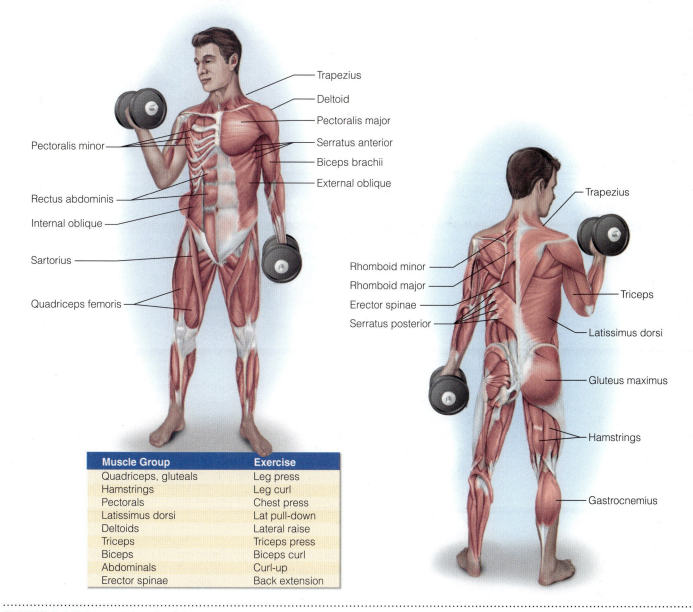

Muscle Group	Exercise
Quadriceps, gluteals	Leg press
Hamstrings	Leg curl
Pectorals	Chest press
Latissimus dorsi	Lat pull-down
Deltoids	Lateral raise
Triceps	Triceps press
Biceps	Biceps curl
Abdominals	Curl-up
Erector spinae	Back extension

FIGURE 6.6 Primary Muscle Groups

Different weight-lifting exercises can strengthen and stretch different muscle groups.

indicate that too-heavy weights have caused tiny tears in the fibers.

Allow no less than 48 hours, but no more than 96 hours, between training sessions, so your body can recover from the workout and you avoid overtraining. Workouts on consecutive days do more harm than good because the body can't recover that quickly. Strength training twice a week at greater intensity and for a longer duration can be as effective as working out three times a week. However, your muscles will begin to atrophy if you let more than 3 or 4 days pass without exercising them.

✓**check-in** How often do you do strength training?

Core Strength Conditioning

"Core strength," a popular trend in exercise and fitness, refers to the ability of the muscles to support your spine and keep your body stable and balanced. The major muscles of your core include:

- The transverse abdominis, the deepest of the abdominal muscles.
- The external and internal obliques on the side and front of the abdomen around your waist.
- The rectus abdominis, a long muscle that extends along the front of the abdomen.

When you have good core stability, the muscles in your pelvis, low back, hips, and abdomen work in harmony. Strengthening all of your core muscles provides stability; improves posture, breathing, appearance, and balance; and protects you from injury. When your core is weak, you become more susceptible to low back pain and injury.

✓**check-in** Do you do exercises to strengthen your core?

Muscle Dysmorphia

Also referred to as "bigorexia" or "reverse anorexia," **muscle dysmorphia** is a condition that primarily affects male bodybuilders. Convinced that they are too small or muscularly insufficient, they spend hours working out at the gym, invest large sums in exercise equipment, take various supplements including potentially harmful drugs, and obsess about their appearance.

Some researchers believe muscle dysmorphia is a form of body dysmorphic disorder; others view it as an eating disorder. Its primary characteristics are as follows:

- Frequently giving up important social, occupational, or recreational activities because of a compulsive need to maintain a workout and diet regimen.

- Avoiding situations that involve bodily exposure (such as swimming) or enduring them only with great distress.

- Preoccupation with body size or musculature that causes significant distress or interferes with work, socializing, or other important aspects of daily life.

- Continued exercise, diet, or use of performance-enhancing substances despite knowledge of their potential for physical or psychological harm.

Drugs Used to Boost Athletic Performance

Sports supplements have exploded into a huge international business expected to generate some $18 billion in revenue by 2025.[67] Both amateur and professional athletes are the greatest users. Some have paid a high price for using drugs to boost their performance, including arrests and convictions. Others have had to end their careers and see their reputation forever tarnished.[68]

The number of college athletes using or at least checking into performance-enhancing drugs is believed to be growing. Some feel the stakes are high enough to outweigh the risks, which include cancer, liver disease, blood diseases, severe arthritis, and sexual dysfunction.

✓**check-in** What do you think of sports doping among college and professional athletes?

Despite the hype, more than 7,500 scientific investigations have found that performance-enhancing drugs do not provide strength benefits. The drugs have been shown to increase lean body mass, heart rate, and metabolic rate, but these do not translate into improved performance.

Here's what we know—and don't know—about the most widely used performance boosters:

- **Anabolic steroids.** These synthetic derivatives of the male hormone testosterone promote the growth of skeletal muscle and increase lean body mass. Taking them to improve athletic performance is illegal. Approximately 1 percent of college students have used steroids for nonmedical purposes. Anabolic steroids have been reported to increase lean muscle mass, strength, and ability to train longer and harder, but they pose serious health hazards, including the following:

  - They may cause liver tumors, jaundice (yellowish pigmentation of skin, tissues, and body fluids), fluid retention, high blood pressure, decreased immune function, and severe acne.

  - Men may experience shrinking of the testicles, reduced sperm count, infertility, baldness, and development of breasts. In men, side effects may be reversible once abuse stops.

  - Women may experience growth of facial hair, acne, changes in or cessation of the menstrual cycle, enlargement of the clitoris, and deepened voice. In women, these changes are irreversible.

  - In adolescents, steroids may bring about a premature halt in skeletal maturation.

  - Anabolic steroid abuse may lead to aggression and other psychiatric side effects, including maniclike symptoms leading to "roid rage," or violent, even homicidal, episodes. Users may suffer from paranoid jealousy, extreme irritability, delusions, and impaired judgment stemming from feelings of invincibility. Stopping the drugs abruptly can lead to depression.

- **Androstenedione ("andro").** This testosterone precursor is normally produced by the adrenal glands and gonads. Despite manufacturers' claims, studies have shown that supplemental androstenedione doesn't increase testosterone, and muscles don't get stronger with andro use. Andro has been classified as a controlled substance, and its use is illegal.

muscle dysmorphia A condition that affects mostly male bodybuilders in which they become obsessed with appearance and size of muscles.

- **Creatine.** This amino acid, which is made by the body and stored predominantly in skeletal muscle, serves as a reservoir to replenish adenosine triphosphate (ATP), a substance involved in energy production. Some studies suggest that creatine may increase strength and endurance. Other effects on the body remain unknown.

  The Food and Drug Administration (FDA) has warned consumers to consult a physician before taking creatine supplements. Creatine may cause dehydration and heat-related illnesses, reduced blood volume, and electrolyte imbalances. Some athletes drink quantities of water hoping to avoid such effects. However, many coaches forbid or discourage creatine use because its long-term effects remain unknown.

- **GBL (gamma butyrolactone).** This unapproved drug is marketed on the Internet and in some professional gyms as a muscle builder and performance enhancer. The FDA has warned consumers to avoid any products containing GBL, noting that they have been associated with at least one death and several incidents in which users became comatose or unconscious.

- **Ergogenic aids.** These substances, some of them very common, are used to enhance energy and provide athletes with a competitive advantage:

  - *Caffeine* (discussed in Chapter 11) may boost alertness in some people but cause jitteriness in others.

  - *Baking soda* (sodium bicarbonate) is believed to delay fatigue by neutralizing lactic acid in the muscles. Its potential drawbacks include explosive diarrhea, abdominal cramps, bloating, and nausea.

  - *Glycerol* is a natural element derived from fats. Some sports-drink manufacturers are testing formulations that include glycerol, which they claim can lower heart rate and stave off exhaustion in marathon events. Glycerol-induced hyperhydration (holding too much water in the blood) may be hazardous to health.

- **Human growth hormone and erythropoietin (EPO).** According to an analysis of all existing research, human growth hormone increases lean body mass but does not affect exercise capacity or aerobic endurance. Previous studies found no beneficial effect on aging in healthy older people. EPO is a hormone that increases red blood cell production and improves endurance. Side effects include blood clots, increased bone growth, increased cholesterol, heart disease, and impotence.

Becoming More Flexible

Flexibility is the characteristic of body tissues that determines the **range of motion** achievable without injury at a joint or group of joints. There are two types of flexibility:

- **Static flexibility**—the type most people think of as flexibility—refers to the ability to assume and maintain an extended position at one end point in a joint's range of motion. Static flexibility depends on many factors, including the structure of a joint and the tightness of the muscles, tendons, and ligaments attached to it.

- **Dynamic flexibility**, by comparison, involves movement. It is the ability to move a joint quickly and fluidly through its entire range of motion with little resistance. Dynamic flexibility is not only influenced by static flexibility but also depends on additional factors, such as strength, coordination, and resistance to movement.

Static flexibility in the hip joint determines whether you can do a split; dynamic flexibility is what would enable you to perform a split leap.

Genetics, age, sex, and body composition all influence how flexible you are. Girls and women tend to be more flexible than boys and men to a certain extent because of hormonal and anatomical differences. The way females and males use their muscles and the activities they engage in can also have an effect. Over time, the natural elasticity of muscles, tendons, and joints decreases in both sexes, resulting in stiffness.

✓**check-in** How would you rate your flexibility?

The Benefits of Flexibility

Just as cardiorespiratory fitness benefits the heart and lungs and muscular fitness builds endurance and strength, a stretching program produces unique benefits, including enhancement of the ability of the respiratory, circulatory, and neuromuscular systems to cope with the stress and demands of our high-pressure world (Figure 6.7).

Among the other benefits of flexibility are the following:

- **Prevention of injuries.** Strong, flexible muscles resist stress better than weak or inflexible ones.[69] Adding flexibility to a training program for sports such as soccer, football, or tennis can reduce the

range of motion The fullest extent of possible movement in a particular joint.

static flexibility The ability to assume and maintain an extended position at one end point in a joint's range of motion.

dynamic flexibility The ability to move a joint quickly and fluidly through its entire range of motion with little resistance.

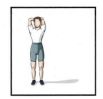

Triceps Stretch
1. Starting position: This exercise may be done while standing or seated. Reach both arms overhead, bend the right elbow, and grasp it with the left hand. The right hand should be pointing straight down the back.
2. Pull the elbow up and slightly back and hold for at least 20 seconds.
3. Repeat on the other side.

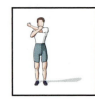

Deltoid Stretch—Rear
1. Starting position: Sit or stand with good posture. Cross the right arm across the front of the body at neck level. Grasp the elbow with the left hand while keeping the shoulders down and relaxed.
2. Press the elbow toward the neck and hold for at least 20 seconds.
3. Repeat on the other side.

Chest Stretch
1. Starting position: Stand beneath a doorway. Bend the left arm and place the forearm against the wall with the elbow at shoulder height.
2. Rotate the body away from the arm and hold for at least 20 seconds.
3. Repeat on the other side.

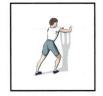

Calf Stretch—Wall
1. Starting position: Stand approximately 2 feet away from a wall and place hands on wall at about shoulder height. Place one foot at the base of the wall with the heel on the floor and toes against the wall.
2. Slowly straighten the knees and press the chest toward the wall to feel a stretch in the back of the lower leg.
3. Hold for at least 20 seconds and repeat on the other side.

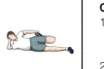

Inner Thigh
1. Starting position: Stand with feet 3 or more feet apart and toes turning outward. Bend one knee and lunge to one side, being careful not to allow the knee to extend beyond the toes.
2. Keeping weight on bent leg, lift the toes of the extended leg to increase the stretch in the inner thigh. Keep torso upright and head lifted.
3. Hold for at least 20 seconds.

Quadriceps Stretch—Lying
1. Starting position: Lie on your side with your legs extended and your lower arm or hand supporting your head. Bend the top knee and grasp the top of the foot with your hand. Knees should be in alignment.
2. Press the top hip forward to feel a stretch along the front of the thigh.
3. Hold for at least 20 seconds and repeat on the other side.

Hamstring Stretch—Lying
1. Starting position: Lie on your back with your legs extended. Lift one leg up and grasp behind the thigh or knee with both hands as you bring the knee to the chest.
2. Press the heel up toward the ceiling as you straighten the leg.
3. Hold for at least 20 seconds and repeat on the other side.

FIGURE 6.7 Basic Stretching Program

Just doing a few minutes of stretching to your major muscle groups can yield many benefits.

rate of injuries by as much as 75 percent. However, stretching before a run has proven neither to prevent nor to cause injury.

- **Relief of muscle strain.** Muscles tighten as a result of stress or prolonged sitting. Stretching helps relieve this tension and enables you

to work more effectively. For certain types of pain, combined strengthening and stretching exercises may be most effective.[70]

- **Relaxation.** Flexibility exercises reduce stress and mental strain, slow the rate of breathing, and reduce blood pressure.

- **Relief of soreness after exercise.** Many people develop delayed-onset muscle soreness (DOMS) 1 or 2 days after they work out. This may be the result of damage to the muscle fibers and supporting connective tissue.

- **Improved posture.** Bad posture can create tight, stressed muscles. If you slump in your chair, for instance, the muscles in the front of your chest may tighten, causing those in the upper spine to overstretch and become loose.

Stretching

When you stretch a muscle, you are primarily stretching the connective tissue. The stretch must be intense enough to increase the length of the connective tissue without tearing it.

Static stretching involves a gradual stretch held for a short time (10 to 30 seconds). A shorter stretch provides little benefit; a longer stretch does not provide additional benefits. Since a slow stretch provokes less of a reaction from the stretch receptors, the muscles can safely stretch farther than usual. Fitness experts most often recommend static stretching because it is both safe and effective.

An example of such a stretch is letting your hands slowly slide down the front of your legs (keeping your knees in a soft, unlocked position) until you reach your toes and holding this final position for several seconds before slowly straightening up. You should feel a pull, but not pain, during this stretch.

In **passive stretching**, your own body, a partner, gravity, or a weight serves as an external force or resistance to help your joints move through their range of motion. You can achieve a more intense stretch and a greater range of motion with passive stretching. There is a greater risk of injury, however, because the muscles themselves are not controlling the stretch.

Active stretching involves stretching a muscle by contracting the opposing muscle (the muscle on the opposite side of the limb). This method allows the muscle to be stretched farther with a low risk of injury.

Dynamic stretching increases the range of motion around a joint or group of joints by using active muscular effort, momentum, and speed. Dynamic stretches, such as walking lunges and arm circles, are considered better alternatives to static stretching for gymnasts, dancers, figure skaters, divers, and hurdlers because they do not decrease muscle strength and power.

Ballistic stretching is characterized by rapid bouncing movements, such as a series of up-and-down bobs as you try again and again to touch your toes with your hands. These bounces can stretch the muscle fibers too far, causing the muscle to contract rather than stretch. They can also tear ligaments and weaken or rupture tendons, the strong fibrous cords that connect muscles to bones. The heightened activity to stretch receptors caused by the rapid stretches can continue for some time, possibly causing injuries during any physical activities that follow. Because of the potential dangers of ballistic stretching, fitness experts generally recommend against it.

Stretching and Warming Up

Warming up means getting the heart beating, breaking a sweat, and readying the body for more vigorous activity. Stretching is a specific activity intended to elongate the muscles and keep joints limber, not simply a prelude to a game of tennis or a 3-mile run. According to a review of recent studies, the value of stretching varies with different activities. While it does not prevent injuries from jogging, cycling, or swimming, stretching may be beneficial in sports, such as soccer and football, that involve bouncing and jumping.

✓**check-in** Did you know that one of the best times to stretch is after an aerobic workout?

After stretching, your muscles will be warm, more flexible, and less prone to injury. In addition, stretching after aerobic activity can help a fatigued muscle return to its normal resting length and may help reduce delayed-onset muscle soreness.

Stretching and Athletic Performance

Conventional wisdom holds that stretching improves athletic performance, but a review of the research finds that this isn't necessarily so. In some cases, active stretching can impede rather than improve performance in terms of muscle force and jumping height. Passive stretching prior to a sprint—a common practice—has also proved to reduce runners' speed. On the other hand, regular stretching can improve athletic performance in a variety of sports.

Pre-exercise stretching is generally unnecessary and may be counterproductive. Static stretching reduces strength in the stretched muscle, especially in people who hold the stretch for 90 seconds or more.

A better choice is to warm up dynamically by moving the muscles that will be used in your workout. Jumping jacks and toy-soldier high leg kicks prepare muscles for many forms of exercise better than stretching.

static stretching A stretching technique in which a gradual stretch is held for a short time of 10 to 30 seconds.

passive stretching A stretching technique in which an external force or resistance (your body, a partner, gravity, or a weight) helps the joints move through their range of motion.

active stretching A technique that involves stretching a muscle by contracting the opposing muscle.

dynamic stretching Stretching that increases the range of motion around a joint or group of joints by using active muscular effort, momentum, and speed.

ballistic stretching Rapid bouncing movements.

- Before you begin, increase your body temperature by slowly marching or running in place. Sweat signals that you're ready to start stretching.

- Don't force body parts beyond their normal range of motion. Stretch to the point of tension, back off, and hold for 10 seconds to 1 minute.

- Do a minimum of four repetitions of each stretch, with equal repetitions on each side.

- Don't hold your breath. Continue breathing slowly and rhythmically throughout your stretching routine.

- Don't attempt to stretch a weak or injured muscle.

- Start small. Work the muscles of the smaller joints in the arms and legs first and then work the larger joints like the shoulders and hips.

- Stretch individual muscles before you stretch a group of muscles; for instance, stretch the ankle, knee, and hip before doing a stretch that works all three at once.

- Don't make any quick, jerky movements while stretching. Stretches should be gentle and smooth.

- Certain positions can be harmful to the knees and lower back. In particular, avoid stretches that require deep knee bends or full squats because they can harm your knees and lower back.

Mind–Body Approaches

Yoga, Pilates, and t'ai chi—increasingly popular on campuses and throughout the country—can help reduce stress, enhance health and wellness, and improve physical fitness, including balance.

Yoga

One of the most ancient of mind–body practices, *yoga* comes from the Sanskrit word meaning "union." Traditionally associated with religion, yoga consists of various breathing and stretching exercises that unite all aspects of a person.

Yoga has grown more popular among Americans of all ages, with the greatest increase in adults ages 18 to 44. Once considered an exotic pursuit, yoga has gained acceptance as part of a comprehensive stress management and fitness program and scientific studies have demonstrated its benefits, which include the following:[71]

- **Improved flexibility,** which may offer protection from back pain and injuries.

- **Protection of joints** because yoga postures take joints through their full range of motion, providing a fresh supply of nutrients to joint cartilage.

- **Stronger, denser bones** from yoga's weight-bearing postures.

- **Enhanced circulation,** which also boosts the supply of oxygen throughout the body.

- **Lower blood pressure.**

- **Relief of stress-related symptoms** and anxiety.

- **Lower blood sugar** in people with diabetes, which reduces the risk of complications.

- **Relief from lower back pain.**[72]

- **Reduced pain** in people with arthritis, carpal tunnel syndrome, fibromyalgia, and other chronic problems.

- **Improved lung function** in people with asthma.

- **Less inflammation, fatigue, and depression** in breast cancer survivors.

- **Eased depression in pregnant women,** serving as an alternative to antidepressants.

The best way to get started is to find a class that appeals to you and learn a few yoga poses and breathing techniques. Once you have mastered these, you can easily integrate yoga into your total fitness program.

The ACSM cautions that yoga should help, not hurt. To prevent injuries to your knees, back, neck, shoulders, wrists, or ankles, avoid forcing your body into difficult postures. Proper technique is essential to safety.

Pilates

Used by dancers for deep-body conditioning and injury rehabilitation, Pilates (pronounced "puh-lah-teez") was developed more than seven decades ago by German immigrant Joseph Pilates. Increasingly used to complement aerobics and weight training or as part of rehabilitation after injury, Pilates exercises improve flexibility and joint mobility and strengthen the core by developing pelvic stability and abdominal control.[73]

Pilates-trained instructors offer "mat" or "floor" classes that stress the stabilization and strengthening of the back and abdominal muscles.[74] Fitness centers may also offer training on Pilates equipment, primarily a device called the Reformer, a wooden contraption with various cables, pulleys, springs, and sliding boards attached that is used for a series of progressive range-of-motion exercises.

According to research from the ACSM, Pilates enhances flexibility and muscular endurance, particularly for intermediate and advanced practitioners, but its potential to increase cardiorespiratory fitness and reduce body weight is limited. The intensity of a Pilates workout increases from basic to intermediate to advanced levels, as does the number of calories burned. For intermediate practitioners, a 30-minute session burns 180 calories, with each additional quarter-hour burning another 90 calories.

T'ai Chi

This ancient Chinese practice, designed to exercise body, mind, and spirit, gently works muscles, focuses concentration, and improves the flow of "qi" (often spelled "chi"), the vital life energy that sustains health. Popular with all ages, from children to seniors, t'ai chi is easy to learn and perform. Because of its focus on breathing and flowing gestures, t'ai chi is sometimes described as "meditation in motion."

According to a recent review of 35 studies involving more than 2,200 people in 10 countries, t'ai chi and other traditional Chinese exercise help lower blood pressure and levels of LDL ("bad") cholesterol and other unhealthy blood fats as well as improve mood and quality of life.[75] Classes are available on campuses and in fitness centers, community centers, and some martial arts schools.

✓**check-in** Have you ever tried any mind-body approaches?

Keeping Your Back Healthy

Low back pain causes more disability than some 300 other conditions worldwide; nearly 1 in 10 people around the globe suffers from an aching lower back.[76] Back pain strikes slightly more women than men and is most common between the ages of 20 and 55. You are at increased risk if you smoke or if you're overstressed, overweight, or out of shape. One of the most effective ways to prevent or recover from back problems is to strengthen the core muscles.

Once bedrest was the primary treatment for back pain, but doctors now urge patients to avoid it. Even 2 to 7 days of bedrest may provide little, if any, benefit. Many people, particularly those experiencing low back pain for the first time, may overestimate the risks of physical activity. Talk with a health professional about the best and safest options.

Psychological approaches, including mindfulness-based stress reduction (discussed in Chapter 4) and cognitive-behavioral therapy (discussed in Chapter 3), have proven effective in relieving low back pain. Acetaminophen (Tylenol) is the first-line medication for pain relief. If it is not effective, doctors recommend nonsteroidal anti-inflammatory drugs, such as ibuprofen (Motrin or Advil). Muscle relaxants seem to be effective for a spasm in the lower back.

The sooner that back patients return to normal activity, the less pain medication they require and the less long-term disability they suffer. The overwhelming majority of patients with chronic low back pain do not benefit from surgeries such as spinal fusion.

✓**check-in** Have you ever experienced back pain?

Sports Nutrition

In general, active people need the same basic nutrients as others. There is no single, superior "athletic diet," since athletes in various competitive sports have different nutritional requirements:[77]

- Athletes generally do not need more protein; the exception may be those engaged in intense strength training. Like most other Americans, athletes typically consume more than the Recommended Daily Allowance for protein.

- Complex carbohydrates are essential in an athlete's diet. (See Chapter 4 for the best sources.)

- Including the right types of fat in the daily diet can actually improve athletic performance—not just by providing calories but by replenishing intramuscular fat stores (fat stored within the muscle and used to fuel extended exercise).

Not just *what* you eat but *when* you eat can affect your exercise performance. If you eat immediately prior to a workout, you may feel sluggish or develop nausea, cramping, or diarrhea. If you don't eat, you may feel weak, faint, or tired.

✓**check-in** Eat and run? Or run and eat? Time your meals so that you exercise 3 to 4 hours after a large meal and 1 to 2 hours after a small one. After a workout, eat a meal containing both protein and carbohydrates within 2 hours to help your muscles recover and to replace fuel stores.

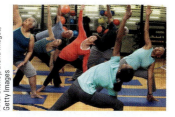

Ariel Skelley/Blend Images/ Getty Images

Mind–body exercises such as yoga provide physical and psychological benefits.

$ HEALTH ON A BUDGET

Low-Cost Fitness Aids

Not all fitness equipment comes with a big price tag. Here are some affordable ways to expand and enhance a home workout:

- **Dumbbells.** You can purchase light weights to carry when walking and jogging to build and firm arm muscles. Training with heavier weights increases muscle strength and endurance, improves balance and body composition, and may reverse some bone loss. An adjustable dumbbell set allows you to add more weight as you build strength.

- **Stability balls.** A large inflatable rubber ball can be a fun, effective way of building core strength, improving posture, and increasing balance. When performing standard exer-

cises like crunches and abdominal curls, the ball provides an additional challenge: maintaining a stable trunk throughout each exercise. You also can sit on the ball while working with hand weights to build core strength and balance. Introductory videos and DVDs are available for rental or purchase.

- **Resistance tubing.** Developed by physical therapists for rehabilitation after injuries, elastic bands and tubing come in different strengths, based on the thickness of the plastic. If you're a beginner, start with a thin band, particularly for the upper body. The lightweight, inexpensive, and easy-to-carry bands aren't particularly risky, but you should check for holes or worn spots, choose a smooth surface, maintain good posture, and perform the exercises in a slow, controlled manner.

Water

Water, which we need more than any other nutrient, is especially important during exercise and exertion. Rather than wait until you're already somewhat dehydrated, you should be fully hydrated when you begin your activity or exercise and, depending on the duration and intensity of your workout, continue to replace fluids both during and afterward.

The ACSM recommends fluid intake before, during, and after exercise to regulate body temperature and replace body fluids lost through sweating. Failure to replace fluids during exercise can lead to dehydration, which can cause muscle fatigue, loss of coordination, heat exhaustion, and an elevation of body-core temperature to dangerously high levels. To avoid this danger, the ACSM advises the following:

- **Consume a nutritionally balanced diet and drink adequate fluids** in the 24 hours before an exercise event.

- **Drink about 17 ounces of fluid** about 2 hours before.

- **During exercise, start drinking early** and at regular intervals to replace all the water lost through sweating (i.e., body weight loss).

- **Drink fluids with carbohydrates and/or electrolytes** for exercise lasting more than an hour. For shorter periods, there is little evidence of differences between drinking a carbohydrate-electrolyte drink and plain water.

Too much water during prolonged bouts of exercise, such as a marathon, can lead to

hyponatremia, or water intoxication. This condition occurs when the body's sodium level falls below normal as a result of salt loss from sweat and dilution of sodium in the bloodstream by overdrinking. Symptoms of hyponatremia include nausea, vomiting, weakness, and, in severe cases, seizures, coma, and death.

✓**check-in** Do you pay attention to proper hydration when working out?

Sports Drinks

In its most recent position stand, the International Society of Sports Nutrition (ISSN) has noted that the primary nutrients in energy and sports drinks are carbohydrates and caffeine. Caffeine's effects have been well studied, but other ingredients added to energy and sports drinks have not been.

Consuming a high-carbohydrate, high-caffeine sports drink 10 to 60 minutes before exercise may improve mental focus, alertness, anaerobic performance, and endurance, but athletes should consider the effects on their metabolic health. Use of more than one serving a day, the ISSN stated, may lead to adverse effects. Individuals with cardiovascular, metabolic, liver, or neurologic disease who are taking medication should avoid all use of energy or sports drinks.

As noted earlier, water best meets the fluid needs of most athletes, but you have other choices. Nonfat milk may be more effective than even a soy protein beverage or sports drink such as Gatorade at burning fat and building lean muscle mass. Most sports drinks contain about 7 percent carbohydrate (about half the sugar of ordinary soft drinks). Less than 6 percent may not enhance performance; more than 8 percent could cause abdominal cramping, nausea, and diarrhea.

Sodium and other electrolytes in sports drinks help replace those lost during physical activity. However, most exercisers do not have to replace minerals lost in sweat immediately. A meal eaten within several hours does so soon enough.

Dietary Supplements

Athletes, particularly elite athletes, are more likely than others to use dietary supplements. A larger proportion of men use vitamin E, protein, and creatine, while iron supplements are more common by women. Those involved in heavy training may need more of several vitamins, such as thiamin, riboflavin, and vitamin B_6, which are involved in energy production. The best source, nutritionists advise, is vitamin-rich foods, such as fruits and vegetables.

Vitamin and mineral supplements, as discussed in Chapter 5, do not provide benefits to healthy, well-nourished individuals. Vitamin supplements marketed for athletes are poorly regulated, and some may be adulterated with banned substances, such as ephedrine.

Mineral deficiencies, such as too little iron in female athletes, can impair athletic performance. Women who exercise rigorously should undergo regular blood testing and, if needed, take iron supplements. In general, calcium, magnesium, iron, zinc, and copper supplements do not enhance sport performance in well-nourished athletes. Chromium, boron, and vanadium have no beneficial effects on body composition or muscular strength and endurance.

Taking salt pills does little to boost performance in endurance exercises. Researchers have found no difference between athletes taking additional salt and those given placebos.

Energy Bars

Little scientific research has studied the benefits of the various types of energy bars, including their effects on blood glucose levels and athletic performance. One nutritional analysis found high-carbohydrate energy bars to be similar to candy bars in their impact on glucose—even though sugars composed 31 percent of the high-carbohydrate energy bar and 86 percent of the candy bar. In fact, the high-carbohydrate energy bar caused a more rapid peak in blood glucose followed by a sharper decline than did the candy bar. This effect may be desirable for athletes involved in short-duration events who want a quick increase in blood glucose.

Energy bars with a lower carbohydrate level produce a more moderate, sustained increase in blood glucose level, possibly because the protein and fat in a 40-30-30 bar diminish blood glucose response. These bars would be a better choice for athletes involved in endurance events. As an alternative, try fiber-rich whole foods, like nuts and fruit, that provide a steady release of energy.

✓**check-in** Do you eat energy bars frequently?

Safe and Healthy Workouts

Whenever you work out, you don't want to risk becoming sore or injured. Starting slowly when you begin any new fitness activity is the smartest strategy. Keep a simple diary to record the time and duration of each workout. Get accustomed to an activity first and then begin to work harder or longer. In this way, you strengthen your musculoskeletal system so you're less likely to be injured, you lower the cardiorespiratory risk, and you build the exercise habit into your schedule.

To prevent exercise-related problems before they happen, use common sense and take appropriate precautions, including the following:

- **Get proper instruction** and, if necessary, advanced training from knowledgeable instructors.

- **Make sure you have good equipment** and keep it in good condition. Know how to check and do at least basic maintenance on the equipment yourself. Always check your equipment prior to each use (especially if you're renting it).

- **Always warm up before and cool down after** a workout.

- Rather than being sedentary all week and then training hard on weekends, try to stay active throughout the week and **don't overdo it on weekends.**

- **Use reasonable protective measures,** including wearing a helmet when cycling or skating.

- For some sports, such as boating, **always go with a buddy.**

- **Take each outing seriously**—even if you've dived into this river a hundred times before, even if you know this mountain like you know your own backyard. Avoid the unknown under adverse conditions (e.g., hiking unfamiliar terrain during poor weather or kayaking a new river when water levels are unusually high or low) or when accompanied by a beginner whose skills may not be as strong as yours.

- **Never combine alcohol or drugs with any workout or sport.**

✓check-in Should you exercise outdoors on a smoggy day? Although health professionals advise people to exercise in low-pollution areas such as parks, the health benefits of outdoor workouts appear o outweigh tthe potential harm of air pollution.[78]

Temperature

Prevention is the wisest approach to heat and cold problems; and knowing what can go wrong is part of that preventive approach.

Heat Cramps
These muscle cramps are caused by profuse sweating and the consequent loss of electrolytes (salts). They occur most often during exercise in hot weather. Salty snacks and sports beverages such as Gatorade can help, but be aware that sports drinks can be very high in calories. Salt tablets usually aren't necessary except in cases of extreme sweating.

Heat Syndromes
More serious temperature-related conditions include heat exhaustion and heat stroke. These are most likely to occur when both temperature and humidity are high because sweat does not evaporate as quickly, preventing the body from releasing heat. Other conditions that limit the body's ability to regulate temperature are old age, fever, obesity, dehydration, heart disease, poor circulation, sunburn, and drug and alcohol use. Some medicines that increase the risk include allergy medicines (antihistamines), some cough and cold medicines, blood pressure and heart medicines, diet pills, laxatives, and psychiatric medications.

Heat Exhaustion
Heat exhaustion is a mild form of heat-related illness that can be caused by exercise or hot weather. The signs of heat exhaustion are heavy sweating, paleness, muscle cramps, tiredness, weakness, dizziness, headache, nausea or vomiting, and/or fainting. Your pulse rate or heart rate may be fast and weak, and your breathing may be fast and shallow.

✓check-in Do you know what to do if you think you may have heat exhaustion? First of all, get out of the heat immediately. Rest in a cool, shady place and drink plenty of water or other fluids. Do *not* drink alcohol, which can make heat exhaustion worse. If you do not feel better within 30 minutes, seek medical attention. If left untreated, heat exhaustion may lead to a heat stroke.

Heat Stroke
A heat stroke can occur when the body temperature rises to 106 degrees Fahrenheit or higher within 10 to 15 minutes. A heat stroke is a medical emergency that can be fatal. The warning signs are extremely high temperature; red, hot, and dry skin; rapid, strong pulse; throbbing headache; dizziness; nausea; and confusion or unconsciousness.

If you think someone might have heat stroke, you should quickly take him or her to a cool, shady place and call a doctor. Remove unnecessary clothing and bathe or spray the victim with cool water. People with heat stroke may seem confused. They may have seizures or go into a coma.

Protecting Yourself from Cold
The tips of the toes, fingers, ears, nose, and chin and the cheeks are most vulnerable to exposure to high wind speeds and low temperatures, which can result in *frostnip*.

Because frostnip is painless, you may not even be aware that it is occurring. Watch for a sudden blanching or lightening of your skin. The best early treatment is warming the area with firm, steady pressure from a warm hand; blowing on it with hot breath; holding it against your body; or immersing it in warm (not hot) water. As the skin thaws, it becomes red and starts to tingle. Be careful to protect it from further damage. Don't rub the skin vigorously or with snow, as you could damage the tissue.

More severe is *frostbite*. There are two types of frostbite:

- *Superficial frostbite*, the freezing of the skin and tissues just below the skin, is characterized by a waxy look and firmness of the skin, although the tissue below is soft. Initial treatment should be to slowly rewarm the area. As the area thaws, it will be numb and bluish or purple, and blisters may form. Cover the area with a dry, sterile dressing and protect the skin from further exposure to cold. See a doctor for further treatment.

- *Deep frostbite*, the freezing of skin, muscle, and even bone, requires medical treatment. It usually involves the tissues of the hands and feet, which appear pale and feel frozen. Keep the victim dry and as warm as possible on the way to a medical facility. Cover the frostbitten area with a dry, sterile dressing.

The center of the body may gradually cool at temperatures above, as well as below, freezing—usually in wet, windy weather. When body temperature falls too low, the body is incapable of rewarming itself because of the breakdown of the internal system that regulates its temperature. This state is known as **hypothermia**. The first sign of hypothermia is severe shivering. Then the victim becomes uncoordinated, drowsy, listless, confused, and is unable to speak properly. Symptoms become more severe as body temperature continues to drop, and coma or death can result.

Hypothermia requires emergency medical treatment. Try to prevent any further heat loss. Move the victim to a warm place, cover him or her with blankets, remove wet clothing, and replace it with dry garments. If the victim is conscious, administer warm liquids, not alcohol.

Here are ways to protect yourself in cold weather (or cold indoor gyms):

- Cover as much of your body as possible but don't overdress.

- Wear one layer less than you would if you were outside but not exercising.

- Don't use warm-up clothes made of waterproof material because they tend to trap heat and keep perspiration from evaporating.

- Make sure your clothes are loose enough to allow movement and exercise of the hands, feet, and other body parts, thereby maintaining proper circulation.

- Choose dark colors that absorb heat.

- Because 40 percent or more of your body heat is lost through your head and neck, wear a hat, turtleneck, or scarf. Make sure you cover your hands and feet as well; mittens provide more warmth and protection than gloves.

- Warm up and cool down. Cold weather constricts muscles, so you need to allow enough time for proper stretching to warm up muscles before you exercise.

Exercise Injuries

According to the American Physical Therapy Association, the most common exercise-related injury sites are the knees, feet, back, and shoulders, followed by the ankles and hips. Types of injuries include the following:

- Acute injuries—sprains, bruises, and pulled muscles—result from sudden trauma, such as a fall or collision.

- Overuse injuries, on the other hand, result from overdoing a repetitive activity, such as running. When one particular joint is overstressed—such as a tennis player's elbow or a swimmer's shoulder—tendinitis, an inflammation at the point where the tendon meets the bone, can develop. Other overuse injuries include muscle strains and aches and stress fractures, which are hairline breaks in a bone, usually in the leg or foot.

The way a runner's foot strikes the ground can affect the risk of injury. In a study of college middle- and long-distance runners, about three in four experienced a moderate or severe injury each year, but those who habitually hit the ground with the rear of their foot had twice the rate of repetitive stress injuries as those who habitually hit with their forefoot.

Although many people worry that running may jeopardize their knees, recent research suggests that jogging and running may benefit the knees. The reason may be that runners tend to weigh less, which reduces the risk for knee arthritis. But jogging and running also may alter the biochemistry within the knee joint in ways to reduce the risk of injury.[79]

✓**check-in** Have you ever suffered a sports-related injury? Sooner or later, most active people do. Although most sports injuries are minor, they all require attention. Ignoring a problem or trying to push through the pain can lead to more serious complications.

PRICE If you develop aches and pains beyond what you might expect from an activity, stop. Never push to the point of fatigue. If you do, you could end up with sprained or torn muscles. Figure 6.8 gives the PRICE prescription for coping with an exercise injury.

Overtraining

About half of all people who start an exercise program drop out within 6 months. One common reason is that they **overtrain**, pushing themselves to work too intensely or too frequently. Signs of overdoing it include persistent

hypothermia An abnormally low body temperature; if not treated appropriately, coma or death could result.

overtrain Working muscles too intensely or too frequently, resulting in persistent muscle soreness, injuries, unintended weight loss, nervousness, and an inability to relax.

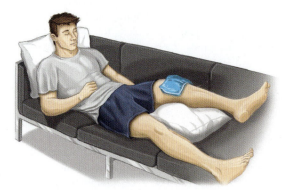

- Protect the area with an elastic wrap, sling, splint, cane, crutches, or air cast.
- Rest to promote tissue healing. Avoid activities that cause pain, swelling, or discomfort.
- Ice the area immediately, even if you're seeking medical help. (Don't put the ice pack directly on the skin.) Repeat every 2 or 3 hours while you're awake for the first 48 to 72 hours. Cold reduces pain, swelling, and inflammation in injured muscles, joints, and connecting tissues and may slow bleeding if a tear has occurred.
- Compress the area with an elastic bandage until the swelling stops. Begin wrapping at the end farthest from your heart. Loosen the wrap if the pain increases, the area becomes numb, or swelling is occurring below the wrapped area.
- Elevate the area above your heart, especially at night. Gravity helps reduce swelling by draining excess fluid. After 48 hours, if the swelling is gone, you may apply warmth or gentle heat, which improves the blood flow and speeds healing.

FIGURE 6.8 PRICE: How to Cope with an Exercise Injury

Just doing a few minutes of stretching to your major muscle groups can yield many benefits.

muscle soreness, frequent injuries, unintended weight loss, nervousness, and inability to relax.

If you develop any of the symptoms of overtraining, reduce or stop your workout sessions temporarily. Make gradual increases in the intensity of your workouts. Allow 24 to 48 hours for recovery between workouts. Make sure you get adequate rest.

Exercise Addiction Excessive exercise can become a form of addiction, and "exercise dependence" is not uncommon among young men and women. Although most physically active college students work out at healthy levels, some exercise to an extent that could signal dependence.

WHAT DID YOU DECIDE?

- What are the dangers of physical inactivity?
- What are the health benefits of physical activity and exercise?
- What would be an ideal workout?
- How can you protect yourself from exercise injuries?

Reflection

Stop and think about the bones that support you, the muscles that carry you, the heart that pumps blood through your arteries and veins, the lungs that sustain your every breath. One simple suggestion for taking the best possible care of your body: Move more!

TAKING CHARGE OF YOUR HEALTH

Shaping Up

This chapter has given you the basic information you need to launch a fitness program. However, you're more likely to succeed if you create a plan and follow it. Check off these basic steps to help you determine where you are now and how to get to where you want to be.

_____ Keep track of your progress in your online journal.

_____ Set fitness goals. Do you have an overall conditioning goal, such as losing weight? Or do you have a training goal, such as preparing for a 5K race or trying out for the volleyball team? Break down your goal into smaller "step" goals that lead you toward it.

_____ Think through your personal preferences. What are your physical strengths and weaknesses? Do you have good upper-body strength but easily get winded? Do you have a stiff back? Do your allergies flare up when you exercise outdoors? By paying attention to your needs, likes, and dislikes, you can choose activities you enjoy—and are more likely to continue.

_____ Schedule exercise into your daily routine. If you can, block out a half-hour for working out at the beginning of the day, between classes, or in the evening. Write it into your schedule as if it were a class or doctor's appointment. If you can't find 30 minutes, look for two 15-minute or three 10-minute slots that you can use for "mini-workouts." Once you've worked out a schedule, write it down. A written plan encourages you to stay on track.

_____ Assemble your gear. Make sure you put your athletic shoes in your car or in the locker at the gym. Lay out the clothes you'll need to shoot hoops or play racquetball.

_____ Start slowly. If you are just beginning regular activity or exercise, begin at a low level. If you have an injury, disability, or chronic health problem, be sure you get medical clearance from a physician.

_____ Progress gradually. If you have not been physically active, begin by incorporating a few minutes of physical activity into each day, building up to 30 minutes or more of moderate-intensity activities. If you have been active but not as often or as intensely as recommended, become more consistent. Continue to increase the frequency, intensity, and duration of your workouts.

_____ Take stock. After a few months of leading a more active life, take stock. Think of how much more energy you have at the end of the day. Ask yourself if you're feeling any less stressed, despite the push and pull of daily pressures. Focus on the unanticipated rewards of exercise. Savor the exhilaration of an autumn morning's walk; the thrill of feeling newly toughened muscles bend to your will; or the satisfaction of a long, smooth stretch after a stressful day. Enjoy the pure pleasure of living in the body you deserve.

SELF-SURVEY

Student Physical Activity Assessment

How Active Are You?

In the past week, did you engage in moderate-intensity cardio or aerobic exercise for at least 30 minutes?

0 days   _____

1–4 days   _____

5–7 days   _____

In the past week, did you engage in vigorous-intensity cardio or aerobic exercise for at least 20 minutes?

0 days   _____

1–2 days   _____

3–7 days   _____

The American College of Sports Medicine and the American Heart Association recommend:

Moderate-intensity cardio or aerobic exercise for at least 30 minutes on 5 or more days per week,

or

Vigorous-intensity cardio or aerobic exercise for at least 20 minutes on 3 or more days per week.

Do you meet the recommended guidelines? If not, use the information in this chapter to develop a plan to incorporate more physical activity into your daily schedule. Be sure to identify and include the types of activity you enjoy most and to block out specific times for your exercise "appointments."

How active are college students?
What do you think?

In the past week, what percentage of college students do you think engaged in moderate-intensity cardio or aerobic exercise for at least 30 minutes?

	Male	Female
0 days	_____	_____
1–4 days	_____	_____
5–7 days	_____	_____

In the past week, what percentage of college students do you think engaged in vigorous-intensity cardio or aerobic exercise for at least 20 minutes?

	Male	Female
0 days	_____	_____
1–2 days	_____	_____
3–7 days	_____	_____

What are the facts?

Percentage of college students who report moderate-intensity cardio or aerobic exercise for at least 30 minutes:

	Male	Female	Average
0 days	21.7	22.3	22.3
1–4 days	53.4	57.2	55.9
5–7 days	24.9	20.5	21.8

Percentage of college students who report vigorous-intensity cardio or aerobic exercise for at least 20 minutes:

0 days	37.2	44.8	42.8
1–2 days	31.1	30.1	30.4
3–7 days	31.8	25.1	26.8

Percentage of students who meet the recommended guidelines for physical activity:

50.9	44.6	46.2

Source: American College Health Association. American College Health Association-National College Health Assessment II: Undergraduate Student Reference Group Executive Summary. Hanover, MD: American College Health Association; Spring 2019.

REVIEW QUESTIONS

(LO 6.1) 1. _____ refers to the ability of the heart to pump blood through the body efficiently.
   a. Cardiorespiratory fitness
   b. Metabolic fitness
   c. Muscular endurance
   d. Muscular strength

(LO 6.1) 2. Which of the following is true of college students' fitness habits?
   a. College women are generally more active than men.
   b. Part-time or employed students exercise less than full-time students.
   c. Married students report more days of vigorous workouts than single students.
   d. Undergraduates living on campus are less active than those living off campus.

(LO 6.2) 3. Regular physical activity can reduce the risk of cancer by _____.
   a. strengthening the bones
   b. maintaining a healthy weight
   c. flushing toxins from the body
   d. enhancing the efficiency of the lungs

(LO 6.3) 4. For substantial health benefits, the government recommends at least _____ minutes of moderate-intensity aerobic exercise a week.
   a. 60
   b. 90
   c. 150
   d. 250

(LO 6.4) 5. The _____ principle states that muscles must work against a greater-than-normal resistance in order to get stronger.
   a. reversibility   c. variation
   b. overload   d. Karvonen

(LO 6.4) 6. Hussain was an athlete throughout high school. However, he stopped exercising once he reached college, and his fitness levels dropped by half. This is an example of the _____ principle.
   a. overload   c. variation
   b. reversibility   d. specificity

(LO 6.5) 7. Which of the following is true of the aerobic activity of spinning?
   a. It is a hybrid of boxing, martial arts, and aerobics.
   b. It combines dance and aerobic elements.
   c. It is a cardiovascular workout for the whole body.
   d. It involves mountain biking.

(LO 6.5) 8. _____ combines dance and aerobic elements with choreography that incorporates hip-hop, samba, salsa, merengue, mambo, martial arts, and belly dancing.
   a. Yoga   c. Zumba
   b. Spinning   d. Pilates

(LO 6.6) 9. In a(n) _____ contraction, the muscle applies force while maintaining an equal length.
   a. isotonic   c. isokinetic
   b. isometric   d. hypotonic

(LO 6.6) 10. Which of the following muscles form a part of the core?
- a. Quadriceps
- c. Pectorals
- b. Deltoids
- d. Obliques

(LO 6.7) 11. Which of the following is true of static flexibility?
- a. It is the ability to move a joint quickly.
- b. It depends on the structure of a joint and the tightness of the muscles.
- c. It refers to the ability to move a joint fluidly through its entire range of motion.
- d. It determines whether one can do a split leap.

(LO 6.7) 12. _____ stretching involves stretching a muscle by contracting the opposing muscle.
- a. Passive
- c. Dynamic
- b. Active
- d. Static

(LO 6.8) 13. Which of the following exercise methods employs a device called the Reformer?
- a. Pilates
- c. T'ai chi
- b. Yoga
- d. Zumba

(LO 6.8) 14. Which of the following Chinese practices is sometimes described as "meditation in motion"?
- a. Shooto
- c. T'ai chi
- b. Karate
- d. Jiu-jitsu

(LO 6.9) 15. An effective treatment for back pain is _____.
- a. surgery
- b. inflammatory medication
- c. bedrest
- d. core muscle strengthening

(LO 6.9) 16. Which of the following groups of people is at increased risk for back pain?
- a. Men
- c. Smokers
- b. Children
- d. Teenagers

(LO 6.10) 17. Which of the following is true in general of athletes' nutritional requirements?
- a. Complex carbohydrates are essential in their diet.
- b. They have higher protein requirements than others, with the exception of those engaged in intense strength training.
- c. Fat should be eliminated entirely from their diet.
- d. They should eat immediately before a workout to avoid feeling weak or tired.

(LO 6.10) 18. Too much water during prolonged bouts of exercise can lead to _____.
- a. fainting
- c. weight gain
- b. low sodium levels
- d. high blood pressure

(LO 6.11) 19. _____ is a medical emergency that can be fatal and occurs when the body temperature rises too quickly.
- a. Frostbite
- c. Heat cramps
- b. Heat exhaustion
- d. Heat stroke

(LO 6.11) 20. Which of the following is a sign of overtraining?
- a. Nervousness
- c. Bruises
- b. Tiredness
- d. Aches and pains

(LO 6.11) 21. If you experience an exercise injury, _____.
- a. immediately apply a heating pad directly on the skin of the injured area for 20 minutes
- b. allow the area to dangle below your heart
- c. ice the area immediately
- d. wrap the area with an elastic bandage tightly until it becomes numb to stabilize the injury

Answers to these questions can be found on page 531.

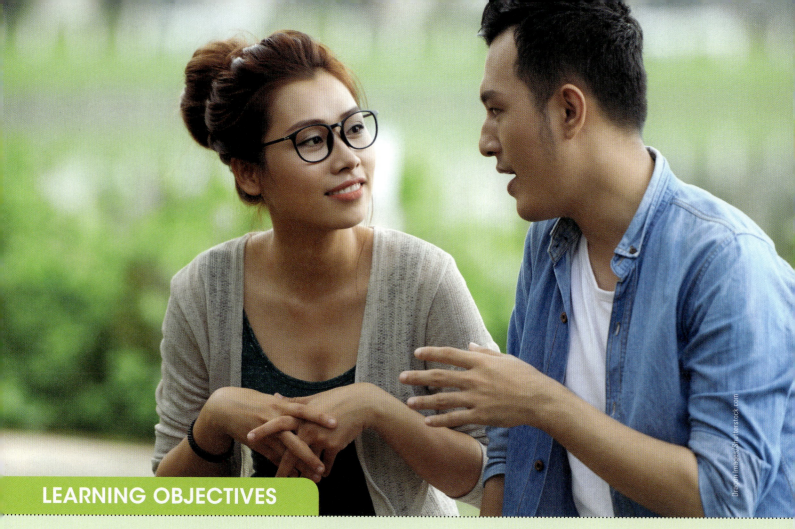

LEARNING OBJECTIVES

After reading this chapter, you should be able to:

7.1 Explain the meaning of the term *social health*, using examples.

7.2 Outline various ways of communicating.

7.3 Examine how relationships contribute to the social health of individuals.

7.4 Evaluate the impact of modern technology on communicating.

7.5 Identify current trends in dating among young people.

7.6 Explain the significance of love to an individual's well-being.

7.7 Summarize the impact of dysfunctional relationships.

7.8 Describe the trends, factors, and forms of long-term partnering in America.

7.9 Summarize the changes that have taken place in the American household over time.

WHAT DO YOU THINK?

- How can you enhance your communication skills?
- How do social media affect the lives of college students?
- What types of relationships are common on college campuses?
- How are healthy and dysfunctional relationships different?

7

Communicating and Connecting

Hannah got her first cell phone on her eighth birthday. She opened an e-mail account when she was 11, joined Facebook at 13, started tweeting and posting YouTube videos at 16, and signed onto LinkedIn after getting her first summer job at 17. Every day Hannah tweets, checks WhatsApp, texts instructors and teaching assistants, and posts photos or videos on Instagram, Pinterest, or Flickr. With more than a thousand friends and followers, Hannah says she can't imagine feeling lonely—as long as she doesn't misplace her smartphone and its battery doesn't die.

Is Hannah the poster child for social health in the 21st century? Or is her virtual socializing somehow undermining her overall well-being? Scientists who study relationships are just beginning to explore the impact of our digital world. Will tweets and emoticons replace conversation? Could online social networking make face-to-face friendships obsolete? <

No one knows the answers to these questions yet, but as much as technology may change our lives, one thing remains constant: We always have craved and always will crave human connection. As individuals and as part of society, we need to care about others and to know that others care about us, to feel for others and have others feel for us, to share what we know and to learn from what others know.

Your relationships with your family, friends, coworkers, and loved ones may amaze, irritate, exhilarate, frustrate, and delight you. Your ability to communicate, to develop satisfying relationships, and to live in harmony with others is an important dimension of health and wellness.

This chapter discusses the need to communicate and connect that we all share, healthy and unhealthy relationships, and the possibilities that exist for coming together from our solitude to warm ourselves in each other's glow.

The Social Dimension of Health

Social health refers to the ability to:

- Communicate and interact effectively with other people and with the social environment.
- Develop satisfying interpersonal relationships.
- Fulfill social roles.

Social health doesn't necessarily mean joining organizations or mingling in large groups, but it does involve participating in your community,

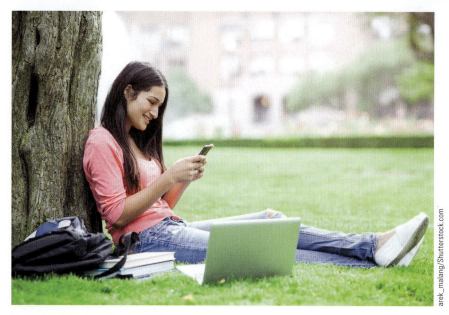

No one yet knows the impact that digital communication may have on relationships. Do you think texting might someday take the place of talking?

living in harmony with others, communicating clearly, and practicing healthy sexual behaviors (discussed in Chapter 8).

✓**check-in** How would you assess your social health? Excellent? Good? Not as good as you'd like?

As huge epidemiological studies have demonstrated beyond any doubt, supportive relationships buffer us from stress, distress, and disease. People with close ties to others have stronger cardiovascular and immune systems, resist colds better, and are less vulnerable to serious illness and premature death.

Specific qualities in a relationship, particularly *social support*, affect physical health. This term refers to the ways in which we provide information or assistance, show affection, comfort, and confide in others. As mounting evidence shows, people of all ages function best in socially supportive environments.

This is particularly true of college students, who report more stress and more physical symptoms when they feel a lack of family support. More than any other component of social support, a sense of belonging may have the greatest impact on college students' health. Because college is a transition time, forming new attachments may be especially important—and beneficial to overall health.

Your social support network might consist of people you see almost every day; more casual acquaintances; and friends, followers, and bloggers you get to know online. Simply staying in touch and sharing each other's lives

social contagion The process by which friends, friends of friends, acquaintances, and others in our social circle influence our behavior and our health—both positively and negatively.

bolster feelings of self-worth, security, and belonging.

✓**check-in** Who is in your social support network?

According to the concept of **social contagion**, friends, friends of friends, acquaintances, and others in our social circle influence our behavior and our health—both positively and negatively. Among the 15,000 people followed over three generations in the Framingham Heart Study, various health-related factors—such as weight gain, drinking, and smoking—changed not just individually over time but among clusters of people. The conclusion: Just as people are connected, so is their health. The reasons may include peer pressure or "mirror neurons" in the brain that automatically mimic what we see in the people around us.

As social scientists have documented, each of us is linked within three degrees (to a friend, a friend of a friend, and that friend's friend) to more than 1,000 people. Think of this social web as an opportunity. By your good health behaviors you can, in theory, influence 1,000 individuals to become healthier, fitter, and happier. And if you choose your friends wisely, they will do the same for you.

✓**check-in** Has your social network influenced any of your health behaviors? How do you think you may have influenced others?

Communicating

Healthy, mutually beneficial relationships add joy to our years and maybe even years to our life. Individuals with poor social skills are more vulnerable to a range of psychosocial problems, especially when confronted with stress, that increase the risk to their mental and physical health.[1]

By mastering skills to communicate more clearly and by being responsible and responsive in your interactions with others, you can cultivate what psychologist Daniel Goleman called "social intelligence" and create relationships worth cherishing.

Learning to Listen

Communication stems from a desire to know and a decision to tell. The first step is learning how to listen. Then you mostly choose what information about yourself to disclose and what to keep private. In opening up to others, you increase your own self-knowledge and understanding.

A great deal of daily communication focuses on facts: on the who, what, where, when, and how. Information is easy to convey and comprehend. Emotions are not. Some people have great difficulty saying "I appreciate you" or "I care about you," even though they are genuinely appreciative and caring. Others find it hard to know what to say in response and how to accept such expressions of affection.

Some people feel that relationships shouldn't require any effort, that there's no need to talk of responsibility between people who care about each other. Yet responsibility is implicit in our dealings with anyone or anything we value—and what can be more valuable than those with whom we share our lives? Friendships and other intimate relationships always demand an emotional investment, but the rewards they yield are great.

✓**check-in** Do you put effort into maintaining and strengthening your close relationships?

Being Agreeable but Assertive

There's an old saying that "nice guys finish last," but that's not the case. Psychologists translate "niceness" into a personality trait called "agreeableness," which includes being helpful, unselfish, generally trusting, considerate, cooperative, sympathetic, warm, and concerned for others. Among the benefits that agreeable people enjoy are strong relationships, less conflict, happy marriages, better job performance, healthier eating habits and behaviors, less stress, and fewer medical complaints.

Agreeable people aren't so "nice" that other people can easily influence or take advantage of them. In situations that call for it, they make their needs and desires clear by being assertive—but not aggressive.

Assertiveness doesn't mean screaming or telling someone off. You can communicate your wishes calmly and clearly. Assertiveness involves respecting your rights and the rights of other people even when you disagree. (See Your Strategies for Change: How to Assert Yourself.

You can change a situation you don't like by communicating your feelings and thoughts in nonprovocative words, by focusing on specifics, and by making sure you're talking with the person who is directly responsible.

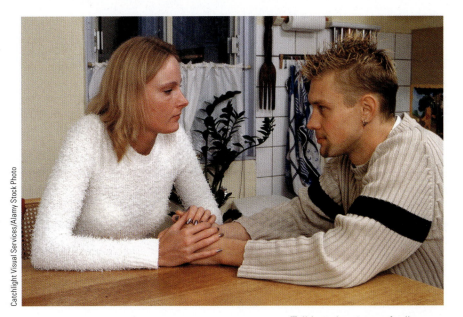

Talking about your feelings and listening intently move a relationship to a deeper and more meaningful level.

✓**check-in** Do you feel comfortable asserting yourself?

How Men and Women Communicate

Sex differences in communication start early. By age 1, boys make less eye contact than girls and pay more attention to moving objects like cars than to human faces. Both mothers and fathers talk less about feelings (except anger) to sons than daughters, and boys' vocabularies include fewer "feeling" words. On the playground, if not at home, boys learn to choke back tears and show

YOUR STRATEGIES FOR CHANGE

How to Assert Yourself

- **Use "I" statements to explain your feelings.** This allows you to take ownership of your opinions and feelings without putting down others for how they feel and think.

- **Listen to and acknowledge what the other person says.** After you speak, find out if the other person understands your position. Ask how he or she feels about what you've said.

- **Be direct and specific.** Describe the problem as you see it, using neutral language rather than assigning blame. Also suggest a specific solution, but make it clear that you'd like the lines of communication and negotiation to remain open.

- **Don't think you have to be obnoxious in order to be assertive.** It's most effective to state your needs and preferences without any sarcasm or hostility.

Catchlight Visual Services/Alamy Stock Photo

no fear. Their faces—once as openly emotional as girls'—become less expressive as they move through the elementary school years. As adults, men use fewer words and talk, at least in public, as a means of putting themselves in a one-up situation—unlike women, who talk to draw others closer. Even with friends, men mainly swap information as they talk shop, sports, cars, and computers.

Although men and women are more similar than different, scientific evidence continues to confirm that sex differences in communication, as well as in some personal qualities and mental abilities, do exist—but should be viewed as neither "better" nor "worse" and as "complementary" rather than "opposite."[2] They include the following differences by sex.

Men

- Speak more often and for longer periods in public.

- Interrupt more, breaking in on another's monologue if they aren't getting the information they need.

- Look into a woman's eyes more often when talking than they would if talking with another man.

- When writing, use more numbers, more prepositions, and articles such as *an* and *the*.

- Write briefer, more utilitarian emails.

- In blogs or chat rooms, are more likely to make strong assertions, disagree with others, and use profanity and sarcasm.

Women

- Speak more in private, usually to build better connections with others.

- Are generally better listeners, facilitating conversation by nodding, asking questions, and signaling interest by saying "uh-huh" or "yes."

- Are more likely to wait for a speaker to finish rather than interrupt.

- Look into another woman's eyes more often than they would if talking with a man.

- When writing, use more words overall; more words related to emotion (positive and negative); more idea words; more hearing, feeling, and sensing words; more causal words (such as *because*); and more modal words (*would, should, could*).

- Write e-mails in much the same way they talk, using words to build a connection with people.

- In blogs or chat rooms, are more prone to posing questions, making suggestions, and including polite expressions. Communication researchers studying the differences between "he-mails" and "she-mails" have also found that people who are not generally verbally expressive—mainly but not exclusively men—often convey more feelings in e-mails than they do in face-to-face conversations.

✓**check-in** What do you feel you can learn from the communication style of the "other" sex?

Nonverbal Communication

More than 90 percent of communication may be nonverbal. While we speak with our vocal cords, we communicate with our facial expressions, tone of voice, hands, shoulders, legs, torsos, and posture. Body language is the building block upon which more advanced verbal forms of communication rest.

Culture has a great deal of influence over body language. In some cultures, for example, establishing eye contact is considered hostile or challenging; in others, it conveys friendliness. A person's sense of personal space—the distance he or she feels most comfortable keeping from others—also varies in different societies.

✓**check-in** What does your body language say about you?

Forming Relationships

We first learn how to relate as children. Our relationships with parents and siblings change dramatically as we grow toward independence. Relationships between friends also change as they move or develop different interests; between lovers, as they come to know more about each other; between spouses, as they pass through life together; and between parents and children, as youngsters develop and mature. But throughout life, close relationships, tested and strengthened by time, allow us to explore the depths of our soul and the heights of our emotions.

Even a relationship with a pet can be beneficial. "Companion animals" have proven beneficial in lessening the symptoms of several mental disorders, easing the sting of rejection, and boosting a sense of well-being. They can also enhance feelings of self-worth and serve as catalysts for forming new relationships with other pet owners and neighbors.[3]

Friendship

Friendship has been described as "the most holy bond of society." Every culture has prized the ties of respect, tolerance, and loyalty that friendship builds and nurtures. An anonymous writer put it well:

> A friend is one who knows you as you are, understands where you've been, accepts who you've become, and still gently invites you to grow.

Friends can be a basic source of happiness, a connection to a larger world, and a source of solace in times of trouble. Although we have different friends throughout life, often the friendships of adolescence and young adulthood are the closest ones we ever form. They ease the normal break from parents and the transition from childhood to independence. Young people report more friends and seeing friends more often, but older individuals report higher levels of satisfaction with their contact with friends.[4]

On average, we devote 40 percent of our limited social time to the five most important people we know, who represent just 3 percent of our social world. Having more than five best friends is impossible when we interact face-to-face because of time constraints. But thanks to social networking online, it's possible to accumulate hundreds, or even thousands, of virtual friends.

Even so, most of us can maintain no more than 150 meaningful relationships online and off—a total called "Dunbar's number," in recognition of the researcher who came up with it. At one time, when almost all humans on Earth lived in small, rural, interconnected communities, everyone in a village may have known the same 150 people.

In our modern mobile society, we move time and again, leaving behind old friends. Emotional closeness, Dunbar found, declines by around 15 percent a year in the absence of face-to-face contact. Social media, at the least, provide us an opportunity to maintain friendships that would otherwise rapidly wither away. Images and messages from faraway friends can provide some of the same benefits as in-person friendship, including enhanced self-esteem and happiness.

✓check-in How many truly close friends do you have? How many "friendly" relationships do you have, both online and offline?

Loneliness

More so than many other countries, ours is a nation of loners. Recent trends—longer work hours, busy family schedules, frequent moves, high divorce rates—have created even more lonely people. In the most recent American College Health Association (ACHA) National College Health Assessment survey, 63 percent of undergraduates—55 percent of men and 66 percent of women—reported feeling very lonely at some time in the past 12 months.[5] (See Snapshot: On Campus Now in this chapter.)

✓check-in Have you felt very lonely at some time in the past 12 months?

Loneliness, defined as "feelings of distress and dysphoria resulting from a discrepancy between a person's desired and achieved social relations," has been identified as a risk factor for depression and poor psychological health. However, it may also threaten physical well-being. In a review of studies involving more than 3 million people, both feeling lonely and social isolation—having few or no social contacts or activities—increased the risk of an earlier death for both men and women, particularly those under the age of 65.[6]

Loneliest of all are adolescents and older adults; those who are divorced, separated, or widowed; and adults who live alone or solely with children. To combat loneliness, people may join groups, fling themselves into projects and activities, or surround themselves with superficial acquaintances. Others avoid the effort of trying to connect, sometimes limiting most of their personal interactions to their computers and mobile devices. The true keys to overcoming loneliness are developing resources to fulfill our own potential and learning to reach out to others. In this way, loneliness can become a means to personal growth and discovery.

Shyness and Social Anxiety Disorder

Many people are uncomfortable meeting strangers or speaking or performing in public. In some surveys, as many as 40 percent of people describe themselves as shy or socially anxious. Some shy people—an estimated 10 to 15 percent of children—are born with a predisposition to shyness. Others become shy because they don't learn proper social responses or because they experience rejection or shame. Some shy people spend excessive amounts of time on their smartphones and computers as a way of easing their anxiety.[7]

Some people are "fearfully" shy; that is, they withdraw and avoid contact with others and experience a high degree of anxiety and fear in social situations. Others are "self-consciously" shy; they enjoy the company of others but become highly self-aware and anxious in social situations.

In studies of college students, men have reported somewhat more shyness than women, and there may be sex differences in the psychosocial factors that trigger anxiety.[8] Some individuals develop symptoms of shyness or social anxiety when they go to a party or are called on in class; others experience symptoms when they try to perform any sort of action in the presence of others, even such everyday activities as eating in public, using a public restroom, or going to the grocery store.

About 7 percent of the population could be diagnosed with a **social anxiety disorder** (social phobia), in which individuals typically fear and avoid various social situations.[9] Childhood shyness, emotional abuse, neglect, and chronic illness increase the likelihood of this problem.[10] Asian cultures typically show the lowest rates; Russian and American, the highest.

Adolescents and young adults with severe social anxiety are at increased risk of major depression. The key difference between social anxiety and normal shyness and self-consciousness is the degree of distress and impairment that individuals experience. Cognitive-behavioral group therapy (discussed later in this chapter) has proven helpful in significantly reducing anxiety and symptoms of social anxiety disorder[11]; mindfulness stress reduction (discussed in Chapter 3) is also beneficial.[12]

social anxiety disorder A fear and avoidance of social situations.

✓**check-in** Do you think of yourself as shy?

If you're shy, you can overcome much of your social apprehensiveness on your own, in much the same way as you might set out to stop smoking or lose weight. For example, you can improve your social skills by pushing yourself to introduce yourself to a stranger at a party or to chat about the weather or the food selections with the person next to you in a cafeteria line. Gradually, you'll acquire a sense of social timing and a verbal ease that will take the worry out of close encounters with others. Those with more disabling social anxiety may do best with psychotherapy and medication, which have been shown to be highly effective.

Building a Healthy Community

"No man is an island," English poet John Donne wrote in 1624. In today's global society, this phrase rings just as true. In addition to our families, friendships, and social networks, we are part of communities—our campus, our neighborhood, our town, or city. (Chapter 19 discusses the community we are all citizens of: planet Earth.)

ⓞ SNAPSHOT: ON CAMPUS NOW

All the Lonely Students

Students who say they felt very lonely:

	Percent (%)		
	Male	Female	Average
No, never	26.2	17.3	19.7
No, not in the past 12 months	18.7	17.2	17.5
Yes, in the past 2 weeks	23.0	28.3	27.1
Yes, in the past 30 days	10.7	14.2	13.2
Yes, in the past 12 months	21.4	23.0	22.5
Anytime within the past 12 months	55.1	65.5	62.8

Source: American College Health Association. American College Health Association-National College Health Assessment II: Reference Group Executive Summary Spring 2018. Silver Spring, MD: American College Health Association, 2018.

Contributing to your community can take many forms, from volunteering at a Habitat for Humanity building project to singing in a church choir. By giving to others, you get a great deal in return. As researchers have documented, **altruism**—helping or giving to others—enhances self-esteem, relieves physical and mental stress, and protects psychological well-being.

✓**check-in** What do you do to contribute to your community?

Doing Good

Helping or giving to others enhances self-esteem, relieves physical and mental stress, and protects psychological well-being. Hans Selye, the father of stress research, described cooperation with others for the self's sake as altruistic egotism, whereby we satisfy our own needs while helping others satisfy theirs. This concept is essentially an updated version of the golden rule: Do unto others as you would have them do unto you. The important difference is that you earn your neighbor's love and help by offering him or her love and help.[13] Simply spending time outdoors may foster "green altruism" and a greater desire to help others.

Volunteerism helps those who give as well as those who receive. People involved in community organizations, for instance, consistently report a surge of well-being called *helper's high*, which they describe as a unique sense of calmness, warmth, and enhanced self-worth. College students who provided community service as part of a semester-long course reported changes in attitude (including a decreased tendency to blame people for their misfortunes), self-esteem (primarily a belief that they can make a difference), and behavior (such as a greater commitment to do more volunteer work).

✓**check-in** Do you volunteer?

The options for giving of yourself are limitless: Volunteer to serve a meal at a homeless shelter. Collect donations for a charity auction. Teach in a literacy program. Perform the simplest act of charity: Pray for others.

Living in a Wired World

Modern technology is changing our social DNA. Today you can use a smartphone to call, text, or video-chat with almost anyone almost anywhere. You also may blog, tweet, follow Facebook or other networking services, upload photos, and give the world (or selected citizens) front-row seats to your life.

Some experts say that with social networking, humans are only doing what comes naturally—but now with 21st-century tools.[14] Our brains seem wired to connect. As neuroimaging studies have shown, the amygdala, a brain region involved in processing emotional reactions, is bigger in individuals with large, complex social networks. These networks are getting bigger than ever—thanks to "computer-mediated communication"—the conveying of written text via the Internet—whether by Facebook, Twitter, Snapchat, Whatsapp, or ever-evolving new apps and sites. Yet researchers have also found that the more time young adults spend on social media the higher their levels of anxiety—and their risk of an anxiety disorder[15] (described in Chapter 2). They also smile less at others when using their smartphones or mobile devices.[16]

✓**check-in** Do you feel a sense of community with your online social network?

Social Networking on Campus

Traditional-age college students, the first "digital natives"—those who have grown up with technology—may be the most active users of online social networks.[17] More than 9 in 10 maintain a profile on a social network.

College students spend the most time on their devices: an average of 37 hours per month, seeking information (including maps and directions), corresponding via e-mail, texts, and other apps, gaming, shopping, flirting, and dating.[18] More than 9 in 10 college students maintain a social networking profile, with Facebook the most popular choice. In various studies college students ages 18 to 24 spend from 32 to 46 hours a month online; those ages 25 to 34 spend 35.8 hours online. Men and women in college also make up the largest percentage (more than 8 in 10) of smartphone owners.[19]

More than 1 in 5 people on the planet (22 percent) use Facebook. About 1 in 3 college students uses Twitter, compared to 1 in 5 high schoolers. About 6 in 10 online adults—most between ages 18 and 29—use Instagram.[20] In international studies of college students, women are more likely than men to use social networks to seek information (researching and learning new things and discussing products and brands) and for convenience (to obtain things with little effort).[21]

altruism Acts of helping or giving to others without thought of self-benefit.

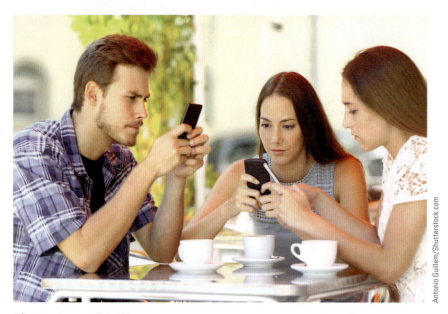

"Computer-mediated communication"—the conveying of written text via the Internet—is changing the ways we relate to others.

The most common motivations undergraduates give for their use of online networks are:

- Nurturing or maintaining existing relationships.
- Seeking new relationships.
- Enhancing their reputation (being cool).
- Avoiding loneliness.
- Keeping tabs on other people.
- Feeling better about themselves.[25]

Students feeling stressed or down report a psychological boost in self-esteem after viewing their Facebook profiles, perhaps because when they do so, they are reminded of the personal traits and relationships that they value most.[26] Simply having a certain number of Facebook friends boosts feelings of happiness, researchers have found. Even more meaningful is getting support from online acquaintances—but only if it comes in response to an honest presentation of oneself.

In general, women tend to use social networking sites to compare themselves with others and search for information. Men are more likely to look at other people's profiles to find friends.[27] The sexes even differ in their profile photos: Women usually add portraits, while men prefer full-body shots. College students of both sexes try to present themselves as positively as possible—but some of the most intense Facebook users attribute others' seeming success and happiness to their personalities. In a study of college women, engaging with attractive peers increased negative feelings about their bodies, while engaging with family had no impact on body image.[28]

More than half of students in one survey said that college social media profiles helped them to feel like part of the community.[29] Students may change their self-presentation on social media when they begin college and reclaim or redefine themselves.[30] In their first year, students become less restricted over the course of their first semester, and deep, positive, and authentic posts were associated with support from friends and higher self-esteem.[31] A class Facebook group may have many benefits. College students in such a group reported a greater sense of social connectedness, better relationships with faculty, and lower course-related stress. It also indirectly enhanced course engagement and satisfaction.[32] Upperclassmen on Facebook show greater positive social adjustment and more attachment to their schools.

✓**check-in** What are your reasons for being on Facebook—or not?

Undergraduates say that social networking is helpful for communication and information gathering, and that it positively influenced their academic work. However, students also reported that social networking had a negative impact on their social interactions, emotional health, and work completion, although younger students reported greater negative effects on work completion. Students also reported that social networking can be addictive, distractive, and a threat to their privacy.[22]

✓**check-in** How much time do you spend online every day?

Facebook has more than 1.23 billion users each month. Many consider it a useful social way to connect with friends, while others suggest that is an "isolating distraction" from creating deeper social interactions.[23]

Although other sites and apps have become popular, users still spend more time on Facebook—an estimated 100 minutes or more a day. Students typically engage in "lurking"—observing content rather than actually posting—and checking on others more often than sending private messages. They also engage in electronic interactions with friends by means of posting, commenting, or replying to messages and in self-presentation through photos, wall posts, "likes," or friend lists. Facebook can have both positive and negative impacts on well-being. In young adults, a higher number of reported Facebook friends was associated with feeling less lonely, but more persistent usage correlated with higher levels of loneliness.[24]

Self-Disclosure and Privacy in a Digital Age

A key element of relationships—whether friendships or romantic relationships—is **self-disclosure**—that is, how much we reveal about ourselves to another person. What you share about yourself is a critical building block that affects the nature and quality of the bonds you establish with others.

Social networking has transformed the issues of privacy and disclosure. Rather than confide in a trusted friend, individuals may go online and reveal highly personal information to a stranger—or, if a comment or video makes its way onto a public site, to many strangers.

Previously personal moments now play out in public—sometimes by choice (as in an engagement announced via a change in status on Facebook) and sometimes by chance (as when someone uploads a video of drunk beer-pong players). College students tend to display "risk behaviors," such as drinking, more often on Facebook than on Twitter.[33] Some view the images (of drinking more than drug use) in positive ways, but parents, friends of parents, siblings, coworkers, and employers often have a very different perspective.

Some social media messages may reveal more than their senders intend to communicate. In an analysis of college freshmen's tweets, researchers found that the tweets of the students reporting the greatest stress contained more negative sentiments, particularly fear. Students reporting a greater sense of love posted happier tweets.[34]

"Sexting"—sending sexually explicit text messages or digital photos—is fairly common among teens and young adults. The reasons for its popularity include peer pressure, the search for romance, and trust that the recipient will respond positively.[35] Despite warnings about potential misuse of such messages, adolescents tend not to consider the potential for negative fallout down the road (see Consumer Alert). Sexual posts can have unanticipated consequences. Sexual references generate powerful "subconscious impressions" that could put female students at risk for unwanted sexual advances.

✓**check-in** How do you react to sexual texts or online posts?

Digital Dating

Online sites and mobile apps allow people to find and introduce themselves to strangers and develop potential relationships. With online dating services, such as Match, eHarmony, and others, members create a "profile" that includes

❗ CONSUMER ALERT

Online Flirting and Dating

Virtual flirtations can be fun, but they also entail some risks, particularly if you decide to go offline and meet in person. Here are some guidelines.

Facts to Know

- Remember that you have no way of verifying whether a correspondent is telling the truth about anything—sex, age, occupation, and marital status. If your online partner seems insincere or strange in any way, stop corresponding.

- Be careful about what you type. Anything you put on the Internet can end up almost anywhere, including with potential employers. To avoid embarrassment, don't say anything you wouldn't want to see in newspaper print.

Steps to Take

- Don't give out your address, telephone number, or any other identifying information. The people you meet online are strangers, and you should keep your guard up.

- Don't "date" on an office or university computer. You could end up supplying your professors, classmates, or coworkers with unintentional entertainment. Also, many organizations and institutions consider e-mail messages company property.

- Don't rely on the Internet as your only method of meeting people. Continue to get out in the real world and meet potential dates the old-fashioned way: live and in person.

- If you do decide to meet someone you met online, make your first face-to-face encounter a double or group date and make it somewhere public, like a café or museum. Don't plan a full-day outing. Coffee or a drink in a crowded place makes the best transition from e-mail.

- Don't let your expectations run wild. Finding Mr. or Ms. Right is no easier in cyberspace than anywhere else, so be realistic about where your relationship might lead.

personal information, as well as photos or videos. Mobile or smartphone dating apps such as Tinder provide similar opportunities to text, chat, flirt, and set up a meeting. In essence, online or mobile dating creates a virtual marketplace in which people "shop" for potential partners and sell themselves in hopes of finding a successful match. Sociologists have identified loneliness, delayed age at marriage, and the high divorce rate as contributors to the popularity of digital dating.

In addition to information on age, sex, and sexual preference, dating sites may specify location so users can connect with someone in close proximity. Some sites are free; others charge for "premium" services or paid subscriptions. Dating services enroll users of any demographic. "Niche" sites are based on age, race, religion, sexual orientation, politics, medical conditions, shared interests, or a specific type of desired relationship. After establishing contact via phone or computer, individuals may or may not choose to meet in person.

The number of online "daters" has skyrocketed in the past decade, particularly among young adults. According to surveys, most view

self-disclosure Sharing personal information and experiences with another that he or she would not otherwise discover; self-disclosure involves risk and vulnerability.

online dating sites as an easy, efficient way to meet a wide range of potential partners. However, many consider online dating as more dangerous than traditional ways of getting to know a potential partner. Site owners may post "bait profiles" to attract new paying members, while advertisers may create "spam profiles" to market services and products.[36] (See Consumer Alert: Online Flirting and Dating.)

Users themselves may post false or misleading information, usually to appear more attractive online or to protect their privacy.[37] According to research, 9 of 10 online "daters" lie about at least one attribute in their profiles. Men are more likely to lie about their height, and women, about their weight.[38]

Others may misrepresent their marital status or health—for instance, not disclosing a history of sexually transmitted infections (STIs). High percentages of both men and women exclude partners on the basis of religion, race, socioeconomic level, or potential disapproval of family and friends.[39]

As researchers have documented, virtual dating typically begins with "pickup" lines to initiate contact and culminates in an offline meeting. Along the way individuals alternate between strategies for attracting and selecting a partner, presenting themselves in a positive but authentic light, creating a shared context for interacting, seeking and revealing information, and adapting to the online dating environment.[40]

✓**check-in** Have you used any online or smartphone dating sites? If so, how would you describe your experience?

Problematic Smartphone and Internet Use

College students primarily use their phones for leisure rather than school or work. Researchers have classified those who are on their phones 10 or more hours a day as "high users," while those who spend 3 hours or less on their phones qualify as low users. In terms of personality characteristics, the low users showed a higher preference for challenge and were least susceptible to boredom. High users may be more susceptible to anxiety and depression.[41] Most Americans say that using a smartphone in a social settings hurts more often than helps conversation—but about 9 in 10 report using their phones in their most recent social interaction.[42]

The concept of Internet "addiction" has evolved over recent years, based on hundreds of individuals whose inability to control their Internet use resulted in academic, financial, occupational and relationship problems.[43] Estimates of problematic Internet use among college students range from 1 to 6 percent. In the ACHA survey, 10 percent of students—more than the percentage citing relationship difficulties or depression—ranked Internet use/computer games as having a negative impact on their academic performance.[44]

Excess use of the Internet seems similar to other addictions in its neurobiological basis, say researchers who are beginning to explore and understand this 21st-century phenomenon. Like other addictions, Internet addiction almost always results from an interaction between many factors, including biological or genetic predisposition, social environment, personality, attitudes, expectations, beliefs, and the nature of the activity itself. Psychosocial factors such as low self-esteem, loneliness, depression, anxiety, and stress are common among those who develop any behavioral addiction.[45]

The characteristics of problematic Internet use include the following[46]:

- Preoccupation with Internet use; tolerance (i.e., the compulsion to use the Internet for ever-increasing amounts of time).

- Repeated but unsuccessful efforts to control, cut back, or stop Internet use.

- Restlessness, irritability, and other signs of withdrawal when unable to use the Internet.

- "Phantom vibration syndrome," which consists of mistakenly feeling a sensation of a vibrating phone—an experience, was reported by 9 in 10 college students in one study).[47]

- Physical symptoms, such as vision problems and "text neck."

- Having jeopardized or lost a relationship, job, or educational or career opportunity because of Internet use.

- Lying to friends, family members, and others to conceal the extent of involvement with the Internet.

- Increased family and personal conflicts and poor academic performance.[48]

- Using the Internet to escape or palliate dysphoric moods such as depression and anxiety.

Online interactions with virtual "friends" can consume users' attention and distract them from spending time with their actual significant others. In one study, social media addiction predicted a great likelihood of online "cheating," particularly among younger individuals.[49]

Neuroimaging studies have shown similarities between the brains of compulsive Internet users and those with other addictive behaviors.[50] Some scholars have argued that people are not addicted to the Internet but to specific activities on the Internet such as online gambling,[51] gaming, shopping, and pornography.[52] This behavior may start early. According to recent surveys, about 4 in 10 boys and 3 in 10 girls in high school reported receiving sexually explicit cell phone pictures, while 16 percent of male students and 14 percent of female students said they had "sexted" revealing photos.[53]

✓**check-in** Has your Internet use ever caused problems for you?

For some the Internet has become an outlet for anger. Various "rant" websites allow anonymous users to adopt a screen name and engage in back-and-forth online screaming. This behavior may seem harmless, but as research shows, individuals who engage in virtual venting may initially feel more relaxed but overall tend to experience more anger in general and express it in maladaptive ways.

Cyberbullying consists of deliberate, repeated, and hostile actions that use information and communication technologies, including online Web pages and text messages, with the intent of harming others by means of intimidation, control, manipulation, false accusations, or humiliation. Cyberbullies may know their victims or strike randomly. About one in five college students reports having been bullied on social networking sites; 46 percent report having been bystanders to social network cyberbullying and 61 percent did not intervene or engage.[54] Its prevalence on college campuses ranges from 8 to 21 percent.[55]

Although more attention has focused on cyberbullying by younger students, undergraduates also can be victims or perpetrators. In a study of more than 1,200 college students between the ages of 18 and 26, a deteriorated family environment increased the probability of being both a victim and an aggressor, while a favorable family environment decreases this probability. In the study, 19 percent of students said they have been victims of cyberbullying; while 19 percent declared they had been cyberbullying aggressors. Higher emotional intelligence lowers cyberbullying.[56]

Cyberstalking, a form of cyberbullying, uses online sites, email messages, and social media to harass victims and try to damage their reputation or turn others against them. Cyberstalking may include false accusations, threats, identity theft,

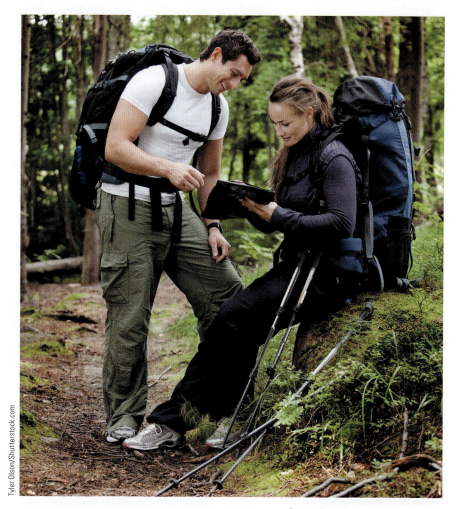

Tyler Olson/Shutterstock.com

damage to data or equipment, or the solicitation of minors for sex. Both cyberbullying and cyberstalking can be criminal offenses punishable by imprisonment. Cyberstalking occurs most often in the context of ex-partner relationships. Most of its perpetrators are male and its victims are female. Its negative psychological impact on a victim's well-being is comparable to real-life stalking.

✓**check-in** Have you ever experienced cyberbullying or cyberstalking?

Loving and Being Loved

You may not think of love as a basic need like food and rest, but it is essential for both physical and psychological well-being. Mounting evidence suggests that people who lack love and

Spending time together gives couples a chance to have fun and share their likes, dislikes, and interests.

cyberbullying Deliberate, repeated, and hostile actions that use information and communication technologies, including online Web pages and text messages, with the intent of harming others by means of intimidation, control, manipulation, false accusations, or humiliation.

cyberstalking A form of cyberbullying that uses online sites, Twitter, e-mail messages, and social media to harass victims and try to damage their reputation or turn others against them.

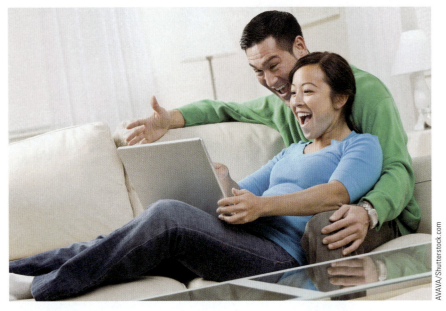

We tend to be attracted to people who are similar to ourselves in age, race, ethnicity, socioeconomic class, and education.

commitment are at high risk for a host of illnesses, including infections, heart disease, and cancer.

Intimate Relationships

The term **intimacy**—the open, trusting, and sharing of close, confidential thoughts and feelings—comes from the Latin word for "within." Intimacy doesn't happen at first sight, or in a day or a week or a number of weeks. Intimacy requires time and nurturing; it is a process of revealing rather than hiding, of wanting to know another and to be known by that other. Although intimacy doesn't require sex, an intimate relationship often includes a sexual relationship, heterosexual or homosexual.

In an intimate relationship, empathy becomes even more important. You can develop your capacity for empathy by pulling back periodically, particularly in moments of stress or conflict, and asking yourself: "What is my partner or spouse feeling right now? What does he or she need?"

✓**check-in** Are you in a committed intimate relationship?

Committed intimate relationships may be beneficial for college students' physical and mental health, just as marriage is for spouses. The reasons may be that these students have less time for risky behavior, that being in a relationship fosters a less impulsive lifestyle, or that partners who use drugs or drink heavily may be unable to keep a romantic partner. Simply having fewer sexual partners lowers general stress as well as the risk of sexual infections or assaults.

intimacy A state of closeness between two people, characterized by the desire and ability to share one's innermost thoughts and feelings with each other either verbally or nonverbally.

What Attracts Two People to Each Other?

Scientists have tried to analyze the combination of factors that attracts two people to each other. In several studies of college students, the following four predictors ranked as the most important reasons for attraction:

- Warmth and kindness.
- Desirable personality.
- Something specific about the person.
- Reciprocal liking.

Economic factors, including money or lack thereof, didn't make the list. Physical attractiveness generally has similar effects on both sexes.

Infatuation

It is tempting to think of love as scenes from a movie script: blazing sunsets and misty nights, fiery glances and passionate embraces, consuming desire and happy-ever-after endings. However, movies last only 2 hours; ideally, love lasts a lifetime. Infatuation falls somewhere in between. Certainly, falling in love is an intense, dizzying experience. A person not only enters our life but also takes possession. We are intrigued, flattered, captivated, and delighted—but is this love or a love of loving?

At the time you're experiencing it, there is no difference between infatuation and lasting love. You feel the same giddy, wonderful way. However, if it's infatuation, it won't last. Infatuation refers only to falling in love. People genuinely in love with each other do more than fall; they start building a relationship together.

Being head over heels in love can have such an impact on the brain that it reduces pain. Stanford University researchers studied 15 undergraduates in the infatuation stage of love and inflicted pain with a handheld thermal probe. Those looking at a photograph of their beloved not only reported less pain but showed the same brain changes as those induced by drugs like cocaine.[57]

The Science of Romantic Love

We like to think of this powerful force, a source of both danger and delight, as something that defies analysis. However, scientists have provided new perspectives on its true nature.

A Psychological View According to psychologist Robert Sternberg, love can be viewed as a triangle with three faces: passion, intimacy, and commitment (Figure 7.1). Each person brings his or her own triangle to a relationship. If they match well, their relationship is likely to be satisfying.

Sternberg also identified six types of love:

- **Liking:** the intimacy friends share.
- **Infatuation:** the passion that stems from physical and emotional attraction.
- **Romantic love:** a combination of intimacy and passion.
- **Companionate love:** a deep emotional bond in a relationship that may have had romantic components.
- **Fatuous love:** a combination of passion and commitment in two people who lack a deep emotional intimacy.
- **Consummate love:** a combination of passion, intimacy, and commitment over time.

An Anthropological View

When you first fall in love, you may be sure that no one else has ever known the same dizzying, wonderful feelings. Yet, while every romance may be unique, romantic love is anything but. Anthropologists have found evidence of romantic love between individuals in most of the cultures they have studied.

As anthropologist Helen Fisher, author of *Anatomy of Love: The Natural History of Monogamy, Adultery and Divorce*, explains, romantic love pulled men and women of prehistoric times into the sort of partnerships that were essential to childrearing. But after about 4 years—just "long enough to rear one child through infancy," says Fisher—romantic love seemed to wane, and primitive couples tended to break up and find new partners.

A Biochemical View

The heart is the organ we associate with love, but the brain may be where the action really is. According to research on neurotransmitters (the messenger chemicals within the brain), love sets off a chemical chain reaction that causes our skin to flush, our palms to sweat, and our lungs to breathe more deeply and rapidly. Neuroimaging studies reveal that viewing images of a romantic partner activates the areas of the brain that produce the so-called "love chemicals"—dopamine, norepinephrine, and phenylethylamine (PEA)—involved in various rewarding experiences, including beauty and love. Falling in love causes changes in the immune system that may have evolved to promote reproduction and preserve the species.[58]

Infatuation may indeed be a natural high, but like other highs, this rush doesn't last—possibly

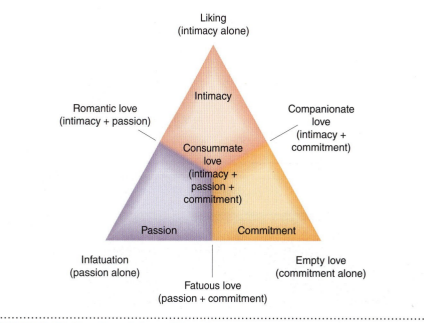

FIGURE 7.1 Sternberg's Love Triangle

The three components of love are intimacy, passion, and commitment. The various kinds of love are composed of different combinations of the three components.

because the body develops tolerance for love-induced chemicals, just as it does with amphetamines. However, as the initial lover's high fades, other brain chemicals may come into play: the endorphins, morphine-like chemicals that can help produce feelings of wellbeing, security, and tranquility. These feel-good molecules may increase in partners who develop a deep attachment.

✓**check-in** Do these theories help you understand love better?

Mature Love

Social scientists have distinguished between *passionate love* (characterized by intense feelings of elation, sexual desire, and ecstasy) and *companionate love* (characterized by friendly affection and deep attachment). Often relationships begin with passionate love and evolve into a more companionate love. Sometimes the opposite happens and two people who know each other well discover that their friendship has "caught fire," and the sparks have flamed an unexpected passion.

Mature love is a complex combination of sexual excitement, tenderness, commitment, and—most of all—an overriding passion that sets it apart from all other love relationships in one's life. This passion isn't simply a matter of orgasm but also entails a crossing of the psychological boundaries between oneself and one's lover. You feel as

Assessing a Relationship

If you're currently involved with someone, read through the following list of positive indicators of a healthy relationship and check all that apply.

___ You feel at ease with your partner.

___ You feel good about your partner when you're together and when you're not.

___ Your partner is open with you about his or her life—past, present, and future.

___ You can say no to each other without feeling guilty.

___ You feel cared for, appreciated, and accepted as you are.

___ Your partner really listens to what you have to say.

The more items you've checked, the more reasons you have to keep seeing each other. Read through the list of negative indicators below and check those that apply. In this case, every check is a warning of dangers ahead.

___ You don't feel comfortable together.

___ You feel angry or let down when you're together or apart.

___ Your partner is very secretive about his or her life.

___ You feel your partner isn't attentive to you.

___ You don't feel cared for and appreciated.

Reflect on the pluses and minuses of your relationship in your online journal.

dysfunctional Characterized by negative and destructive patterns of behavior between partners or between parents and children.

if you're becoming one with your partner while simultaneously retaining a sense of yourself.

Dysfunctional Relationships

Mental health professionals define a **dysfunctional** relationship as one that doesn't promote healthy communication, honesty, and intimacy and here either person is made to feel worthless or incompetent. Individuals with addictive behaviors or dependence on drugs or alcohol (see Chapters 15 and 16), and the children or partners of such people, are especially likely to find themselves in a dysfunctional relationship.

Often partners have magical, unrealistic expectations (e.g., they expect that a relationship with the right person will make their life okay), and one person uses the other almost as if he or she were a mood-altering drug. The partners may compulsively try to get the other to act the way they want. Both persons may distrust or may deceive each other. Often they isolate themselves from others, thus trapping themselves in a recurring cycle of pain.

Physical symptoms, such as headaches, digestive troubles, tics, and inability to sleep well, can be signs of a destructive relationship. Yet, although one person may repeatedly attack, abandon, betray, badger, bully, criticize, deceive, dominate, or demean the other, the responsibility for changing the unhealthy dynamic belongs to both.

Intimate Partner Violence

Dysfunction can lead to violence, discussed in Chapter 14. Nearly half of all couples experience some form of physical aggression. Couples who are cohabiting (see page 201) experience more aggression than married partners and those who are dating but living separately. In the most recent ACHA survey, about 2 percent of students had been in a physically abusive relationship in the preceding 12 months and about 10 percent reported being in an emotionally abusive intimate relationship[59] (see Table 7.1).

Women attending urban commuter colleges may be at particular risk if they have partners who seek to control or limit their college experience or who feel threatened by what they may achieve by attending college.[60] Minority stress (discussed in Chapter 4) may contribute

to violence among lesbian, gay, bisexual, transgender, and queer or questioning (LGBTQ) partners, who are much less likely than other couples to disclose what happened. In one recent study, only about a third (compared to roughly three-quarters of heterosexuals) revealed a violent episode to any person, most often a friend. The reasons for nondisclosure include a feeling that it was "not a big deal," a desire for privacy, and concern about others' reactions.[61]

An estimated one in three women have been sexually assaulted; one in four have been victims of intimate partner violence. The consequences include increased risk for mental and physical health problems, such as injury, chronic pain, disability, depression, anxiety, eating disorders, posttraumatic stress disorder (PTSD), and addiction.[62] Some perpetrators of interpersonal domestic violence are aggressive only with family, while some also become violent with others and present a higher risk for severe or deadly violence.[63]

Mental health problems are often linked with interpersonal violence. Women who suffer from depression or PTSD are more vulnerable to victimization. Anxiety and antisocial personality disorder correlated with a greater likelihood of perpetrating violence in men.[64] Intimate partner violence also increases the incidence of depression in married women.[65] (See Chapter 18 for an in-depth discussion of sexual victimization and violence.)

Emotional Abuse

Abuse consists of any behavior that uses fear, humiliation, or verbal or physical assaults to control and subjugate another human being. Rather than being physical, emotional abuse takes many forms:

- Berating.
- Belittling or demeaning.
- Constant criticism.
- Name calling.
- Blaming.
- Threatening.
- Accusing.
- Judging.
- Trivializing, minimizing, or denying what a person says or feels.

Even if done for the sake of "teaching" or "helping," emotional abuse wears away at self-confidence, sense of self-worth, and trust and belief in oneself. Because it is more than skin deep, emotional abuse can leave deeper, longer-lasting scars.

No one wants to get into an abusive relationship, but often people who were emotionally abused in childhood find themselves in similar circumstances as adults. Dealing with an emotional abuser, regardless of how painful, may feel familiar or even comfortable. Individuals who think very little of themselves may also pick partners who treat them as badly as they believe they deserve.

Abusers may also have grown up with emotional abuse and view it as a way of coping with feelings of fear, hurt, powerlessness, or anger. They may seek partners who see themselves as helpless and who make them feel more powerful.

Among the signs of emotional abuse are the following:

- **Attempting to control various aspects of your life**, such as what you say or wear.
- **Frequently humiliating you** or making you feel bad about yourself.
- **Making you feel as if you are to blame** for what your partner does.
- **Wanting to know where you are** and whom you're with at all times.
- **Becoming jealous or angry** when you spend time with friends.
- **Threatening to harm you** if you break up.
- **Trying to coerce you** into unwanted sexual activity with statements such as "If you loved me, you would. . . ."

If you can never get what you need or if you're afraid, you need to get out of the relationship. Take whatever steps necessary to ensure your safety. Find a trusted friend who can help. Don't isolate yourself from family and friends. This is a time when you need their support and often the support of a counselor, minister, or doctor as well. (See Your Strategies for Change: How to Cope with an Unhealthy Relationship.)

Codependency

The definition of **codependency** has expanded to include any maladaptive behaviors learned by family members in order to survive great emotional pain and stress, such as an addiction, chronic mental or physical illness, and abuse. Some therapists refer to codependency as a "relationship addiction" because codependent people often form or maintain relationships that are one-sided, emotionally destructive, or abusive. First identified in studies of the relationships in families of alcoholics, codependent behavior can occur in any dysfunctional family.

TABLE 7.1 Abusive Relationships on Campus

Within the past 12 months, college students reported experiencing:			
	Men	Women	Average
An emotionally abusive intimate relationship	6.5	10.7	9.6
A physically abusive intimate relationship	1.7	1.9	1.9
A sexually abusive intimate relationship	1.1	3.0	2.5

Source: American College Health Association. American College Health Association-National College Health Assessment II: Reference Group Executive Summary Spring 2018. Silver Spring, MD: American College Health Association, 2018.

Signs of Codependency Among the characteristics of codependency are:

- An exaggerated sense of responsibility for the actions of others.
- An attraction to people who need rescuing.
- Always trying to do more than one's share.
- Doing anything to cling to a relationship and avoid feeling abandoned.
- An extreme need for approval and recognition.
- A sense of guilt about asserting needs and desires.
- A compelling need to control others.
- Lack of trust in self and/or others.
- Fear of being alone.
- Difficulty identifying feelings.
- Rigidity/difficulty adjusting to change.
- Chronic anger.
- Lying/dishonesty.
- Poor communications.
- Difficulty making decisions.

Because the roots of codependency run so deep, people don't just "outgrow" this problem or magically find themselves in a healthy relationship. Treatment to resolve childhood hurts and deal with emotional issues may take the form of individual or group therapy, education, or programs such as Co-Dependents Anonymous (www.coda.org). The goal is to help individuals get in touch with long-buried feelings and build healthier family and relationship dynamics.

Enabling Experts on the subject of addiction first identified traits of codependency in spouses of alcoholics, who followed a predictable pattern of behavior: While intensely trying to control the drinkers, the codependent mates would act in

codependency An emotional and psychological behavioral pattern in which the spouses, partners, parents, children, and friends of individuals with addictive behaviors allow or enable their loved ones to continue their self-destructive habits.

ways that allowed the drinkers to keep drinking. For example, if an alcoholic found it hard to get up in the morning, his wife would wake him up, pull him out of bed and into the shower, and drop him off at work. If he was late, she made excuses to his boss. The husband was the one with the alcohol-abuse problem, but without realizing it, his wife was enabling him to continue drinking. In fact, he might not have been able to keep up his habit without her unintentional cooperation.

Codependency progresses just as an addiction does, and codependents excuse their own behavior with many of the same defense mechanisms used by addicts, such as rationalization ("I cut class so I could catch up on my reading, not to keep an eye on my partner") and denial ("He likes to gamble, but he never loses more than he can afford"). In time, codependents lose sight of everything but their loved one. They feel that if they can only "fix" this person, everything will be fine.

When Love Ends

As the old song says, breaking up is indeed hard to do. Sometimes two people grow apart gradually, and both of them realize that they must go their separate ways. More often, one person falls out of love first. It hurts to be rejected; it also hurts to inflict pain on someone who once meant a great deal to you.

In surveys, college students say it's more difficult to initiate a breakup than to be rejected. Those who decide to end a relationship report greater feelings of guilt, uncertainty, discomfort, and awkwardness than their girlfriends or boyfriends. However, students with high levels of jealousy are likely to feel a desire for vengeance that can lead to aggressive behavior.

Research suggests that people do not end their relationships because of the disappearance of love. Rather, a sense of dissatisfaction or unhappiness develops, which may then cause love to stop growing. The fact that love does not dissipate completely may be why breakups are so painful.

While the pain does ease over time, it can help both parties if they end their relationship in a way that shows kindness and respect. Your basic guideline should be to think of how you would like to be treated if someone were breaking up with you:

- Would it hurt more to find out from someone else?

- Would it be more painful if the person you cared for lied to you or deceived you, rather than admitting the truth?

Saying "I don't feel the way I once did about you; I don't want to continue our relationship" is hard, but it's also honest and direct.

✓check-in Have you ever broken up with someone? Has someone ever broken up with you?

Partnering across the Lifespan

Even though men and women today may have more sexual partners than in the past, most still yearn for an intense, supportive, exclusive relationship, based on mutual commitment and enduring over time. In our society, most such relationships take the form of heterosexual marriages, but partners of the same sex or heterosexual partners who never marry may also sustain long-lasting, deeply committed relationships.

These couples are much like married people: They make a home, handle daily chores, cope with problems, celebrate special occasions, plan for the future—all the while knowing that they are not alone, that they are part of a pair that adds up to far more than just the sum of two individual souls.

The New Transition to Adulthood

Growing up is not what it used to be. Social scientists have identified "emerging adulthood" as a unique developmental period that spans the late teens and the 20s, marked by volatility and identity formation. Traditionally the milestones of this life stage were completing school, leaving home, becoming financially independent, marrying, and having a child.

Today more than 95 percent of Americans consider the most important markers of adulthood to be completing school, establishing an independent household, and being employed full time. Only about half consider it necessary to marry or have children to be regarded as an adult. Unlike their parents and grandparents, young people view these markers as life choices rather than requirements.

✓check-in Do you think of graduation, living on your own, or getting a full-time job as a marker of maturity or a life choice?

The changing time table for adulthood has affected the timing and nature of intimate relationships or, as sociologists describe them, "partnerships." Although just as eager for intimacy—emotional and sexual—younger adults are following a different pattern than past generations. Among a smorgasbord of romantic options, they may:

- Enter into casual, short-term relationships.
- Commit to a long-term monogamous relationship.
- Live with a partner with or without the intent of getting married.
- View marriage as the final step in a relationship that may take place after sexual involvement, shared living, and even childbearing and parenting.

Nearly half of young people live with their parents. This percentage drops below 1 in 7 by the late 20s and below 1 in 10 by the early 30s. Women are typically younger than men when they leave home because they complete college earlier, form cohabiting unions earlier, and marry about 2 years earlier. In 1970, two-thirds of 20-somethings were married. Now just about one-quarter are.

Cohabitation

Although couples have always shared homes in informal relationships without any official ties, "living together," or **cohabitation**, has become more common. The majority of young adults have lived with a partner by their mid-20s, but they do not view it as a permanent alternative to marriage. Although cohabitation has been increasing steadily for decades, the number of couples living together has spiked in recent years.

One reason may be economic. Partners may not have enough money to live alone but don't plan to get married until they have more money—which is harder to get in a bad economy. Social acceptance may also contribute. A few generations ago, "shacking up" seemed shocking. Today fewer than half of Americans think living together is a bad idea.

··
✓check-in What do you think of cohabitation?
··

About one-quarter of unmarried women ages 25 to 39 are currently living with a partner; an additional one-quarter lived with a partner in the past. Couples live together before more than half of all marriages, a practice that was practically unknown 50 years ago. In addition, the proportion of cohabiting women between the ages of 20 and 50 has tripled in the past 50 years.

YOUR STRATEGIES FOR CHANGE

How to Cope with an Unhealthy Relationship

- **Start a dialogue.** Focus on communication, not confrontation. Start with a positive statement, for instance, saying what you really value in the relationship. Volunteer what you might do to make it better and state what you need from the other person.

- **Distance yourself.** Take a vacation from a toxic friendship. Skip the family reunion or Thanksgiving dinner. When forced into proximity, be polite. If you refuse to engage—not arguing, not getting angry, not trying to make things better—toxic people give up trying to get under your skin.

- **Consult a professional.** A therapist or minister can help people recognize and change toxic behavior patterns. Changes you make in how you act and react may trigger changes in others.

- **Save yourself.** If you can never get what you need in a relationship, you may need to let it go. Nothing is worth compromising your mental or physical health.

Cohabitation can be a prelude to marriage, an alternative to living alone, or an alternative to marriage. Couples choose to cohabit for different reasons. Couples who move in together to "test" their relationship report more problems—including more negative communication, physical aggression, and symptoms of depression and anxiety—than others. Cohabitation is associated with better health for men in same-sex relationships but with poorer health for men and women in different-sex relationships.[66]

The timing of a decision to move in together also matters. Couples who cohabited before getting engaged later reported less marital satisfaction, dedication, and confidence as well as more negative communication and greater potential for divorce than those who lived together after engagement or after getting married.

Asians and non-Hispanic white couples are the least likely to cohabit. A higher percentage of Native American, black, and Hispanic couples are unmarried. "Cohabiters" tend to have lower income and education levels. They are also younger—on average, some 12 years younger than married men and women.

Committed couples, both heterosexual and homosexual, can register as domestic partners in certain areas. This may enable them to qualify for benefits such as health insurance. Recent court rulings have placed domestic partners on the same legal footing as married couples in dealings with businesses.

cohabitation Two people living together as a couple, without official ties such as marriage.

Long-Term Relationships

Both heterosexual ("straight") and same-sex couples progress through various stages as their relationships develop:

- Blending, a time of intense passion and romantic love.

- Nesting (starting a home together).

- Building trust and dependability.

- Merging assets.

- Establishing a strong sense of partnership.

Gay and lesbian relationships are comparable to straight relationships in other ways.[67] However, because there are no social norms for same-sex unions, researchers describe these relationships as more egalitarian. Each partner tends to be more self-reliant, and homosexual men and women tend to be more willing to communicate and experiment in terms of sexual behaviors.

But many same-sex couples have to deal with everyday ups-and-downs in a social context of isolation from family, workplace prejudice, and other social barriers. Individuals in interracial and same-sex relationships often encounter stigma from different sources, including family, friends, and the general public, which can lead to symptoms of anxiety and depression and poorer health.[68]

Compared to straight couples, gay and lesbian couples use more affection and humor when they bring up a disagreement and remain more positive after a disagreement. They also display less belligerence, domineering, and fear with each other than straight couples do. When they argue, they are better able to soothe each other, so they show fewer signs of physiological arousal, such as an elevated heart rate or sweaty palms, than heterosexual couples.

Regardless of sexual orientation, couples influence—or try to influence—a partner's health behaviors. In straight couples, women are most likely to play this role. In gay and lesbian couples, partners mutually influence each other's health choices and habits.

Marriage

A generation ago, nearly 70 percent of Americans were married; now only about half are. The proportion of married people, especially among younger age groups, has been declining for decades. Here are the most recent statistics on Americans' unions:

- The median age for first marriage, which has gone up about a year every decade since the 1960s, has risen to 28.2 years for men and 26.1 years for women.

- Men in every age bracket through age 34 are more likely to be single than are women.

- Black men and women are less likely to be married than whites, with Hispanics between the two.

- Most young adults view marriage positively, and 95 percent expect to marry in the future—except for young African Americans, who have significantly lower expectations of being wed than their white counterparts.

If you aren't already married, simply getting a college degree increases your odds of entering into matrimony in the future. College-educated women are most likely to be currently married, in part because they are more likely to stay married or remarry after divorce or widowhood. Less well-educated Americans are less likely to marry; in addition, if they do, their unions are more likely to end in divorce.

✓**check-in** If you aren't married, do you expect to get married in the future?

Preparing for Marriage Most people say they marry for one far-from-simple reason: love. However, with more than half of all marriages ending in divorce, there's little doubt that modern marriages aren't made in heaven. Common predictors of marital discord, unhappiness, and separation are:

- A high level of arousal during a discussion.

- Defensive behaviors such as making excuses and denying responsibility for disagreements.

- A wife's expressions of contempt.

- A husband's stonewalling (showing no response when a wife expresses her concerns).

By looking for such behaviors, researchers have been able to predict with better than 90 percent accuracy whether a couple will separate within the first few years of marriage.

The Benefits of Marriage Despite its problems, marriage endures because it is a fulfilling way for two people to live. As researchers have proved, saying "I do" can do wonders for health. Compared to those who are divorced, widowed, never married, or living with a partner, married people:

- Are healthier.

- Live longer.

- Have lower rates of coronary disease and cancer.

- Are less likely to suffer back pain, headaches, and other common illnesses.
- Recover faster and have a better chance of surviving a serious illness.
- Have lower rates of most mental disorders than single or divorced individuals.

For years researchers thought that marriage was especially beneficial to men. Married men have lower rates of alcohol and drug abuse, depression, and risk-taking behavior than divorced men. They also earn more money—possibly because they have more incentive to do so. However, newer research indicates that a happy marriage boosts mental health and well-being in both spouses.

Among the theories of why marriage benefits health are the following:

- **Selection.** People in better physical and psychological health may be more likely to get married in the first place and to remain married.
- **Social support.** Marriage may provide people with emotional satisfaction that buffers them against daily life stressors.
- **Behavioral regulation.** Marriage partners may monitor each other's behaviors, discourage risky behaviors like smoking, and encourage healthier ones such as driving safely.

Same-Sex Marriage   Gay or single-sex or gender-neutral marriage refers to a governmentally, socially, or religiously recognized marriage in which two people of the same sex live together as a family. In a landmark decision in 2015, the U.S. Supreme Court ruled that the Constitution guarantees a right to marriage for all Americans, regardless of their sexual orientation or gender. Marriage is a "keystone of our social order," the majority of justices ruled, noting that all citizens are entitled to "equal dignity in the eyes of the law."

Same-sex marriage triggered intense controversy for decades. Some people opposed gay unions on religious and moral grounds, while others argued that marriage is a right based on procreation and designed to protect the children of a man and a woman. Advocates of single-sex marriage campaigned for years to win the same civil rights and legal protections as heterosexual couples.

Same-sex marriages have accounted for about 2 to 7 percent of all marriages contracted in a single year in the United States. The median age at marriage tends to be higher for persons in gay marriages, followed by those in lesbian marriages, and then in heterosexual marriages.

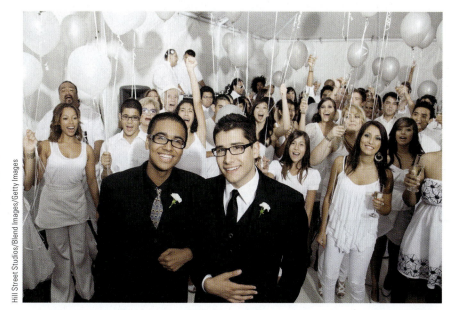

Hill Street Studios/Blend Images/Getty Images

With the Supreme Court's historic ruling on marriage equality, same-sex partners won the legal right to marry anywhere in the United States.

Same-sex couples live together and marry for similar reasons as heterosexual couples: At least a half million same-sex couples live together in the United States, and their numbers are expected to grow. More than 9 in 10 lesbians and 8 in 10 gay youth expect to have monogamous partners by age 30. Because access to legal marriage was long denied, marriage may take on special significance for gay couples, although their reasons for marrying are similar to those of heterosexuals: to indicate long-term commitment, provide emotional support, establish a family, and share life together.[69] Just as for heterosexual couples, marriage brings not only economic and psychosocial benefits but also improved health.[70] The married are in better health than the unmarried—for both same-sex and opposite-sex marriages.[71]

Issues Couples Confront

No two people can live together in perfect harmony all the time. Some of the issues that crop up in any long-term relationship include expectations, money, sex, and careers.

Money   Money may make the business world go around, but it has the opposite effect on relationships: It knocks them off their tracks, brings them to a halt, and twists them upside down. However, even though almost all couples quarrel about money, they rarely fight over how much they have. What matters more—whether they make $10,000 or $100,000 a year—is what money means to both partners.

✓**check-in** Have you ever had to deal with money issues in an intimate relationship?

same-sex marriage
Governmentally, socially, or religiously recognized marriage in which two people of the same sex live together as a family.

To avoid fighting over money, understand that having different money values or expectations doesn't make one of you right and the other wrong:

- Recognize the value of unpaid work. A partner who's finishing school or taking care of the children is making an important contribution to the family and its future.
- Go over your finances together so that you have a firm basis in reality for what you can and can't afford.
- Talk about the financial goals you hope to attain 5 years from now.
- Set aside money for each of you to spend without asking or answering to the other. Even a small amount can make each partner feel more independent.

Sex Like every other aspect of a relationship, sex evolves and changes over the course of marriage. The red-hot sexual chemistry of the early stages of intimacy invariably cools down. Even so, the happiest couples have sex more often than unhappily married pairs do.

What matters most isn't quantity alone, but the quality of sexual activity and intimacy. Here are some common questions that arise in a marriage:

- Are both partners satisfied with their sexual relationship?
- Does one partner always initiate sex?
- Do the partners talk about their preferences and pleasures?

- Do the partners acknowledge and adapt to the changes in sexuality that time brings?
- Do they feel sufficiently at ease with each other to discuss anxieties about sex?

The answers to these questions can determine how sexually gratifying a marriage is for both spouses.

Extramarital Affairs How faithful are American mates? The answer depends on the questions researchers ask and who they ask. In face-to-face interviews, University of Chicago researchers found that 25 percent of men and 15 percent of women had had affairs and that 94 percent of the married subjects had been monogamous in the past year. Another survey of Americans found that one of six Americans had had an extramarital relationship.

High or low, numbers are little comfort when affairs do occur. A husband or wife who learns about a spouse's affair typically feels a devastating sense of betrayal as well as deep feelings of shame, fear of abandonment, depression, and anger. Two crucial questions determine whether a marriage can survive: Do the spouses still feel a serious commitment to each other? Do they love each other and want to remain together?

Two-Career Couples More than 75 percent of women with children work—a dramatic increase from the 1960s, when only 30 percent of mothers worked outside the home. Two careers can bring pressure to a relationship: Both individuals may come home tired and

---

$ HEALTH ON A BUDGET

Money Can't Buy Love

The things that matter most in a healthy relationship don't come with a price tag. Here are some guidelines for what you should invest in to have a healthy, happy relationship:

- **Recognize that both people in the relationship have the right to be accepted as they are,** to be treated with respect, to feel safe, to ask for what they want, to say no without feeling guilty, to express themselves, to give and receive affection, and to make some mistakes and be forgiven.

- **Remember that no one in a relationship has the right to force the other to do anything,** to tell the other where or when to speak up or go out, to humiliate the other in public or private, to isolate the other from friends and family, to read personal material without permission, to pressure the other to give up goals or interests, or to abuse the other person verbally or physically.

- **Be willing to open up.** The more you share, the deeper the bond between you and your friend will become.

- **Be sensitive to your friend's or partner's feelings.** Keep in mind that, like you, he or she has unique needs, desires, and dreams.

- **Express appreciation.** Be generous with your compliments. Let your friends and family know you recognize their kindnesses.

- **Know that people will disappoint you from time to time.** We are only human. Accept your loved ones as they are. Admitting their faults need not reduce your respect for them.

- **Talk about your relationship.** If you have any gripes or frustrations, air them.

irritable; both may have to spend a great deal of time on their jobs; both may have to travel or work on weekends. Two-career couples must be able to discuss their problems openly to resolve these pressures.

✓**check-in** Couples pursuing individual careers sometimes face difficult choices. What if you or your partner is offered a promising job in another city? Would you quit your job, pack up, and move?

Some couples resolve such dilemmas by working in different cities and spending weekends together. Others try to alternate career and home priorities. However imperfect these arrangements may be, they work for some couples.

Conflict in Marriage
While all couples may wish to live happily and peacefully ever after, sooner or later, they disagree. In a 5-year study of newly married couples, 36 percent sought some form of help for their relationship, most often from books on relationships and marital therapy.[72] Years of research have shown that while conflict is inevitable, the key difference between happy and unhappy couples is the way they handle disagreements.

Happier couples interject positive interactions, like a joke or a smile, into their arguments. As long as the ratio of positive to negative interactions remains at least five to one, the relationship remains intact. By comparison, unhappy couples unfurl a barrage of negative words, gestures, criticisms, and hostility at their mates, with hardly any positive interactions.

Saving Marriages
Fewer than two-thirds of couples—64 percent of husbands and 60 percent of wives—say their marriages are very happy (down from 70 percent of men and 66 percent of women a generation ago).

According to research, happy marriages allow both partners to self-actualize (discussed in Chapter 2) and develop to their fullest potential. Some refer to this mutual benefit as "coactualization." Others refer to the process of using a relationship to accumulate knowledge and experiences as "self-expansion." The more self-expansion that people experience from their partner, the more committed and satisfied they are in the relationship.

Among the other suggestions therapists offer couples are the following:

- **Focus on friendship.** If a marriage is not built on a strong friendship, it may be difficult to stay connected over time.

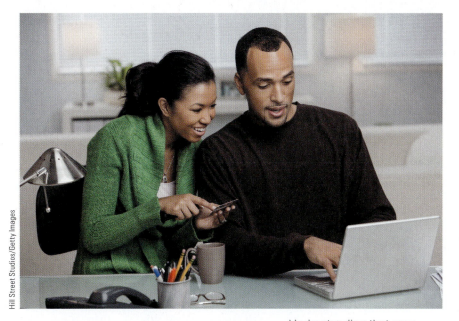

- **Remember what you loved and admired in your partner in the first place.** Focusing on these qualities can foster a much more positive attitude toward your mate.
- **Show respect.** Your spouse deserves the same courtesy and civility that your colleagues do. Without respect, love cannot survive.
- **Compliment what your partner does right.** Noticing the positive can change how both of you feel about each other.
- **Forgive each other.** When your partner hurts your feelings but then reaches out, don't reject his or her attempts to make things better.

Each year, hundreds of thousands of couples go into counseling in an effort to make their unions happier. Marriage education consists of workshops that teach couples practical skills so they get along better. Some studies indicate that graduates of these programs have a lower divorce rate than unhappy couples who do not enroll in them.

Divorce

According to the most recent estimates, 40 to 50 percent of first marriages end in divorce, affecting about 2.5 million adults a year. The leveling of divorce among persons born since 1980, especially college-educated women, may reflect a delay in getting married, increasing selectivity when choosing partners, or a preference for cohabitation rather than marriage.[73]

In addition to age, other factors lower the risk of divorce, including:

- Having some college education.
- Earning an income higher than $50,000 a year.

Understanding that your partner may have a different perspective on saving and spending money can help avoid arguments.

- Marrying at age 25 or older.
- Not having a baby during the first 7 months after the wedding.
- Coming from an intact family.
- Having some religious affiliation.

College students from divorced homes are not as close with their parents and report decreased religiosity as compared with those from nondivorced homes.[74] [Shimkowski] Parental divorce also affects college students' expectations for love, romance, and marriage.[75]

Children whose parents divorced are less likely to marry and to stay married. Race also influences marriage and divorce rates. African American couples are more likely to break up than white couples, and black divorcées are less likely to marry again. Researchers have found that African Americans place an equally high value on marriage. However, there is a smaller "marriageable pool" of black men for a variety of reasons, including a higher mortality rate. An analysis of marital stability in interracial marriages found higher divorce rates for Latino/white intermarriages but not for black/white intermarriages.

Many marriages dissolve simply because one partner's commitment to maintaining the relationship declines. Even couples who are initially very happy can go on to divorce if they begin to engage in more negative communication and emotion and provide less mutual support.

Divorce can have long-term consequences for mental and physical health, including:

- Long-term decreases in life satisfaction.
- Heightened risk for a range of illnesses.
- Poor prognosis for those already ill.
- Increased risk of early death.[76]
- Higher chance of heart attack.[77]

✓**check-in** How would you assess your "risk" of divorce?

families Groups of people united by marriage, blood, or adoption—each residing in the same household; maintaining a common culture; and interacting with one another on the basis of their roles within the group.

blended families Families formed when one or both of the partners bring children from a previous union to the new marriage.

Family Ties

A century ago, most households contained children under age 18. In 1960, slightly fewer than half did. Only about one-third of households now include children. Attitudes have also changed. While many traditionally viewed having children as the primary purpose for getting married, nearly 70 percent of Americans now cite another reason.

In 1960, the average woman had 3.5 children (statistically speaking) over the course of her life. Today's woman has an average of about two children, which is lower than the "replacement level" of 2.1 children per woman—that is, the level at which the population would be replaced by births alone. In most European and several Asian countries, fertility has dropped even lower.

✓**check-in** Do you have children? Do you want to have children someday?

Diversity within Families

Families have become as diverse as the American population and reflect different traditions, beliefs, and values:

- Within African American families, for instance, traditional sex roles are often reversed, with women serving as head of the household, a kinship bond uniting several households, and a strong religious commitment or orientation. As researchers have noted, black families reflect the sociological and historical experience of African Americans under slavery.[78]

- In Chinese American families, both spouses may work and see themselves as breadwinners, but the wife may not have an equal role in decision making.

- In Hispanic families, wives and mothers are acknowledged and respected as healers and dispensers of wisdom. At the same time, they are expected to defer to their husbands, who see themselves as the strong, protective, dominant head of the family.

As time passes and families from different cultures become more integrated into American life, traditional sex roles and decision-making patterns often change, particularly among the youngest family members.

American families are diverse in other ways. *Multigenerational families*—with children, parents, and grandparents—make up about 4 percent of households. They occur most often in areas where new immigrants live with relatives, where housing shortages or high costs force families to double up their living arrangements, or where high rates of out-of-wedlock childbearing force unwed mothers to live with their children in their parents' home.

Three of every 10 households consist of **blended families**, formed when a biological parent cohabits with or marries a partner who is not the biological parent of his or her child.[79]

In the future, social scientists predict, American families will become even more diverse, or pluralistic. But as norms or expectations about the configurations of families have changed, values or ideas about the intents and purposes of families have not. American families of every type still support each other and strive toward values such as commitment and caring.

The traditional family with a breadwinner and a homemaker has been replaced by what some call "the juggler family." Two working parents or an unmarried working parent head 70 percent of American families with children. As a result, American parents have fewer hours to spend with their children. Women, balancing multiple roles as parents, spouses, caregivers, and employees, often give their own personal needs the lowest priority.

✓**check-in** How would you describe the family you grew up in?

Fathers as well as mothers often find themselves juggling the needs of their children and the demands of their jobs.

Unmarried Parents

The proportion of babies born to unmarried parents has grown from about 4 percent in 1940 to about 40 percent today. About 7 in 10 African American babies and half of Hispanic babies are born out of wedlock. African American mothers have the lowest rates of marriage and cohabitation and the highest breakup rates. Mexican immigrant mothers have the highest rates of marriage and cohabitation and the lowest breakup rates.

Many unmarried parents are in a romantic relationship when their baby is born, with about half cohabiting and the others living apart. The majority are not able to establish stable unions. One-third of fathers virtually disappear from their children's lives within 5 years.

An increasing number of college students have children. The percentage of undergraduates who are unmarried parents has nearly doubled over the past 20 years, from 7 percent to just over 13 percent. Overall, 8 percent of male undergraduates and 17 percent of female undergraduates are unmarried parents.

Even though they earn higher GPAs on average, students with preschool-aged children have a significantly lower quantity and quality of time for college than peers with older or no children. Time spent on childcare is the primary reason for this difference.[80] Single parents who received scholarships have shown higher levels of academic achievement, greater progress toward a degree, and higher degree completion rates than those who did not receive financial aid.[81]

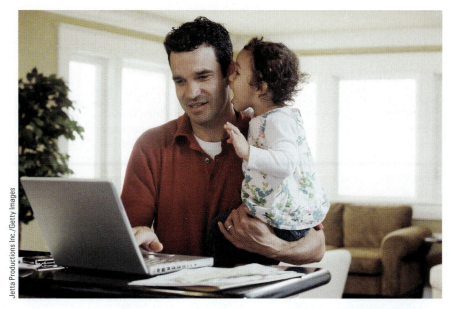

Jetta Productions Inc./Getty Images

Fathers as well as mothers often find themselves juggling the needs of their children and the demands of their jobs.

WHAT DID YOU DECIDE?

- How can you enhance your communication skills?
- How do social media affect the lives of college students?
- What types of relationships are common on college campuses?
- How are healthy and dysfunctional relationships different?

Reflection

This chapter provides information that can strengthen your communication skills and your relationships. Think of the most important relationship in your life at this moment. Can you apply what you've learned to make it stronger and more fulfilling?

TAKING CHARGE OF YOUR HEALTH

Creating Better Relationships

We are born social. From our first days of life, we reach out to others, struggle to express ourselves, and strive to forge connections. The fabric of our lives becomes richer as family and friends weave through it the threads of their experiences. No solitary pleasure can match the gifts that we gain by reaching out and connecting with others.

As with other significant endeavors, good relationships require work—through hard times, despite conflicts, over months and years and decades. As you strive to improve the ties that bind you to others, keep in mind the characteristics of a good relationship. Check the ones that are most important to you.

____ **Trust.** Partners are able to confide in each other openly, knowing their confidences will be respected.

____ **Togetherness.** In a healthy relationship, two people create a sense of both intimacy and autonomy. They enjoy each other's company but also pursue solitary interests.

____ **Expressiveness.** Partners in healthy relationships say what they feel, need, and desire.

____ **Staying power.** People in committed relationships keep their bond strong through tough times by proving that they will be there for each other.

____ **Security.** Because a good relationship is strong enough to absorb conflict and anger, partners know they can express their feelings honestly. They are also willing to risk vulnerability for the sake of becoming closer.

____ **Laughter.** Humor keeps things in perspective—always crucial in any sort of ongoing relationship or enterprise.

____ **Support.** Partners in good relationships continually offer each other encouragement, comfort, and acceptance.

____ **Physical affection.** Sexual desire may fluctuate or diminish over the years, but partners in loving, long-term relationships usually retain some physical connection.

____ **Personal growth.** In the best relationships, partners are committed to bringing out the best in each other and have the other's best interests at heart.

____ **Respect.** Caring partners are aware of each other's boundaries, need for personal space, and vulnerabilities. They do not take each other or their relationship for granted.

SELF-SURVEY

What's Your Intimacy Quotient?

Creating and maintaining close relationships require essential skills, including those listed here. Read through the following brief descriptions, and answer the questions at the end of each with a "yes" or "no."

Scoring

Count up the number of "yes" responses to calculate your score from 0 to 10. A higher score indicates that you have mastered some of the key skills for establishing significant relationships. But focus on the "no" responses as well as the "yes" responses so you can identify the skills that require greater attention. You might want to focus on a specific skill to strengthen during this term. However, it's important to keep working to deepen and enrich your relationships throughout life.

1. Self-love.

Self-love means being at ease with your positive qualities and forgiving yourself for your faults and failings. Don't confuse this with narcissism, or excessive admiration of one's self. *Self-intimacy*, getting to know and feel comfortable with yourself, is the cornerstone of intimacy with others. If you do not understand and accept yourself, how can you expect to understand and accept others and how can you expect others to think that you will be any more interested in or accepting of them? When you know and like yourself, you can reach out to connect with others. And you can extend to them the same care and appreciation you extend to yourself.

Do you spend time often keeping in touch with yourself by journaling or another structured activity? ____

2. Receptivity.

If you are text messaging or checking email while talking to your partner, friend, or child, you're not really tuning in to what the other person has to say. In fact, the message you're sending is, "Don't bother me. I've got something better to do." You signal genuine receptivity by smiling, making eye contact, and turning away from other distractions. Be open and attentive to another's requests for attention.

Do you spend some time every day simply sitting and reconnecting with your partner? Do you spend some time every day simply sitting and reconnecting with yourself? ____

3. Listening.

The greatest gift you can give another person is your full attention. Ask questions. Look into your partner's eyes. Nod your head. Don't interrupt or judge. See things from your partner's perspective. (See the Listen Up lab for more suggestions.)

Do you spend time every day listening to your partner? ____

Do you spend time every day listening to yourself? ____

4. Expressing yourself.

Relationships begin with signals: "yes," "no," and "maybe" responses. It's your responsibility to make the signals and messages you send as clear as possible. Don't expect your partner to read your mind. Avoid the "if you loved me, you'd know" trap. Make sure your words and actions match your feelings. Pay attention to your body language. Use "I" statements, such as "I feel sad because I missed you." Avoid fuzzy expressions like "sort of," "kind of," and "maybe."

Do you spend time every day communicating your thoughts, needs, and wishes to yourself and to your partner? ____

5. Support and acceptance.

When you love someone, support that person. When you become truly intimate, the nature of the support becomes more complex and less conventional. Being willing to say difficult things without aggression, to tell the truth in the least accusatory and most tender way, is an art worth achieving. Only by being willing to reveal your own weaknesses do you create an island of safety where intimacy flourishes. Only by being willing to reveal the truth about yourself can you request the truth from your partner and achieve the utmost intimacy. Only by knowing and acknowledging the intentions behind each act you make can you create a safe place in which your and your partner's faults and foibles are acknowledged without attack or scolding. Do not seek perfection, in the sense of banishing every false step or idiosyncrasy, in your partner or in yourself.

Do you consciously create this special support and acceptance every day? ____

6. Affection.

Infinite possibilities exist for expressing affection. Some are obvious, like a handwritten note. The more subtle ones may go unnoticed but stem from serious contemplation of your partner's nature and needs. When you know and care for someone deeply, you sense when to approach and when to retreat, when to speak and when to be silent. You also communicate, in ways beyond mere words, that you are and always will be there for your partner.

Love is a noun. Love is a verb. Do you seek, create, and act on opportunities to "verb" your love every day? ____

7. Touch.

As humans, we're wired to respond to loving touches. Watch doting parents with their babies or toddlers. They can't keep their hands off them: They hug, hold, kiss, cuddle, and enfold them in their arms. Physical displays of affection show that you feel a sense of warmth and security with your partner.

Do you spend time often kissing or caressing your partner or simply lying in each other's arms? ____

8. Trust.

Love—or at least infatuation—can strike in a heart-pounding, head-spinning moment, but trust builds as slowly as a coral reef. With each promise kept, each secret safeguarded, and each inch of soul exposed, something soft and squishy between two people grows stronger and firmer. In an intimate relationship, trust creates a safe harbor where you can be who you are without being attacked, rejected, or abandoned—and without attacking, rejecting, or abandoning.

Do you honor the trust between you and your partner every day by following a basic rule: no secrets, no lies, no deceptions, no excuses, no illusions? ____

9. Respect.

Your partner in an intimate relationship may like the same music, pursue the same interests, and even share the same favorite ice cream flavor. However, your partner is not you but a unique individual with his or her own desires, needs, and—face it—quirks. Respect means acknowledging, understanding, and accepting what makes your partner different from you and you different from your partner.

Do you show respect for your partner every day? ____

Source: Hales D, Christian KW. *Labs for an Invitation to Personal Change*, Belmont, CA: Wadsworth, 2009.

REVIEW QUESTIONS

(LO 7.1)   1. Which of the following statements is true of social health?
  a. It involves being sexually active.
  b. It involves periodic withdrawal from large groups.
  c. It primarily involves joining large social organizations.
  d. It involves developing interpersonal relationships.

(LO 7.1)   2. The process by which friends, friends of friends, acquaintances, and others in our social circle influence our behavior and our health—both positively and negatively—is termed ____.
  a. social connection
  b. social contagion
  a. social adjustment
  b. cyberbullying

(LO 7.2)   3. Which of the following traits is essential to communicate clearly?
  a. Being assertive
  b. Being aggressive
  c. Being loud
  d. Being humble

(LO 7.2)   4. Which of the following statements is true regarding the sex differences in communication?
  a. Men are generally better listeners.
  b. Women speak more in private, usually to build better connections with others.
  c. Men facilitate conversation better by nodding, asking questions, and signaling interest.
  d. Women interrupt more if they aren't getting the information they need.

(LO 7.3)   5. Which of the following is true of friendship?
  a. It is not as important for men's well-being as it is for women
  b. It is not possible to have more than five best friends through face-to-face contact.
  c. Younger people report higher levels of satisfaction in their interactions with friends.
  d. Online interactions do not provide any of the same benefits as in-person friendships.

(LO 7.3)   6. What is social anxiety disorder?
  a. A mental illness requiring medication.
  b. Feeling self-conscious in social situations.
  c. Fear and avoidance of social situations.
  d. Shyness around people one does not know well.

(LO 7.4)   7. Possible unintended negative consequences of sexting include _____.
  a. a risk of unwanted sexual advances
  b. sexually transmitted infections
  c. the spread of misinformation about sexual health
  d. the sharing of private negative emotions

(LO 7.4)   8. Which of the following uses online sites, forums, and social media to harass victims, and also tries to damage their reputation or turn others against them?
  a. Cyberterrorism
  b. Facebook "lurking"
  c. Cybersquatting
  d. Cyberstalking

(LO 7.5)   9. Online dating is on the rise. Which of the following is true about this form of meeting a potential partner?
  a. Ten percent of people lie about at least one attribute in their profiles.
  b. In general, people do not lie about their marital status, health, or height/weight.
  c. One positive aspect of this type of dating is that you can rely on the company who sponsors the site to do some background checking.
  d. Many consider online dating to be a bit more dangerous than the traditional forms of meeting a potential partner.

(LO 7.6) 10. ____ is a state of closeness between two people, characterized by the desire and ability to share one's innermost thoughts and feelings with each other either verbally or nonverbally.
  a. Intimacy
  b. Marriage
  c. Infatuation
  d. Falling in love

(LO 7.6) 11. Which of the following have studies shown to be among the most important reasons for attraction among college students?
  a. Physical attraction
  b. Mutual interests
  c. Warmth and kindness
  d. Social status

(LO 7.7) 12. Which of the following is true about intimate partner violence?
  a. It occurs more often among married couples.
  b. It occurs more often among cohabiting couples.
  c. It tends not to be disclosed to others mostly out of fear
  d. It is most often initiated by a partner with a criminal record.

(LO 7.7) 13. Which of the following terms refers to unwittingly contributing to a person's addictive or abusive behavior?
a. Blending
b. Enabling
c. Cohabiting
d. Coercing

(LO 7.8) 14. Which of the following is the first stage of a relationship?
a. Establishing a strong sense of partnership
b. Building trust and dependability
c. Nesting
d. Blending

(LO 7.8) 15. Which of the following statements is true of marriages and divorces among Americans?
a. Children whose parents are divorced are more likely to marry.
b. Married people have lower rates of coronary disease and cancer.
c. Well-educated Americans are less likely to marry and, if they do, their unions are more likely to end in divorce.
d. Having a baby during the first seven months after getting married lowers the risk of divorce.

(LO 7.9) 16. Which of the following statements is true of American families?
a. The average household has more children under age 18 now than a century ago.
b. In white American families, wives and mothers are acknowledged and respected as healers and dispensers of wisdom.
c. The primary purpose cited by the current American population for getting married is having children.
d. In African American families, traditional gender roles are often reversed.

(LO 7.9) 17. Blended families are families ____.
a. in which one or both of the partners bring children from a previous union
b. in which children, parents, and grandparents live in the same house
c. with two working parents or an unmarried working parent
d. with same-sex parents

Answers to these questions can be found on page 531.

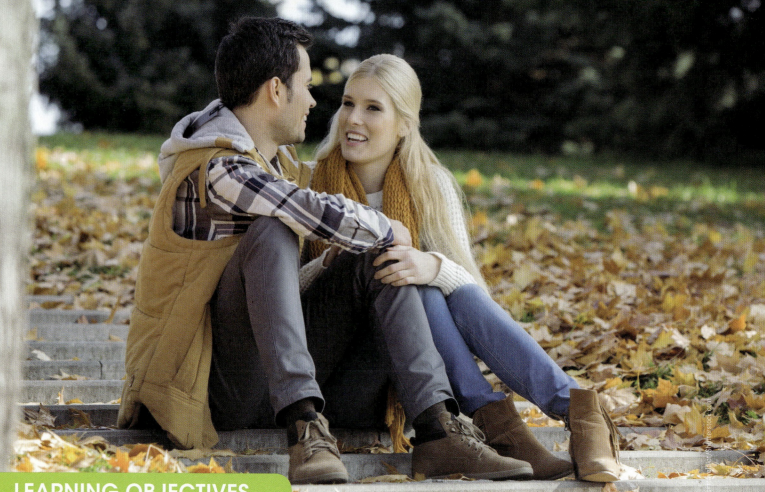

Monkey Business Images/Shutterstock.com

LEARNING OBJECTIVES

After reading this chapter, you should be able to:

8.1 Describe women's and men's sexual health, their sexual anatomy, and the role of sex hormones in the development of gender identities.

8.2 Specify the aspects of healthy sexual relationships that lead toward responsible sexuality.

8.3 Summarize the sexual practices of college students.

8.4 Discuss sexual diversity in human beings.

8.5 Outline the major types of sexual activity.

8.6 Describe the stages of sexual response in men and women.

8.7 Identify the risk factors and characteristics of sexually transmitted infections and diseases.

8.8 Review the signs, symptoms, and treatment of common sexually transmitted diseases.

WHAT DO YOU THINK?

- What are the basic hormonal and anatomical differences between men and women?

- What should college students know about hooking up?

- What are the sexual preferences and behaviors of American adults?

- What do you know about the incidence, signs, symptoms, and treatments for the most common sexually transmitted infections (STIs)?

8

Sexual Health

Alex, several years older than the typical college freshman, usually doesn't think much about the age difference—until the conversation turns to sex. He understands his younger classmates' seemingly endless fascination with sex, but his perspective is different. As a teenager, he had plunged recklessly into dangerous territory of every type. Sex—casual and sometimes unprotected—was one of them.

"Looking back," Alex muses, "I feel lucky that I didn't end up a statistic." But he still regrets the irresponsible ways he acted—and the chronic sexually transmitted infection (STI) acquired along the way.

Now 28, Alex is a veteran of military service, a married man, and an expectant father. His enjoyment of sex hasn't faded; in many ways, it has deepened and become more gratifying. He now realizes that sexual choices have consequences and effects on one's own life and on other people. These are the lessons he hopes someday to pass on to his own children.

As Alex learned with time and experience, you are ultimately responsible for your sexual health and behavior. You make decisions that affect how you express your sexuality, how you respond sexually, and how you give and receive sexual pleasure. Yet most sexual activity involves another person. Therefore, your

decisions about sex—more so than those you make about nutrition, drugs, or exercise—have important effects on other people.

All human beings are sexual from birth to death. Whether you are male or female, single or married, straight, gay, lesbian, bisexual, or transgender, sexuality is a normal, natural part of your life. You are just as responsible for your sexual health as for any other aspect of your well-being. To safeguard your sexual health, you need to be aware of and protect yourself from sexually transmitted infections and diseases.

Sexual responsibility begins with learning about your body, your partner's body, your sexual development and preferences, and the health risks associated with sexual activity, including STIs. This chapter provides information and insight you can use in making decisions and choosing sexually responsible behaviors.<

Sexual Health

Human **sexuality**—the quality of being sexual—is as rich, varied, and complex as life itself. Along with our **sex**, or biological maleness or femaleness, it is an integral part of who we are, how we see ourselves, and how we relate to others. Of all of our involvements with others, sexual **intimacy**, or physical closeness, can be the most rewarding. But while sexual expression and experience can provide intense joy, they also can involve great emotional turmoil.

Sexual health refers, by simplest definition, to a state of optimal well-being related to sexuality throughout the lifespan. The World Health Organization (WHO) describes it more comprehensively as "a state of physical, emotional, mental, and social well-being related to sexuality; it is not merely the absence of disease, dysfunction, or infirmity. Sexual health requires a positive and respectful approach to sexuality and sexual responses, as well as the possibility of having pleasurable and safe sexual experiences, free of coercion, discrimination, and violence."

The sexual health of college students, particularly those in the period termed "emerging adulthood" (ages 18–25), is at greater risk than that of the rest of the population. Less likely to use condoms or practice birth control, young adults in this age group face a greater likelihood of STIs and, if heterosexual, unwanted pregnancy. Older students also engage in a range of sexual experiences, depending on their gender identity, sexual orientation, and relationship status, but are more likely to protect against pregnancy and sexually transmitted infections.

···
✓**check-in** How would you describe your sexual health: excellent, average, poor?
···

Sexuality and the Dimensions of Health

Our sexuality both affects and is affected by the various dimensions of health. Responsible sexuality and high-level sexual health contribute to the fullest possible functioning of body, mind, spirit, and social relationships. In turn, other aspects of health enhance our sexuality. Here are some examples:

- **Physical.** Safer sex practices reduce the risk of STIs that can threaten sexual health, physical health, and even survival. When

our bodies are healthy and well, we feel better about ourselves, which enhances both self-esteem and healthy sexuality.

- **Emotional.** By acknowledging and respecting the intimacy of a sexual relationship, responsible sexuality builds trust and commitment. When our emotional health is high, we can better understand and cope with the complex feelings related to being sexual.

- **Social.** From dating to mating, we express and fulfill our sexual identities in the context of families, friends, and society as a whole. Having strong friendships, intimate relationships, and caring partnerships enables us to explore our sexuality in safe and healthy ways.

- **Intellectual.** Our most fulfilling relationships involve a meeting of minds as well as bodies. High-level intellectual health enables us to acquire and understand sexual information, analyze it critically, and make healthy sexual decisions.

- **Spiritual.** At its deepest, most fulfilling level, sexuality uplifts the soul by allowing us to connect to something greater than ourselves. Individuals who have developed their spirituality bring to their most intimate relationships an awareness and appreciation that lifts them beyond the physical.

- **Environmental.** Responsible sexuality makes people more aware of the impact of their decisions on others. Protecting yourself from sexual threats and creating a supportive environment in which to study and work are crucial to high-level health and to healthy sexuality.

Women's Sexual Health

All women of childbearing age should undergo regular "health maintenance" exams to monitor their sexual and reproductive well-being, detect infections and other medical problems, and prevent unwanted pregnancy. These should include:

- Counseling on contraception for women who do not want to get pregnant.

- Counseling on pre-pregnancy health care for women who are attempting to conceive.

- Counseling for all women who may become pregnant to take a daily folic acid supplement of 400 to 800 mcg.

sexuality The behaviors, instincts, and attitudes associated with being sexual.

sex Maleness or femaleness, resulting from genetic, structural, and functional factors.

intimacy A state of closeness between two people, characterized by the desire and ability to share one's innermost thoughts and feelings with each other either verbally or nonverbally.

sexual health The integration of the physical, emotional, intellectual, social, and spiritual aspects of sexual being in ways that are positively enriching and that enhance personality, communication, and love.

- Counseling on reducing the risks of STIs.

- Screening of all women age 24 or younger for chlamydia.

- Screening of all women at high risk for chlamydia, gonorrhea, and syphilis and of all women for HIV.

- Screening for domestic violence and sexual or reproductive coercion.

In the past, gynecologists recommended annual pelvic exams for all women age 21 and older. However, some physicians question the need for pelvic exams in women who do not have symptoms such as pelvic pain, menstrual problems, or vaginal discharge. Other, less expensive and less invasive forms of testing can detect STIs, and a pelvic exam is usually not required before initiation of many forms of birth control.[1]

✓**check-in** If you are a woman, have you asked your doctor how often you need a pelvic exam?

Female Sexual Anatomy

As illustrated in Figure 8.1a, the **mons pubis** is the rounded, fleshy area over the junction of the pubic bones. The folds of skin that form the outer lips of a woman's genital area are called the **labia majora**. They cover soft flaps of skin (inner lips) called the **labia minora**. The inner lips join at the top to form a hood over the **clitoris**, a small elongated erectile organ, and the most sensitive spot in the entire female genital area. Below the clitoris is the **urethral opening**, the outer opening of the thin tube that carries urine from the bladder. Below that is a larger opening, the mouth of the **vagina**, the canal that leads to the primary internal organs of reproduction. The **perineum** is the area between the vagina and the anus (the opening to the rectum and large intestine).

At the back of the vagina is the **cervix**, the opening to the womb, or **uterus** (see Figure 8.1b). The uterine walls are lined with a layer of tissue called the **endometrium**. The ovaries, about the size and shape of almonds, are located on either side of the uterus and contain egg cells called ova (singular, **ovum**). Extending outward and back

mons pubis The rounded, fleshy area over the junction of the female pubic bones.

labia majora The fleshy outer folds that border the female genital area.

labia minora The fleshy inner folds that border the female genital area

clitoris A small erectile structure on the female, corresponding to the penis on the male.

urethral opening The outer opening of the thin tube that carries urine from the bladder.

vagina The canal leading from the exterior opening in the female genital area to the uterus.

perineum The area between the anus and vagina in the female and between the anus and scrotum in the male.

cervix The narrow, lower end of the uterus that opens into the vagina.

uterus The female organ that houses the developing fetus until birth.

endometrium The mucous membrane lining the uterus.

ovum (plural, ova) The female gamete (egg cell).

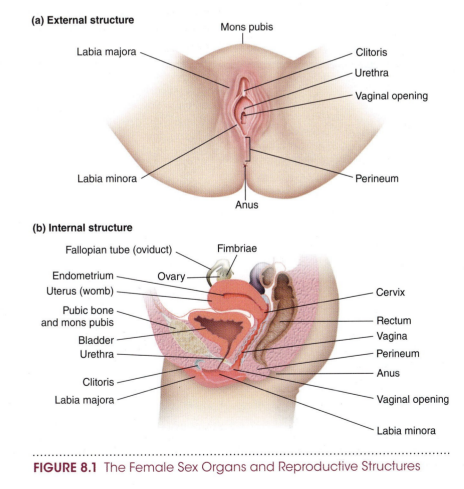

(a) External structure

Mons pubis
Labia majora
Clitoris
Urethra
Vaginal opening
Labia minora
Perineum
Anus

(b) Internal structure

Fallopian tube (oviduct)
Fimbriae
Endometrium
Ovary
Uterus (womb)
Pubic bone and mons pubis
Bladder
Urethra
Clitoris
Labia majora
Cervix
Rectum
Vagina
Perineum
Anus
Vaginal opening
Labia minora

FIGURE 8.1 The Female Sex Organs and Reproductive Structures

from the upper uterus are the **fallopian tubes**, the canals that transport ova from the ovaries to the uterus. When an egg is released from an ovary, the fingerlike ends of the adjacent fallopian tube "catch" the egg and direct it into the tube.

Discharge and changes in odor normally occur in a healthy vagina. They typically fluctuate through the menstrual cycle, depending on hormone level. In the past, many women practiced douching, the introduction of a liquid into the vagina, to cleanse the vagina. However, particularly if done frequently, douching may increase the risk of pelvic inflammatory disease (discussed later in this chapter) and ectopic (out-of-uterus) pregnancy. As discussed in Chapter 14, physicians no longer recommend annual pelvic exams for all women, but some women continue to view them as reassuring or necessary to detect ovarian cancer or sexually transmitted infections.[2]

The Menstrual Cycle

A women's reproductive lifespan begins at menarche, with her first menstrual period, and ends at menopause, when her periods end. Women with more than 40 reproductive years—who may begin menstruating at age 12 and continue to do so until their early 50s—are likely to outlive women who menstruate for less than 33 years.[3]

Every menstrual cycle begins in the brain with the production of gonadotropin-releasing hormone (GnRH) and then proceeds through the following steps:

- GnRH sets into motion the sequence of steps that lead to ovulation, the potential for conception, and, if conception doesn't occur, menstruation. The hypothalamus monitors hormone levels in the blood and sends messages to the pituitary gland to release follicle-stimulating hormone (FSH) and luteinizing hormone (LH).

- As shown in Figure 8.2, in the ovaries, these hormones stimulate the growth of a few of the immature eggs, or ova, stored in follicles in every woman's body. Usually, only one ovum matures completely during each monthly cycle. As it does, it increases its production of the female sex hormone estrogen, which in turn triggers the release of a larger surge of LH.

- At midcycle, the increased LH hormone levels trigger **ovulation**, the release of the egg cell, or ovum, from the follicle. Estrogen levels drop, and the remaining cells of the follicle then enlarge, change character, and form the corpus **luteum**, or yellow body.

- In the second half of the menstrual cycle, the corpus luteum secretes estrogen and larger amounts of progesterone. The endometrium (uterine lining) is stimulated by progesterone to thicken and become more engorged with blood in preparation for nourishing an implanted, fertilized ovum.

- If the ovum is not fertilized, the corpus luteum disintegrates. As the level of progesterone drops, **menstruation** occurs; the uterine lining is shed during the course of a menstrual period.

- If the egg is fertilized and pregnancy occurs, the cells that eventually develop into the placenta secrete *human chorionic gonadotropin (HCG)*, a messenger hormone that signals the pituitary not to start a new cycle. The corpus luteum then steps up its production of progesterone.

Many women experience physical or psychological changes, or both, during their monthly cycles. Usually the changes are minor, but more serious problems can occur.

Women's attitudes toward menstruation may reflect how positively or negatively they view their own body in general.[4]

Premenstrual Syndrome Women with **premenstrual syndrome (PMS)** experience bodily discomfort and emotional distress for up to 2 weeks, from ovulation until the onset of menstruation. As many as 95 percent of menstruating women report one or more premenstrual symptoms; fewer than 10 percent experience disabling, incapacitating symptoms.[5] Among the factors linked with premenstrual symptoms in college students are stress, sleep quality, and higher rates of psychological disorders.

Once dismissed as a psychological problem, PMS has been recognized as a very real physiological disorder that may be caused by various factors, including:

- A hormonal deficiency.
- Abnormal levels of thyroid hormone.
- An imbalance of estrogen and progesterone.
- Social and environmental factors, particularly stress.
- Vitamin D deficiency[6]

The most common symptoms of PMS are as follows:

- Mood changes.
- Anxiety.
- Irritability.
- Difficulty concentrating.

fallopian tubes The pair of channels that transport ova from the ovaries to the uterus; the usual site of fertilization.

ovulation The release of a mature ovum from an ovary approximately 14 days prior to the onset of menstruation.

luteum A yellowish mass of tissue that is formed, immediately after ovulation, from the remaining cells of the follicle; it secretes estrogen and progesterone for the remainder of the menstrual cycle.

menstruation Discharge of blood from the vagina as a result of the shedding of the uterine lining at the end of the menstrual cycle.

premenstrual syndrome (PMS) A disorder that causes physical discomfort and psychological distress prior to a woman's menstrual period.

FIGURE 8.2 Menstrual Cycle

(a) In response to the hypothalamus, the pituitary gland releases the gonadotropins FSH and LH. Levels of FSH and LH stimulate the cycle (and in turn are affected by production of estrogen and progesterone).

(b) FSH does what its name says: It stimulates follicle development in the ovary. The follicle matures and ruptures, releasing an ovum (egg) into the fallopian tube.

(c) The follicle produces estrogen, and the corpus luteum produces estrogen and progesterone. The high level of estrogen at the middle of the cycle produces a surge of LH, which triggers ovulation.

(d) Estrogen and progesterone stimulate the endometrium, which becomes thicker and prepares to receive an implanted, fertilized egg. If a fertilized egg is deposited in the uterus, pregnancy begins. If the egg is not fertilized, progesterone production decreases, and the endometrium is shed (menstruation). At this point, both estrogen and progesterone levels have dropped, so the pituitary responds by producing FSH, and the cycle begins again.

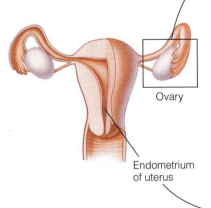

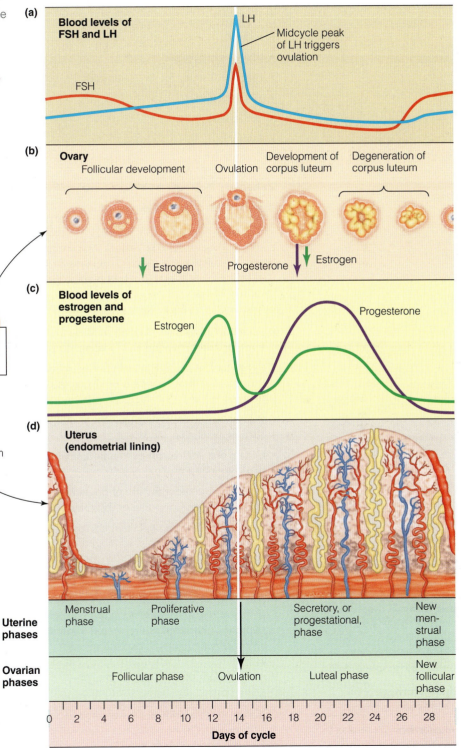

- Forgetfulness.
- Impaired judgment.
- Tearfulness.
- Digestive symptoms (diarrhea, bloating, and constipation).
- Hot flashes.
- Palpitations.
- Dizziness.
- Headache.
- Fatigue.
- Changes in appetite.
- Cravings (usually for sweets or salt).
- Water retention.
- Breast tenderness.
- Insomnia.

✓**check-in** If you are a woman, have you experienced any of these symptoms of PMS?

For a diagnosis to be made, women must report troubling premenstrual symptoms in the days before menstruation in at least two successive menstrual cycles.

Treatments for PMS symptoms include:

- Diuretics (drugs that speed up fluid elimination) for water retention and bloating.
- Psychotherapy, including cognitive-behavioral therapy, to relieve symptoms of anxiety and depression.[7]
- Relaxation and stress management techniques such as meditation and yoga.[8]
- Certain oral contraceptives to relieve mild to moderate physical symptoms.[9]
- Sleep deprivation or the use of bright light to adjust a woman's circadian or daily rhythm.
- Certain oral contraceptives that effectively relieve physical but not psychological symptoms.[10]
- Charting of cycles to identify vulnerable periods.
- Low doses of medications known as *selective serotonin reuptake inhibitors* (*SSRIs*), such as fluoxetine (marketed as Prozac and Sarafem and in generic forms), for symptoms such as tension, depression, irritability, and mood swings, taken only during the premenstrual phase or daily throughout the month.

Other treatments with some reported success include exercise; lower caffeine, alcohol, salt, and sugar intake; and acupuncture.

premenstrual dysphoric disorder (PMDD) A disorder that causes symptoms of psychological depression during the last week of the menstrual cycle.

dysmenorrhea Painful menstruation.

amenorrhea The absence or suppression of menstruation.

Premenstrual Dysphoric Disorder Not related to PMS, **premenstrual dysphoric disorder (PMDD)** occurs in an estimated 3 to 5 percent of all menstruating women. It is characterized by regular symptoms of depression (depressed mood, anxiety, mood swings, and diminished interest or pleasure) as well as physical symptoms, such as changes in appetite, energy, weight, or sleep during the last week of the menstrual cycle.

Women with PMDD cannot function as usual at work, school, or home. They feel better a few days after menstruation begins. Certain birth control pills can help by stopping ovulation and stabilizing hormone fluctuations. SSRIs, which are often used to treat PMS, are also effective in relieving symptoms of PMDD.[11] Some women may benefit from exercise, relaxation, or cognitive-behavioral therapy.[12]

Menstrual Cramps The medical name for menstrual cramps is **dysmenorrhea**, which may involve abdominal cramps and pain, back and leg pain, diarrhea, tension, water retention, fatigue, and depression during menstruation. About half of all menstruating women suffer from dysmenorrhea. The cause seems to be overproduction of bodily substances called prostaglandins, which typically rise during menstruation. Medications that inhibit prostaglandins can reduce menstrual pain, and exercise can also relieve cramps.

✓**check-in** If you are a woman, have you ever experienced dysmenorrhea?

Amenorrhea Women may stop menstruating—a condition called **amenorrhea**—for a variety of reasons, including a hormonal disorder, drastic weight loss, strenuous exercise, or change in the environment. "Boarding-school amenorrhea" is common among young women who leave home for school. Distance running and strenuous exercise can also lead to amenorrhea. The reason may be a drop in body fat from the normal range of 18 to 22 percent to a range of 9 to 12 percent.

To be considered amenorrheic, a woman's menstrual cycle is typically absent for 3 or more consecutive months. Prolonged amenorrhea can have serious health consequences, including a loss of bone density that may lead to stress fractures or osteoporosis. Scientists have developed chemical mimics, or analogues, of GnRH—usually administered by nasal spray—that trigger ovulation in women who don't ovulate or menstruate normally.

Toxic Shock Syndrome This rare, potentially deadly bacterial infection primarily strikes menstruating women under age 30 who use tampons. Both *Staphylococcus aureus* and group A *Streptococcus pyogenes* can produce **toxic shock syndrome (TSS)**. Symptoms include a high fever; a rash that leads to peeling of the skin on the fingers, toes, palms, and soles; dizziness; dangerously low blood pressure; and abnormalities in several organ systems (the digestive tract and the kidneys) and in the muscles and blood. Treatment usually consists of antibiotics and intense supportive care; intravenous administration of immunoglobulins that attack the toxins produced by these bacteria may also be beneficial.

Men's Sexual Health

Because the male reproductive system is simpler in many ways than the female, it is often ignored—especially by healthy young men. However, men should make regular self-exams (including checking the penis and testes) part of their routine.

Male Sexual Anatomy

The visible parts of the male sexual anatomy are the **penis** and the **scrotum**, the pouch that contains the **testes** (Figure 8.3a). The testes manufacture testosterone, the hormone that stimulates the development of a male's secondary sex characteristics, and **sperm**, the male reproductive cells. Immature sperm are stored in the **epididymis**, a collection of coiled tubes adjacent to each testis.

The penis contains three hollow cylinders loosely covered with skin. The two major cylinders, the corpora cavernosa, extend side by side through the length of the penis. The third cylinder, the corpus spongiosum, surrounds the urethra, the channel for both seminal fluid and urine (see Figure 8.3b).

Men of all ages may have concerns about the size of their penis. In a recent scholarly analysis titled "Am I Normal?" researchers analyzed 20 studies of the penis size of more than 15,000 men around the world—all measured by physicians in clinical settings. The mean length of a flaccid penis was 3.6 inches; of both a stretched flaccid penis or an erect penis, about 5.2 inches. Penile lengths varied by 1 to 1.5 inches, and the analysis found no indications of size variability based on race.[13]

Does penis size matter? In surveys of heterosexual men and women, 85 percent of women typically report satisfaction with their partner's penis size, but only about 55 percent of the men say they are satisfied. Some men's anxiety is so distressing that they develop what therapists term "small penis anxiety" or "small penis disorder." Among those who consult physicians, almost all learn that their penis is within the normal size range. Fewer than 2 percent of men

toxic shock syndrome (TSS) A disease characterized by fever, vomiting, diarrhea, and often shock, caused by a bacterium that releases toxic waste products into the bloodstream.

penis The male organ of sex and urination.

scrotum The external sac or pouch that holds the testes.

testes (singular, testis) The male sex organs that produce sperm and testosterone.

sperm The male gamete produced by the testes and transported outside the body through ejaculation.

epididymis The portion of the male duct system in which sperm mature.

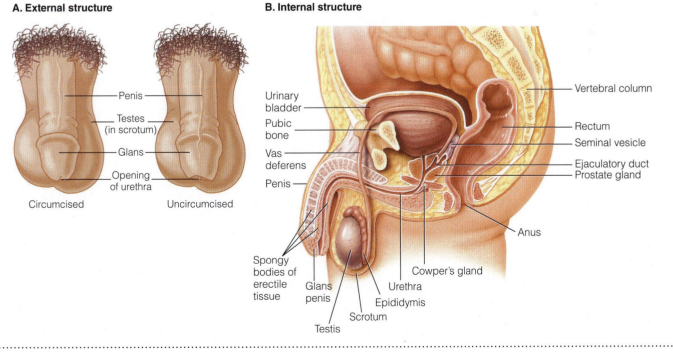

A. External structure

Penis
Testes (in scrotum)
Glans
Opening of urethra

Circumcised   Uncircumcised

B. Internal structure

Urinary bladder
Pubic bone
Vas deferens
Penis
Spongy bodies of erectile tissue
Glans penis
Testis
Scrotum
Epididymis
Urethra
Cowper's gland
Anus
Prostate gland
Ejaculatory duct
Seminal vesicle
Rectum
Vertebral column

FIGURE 8.3 Male Sex Organs and Reproductive Structures

semen The viscous whitish fluid that is the complete male ejaculate; a combination of sperm and secretions from the prostate gland, seminal vesicles, and other glands.

vas deferens Two tubes that carry sperm from the epididymis into the urethra.

urethra The canal through which urine from the bladder leaves the body; in the male, also serves as the channel for seminal fluid.

seminal vesicles Glands in the male reproductive system that produce the major portion of the fluid of semen.

ejaculatory ducts The canal connecting the seminal vesicles and vas deferens.

prostate gland A structure surrounding the male urethra that produces a secretion that helps liquefy the semen from the testes.

Cowper's glands Two small glands that discharge into the male urethra; also called bulbourethral glands.

circumcision The surgical removal of the foreskin of the penis.

gender identity An individual's perception of having a particular gender, which may or may not correspond with the person's birth sex.

cisgender A person whose sense of personal identity and gender corresponds with the individuals birth sex.

transgender Having a gender identity opposite one's biological sex.

have a "micropenis," measuring 2 inches or less in flaccid state and less than 3.3 inches when stretched.[14]

Inside the body are several structures involved in the production of seminal fluid, or **semen**, the liquid in which sperm cells are carried out of the body during ejaculation. The **vas deferens** are two tubes that carry sperm from the epididymis into the **urethra**. The **seminal vesicles**, which make some of the seminal fluid, join with the vas deferens to form the **ejaculatory ducts**.

The **prostate gland** produces some of the seminal fluid, which it secretes into the urethra during ejaculation. The **Cowper's glands** are two pea-sized structures on either side of the urethra (just below where it emerges from the prostate gland) and are connected to it via tiny ducts. When a man is sexually aroused, the Cowper's glands often secrete a fluid that appears as a droplet at the tip of the penis. This fluid is not semen, although it occasionally contains sperm.

Circumcision In its natural state, the tip of the penis is covered by a fold of skin called the *foreskin*. About 60 percent of baby boys in the United States undergo **circumcision**, the surgical removal of the foreskin, for reasons that vary from religious traditions to preventive health measures.

....
✓check-in If you are a man, have you been circumcised?
....

The first federal guidelines affirmed that circumcision is a personal decision that may involve religious or cultural preferences. Based on the scientific evidence, circumcision provides numerous health benefits that outweigh its risks, including[15]:

- Less risk of urinary tract infections during the first year of life. (An uncircumcised baby boy has a 1 in 100 chance of getting a urinary tract infection, compared with a 1 in 1,000 chance for a circumcised baby boy.)

- Prevention of foreskin infections and retraction.

- Easier genital hygiene.

- Reduced risk of acquiring an STI from an infected female partner.[16]

- Less risk of cancer of the penis and possibly of the prostate gland.

- Less risk to female partners of human papillomavirus (HPV), cervical cancer, *Trichomonas vaginalis* infection, bacterial vaginosis, and possibly genital ulcer disease.[17]

Critics of circumcision emphasize the pain, bleeding, and risk of infections. In newborns, the estimated complication rate is 0.5 percent. Complications may include bleeding, infection, improper healing, or cutting the foreskin too long or too short. Analgesic creams or anesthetic shots are typically used to minimize discomfort. There is little consensus on what impact the presence or absence of a foreskin has on sexual function or satisfaction.

The Gender Spectrum

The way we think and talk about gender continues to evolve beyond the binary (limited to two options) view of individuals as either male or female. Unlike biological sex, which is assigned at birth based on genes, anatomy, and reproductive organs, **gender identity**, an individual's internal sense of being male, female, both, or neither, is a product of both innate and external influences and can shift over time.

The vast majority of people identify as **cisgender**, which means that their biological sex and gender identity match—for example, someone born with male genes and sex organs identifies as a man. **Transgender** individuals have a gender identity that does not match their assigned sex—for example, a birth-assigned female identifies as a male.[18]

Rather than the labels of male or female, individuals may identify as:

- Gender-fluid (a person with a gender identity that shifts between masculine and feminine at varying times).

- Gender-neutral (a person who prefers not to be described by a specific gender).

- Gender nonbinary (a person who identifies as neither male nor female but as outside the gender binary, sometimes shortened to NB).

- Gender nonconforming, or GNC (a person who expresses gender outside the traditional norms associated with masculinity or femininity). Some, but not all, gender-nonconforming individuals are transgender.

- Genderqueer (a term often chosen by people who do not identify with the gender binary of male or female).

- Intersex (a person born with biological sex characteristics that aren't traditionally associated with male or female bodies). Intersexuality does not refer to gender identity.

- MAAB/FAAB/UAB (male assigned at birth, female assigned at birth, unassigned at birth).

- Trans* or trans+ (umbrella terms for non-cisgender identities).

   The transgender community includes:

- Transyouth (young people experiencing issues related to gender identity or expression).

- Transsexuals (who identify with a gender other than the one they were given at birth).

- Transwomen (a term for male-to-female transsexuals to signify that they are female with a male history).

- Transmen (a term for female-to-male transsexuals to signify that they are male with a female history).

   Gender expression, an outward presentation of gender, includes clothes, makeup, piercings, or hairstyles that may be perceived as feminine, masculine, or androgynous. Transgender individuals may be happy with the biological sex in which they are born but enjoy dressing up and behaving like the other sex. Most do so for psychological and social pleasure rather than sexual gratification.

   Some transsexuals feel trapped in the body of the wrong gender—a phenomenon called gender dysphoria. In general, more men than women have this experience. Gender transition is the process of shifting one's outward gender expression to match one's internal sense of gender—from masculine to feminine or from feminine to masculine. For transgender individuals, this may include gender-affirming hormones and surgical procedures.

   The decision to go through a gender transition is usually made after months or years of weighing the risks, benefits, and impact on loved ones. The complex process remains controversial but can lead to greater emotional well-being and healthier post-operative functioning.[19]

   Transgender and gender-nonconforming individuals face varied health risks. They are more likely to use drugs and alcohol, smoke, be diagnosed with HIV or other sexually transmitted infections, experience depression, or attempt suicide. Recent research suggests that early recognition may lessen these risks.[20] However, violence—including harassment, rape, sexual abuse, physical abuse, and suicide—remains a major threat.[21]

Responsible Sexuality

Most people grow up with a lot of myths and misconceptions about sex. Than rely on what peers say or what you've always thought was true, find out the facts.

✓**check-in** How would you rate your knowledge about sex and sexuality?

   This textbook is a good place to start expanding your sexual literacy. The student health center and the library can provide additional materials on sexual identity, orientation, behavior, and health, as well as on options for reducing your risk of acquiring STIs or becoming pregnant.

Creating a Sexually Healthy Relationship

A sexually healthy relationship, as defined by the Sexuality Information and Education Council of the United States (SIECUS), is based on shared values and has five characteristics:

- Consensual.

- Nonexploitative.

- Honest.

- Mutually pleasurable.

- Protected against unintended pregnancy and STIs.

✓**check-in** If you are in a sexual relationship, does it have these five characteristics?

   The key to a healthy, happy sexual relationship is open, honest communication—even when you and your partner have different points of view. All individuals also have sexual rights, which include the right to the information, education, skills, support, and services they need to make responsible decisions about their sexuality, consistent with their own values, as well as the right to express their sexual orientation without violence or discrimination.

   Communication is vital in a sexually healthy relationship, even though these discussions can be awkward. Yet if you have a need or a problem that relates to your partner, it is your responsibility to bring it up (see Health on a Budget in this chapter).

HEALTH NOW!

Developing Sexual Responsibility

The Sexuality Information and Education Council of the United States (SIECUS) has worked with nongovernmental organizations around the world to develop a consensus about the life behaviors of a sexually healthy and responsible adult. These include the following:

- Appreciating one's own body
- Seeking information about reproduction as needed
- Affirming that sexual development may or may not include reproduction or genital sexual experience
- Interacting with both genders in respectful and appropriate ways
- Affirming one's own sexual orientation and respecting the sexual orientation of others
- Expressing love and intimacy in appropriate ways
- Developing and maintaining meaningful relationships
- Avoiding exploitative or manipulative relationships
- Making informed choices about family options and lifestyles
- Enjoying and expressing one's sexuality throughout life
- Expressing one's sexuality in ways congruent with one's values
- Discriminating between life-enhancing sexual behaviors and those that are harmful to oneself and/or others

From the preceding list, choose three characteristics that you would like to improve in your intimate relationships. Why did you choose these three? Do they have special significance for you? How will you go about strengthening them? Do you have other goals for responsible sexuality? Record your reflections in your online journal.

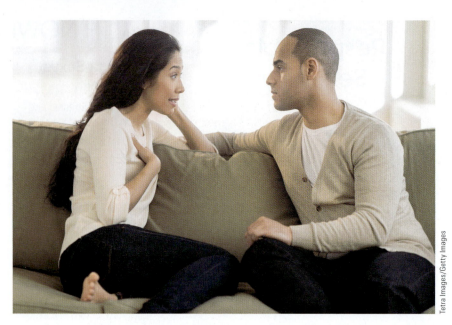

The key to a healthy, happy sexual relationship is open, honest communication—even when you and your partner have different points of view.

Making Sexual Decisions

Sexual decision making should always take place within the context of an individual's values and perceptions of right and wrong behavior. Making responsible sexual decisions means considering all the possible consequences—including emotional consequences—of sexual behavior for both yourself and your partner. (See Health Now in this chapter.)

Culture can influence sexual attitudes and activities through the messages young people receive. In a recent study, Latino college students described four types of messages from parents and friends:

- Sex is only for marriage (procreational).

- Sex is only appropriate in a loving relationship (relational).

- Sex is for pleasure (recreational).

- There is a gender-based double standard for male and female sexual behavior.

The students who received fewer procreational sex messages from parents and more recreational sex messages from friends reported higher levels of sexual exploration and assertiveness.[22]

✓**check-in** How would you describe the messages about sex you have received from parents and friends?

Prior to any sexual activity that involves a risk of STI or pregnancy, both partners should talk about their prior sexual histories (including number of partners and exposure to STIs) and other high-risk behavior, such as the use of injection drugs. They should also discuss the issue of birth control and which methods might be best for them to use. If you know someone well enough to consider having sex with that person, you should be able to talk about such sensitive subjects. If a potential partner is unwilling to talk or hedges on crucial questions, you shouldn't be engaging in sex.

Here are some questions to consider as you think and talk about the significance of becoming sexually intimate with a partner:

- **What role do we want relationships and sex to have in our life at this time?**

- **What are my values and my potential partner's values as they pertain to sexual relationships?** Does each of us believe that intercourse should be reserved for a permanent partnership or committed relationship?

- **Will a decision to engage in sex enhance my positive feelings about myself or my partner?** Does either of us have questions about sexual orientation or the kinds of people we are attracted to?

- **Do my partner and I both want to have sex?** Is my partner pressuring me in any way? Am I pressuring my partner? Am I making this decision for myself or for my partner?

- **Have my partner and I discussed our sexual histories and risk factors?** Have I spoken honestly about any STIs I've had in the past? Am I sure that neither my partner nor I have an STI?

- **Have we taken precautions against unwanted pregnancy and STIs?**

Saying No to Sex

Whether couples are on a first date or have been married for years, each partner always has the right not to have sex. Sometimes partners have differing intentions and can make incorrect assumptions that the other is willing to engage in sexual acts.

The following strategies can help you assert yourself when saying no to sex:

- **Recognize your own values and feelings.** If you believe that sex is something to be shared only by people who've already become close in other ways, be true to that belief.

- **Be direct.** Look the person in the eyes, keep your head up, and speak clearly and firmly.

Tetra Images/Getty Images

Seven Secrets to a Good Sexual Relationship

The secret to a healthy, happy sexual relationship isn't a hot car or sexy outfit. It's the ability to communicate openly, honestly, and respectfully with your partner. Here are some specific suggestions:

- **Choose an appropriate time and place for an intimate discussion.** In a new relationship, talking in a public place, such as a park bench or a quiet table at a coffeehouse, can seem safer. If you're in an established relationship, choose a time when you can give each other complete attention and a setting in which you can both relax.

- **Ask open-ended questions that encourage a dialogue—for instance, "How do you feel about . . . ?"** or "What are your thoughts about . . . ?"

- **Listen actively rather than passively when your partner speaks.** Show that you're paying attention by nodding, smiling, and leaning forward. Paraphrase what he or she says to show you understand it fully.

- **Use "I" statements, such as "I really enjoy making love, but I'm so tired right now that I won't be a responsive partner.** Why don't we get the kids to bed early tomorrow so we can enjoy ourselves a little earlier?"

- **If you would like to try something different, say so.** Practice saying the words first if they embarrass you. If your partner feels uncomfortable, don't force the issue, but do try talking it through.

- **If you want to request changes or tackle a touchy topic, start with positive statements.** Let your partner know how much you enjoy having sex, and then express your desire to enjoy lovemaking more often or in different ways.

- **Encourage small changes.** If you want your partner to be less inhibited, start slowly, perhaps by suggesting sex in a different room or place.

- **Just say no.** Make it clear you're rejecting the offer, not the person. You don't owe anyone an explanation for what you want, but if you want to expand on your reasons, you might say, "I enjoy your company, and I'd like to do something together, but no," or "Thank you. I appreciate your interest, but no."

- **If you're still at a loss for words,** try these responses: "I like you a lot, but I'm not ready to have sex," "You're a great person, but sex isn't something I do to prove I like someone," or "I'd like to wait until I'm in a committed relationship to have sex."

- **If you're feeling pressured,** let your date know that you're uncomfortable. Be simple and direct. Watch out for emotional blackmail. If your date says, "If you really liked me, you'd want to make love," point out that if he or she really liked you, he or she wouldn't try to force you to do something you don't want to do.

- **Communicate your feelings** to your date sooner rather than later. It's far easier to say, "I don't want to go to your apartment" than to fight off unwelcome advances once you're there.

- **Remember that if saying no to sex** puts an end to a relationship, it wasn't much of a relationship in the first place.

Sexual Behavior

From birth to death, we are sexual beings. Our sexual identities, needs, likes, and dislikes emerge in adolescence and become clearer as we enter adulthood, but we continue to change and evolve throughout our lives. In men, sexual interest is most intense at age 18; in women, it reaches a peak in the 30s. Although age brings changes in sexual responsiveness, we never outgrow our sexuality.

Sexuality may be timeless, but sexual behaviors change over time. Acceptance of nonmarital sex rose steadily between those born between 1901 to 1924 and baby boomers (born from 1946 to 1964), dipped slightly among early Generation X-ers (born from 1965 to 1981), and then rose again with Millennials (born 1982 to 1999) (Table 8.1). Generational shifts for men and for blacks are greater for men and black, as compared with whites and women.

The sex lives of Americans born after 1980 are quite different from those of Americans born in preceding decades. Among the key changes:

- Younger age for sexual initiation. The median age at first intercourse for today's "emerging adults" is 16.1 years for males and 16.2 years for females.

TABLE 8.1 Sex in America

For Men and Women	Lifetime Other-Sex Partners
Born in the 1910s to 1920s:	1
Born in the 1930s:	2
Born in the 1940s:	3
Born in the 1950s to 1960s:	4
Born in the 1970s to 1990s:	3
	Other-Sex Partners in Last Year (all ages)
Men	1
Women	1
Top 5% of Most Sexually Active Men	3
Top 5% of Most Sexually Active Women	2

Source: Harper CR et al. Changes in the distribution of sex partners in the United States: 2002 to 2011–2013. *Sex Transm Dis.* 2017; 44(2)96–100. doi:10.1097/OLQ.0000000000000554.

- The percentage of sexually active adolescents increases with age, from 13.1 percent of males and 12.5 percent of females at age 14 to more than 75 percent for both sexes at age 19.[23]

- More sexual partners. The median number of lifetime partners has risen to 8.8 for males and 5.3 for females.

- More women with same-sex partners. Among women ages 20 to 24, 14.9 percent report having had sex with another woman. The percentage of men having sex with men did not change over recent decades.

- Less of a gender gap in sexual activity. Female respondents report initiating sexual activity at about the same age as males. Men report more lifetime partners than women, but the difference has narrowed over time.[24]

Sexual Initiation: "Having Sex" for the First Time

✓**check-in** What does "having sex" mean to you?

This widely used term has different meanings to different people. In an online survey of more than 500 men and women, 97 percent defined "having sex" as "penile—vaginal intercourse." Far fewer use these words to indicate manual stimulation of genitals, oral sex, or anal sex.[25]

According to longitudinal studies, most people engage in vaginal intercourse for the first time between the ages of 15 and 17, with 70 to 90 percent engaging in sexual behavior by age 18.

hooking up An experience in which partners engage in intimate behaviors without explicit expectation of future romantic commitment.

First-time sexual experiences can affect a variety of health outcomes. For instance, individuals who use condoms during first intercourse are more likely to continue to do so.

The circumstances of losing one's virginity also have psychological effects. According to research, women who did not lose their virginity with a steady dating or committed partner have greater feelings of guilt and remain less comfortable with their sexuality and less sexually satisfied. Men generally have higher levels of physical and emotional satisfaction with their initial sexual experience and less anxiety and negativity than do women.

Sex on Campus

"Casual" sex, defined as any sexual experience outside a committed relationship, is common on college campuses. However, students often define casual sex differently, depending on the nature of the sexual encounter (e.g., kissing vs. intercourse), perceived intimacy, commitment level, and length of the acquaintance or relationship.

Although college students see sexual activity as normal behavior for their peer group, they tend to overestimate how much sex their peers are having. According to the American College Health Association, a third of undergraduates report having had no sexual partners within the past 12 months. Among sexually active students, the mean number of partners is two.[26] (See Snapshot: On Campus Now: The Sex Lives of College Students.) In a study that compared young adults (ages 18–24) attending 2-year colleges, attending 4-year colleges, and not in college, those not enrolled in school were more likely than full- or part-time students to have multiple lifetime sexual partners and to report never using a condom. Undergraduates at 2-year colleges reported more partners than their counterparts at 4-year schools.[27] Men generally report more lifetime sex partners than women, but this difference has narrowed over time.

Hooking Up

Hooking up can be defined as an experience in which partners engage in physically intimate behaviors (such as kissing, oral sex, or sexual intercourse) without explicit expectation of future romantic commitment. Some students describe it more informally as "making out with no future" or "a one-time experience without any kind of responsibility to each other."

Although popular media have described a pervasive "hookup culture" on campuses, its true prevalence remains unknown. The average graduating senior reports hooking up eight times in the past 4 years. Almost one-third of college

The Sex Lives of College Students

Students report having:

Oral sex within the past 30 days:	Percent (%)		
	Male	Female	Average
No, have never done this sexual activity	30.2	30.3	30.4
No, have done this sexual activity but not in the past 30 days	27.3	25.1	25.8
Yes	42.5	44.5	43.8

Anal sex within the past 30 days:	Percent (%)		
	Male	Female	Average
No, have never done this sexual activity	70.5	75.2	73.5
No, have done this sexual activity but not in the past 30 days	22.1	20.3	20.9
Yes	7.4	4.5	5.5

Vaginal sex within the past 30 days:	Percent (%)		
	Male	Female	Average
No, have never done this sexual activity	36.4	31.5	33.1
No, have done this sexual activity but not in the past 30 days	21.3	18.1	19.1
Yes	42.3	50.4	47.8

College students reporting having the following number of sexual partners (oral sex, vaginal, or anal intercourse) within the past 12 months:

	Percent (%)		
	Male	Female	Average
None	34.7	31.4	32.5
1	40.5	46.1	44.2
2	8.3	9.0	8.8
3	5.4	5.0	5.1
4 or more	11.1	8.5	9.3

Most college students assume that their classmates are more sexually active than they are. As the preceding data indicate, a significant percentage have never had sexual intercourse. Those who are sexually active report a median of two partners. Do these statistics change your perception of sexual activity on campus? Do they have any influence on your own intimate relationships?

Source: American College Health Association. American College Health Association-National College Health Assessment II: Reference Group Executive Summary Spring 2018. Silver Spring, MD: American College Health Association, 2018.

students never hook up at all. In one study, both college men and women reported twice as many hookups as first dates.[28]

Students may engage in or endorse casual, commitment-free sexual encounters for various reasons, including a belief that hooking up is harmless because it requires no emotional commitment, will enhance their status in a peer group, allows them to assert control over their sexuality, or reflects sexual freedom.

A college hookup usually involves two people who have met online or previously, often at a bar, fraternity house, club, or party, and agree to engage in some sexual behavior for which there is little or no expectation of future commitment. There is often minimal communication, and the hookup ends when one partner leaves, falls asleep, or passes out.

The students most likely to engage in hookups tend to:

- Be white.
- Be attractive.
- Be outgoing.
- Be nonreligious.
- Have high-income and/or divorced parents.
- Have a history of middle and high school hookups.
- Use marijuana
- Engage in heavy or binge drinking.[29]
- Be in a situation, such as studying abroad or spring break, that encourages hookups.[30]
- More frequently view pornography.
- Belong to athletic or certain social groups.

High school sexual norms have a strong influence on college sexual experiences. In a study that categorized female students as placing priority on religion, relationships, partying, or careers, these values influenced their behavior in college much as they did in high school.[31]

College norms also have an effect. Women at an elite academic college and those at a state

How to Stay Safe in the "Hookup Era"

- Avoid drugs and excess alcohol. Alcohol or drugs are involved in at least one-third of hookups—sometimes consumed on purpose to facilitate hooking up and sometimes the reason why a hookup went farther than was expected or wanted. When either or both partners drink too much, what starts off as a consensual hookup situation can get out of control and culminate in date rape (discussed in Chapter 18).

- Plan ahead. Think through a strategy for a situation that might lead to casual sex, whether it's deciding to leave with a friend at a certain hour or always carrying a condom if you get caught in the heat of the moment.

- Prepare for talking to a potential partner about safe sex. Rehearse in your mind what you want—and need—to say to protect yourself. Inform yourself about condoms so you know how to use them correctly and can refute myths such as the assertion that they interfere with sexual pleasure.

- Don't assume that "friends" who care about you are safe sexual partners. They may not realize that they have an STI or may assume that they aren't infectious at the moment. Keep in mind that real friends look out for each other and take steps to ensure each other's well-being.

- Don't let looks fool you. Attractiveness may make someone desirable but tells you nothing about his or her sexual history and riskiness. Don't shut down your brain just because your body is aroused.

university reported different reasons for engaging in hookups. At "Ivy U," hook ups and long-distance relationships were seen as advantageous for time-crunched "preprofessional students." At a public school with a party reputation, women described hookups as part of the "fun of college life," while women seeking or involved in committed relationships negotiated the effects of a party culture in their partnerships.[32]

About a third of students who've reported hooking up have described the experiences as "traumatic" or "very difficult to handle." The negative consequences include unprotected sex, unwanted sex, and emotional distress, including sexual regret, loss of self-respect, and embarrassment.

✓ **check-in** What is your opinion of hooking up?

Friends with Benefits

Like hookups, relationships between "friends with benefits" include varied sexual behaviors but occur between two individuals who do not identify their relationship as romantic but engage in sexual interaction (ranging from kissing to sexual intercourse) on repeated occasions. About half of college students report having engaged in a friends-with-benefits relationship in the preceding 12 months. A significant number were also involved in other friends-with-benefits relationships simultaneously.

Researchers have found differences between platonic (nonsexual) friendships and those that mixed friendship and sex. In one study, those in casual-sex friendships did less to maintain the relationship as compared with platonic friends.[33] Men are more likely to desire no change in a friends-with-benefits relationship, while women typically prefer either to go back to being "just friends" or to move into a committed romantic relationship.

✓**check-in Do** you think sexual "benefits" affect a friendship?

Choosing Sexual Partners

How do students choose partners (researchers sometimes use the term *targets*) for casual sex? Physical attraction may matter most. Men, according to numerous studies, are more likely to judge an attractive woman as less risky because she looks healthy. Even when men acknowledge that an attractive woman has probably had more sexual encounters, including one-night stands, they still say they would have sex with her.

Women also see physically attractive men as more desirable short-term sexual partners than those who look less appealing. Some say they would be willing to have sex with a physically attractive man, even if he seemed more likely to have an STI and if the sexual encounter would be unprotected. The reasons, researchers theorize, may be that sexual arousal lowers inhibitions and impairs decision making or that "sociosexuality"—the willingness to engage in casual sexual encounters—decreases perception of risk.

Romantic Relationships

Most college students still engage in sex in the context of a romantic relationship. In one study of first-year female undergraduates, romantic sexual encounters—including oral and vaginal sex—were approximately twice as common as hookup sex.

The context of sexual activity can affect sexual enjoyment in both sexes. In a recent study, young adults who saw themselves in more committed relationships reported enjoying their "partnered sex acts" more, on average, than those in less committed relationships. However, there was no consistent association between sexual enjoyment and formal relationship status. The reasons may be that people who feel a commitment experience fewer inhibitions and less anxiety, are more motivated to invest time and energy in learning to please each other sexually, and communicate more successfully, ultimately providing each other with greater sexual satisfaction.

Ethnic Variations

As with other aspects of health, cultural, religious, and personal values affect students' sexual behaviors. Researchers raised concern about young Latina women, who have the highest teen birth rate in the United States (twice the national rate) and are at greater risk of STIs. Although Latinas represent about 10 percent of women over age 21, they account for 20 percent of female AIDS cases. Among college students and other populations, Latinas are more likely to engage in unprotected intercourse than women from other ethnic groups.

Acculturation—the process of adaptation that occurs when immigrants enter a new country—also affects sexual behavior. As Latina immigrants become more acculturated in the United States, some aspects of their sexual behavior become more Americanized; for instance, they become more likely to engage in nonmarital sexual activity and to have multiple partners. In a study of Cuban American college women, older, less religious, and U.S.-born Latinas were more likely to be sexually active and to engage in risky sexual behavior than other Latinas.

Sex in America

The average American adult reports having sex about once a week. However, one in five Americans has been celibate for at least a year, and 1 in 20 engages in sex at least every other day. Men report more sexual frequency than women—probably because more older women are widowed or do not have healthy partners.

Although many people assume that Americans today have more sexual partners than in the past, this isn't necessarily the case. According to recent research, men and women born in the 1970s to 1990s report three lifetime other-sex partners, the same as those born in the 1940s—although this number may rise as this cohort of individuals grows older. Among Americans of all ages, both men and women report an average of one other-sex partner in the last year (see Table 8.1).[34]

Among married people, husbands and wives report having sex 58 to 59 times a year. If other differences between men and women are statistically controlled (such as sexual preference, age, and educational attainment), married women report a slightly higher frequency than men.

According to a national survey of about 9,000 adults ages 18 to 44:

- 94.2 percent of women and 92.0 percent of men had vaginal intercourse.

- 86.2 percent of women and 87.4 percent of men had oral sex.

- 35.9 percent of women and 42.3 percent of men had anal sex.

- 92.3 percent of women and 95.1 percent of men said they were "heterosexual or straight."

- 17.4 percent of women and 6.2 percent of men reported any same-sex contact in their lifetime.

- 1.3 percent of women and 1.9 percent of men said they were "homosexual, gay, or lesbian."

- 5.5 percent of women and 2.0 percent of men said they were bisexual.

- 0.9 percent of women and 1 percent of men said "don't know" or did not report their sexual orientation.

- 81 percent of women and 92.1 percent of men reported feelings of attraction "only to the opposite sex."[35]

Sexual frequency peaks among those with some college education, then decreases among 4-year college graduates, and declines even further among those with professional degrees. Americans who have attended graduate school are the least sexually active educational group in the population. These respondents may be more honest than others in reporting sexual activity, or they may be more precise in their definition of what counts as sex.

✓**check-in** Do you think that sex makes people happier or healthier?

Researchers have concluded that the more sex a person has, the more likely he or she is to report having a happy life and marriage. This connection is stronger among women than among men. A second and more important predictor of sexual frequency is the feeling that one's life is exciting rather than routine or dull. As researchers have noted, "Increased sexual activity is one of the many benefits of having a positive attitude."

Sexual Diversity

Human beings are diverse in all ways, including sexual preferences and practices. Sexual orientation refers to the gender(s) to which someone feels sexually attracted. The acronym LGBTQIA is an acronym for lesbian, gay, bisexual, transgender, queer/questioning, intersex, asexual (or allied individuals). Transgender people, like their cisgender counterparts, might identify as gay, straight, queer, bisexual, or gender-fluid.[36] **Sexual orientation** can indicate whether an individual:

- Engages in sexual behavior with men, women, both, or neither.
- Feels sexual desire for men, women, both, or neither.
- Falls in love with men, women, both, or neither.
- Identifies with a specific sexual orientation: **heterosexual**, for individuals whose primary attraction is toward members of the other sex; **homosexual**, for those preferring partners of their own sex; **bisexual**, for those attracted to both men and women; and **asexual**, for those who do not feel a sexual attraction to either sex. Some individuals describe themselves as pansexual, polysexual, or omnisexual because they are attracted to individuals who identify themselves as men, women, transgender, or intersex—terms defined and discussed on page 220. Asexual individuals, according to the Asexual Visibility and Education Network, do not experience sexual attraction.

Sexual orientation represents only one aspect of a person's life rather than a complete identity. The term "sexual fluidity" describes variability in same-sex and other-sex attraction and experiences throughout the life span. As longitudinal research has shown, sexual self-identity and the biological sex of preferred sexual partners vary over time. Generally more women than men experiment sexually with the same sex, while sexual fluidity among men is less common.[37]

Neither sexual orientation nor attraction necessarily correlates with reported sexual behavior. Researchers use the terms *heteroflexibility* and *homoflexibility* to describe individuals who are primarily heterosexual or homosexual, yet report some sexual interest in or experience with both sexes.

Sexual orientation influences various risky behaviors among college students, including smoking and substance use.[38] According to recent research, lesbian and bisexual females drink heavily more often than heterosexual women, while heterosexual men engage in heavy drinking more than gay men.[39] Although there has been an increase in legal recognition, social acceptance, and visibility for LGBTQIA people, sexual prejudice and intolerance persist, particularly toward LGBTQIA individuals.[40] Compared to heterosexuals, LGBTQIA youth experience higher rates of harassment, abuse, and violence.[41]

Heterosexuality

Heterosexuality, the most common sexual orientation, refers to sexual or romantic attraction between different sexes. The adjective *heterosexual* describes intimate relationships and/or sexual relations between a man and a woman. The term *straight* is used predominantly for self-identified heterosexuals of either sex. In his landmark research in the 1940s, Alfred Kinsey reported that while many men and women were exclusively heterosexual, a significant number (37 percent of men and 13 percent of women) had at least one adult sexual experience with a member of the same sex.

Bisexuality

Bisexuality—sexual attraction to both males and females—can develop at any point in one's life. Individuals may identify themselves as bisexual even if they don't behave bisexually. Some individuals are sexually involved with same-sex partners for a while and then with partners of the other sex or vice versa. Individuals who experience emotional, physical, sexual, and/or romantic attraction for members of all gender identities/expressions may also be referred to as pansexual.

Bisexuality can be viewed on the basis of behavior, attraction, or identity. An individual who has been erotically attracted to or who has had sexual experiences with persons of more than one gender can be described as bisexual, but may not identify as such. Other individuals may identify as bisexual, whether or not they've ever engaged in sexual behaviors with partners of more than one gender. Gender identities and expressions also are fluid and can change over time or in different contexts.

An estimated 7 to 9 million men, about twice the number thought to be exclusively homosexual, could be described as bisexual during some extended period of their lives. Until relatively recently, many bisexual men were married and had secret sexual relationships with men. As HIV became more prevalent, an estimated 20 to 30 percent of cases of AIDS in women were attributed to bisexual partners.

Homosexuality

Homosexuality—social, emotional, and sexual attraction to members of the same sex—exists in almost all cultures. Men and women attracted to

sexual orientation The direction of an individual's sexual interest, either to members of the opposite sex or to members of the same sex.

heterosexual Primary sexual orientation toward members of the other sex.

homosexual Those with primary sexual orientation toward members of the same sex.

bisexual Sexual attraction to both males and females.

asexual Without sexual feelings or desires.

bisexuality Sexual attraction to both males and females

same-sex partners are commonly referred to as *gay*; female homosexuals are also called *lesbian*.

Like other aspects of human identity and experience, homosexuality is complex and diverse. Researchers have analyzed sexual orientation from many difference perspectives, including genetics, hormones, physiology, development, and behavior. "Interactional" theory proposes that homosexuality results from an interaction of biological, psychological, and social factors.

Before 1973, homosexuality was classified as a mental disorder, and research focused on its sources and associated psychological issues. Only in recent decades have we learned more about the development of lesbian, gay and bisexual identities and about the strengths and rewards of LGBTQ relationships.

Homosexuality threatens and upsets many people, perhaps because homosexuals are viewed as different, or perhaps because no one understands why some people are heterosexual and others homosexual. *Homophobia* has led to *gay bashing* (attacking homosexuals) in many communities, including college campuses.

Different ethnic groups respond to homosexuality in different ways. To a greater extent than white homosexuals, gays and lesbians from ethnic groups tend to stay in the closet longer rather than risk alienation from their families and communities. LGBTQ individuals develop and live in the context of other social identities. According to intersectionality theory, those who are also members of racial or ethnic minorities may confront additional challenges associated with being in two stigmatized minority groups.

Among men, more masculine gender identity and less spiritual meaning in life are associated with greater homophobia.[42] Young black men who have sex with men report greater gender role strain arising from conflict between homosexuality and rigid, often antihomosexual expectations of masculinity from their families, peers, and communities. As a result, they may feel greater psychological distress, try to camouflage their homosexuality, or attempt to prove their masculinity in ways that damage their self-esteem and increase social isolation.[43]

Hispanic culture, with its emphasis on *machismo*, also has a very negative view of male homosexuality. Asian cultures, which tend to view an individual as a representative of his or her family, tend to view open declarations of sexual orientation as shaming the family and challenging their reputation and future.

Roots of Homosexuality

Nobody knows what causes a person's sexual orientation. Research has discredited theories tracing homosexuality to troubled childhoods or abnormal psychological development. Sexual orientation probably emerges

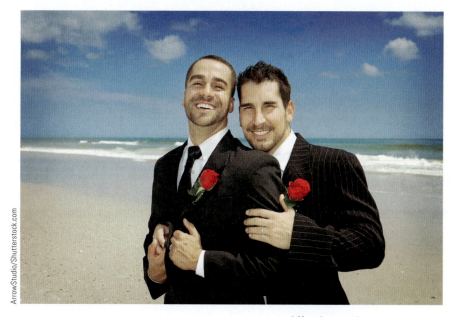

ArrowStudio/Shutterstock.com

Affection and romance are significant for partners in same-sex as well as heterosexual relationships.

from a complex interaction that includes biological and environmental factors.

Coming Out

Many young people have questions about their sexuality, but relatively few gay adolescents declare their homosexuality, or *come out*, while in a state of identity confusion. Many lesbian and bisexual women report that their first sexual experience occurred with a man (at the median age of 18) and that sex with a woman followed a few years later (at median age 21).

Most homosexual individuals progress through several stages,[44] although men may reach these milestones sooner[45]:

- **Stage 1: "I feel different from other kids . . ."** Many gay and lesbian teens say they sensed something "different" about themselves early in life, sometimes as far back as age 5. A boy may have liked to play house instead of sports, and vice versa for a girl. Patterns of social isolation from peers frequently start very young.

- **Stage 2: "I think I might be gay, but I'm not sure, and if I am, I'm not sure that I want to be . . ."** Many homosexual youngsters first realize that they are attracted to members of their own sex at puberty. A common response is to try to bury those feelings or to isolate themselves from other teens for fear of being exposed, or "outed."

- **Stage 3: "I accept the fact that I'm gay, but what's my family going to say?"** Homosexual men and women often do not accept their sexual orientation until their late teens or their 20s. Even then, they often fear their family's rejection or disapproval. As societal prejudice against gays and lesbians abates, boys and girls may arrive at this point somewhat earlier.

- **Stage 4: "I finally told my parents I'm gay."** In an online survey of nearly 2,000 gay and bisexual young people age 25 and under, the respondents were 16 the first time they revealed their sexuality to anyone, including their parents. Many homosexual teens don't begin to date until they're on their own—possibly on a campus or in a city with a sizable gay population. Only then do they begin having the experiences that straight kids encounter earlier in their sexual development.

✓**check-in** How would you describe the experience of LGBTQIA students on your campus?

Sexual Activity

Part of learning about your own sexuality is having a clear understanding of human sexual behaviors. Understanding frees us from fear and anxiety so that we can accept ourselves and others as the natural sexual beings we all are.

Celibacy

A celibate person does not engage in sexual activity. Complete **celibacy** means that the person doesn't masturbate (stimulate him- or herself sexually) or engage in sexual activity with a partner. In partial celibacy, the person masturbates but doesn't have sexual contact with others. Many people decide to be celibate at certain times of their lives. Some don't have sex because of concerns about pregnancy or STIs; others haven't found a partner for a permanent, monogamous relationship. Many simply have other priorities, such as finishing school or starting a career, and realize that sex outside a committed relationship is a threat to their physical and psychological well-being.

Abstinence

The Centers for Disease Control and Prevention (CDC) defines **abstinence** as "refraining from sexual activities which involve vaginal, anal, and oral intercourse." The definition of abstinence remains a subject of debate and controversy, with some emphasizing positive choices and others avoidance of specific behaviors. In reality, abstinence means different things to different people, cultures, and religious groups.

Increasing numbers of adolescents and young adults are choosing to remain virgins and abstain from sexual intercourse until they enter a permanent, committed, monogamous relationship. About 2.5 million teens have taken pledges to abstain from sex.

People who were sexually active in the past may choose abstinence because the risk of medical complications associated with STIs increases with the number of sexual partners a person has. Practicing abstinence is the safest, healthiest option for many. However, there is confusion about what it means to abstain, and individuals who think they are abstaining may still be engaging in behaviors that put them at risk for HIV and STIs. (See Chapter 9 for more on abstinence as a form of birth control.)

✓**check-in** What do you think are good reasons for abstaining from sex?

Among the reasons students give for abstaining are:

- Remaining a virgin until you meet someone you love and see as a life partner.
- Being true to your religious and moral values.
- Getting to know a partner better.
- Avoiding pregnancy.
- Ensuring you're safe from STIs.

Abstinence education programs, which received federal support and became widespread in American schools, have had little, if any, impact on teen sexual behavior.

Fantasy

The mind is the most powerful sex organ in the body, and erotic mental images can be sexually stimulating. Sexual fantasies can accompany sexual activity or be pleasurable in themselves.

Fantasies generally enhance sexual arousal, reduce anxiety, and boost sexual desire. They're also a way to anticipate and rehearse new sexual experiences, as well as to bolster a person's self-image and feelings of desirability. Part of what makes fantasies exciting is that they provide an opportunity for expressing forbidden desires, such as sex with a different partner or with a past lover.

Men and women have different types of sexy thoughts, with men's fantasies containing more explicit genital images and culminating in sexual acts more quickly than women's. For many women, fantasy helps in reaching orgasm during intercourse; a loss of fantasy is often a sign of low sexual desire.

celibacy Abstention from sexual activity; can be partial or complete, permanent or temporary.

abstinence Voluntarily refraining from sexual intercourse.

Fantasies lived out via the Internet are becoming more common but may also be harmful to psychological health. (See Consumer Alert.)

Pornography

The explosive growth of the Internet has made pornography more available, affordable, and accessible almost anywhere on computers and mobile devices. Although, as researchers put it, "the effects of pornography are probably not uniformly negative," a considerable amount of research suggests potentially negative impacts, including:

- Increased viewing of women as sex objects.
- Increased aggression toward women.
- Greater acceptance of rape.
- Decreased sexual satisfaction within romantic relationships.[46]
- Partner's feelings of betrayal.
- More infidelity among college students in committed relationships.
- Increased hooking up, with more risky behaviors (oral sex and intercourse rather than kissing and petting).
- Increased number of hookup partners.[47]

Another negative effect of pornography is its seemingly addictive nature. Therapists debate whether some individuals, usually men, develop a specific compulsion for pornography or whether their behavior is a manifestation of sexual addiction.[48] Yet those unable to curtail or limit their use of pornography can suffer intense psychological distress, including a deep sense of guilt and shame.

Masturbation

Not everybody masturbates, but most people do. Kinsey estimated that 7 of 10 women and 19 of 20 men masturbate (and admit they do). Their reason is simple: It feels good. **Masturbation** produces the same physical responses as sexual activity with a partner and can be an enjoyable form of sexual release.

Masturbation has been described as immature; unsocial; tiring; frustrating; and a cause of hairy palms, warts, blemishes, and blindness. None of these myths is true. Sex educators recommend masturbation to adolescents as a means of releasing tension and becoming familiar with their sexual organs.

In a recent survey of college students, nearly all learned about masturbation through the media or from peers rather than from parents or teachers. Most of the women reported struggling with feelings of stigma and taboo

---

⚠ CONSUMER ALERT

Safe Sex in Cyberspace

Sex is the number one word searched for online. About 15 percent of Americans logging onto the Internet visit sexually oriented sites. Most people who check out sex sites on the Internet do not suffer any negative impact, but be aware of some potential risks.

Facts to Know

- Men are the largest consumers of sexually explicit material and outnumber women by a ratio of six to one. However, while men look for visual erotica, women are more likely to visit chat rooms, which offer more interactions.

- While most individuals use their home computers when surfing the Internet for sex-related sites, one in ten has used a school computer. Some universities have strict policies barring such practices and may take punitive actions against students or employees who violate the rules.

Steps to Take

- **Limit time online.** Individuals who spend 11 hours or more a week online in sexual pursuits show signs of psychological distress and admit that their behavior interferes with some areas of their lives.

- **Be skeptical.** Most Internet surfers admit that they occasionally "pretend" about their age on the Internet. Most keep secret how much time they spend on sexual pursuits in cyberspace.

- **Monitor yourself for signs of compulsivity.** A small but significant number of users are at risk of a serious problem as a result of their heavy Internet use.

- **Don't do anything virtually that you wouldn't do in real life.** For instance, "sexting" a photo of yourself nude or partially nude to your boyfriend or girlfriend might seem funny and flirty at the time. But would you flash your body on the quad or at a mall? Remember that nothing remains totally private once it makes its way into cyberspace.

---

and enjoying this pleasurable act. Most of the men saw masturbation as part of healthy sexual development.

Throughout adulthood, masturbation is often the primary sexual activity of individuals not involved in a sexual relationship and can be particularly useful when illness, absence, divorce, or death deprives a person of a partner. In a University of Chicago survey, about 25 percent of men and 9 percent of women said they masturbate at least once a week.

··
✓**check-in** How do you compare with this statistic?
··

White men and women have a higher incidence of masturbation than African American men and women. Latina women have the lowest rate of masturbation, compared with Latino men, white men and women, and African American men and women. Individuals with a higher level of education are more likely to masturbate than those with less schooling, and people living with sexual partners masturbate more than those who live alone.

masturbation Manual (or nonmanual) self-stimulation of the genitals, often resulting in orgasm.

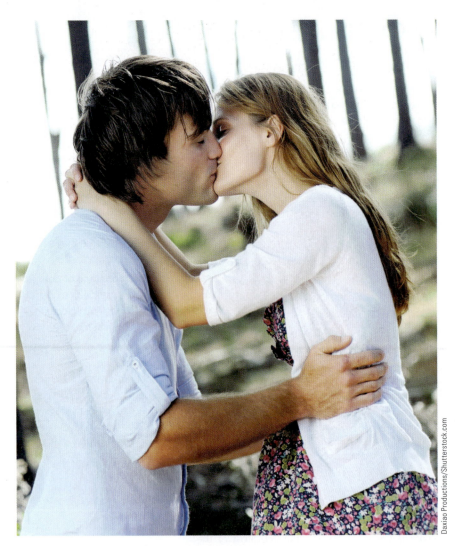

In a loving, committed relationship, every form of physical contact can serve as an intimate form of expressing deep emotion.

Daxiao Productions/Shutterstock.com

Nonpenetrative Sexual Activity (Outercourse)

Various pleasurable behaviors can lead to orgasm with little risk of pregnancy or STI. The options for "outercourse" include kissing, hugging, and touching but do not involve genital-to-genital, mouth-to-genital, or insertive anal sexual contact.

A kiss can be just a kiss—a quick press of the lips—or it can lead to much more. Usually kissing is the first sexual activity that couples engage in, and even after years of sexual experimentation and sharing, it remains an enduring pleasure for partners.

Touching is a silent form of communication between friends and lovers. Although a touch to any part of the body can be thrilling, some areas, such as the breasts and genitals, are especially sensitive. Stimulating these **erogenous** regions can lead to orgasm in both men and women. Though such forms of stimulation often accompany intercourse, more couples are gaining an

erogenous Sexually sensitive.

intercourse Sexual stimulation by means of entry of the penis into the vagina; coitus.

cunnilingus Sexual stimulation of a woman's genitals by means of oral manipulation.

fellatio Sexual stimulation of a man's genitals by means of oral manipulation.

appreciation of these activities as primary sources of sexual fulfillment—and as safer alternatives to intercourse.

Intercourse

Vaginal **intercourse** or coitus, refers to the penetration of the vagina by the penis (Figure 8.4). This is the preferred form of sexual intimacy for most heterosexual couples, who may use a wide variety of positions. The most familiar position for intercourse in our society is the so-called missionary position, with the man on top, facing the woman. An alternative is the woman on top, either lying down or sitting upright. Other positions include lying side by side (either face-to-face or with the man behind the woman, his penis entering her vagina from the rear); lying with the man on top of the woman in a rear-entry position; and kneeling or standing (again, in either a face-to-face or rear-entry position). Many couples move into several different positions for intercourse during a single episode of lovemaking; others may have a personal favorite or may choose different positions at different times.

Sexual activity, including intercourse, is possible throughout a woman's menstrual cycle. However, some women prefer to avoid sex while menstruating because of uncomfortable physical symptoms, such as cramps, or concern about bleeding or messiness. Others use a diaphragm or cervical cap (see Chapter 9) to hold back menstrual flow. Since different cultures have different views on intercourse during a woman's period, partners should discuss their own feelings and try to respect each other's views. If they choose not to have intercourse, there are other gratifying forms of sexual activity.

Vaginal intercourse, like other forms of sexual activity involving an exchange of body fluids, carries a risk of STIs, including HIV infection. In many other parts of the world, heterosexual intercourse is the most common means of HIV transmission (discussed later in this chapter).

Oral Sex

The formal terms for oral sex are **cunnilingus**, which refers to oral stimulation of the woman's genitals, and **fellatio**, oral stimulation of the man's genitals. For many couples, oral sex is a regular part of their lovemaking. For others, it's an occasional experiment. Oral sex with a partner infected with herpes, HIV, or other pathogens can transmit an STI, so a condom should be used (with cunnilingus, a dental dam can be used).

In a recent study of sexually active first-year college students, oral sex led to fewer positive consequences (such as intimacy or physical satisfaction) than negative ones (such as guilt or worry about health) compared to vaginal sex. Female freshmen generally found vaginal sex more satisfying than oral sex, whereas males found them equally pleasurable.[49]

Sperm are formed in each of the testes and stored in the epididymis. When a man ejaculates, sperm carried in semen travel up the vas deferens. (The prostate gland and seminal vesicles contribute components of the semen.) The semen is expelled from the penis through the urethra and deposited in the vagina, near the cervix. During sexual excitement and orgasm in a woman, the upper end of the vagina enlarges and the uterus elevates. After orgasm, these organs return to their normal states, and the cervix descends into the pool of semen.

Anal Stimulation and Intercourse

Because the anus has many nerve endings, it can produce intense erotic responses. Stimulation of the anus by the fingers or mouth can be a source of sexual arousal; anal intercourse involves penile penetration of the anus. An estimated 25 percent of adults have experienced anal intercourse at least once. However, anal sex involves important health risks, such as damage to sensitive rectal tissues and the transmission of various intestinal infections, hepatitis, and STIs, including HIV.

Sexual Response

Sexuality involves every part of you: mind and body, muscles and skin, glands and genitals. The pioneers in finding out exactly how human beings respond to sex were William Masters and Virginia Johnson, who first studied more than 800 individuals in their laboratory in the 1950s. They discovered that sexual response is a well-ordered sequence of events, so predictable it could be divided into four phases: excitement, plateau, orgasm, and resolution (Figure 8.5). In real life, individuals don't necessarily follow this well-ordered pattern. But the responses for both sexes are remarkably similar. And sexual response always follows the same sequence, whatever the means of stimulation.

Excitement Stimulation is the first step: a touch, a look, a fantasy. In men, sexual stimuli set off a rush of blood to the genitals, filling the blood vessels in the penis. Because these vessels are wrapped in a thick sheath of tissue, the penis becomes erect. The testes lift.

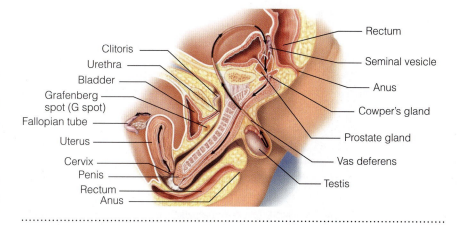

FIGURE 8.4 A Cross-Sectional View of Sexual Intercourse

Sperm are formed in each of the testes and stored in the epididymis. When a man ejaculates, sperm carried in semen travel up the vas deferens. (The prostate gland and seminal vesicles contribute components of the semen.) The semen is expelled from the penis through the urethra and deposited in the vagina, near the cervix. During sexual excitement and orgasm in a woman, the upper end of the vagina enlarges and the uterus elevates. After orgasm, these organs return to their normal states, and the cervix descends into the pool of semen.

Women respond to stimulation with vaginal lubrication within 10 to 20 seconds of exposure to sexual stimuli. The clitoris becomes larger, as do the vaginal lips (the labia), the nipples, and later the breasts. The vagina lengthens, and its inner two-thirds increase in size. The uterus lifts, further increasing the free space in the vagina.

Plateau During this stage, the changes begun in the excitement stage continue and intensify. The penis further increases in both length and diameter. The outer one-third of the vagina swells. During intercourse, the vaginal muscles grasp the penis to increase stimulation for both partners. The upper two-thirds of the vagina become wider as the uterus moves up; eventually its diameter is 2.5 to 3 inches.

Orgasm Men and women have remarkably similar **orgasm** experiences. Both men and women typically have 3 to 12 pelvic muscle contractions approximately four-fifths of a second apart and lasting up to 60 seconds. Both undergo contractions and spasms of other muscles, as well as increases in breathing and pulse rates, and blood pressure. Both can sometimes have orgasms simply from kisses, stimulation of the breasts or other parts of the body, or fantasy alone.

The process of **ejaculation** (the discharge of semen by a male) requires two separate events. First, the vas deferens, the seminal vesicles, the prostate, and the upper portion of the urethra contract. The man perceives these subtle

orgasm A series of contractions of the pelvic muscles occurring at the peak of sexual arousal.

ejaculation The expulsion of semen from the penis.

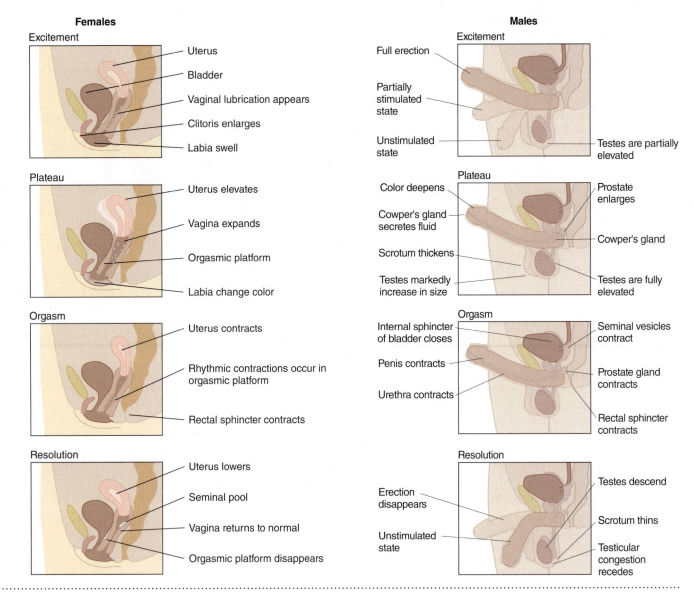

FIGURE 8.5 Human Sexual Response

The four stages of sexual response are excitement, plateau, orgasm, and resolution.

contractions deep in his pelvis just before the point of no return—which therapists refer to as the point of "ejaculatory inevitability." Then, seconds later, muscle contractions force semen out of the penis via the urethra.

Female orgasms follow several patterns. Some women experience a series of mini-orgasms—a response sometimes described as "skimming." Another pattern consists of rapid excitement and plateau stages, followed by a prolonged orgasm. This is the most frequent response to stimulation by a vibrator.

Female orgasms are primarily triggered by stimulating the clitoris. When stimulation reaches an adequate level, the vagina responds by contracting. Although it sometimes seems that vaginal stimulation alone can set off an orgasm, the

clitoris is usually involved—at least indirectly during full penile penetration.

Some researchers have identified what they call the *Grafenberg* (or G) *spot* (or area) just behind the front wall of the vagina, between the cervix and the back of the pubic bone (see Figure 8.4). When this region is stimulated, women report various sensations, including slight discomfort, a brief feeling that they need to urinate, and increasing pleasure. Continued stimulation may result in an orgasm of great intensity, accompanied by ejaculation of fluid from the urethra. However, other researchers have failed to confirm the existence and importance of the G spot, and sex therapists disagree about its significance for a woman's sexual satisfaction.

As part of their sexual response, some women experience female ejaculation, the expulsion from the urethra of a fluid that is different from urine. Hundreds of studies over more than 20 years have confirmed this phenomenon and identified the chemical composition of the ejaculated fluid. G spot stimulation, orgasm, and female ejaculation are not always related. Some women report experiencing ejaculation with orgasm from clitoral stimulation; others experience ejaculation without orgasm.[50]

Resolution

The sexual organs of men and women return to their normal, nonexcited state during this final phase of sexual response. Heightened skin color quickly fades after orgasm, and the heart rate, blood pressure, and breathing rate soon return to normal. The clitoris also resumes its normal position and appearance very shortly thereafter, whereas the penis may remain somewhat erect for up to 30 minutes.

After orgasm, men typically enter a **refractory period** during which they are incapable of another orgasm. The duration of this period varies from minutes to days, depending on age and the frequency of previous sexual activity. If either partner doesn't have an orgasm after becoming highly aroused, resolution may be much slower and may be accompanied by a sense of discomfort.

Other Models of Sexual Response

Since Masters and Johnson's pioneering work, other researchers have challenged and expanded their theories. Some argue that their model neglects the importance of desire in sexual response and that the plateau stage is virtually indistinguishable from excitement. Others note that arousal may come before desire, particularly for women who may not have spontaneous feelings of sexual desire.

As many experts have concluded, physiology alone can never explain the complexity of human sexual response. Desire, arousal, pleasure, and satisfaction are highly subjective. Positive feelings like trust and happiness enhance them. Negative emotions such as anger and anxiety can undermine them. For women, sexual satisfaction cannot be defined, as it typically is for men, by whether or not they achieved orgasm.

Sexual Concerns

Many sexual concerns stem from myths and misinformation. There is no truth, for instance, behind these misconceptions: Men are always capable of erection, sex always involves intercourse, partners should experience simultaneous orgasms, or people who truly love each other always have satisfying sex lives.

Cultural and childhood influences can affect our attitudes toward sex. Even though America's traditionally puritanical values have eased, our society continues to convey mixed messages about sex. Some children, repeatedly warned of the evils of sex, never accept the sexual dimensions of their identity. Others—especially young boys—may be exposed to macho attitudes toward sex and feel a need to prove their virility. Young girls may feel confused by media messages that encourage them to look and act provocatively and a double standard that blames them for leading boys on. In addition, virtually everyone has individual worries. A woman may feel self-conscious about the shape of her breasts; a man may worry about the size of his penis; both partners may fear not pleasing the other.

The concept of sexual normalcy differs greatly in different times, cultures, or racial and ethnic groups. In certain times and places, only sex between a husband and wife has been deemed normal. In other circumstances, "normal" has been applied to any sexual behavior—alone or with others—that does not harm others or produce great anxiety and guilt. The following are some of the most common contemporary sexual concerns.

✓**check-in** What do you think is the most common sexual concern of people your age?

Sexually Transmitted Infections and Diseases

In medical terms, **sexually transmitted infection (STI)** refers to the presence of an infectious agent that can be passed from one sexual partner to another. In public health, this term is replacing **sexually transmitted disease (STD)** because sexual infections can be—and often are—transmitted by people who do not have symptoms. Again, the odds of acquiring an STI in the course of a lifetime are one in four. These diseases cannot be prevented in a laboratory. Only you, by your behavior, can prevent and control them.

refractory period The period of time following orgasm during which a male cannot experience another orgasm.

sexually transmitted infection (STI) The presence in the human body of an infectious agent that can be passed from one sexual partner to another.

sexually transmitted disease (STD) A disease that is caused by a sexually transmitted infection that produces symptoms.

✓**check-in** Do you consider yourself well informed about STIs and STDs?

STIs can:

- Last a lifetime.
- Put stress on relationships.
- Cause serious medical complications.
- Impair fertility.
- Cause birth defects.
- Lead to major illness and death.

Although each STI is distinct, they are all transmitted mainly through:

- Direct sexual contact with someone's symptoms (e.g., genital ulcers) or sexual contact with someone's infected semen, vaginal fluids, blood, and other body fluids.
- Sharing contaminated needles through injectable drug use.
- Maternal transfer (mother to fetus during pregnancy or childbirth).

All STI pathogens like dark, warm, moist body surfaces, particularly the mucous membranes that line the reproductive organs; they hate light, cold, and dryness. Figure 8.6 shows how STIs in body fluids spread from person to person and how a barrier can help prevent their entry. It is possible to catch or have more than one STI at a time. Curing one doesn't necessarily cure another, and treatments don't prevent another bout with the same STI.

Many STIs, including early HIV infection, may not cause any symptoms. As a result, infected individuals may continue their usual sexual activity without realizing that they're jeopardizing another's well-being.

Globally more than a million STIs are acquired every day.[51] More Americans are infected with STIs now than at any other time in history. Almost half of STIs occur in young people ages 15 to 24.[52] Within 2 years of having sex for the first time, half of teenage girls may acquire an STI. The three most common are chlamydia, gonorrhea, and trichomoniasis. (See Table 8.2 for a list and description of common STDs.)

Risk Factors for Sexually Transmitted Infections

Various factors put young people at risk of STIs, including:

- **A sexual partner who has an STI.**
- **A history of STIs.**
- **Feelings of invulnerability,** which lead to risk-taking behavior. Even when they are well informed of the risks, adolescents and young adults may remain unconvinced that anything bad can or will happen to them.

- **Use of injection drugs or a sexual partner who uses them.**
- **Multiple partners or a partner who has had more than one sexual partner.** Figure 8.7 illustrates how STI risks increase as relationships become less familiar and exclusive. In surveys of students, a significant number report having had four or more sexual partners during their lifetime. Individuals with more than one concurrent partner are also at greater risk.
- **Meeting sex partners through the Internet.** Individuals who find sex partners online are more likely to report unprotected sex, higher rates of drug use in the past 12 months, more sexual partners, and failure to discuss sexual histories—all behaviors that increase the risk of STIs.[53]
- **Failure to use condoms.** Among students who reported having had sexual intercourse in the previous 3 months, fewer than half report condom use.[54]

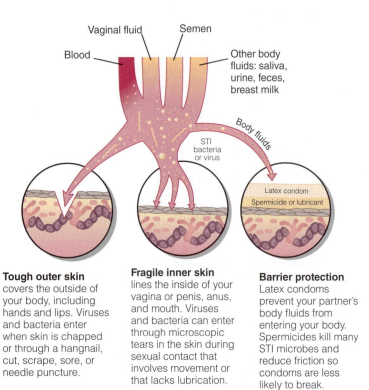

Tough outer skin covers the outside of your body, including hands and lips. Viruses and bacteria enter when skin is chapped or through a hangnail, cut, scrape, sore, or needle puncture.

Fragile inner skin lines the inside of your vagina or penis, anus, and mouth. Viruses and bacteria can enter through microscopic tears in the skin during sexual contact that involves movement or that lacks lubrication.

Barrier protection Latex condoms prevent your partner's body fluids from entering your body. Spermicides kill many STI microbes and reduce friction so condoms are less likely to break.

FIGURE 8.6 How STIs Spread

Most STIs are spread by viruses or bacteria carried in certain body fluids.

TABLE 8.2 Common Sexually Transmitted Infections (STIs)

STI	Transmission	Signs and Symptoms
Human papillomavirus (HPV) (genital warts) (p. 241)	Spread primarily through vaginal, anal, or oral sex	Cauliflower-like growths in genital and rectal areas
Herpes simplex (p. 244)	Genital herpes virus (HSV-2) transmitted by vaginal, anal, or oral sex. Oral herpes virus (HSV-1) transmitted primarily by kissing.	Small, painful red bumps (papules) to the genital region (genital herpes) or mouth (oral herpes). The papules become painful blisters that eventually rupture to form wet, open sores.
Chlamydia (p. 245)	*Chlamydia trachomatis* bacterium transmitted primarily through sexual contact (can also be spread by fingers from one body site to another)	Men: Watery discharge; pain when urinating Women: Usually asymptomatic; sometimes a similar discharge to men's; leading cause of pelvic inflammatory disease (PID)
Gonorrhea ("clap") (p. 247)	*Neisseria gonorrhoeae* bacterium ("gonococcus") spread through genital, oral–genital, or genital–anal contact	Men: Pus discharge from urethra; burning during urination Women: Usually asymptomatic; can lead to PID and sterility in both men and women
Nongonococcal urethritis (NGU) (p. 248)	Bacteria, most commonly transmitted through sexual intercourse	Men: Discharge from the penis and irritation during urination Women: Mild discharge of pus from the vagina but often no symptoms
Syphilis (p. 248)	*Treponema pallidum* bacterium ("spirochete") transmitted from open lesions during genital, oral–genital, or genital–anal contact	Primary: Chancre Secondary: Rash Latent: Asymptomatic Late: Irreversible damage to central nervous system, cardiovascular system
Chancroid (p. 249)	*Haemophilus ducrevi* bacterium transmitted by sexual interaction	Men: Painful irregular chancre on penis Women: Chancre on labia
Pubic lice ("crabs") (p. 249)	*Pthirus pubis* spread easily through body contact or through shared clothing or bedding	Persistent itching; visible lice often located in pubic hair or other body hairs
HIV/AIDS (p. 250)	HIV transmitted in blood and semen, primarily through sexual contact or needle sharing among injection drug users	Asymptomatic at first; opportunistic infections

- **Alcohol and substance abuse.** Drinking in almost all contexts (Greek parties, off-campus parties, campus events, dorms, and bars) is associated with a greater number of sexual partners, unplanned sex, and unprotected sex.[55] The more alcohol or substance use that students report, the more likely they are to engage in risky sexual behavior and to acquire an STI.[56]

- **Failure of a partner to be notified and treated.** Although physicians and health officials urge infected individuals to notify all their sexual partners, only an estimated 40 to 60 percent are notified and seek treatment.

  The CDC has endorsed "expedited partner therapy" (giving medications to the infected

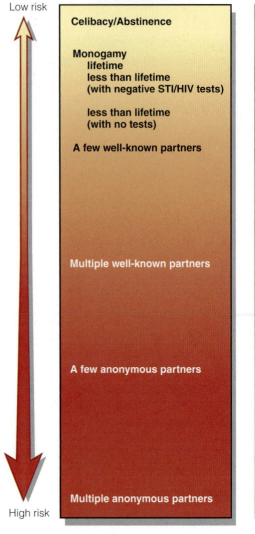

RELATIONSHIPS

Low risk

Celibacy/Abstinence

Monogamy
  lifetime
  less than lifetime
  (with negative STI/HIV tests)

  less than lifetime
  (with no tests)

A few well-known partners

Multiple well-known partners

A few anonymous partners

Multiple anonymous partners

High risk

BEHAVIORS

Noninsertive

Kissing/Making out
Petting/Fondling
Masturbation
Sex toy use
Outercourse

Insertive and protected
(condoms, other barriers)
Cunnilingus
Fellatio
Vaginal intercourse (i)
Vaginal intercourse (r)
Anal intercourse (i)
Anal intercourse (r)

Insertive and
not protected
(withdrawal)

Fellatio
Cunnilingus
Anilingus
Vaginal intercourse (i)
Vaginal intercourse (r)
Anal intercourse (i)
Anal intercourse (r)

Insertive, not protected,
including ejaculation
Fellatio
Vaginal intercourse (r)
Anal intercourse (r)

i = insertive partner
r = receptive partner

FIGURE 8.7 Continuum of Risk for Sexual Relationships and Behaviors
STI risks increase as relationships become less familiar and exclusive and as sexual activities become unprotected and receptive.

person to give to partners) for cases of gonorrhea, chlamydia, and trichomoniasis. This approach is permissible or potentially allowable in most states, but prohibited in Arkansas, Florida, Kentucky, Michigan, Ohio, Oklahoma, South Carolina, Vermont, and West Virginia.

Various factors influence an individual's willingness to disclose an STI to a prospective sexual partner, including age, masculinity-related values, interpersonal violence, partner cell phone monitoring, alcohol and/or drug use, condom use, number and characteristics of sexual partners, and previous STIs. Among college-age men, type of sex partner and masculinity-related values are key determinants in predicting whether an individual is willing to reveal having an STI.[57]

Screening for Sexually Transmitted Infections

The U.S. Preventive Services Task Force (USP-STF) recommends that health-care providers routinely ask about the sexual history of adolescents and young adults in order to screen for specific STIs, including:

- Chlamydia and gonorrhea in all sexually active and pregnant women younger than 25 and in older women at increased risk because of new or multiple sex partners.

- Human immunodeficiency virus (HIV) infection in all patients 15 to 65 years of age regardless of risk.

- Hepatitis B virus infection and syphilis in persons at increased risk.

- Hepatitis B virus infection, HIV infection, gonorrhea, chalmydia, and syphilis in pregnant women at risk.

- Testing for syphilis, gonorrhea, chlamydia, and HIV at least once a year for men having sex with men. Those with multiple partners are advised to seek testing more frequently, such as every three to six months.[58]

✓**check-in** Are you at risk of getting an STI? Take the Self-Survey "Assessing Your STI Risk."

The ABCs of Safer Sex

Although there are many specific steps to take to safeguard your sexual health, the three key fundamentals are as simple as A, B, C.

A Is for Abstain

Abstinence from vaginal and anal intercourse and oral sex is free, available to everyone, extremely effective at preventing both pregnancy and STIs, and has no medical or hormonal side effects.

If you decide to abstain only from vaginal or anal penetration, remember that other sexual activity such as oral sex can also expose you to STIs. If you have oral sex, make it safer by using effective barrier methods such as condoms or latex dental dams. (A dental dam is a square piece of latex that can be stretched across the vulva or anus to prevent the transmission of STIs.) In the absence of barrier methods, men should avoid ejaculating in their partner's mouth. Also:

- Be aware of sores and discharge or unpleasant odors from your partner's genitals. These are signs to avoid oral sex.
- Don't floss or brush teeth before oral sex. It might tear the lining of the mouth, increasing exposure to viruses.
- Avoid aggressive and deep thrusting in oral sex, which can damage throat tissues and increase susceptibility for throat-based gonorrhea, herpes, and abrasions.
- Remember that oral sex can transmit various STIs, including HPV, herpes, gonorrhea, syphilis, and HIV.

B Is for Be Faithful

For men and women who are sexually active, a mutually faithful sexual relationship with just one healthy partner is the safest option. Women and men in a committed relationship don't need to worry about getting STIs if:

- Neither partner ever had sex with anyone else.
- Neither partner ever shared needles.
- Neither partner currently has or ever had an STI.

If these criteria fail to apply, two partners should be sure that neither has an STI before giving up on safer sex practices. Some infections, such as HIV, may take years to develop symptoms. The only way to know is by being tested.

In the American College Health Association (ACHA) survey, 28.8 percent of college students reported being tested for HIV.[59] After testing, a committed relationship remains safe only as long as both partners remain committed. Most women who get HIV from having sex believe that they are their sex partner's only lover and never suspect that their partner's other lovers are men or women with HIV.

C Is for Condoms

Condoms are the only contraceptive that helps prevent both pregnancy and STIs when used properly and consistently. Male condoms reduce the risk of transmission of an STI by 50 to 80 percent. They are more effective against STIs transmitted by bodily fluids (chlamydia, gonorrhea, HIV, etc.) than those transmitted by skin-to-skin contact (HPV, syphilis, herpes, and chancroid). Inexpensive and widely available in pharmacies, supermarkets, and convenience stores, condoms don't require a doctor visit or a prescription. Contrary to a common

misconception, condoms do not interfere with sexual enjoyment. (See Chapter 10 for a comprehensive discussion of condoms.) Here are some essential guidelines to keep in mind:

- Most physicians recommend American-made latex condoms. Check the package for FDA approval.
- Also check the expiration (Exp) or manufacture (MFG) date on the box or individual package to make sure the condom is still effective.
- Make sure the package and the condom appear in good condition. If the package does not state that the condoms are meant to prevent disease, they may not provide adequate protection, even if they are the most expensive ones on the shelf.
- Get the right size. Ill-fitting condoms lead to more problems with slippage and breakage, as well as diminished sexual pleasure. Men also may be more likely to remove a condom that doesn't fit well before ejaculation.
- Condoms can deteriorate if not stored properly, because they are affected by both heat and light. Don't use a condom that has been stored in your back pocket, your wallet, or the glove compartment of your car. If a condom feels sticky or very dry, don't use it; the packaging has probably been damaged.

✓**check-in** Have you ever felt embarrassed about getting condoms? If you answered yes, you're not alone. In a recent study, college students were less embarrassed about obtaining free condoms distributed by their schools than purchasing condoms at a store.[60] More women than men reporting being embarrassed when purchasing condoms.[61]

STIs and Sex

Both men and women can develop STIs, but their risks are not the same. Here is what you need to know about your risks. (See Health on a Budget for more ways of reducing the risks of STIs.)

If You Are a Woman

- Keep in mind that your risk of getting an infection is greater than a man's. STIs can be transmitted through breaks in the mucous membranes, and women have more mucosal area exposed and experience more trauma to these tissues during sexual activity than men.

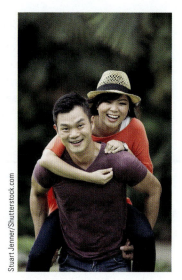

Following the ABCs of safer sex—*Abstain, Be* Faithful, use *Condoms*—doesn't mean you can't have an intimate, loving relationship.

YOUR STRATEGIES FOR CHANGE

If You Have an STI

- **If you suspect that you have an STI, don't feel too embarrassed to get help through a physician's office or a clinic.** Treatment relieves discomfort, prevents complications, and halts the spread of the disease.

- **Following diagnosis, take oral medication** (which may be given instead of or in addition to shots) exactly as prescribed.

- **Try to figure out from whom you got the STI.** Be sure to inform that person, who may not be aware of the problem.

- **If you have an STI, never deceive a prospective partner about it.** Tell the truth—simply and clearly. Be sure your partner understands exactly what you have and what the risks are.

- Don't think you don't have to worry just because you have no symptoms. Symptoms of STIs also tend to be more "silent" in women, so they often go undetected and untreated, leading to potentially serious complications. For instance, pelvic inflammatory disease has no symptoms but puts you at risk of infertility and ectopic pregnancy.

- At your checkup, talk to your doctor about whether you should be tested for STIs. You may need to ask for these tests.

- Be aware that frequent Brazilian bikini waxing and similar forms of pubic grooming may increase the risk of STIs, including herpes, HPV, and syphilis. At highest risk are "extreme" groomers who remove all their pubic hair more than eleven times a year and "high frequency" groomers who trim their pubic hair daily or weekly.[62]

If You Are a Man

- Involve your partner. Men are more likely to avoid common errors, such as removing condoms before sexual contact ends or slippage during withdrawal, when both partners mutually decide on their use.

- After potential exposure to an STI, give yourself a little extra protection by urinating and washing your genitals with an antibacterial soap.

- At your checkup, talk to your doctor about whether you should be tested for STIs.

- Although it can be awkward to bring up the subject of condoms, don't let your embarrassment put your health at risk. Discuss using a condom before having sex; don't wait until you're on the brink of a sexual encounter.

See Chapter 10 for instructions on condom use. Here are some additional guidelines:

- **Use a new condom** each and every time you engage in any form of intercourse.

- **Do not open the wrapper** of a condom with your teeth or fingernails since this can weaken or tear the condom.

- **Squeeze the air out of a condom** before putting it on.

- **Do not use spermicide containing nonoxynol-9**. Frequent use of nonoxynol-9 (N-9) may increase the risk of HIV by creating vaginal or rectal ulceration. N-9 does not offer protection from gonorrhea, chlamydia, or HIV. The FDA has required that products containing N-9 state that they do not protect against HIV and other STIs and may increase the risk of getting HIV from an infected partner.

- **If a condom fails** during vaginal or anal intercourse, remove it carefully. If you continue sexual activity, use a new condom.

$ HEALTH ON A BUDGET

Reducing Your Risk of STIs

- Abstain from sex until you are in a relationship with only one person, you are having sex only with each other, and each of you knows the other's health.
- Talk about STIs with every partner before you have sex.
- Learn as much as you can about each partner's past behavior, including sexual activity and drug use.
- Ask prospective partners if they have recently been tested for STIs.

- If you think you may have been exposed to an STI, get tested and treated.
- Do not inject illicit drugs.
- Do not put yourself in situations where sexual activity could occur when you are drunk or high because your judgment may be impaired.

STIs on Campus

Young people of traditional college ages acquire half of all new sexually transmitted infections One in four sexually active adolescent females has an STI, such as chlamydia or human papillomavirus (HPV). Why are young people at higher risk? Researchers have identified biological, cultural, and behavioral reasons:

- Young women naturally have higher levels of certain cells particularly susceptible to infection on the outer surface of the cervix. Such "cervical ectopy" is normal but increases their risk of infections such as chlamydia.

- Inability to pay

- Lack of transportation

- Long waiting times

- Conflict with work and school schedules

- Embarrassment and stigma

- Concerns about confidentiality and privacy.[63]

About two-thirds of undergraduates report engaging in oral sex or vaginal or anal intercourse within the last year, but only about half (44.4 percent) used condoms most or all of the time they engaged in vaginal intercourse in the last 30 days. Fewer (26.6 percent) used condoms the last time they engaged in anal sex; only 5.1 percent used condoms for oral sex.[64]

Contracting an STI may increase the risk of being infected with HIV. Because college students have more opportunities to engage in sex with different partners and may use drugs and alcohol more often before sex, they are at greater risk for all STIs, including HIV.

About 60 percent of colleges with a student health center provide some STI testing and treatment. However, in various studies, fewer than a third of students report that they've been tested for HIV or other STIs.[65] The reasons may include shame, stigma, fear, denial, concern about social consequences, inaccurate beliefs about STIs, privacy concerns, and inconveniences such as long waiting times.

What College Students Don't Know about STIs

"At my age, I know everything already and believe that my classmates do, too."

That's what an entering freshman said in a survey of undergraduates' sexual health knowledge. Many undergraduates would echo the same words, yet often they think that they know more than they actually do. This is particularly true of STIs. Although they often can name common STIs, such as HIV, genital herpes, gonorrhea, and chlamydia, undergraduates are less familiar with human papillomavirus (HPV) and syphilis, the symptoms associated with STIs, and the ways in which STIs are transmitted or diagnosed. Many do not realize that STIs can exist without symptoms, so they don't take steps to protect themselves or to avoid risky sexual behaviors.

College students often report never using a condom or using condoms inconsistently during sex. The reasons may have more to do with emotions and attitudes than with availability or cost. Some fear that bringing up condom use might jeopardize the relationship or cause embarrassment. Even if partners believe that condoms could help prevent an STI, those hoping for or seeing themselves as already in a long-term relationship may feel that condoms are not necessary because they and their partners know each other well. (See Health Now! for suggestions about how to tell a partner you have an STI.)

✓**check-in** Why do you think students don't use condoms consistently?

Common STIs and STDs

Human Papillomavirus

Human papillomavirus (HPV) is the most common STI in the world and a necessary cause of all cases of cervical cancer.[66] Of the 100 or more different strains, or types, of HPV, approximately 40 are sexually transmitted, and 15 have been identified as "oncogenic," or cancer-causing. Some "high-risk" HPV strains may lead to cancer of the cervix, vulva, vagina, anus, or penis. If transmitted via oral sex, they significantly increase the risk of mouth and throat cancers.[67] The risk to an individual increases along with the number of oral sex partners.

The "low-risk" types of HPV may trigger changes in cervical cells that cause Pap test abnormalities or genital warts. Genital warts are single or multiple growths or bumps, sometimes shaped like cauliflower, that appear in the genital area.

human papillomavirus (HPV) A pathogen that causes genital warts and increases the risk of cervical cancer.

Students and STIs

Students	Percent	Students	Percent
Vaccinated against hepatitis B	68.6	Diagnosed with chlamydia	1.7
Vaccinated against HPV	56.1	Diagnosed with genital herpes	0.8
Diagnosed with HPV	0.9	Diagnosed with PID	0.3

What have you done to protect yourself from STIs? Have you been vaccinated against HPV? Have you been tested for HIV? The incidence of diagnosed STIs on campuses is low, but many individuals are not aware that they have these infections. Write down your feelings about how getting an STI might affect your health and your life in your online journal.

Source: American College Health Association. American College Health Association-National College Health Assessment II: Reference Group Executive Summary Spring 2018. Silver Spring, MD: American College Health Association, 2018.

Condoms provide only limited protection. Most people who become infected with HPV do not have any symptoms, and the infection clears on its own. However, HPV infection can cause cervical cancer in women and genital warts and other types of cancers in both sexes.

The primary risk factors for oral HPV infection include:

- Number of sex partners.
- Smoking.
- Heavy drinking.
- Marijuana use.

✓**check-in** Do you think you are at risk for HPV infection?

Incidence Approximately 20 million people in the United States—almost 7 percent of those between ages 14 and 69—are currently infected with HPV, and 6.2 million Americans get a new HPV infection each year. Worldwide, more than 440 million individuals are infected with HPV.

As many as 80 percent of sexually active women acquire HPV by age 50. However, 44 percent of women ages 20 to 24 have HPV. Approximately 70 percent of sexually active women contract HPV, most within 5 years of their first sexual encounter.

Young women who engage in sexual intercourse at an early age are more likely than those with later sexual debuts to become infected with HPV. Their risk also increases if they are black, have multiple sexual partners or a history of an STI, use drugs, or have partners with multiple sexual partners. College-age women are among those at greatest risk

of acquiring HPV infection. In various studies conducted in college health centers, 10 to 46 percent of female students (mean age, 20 to 22) had positive HPV tests.

Men who have sex with men and men who have sex with both men and women have the highest rates of HPV. Men who have had more than 16 sex partners have about three times the HPV risk of those with fewer sex partners and are nearly 10 times more likely to contract a potentially cancer-causing strain. Once infected, men who have been circumcised are more likely to have their immune systems "clear" the virus. Circumcised men are also less likely to transmit the virus to female partners. HPV has also been linked to penile cancer.[68]

✓**check-in** Have you ever been tested for HPV?

HPV Vaccination Federal authorities and the American Academy of Pediatrics recommend HPV vaccination for:

- All girls ages 11 or 12, with catch-up vaccinations for those through age 26.
- Males ages 11–12 years, with catch-up vaccinations through age 21.
- Gay, bisexual, and other men who have sex with men (collectively referred to as MSM) and persons who are immunocompromised (including those infected with HIV), through age 26.

Initially, doctors had targeted girls because the vaccination is highly effective in preventing cervical cancer. However, other cancers linked to HPV, including anal cancer and some head and neck cancers, have been increasing, especially among men.

Three FDA-approved vaccines—Gardasil, Gardasil 9, and Cervarix—are effective in preventing cervical cancer caused by the two types of high-risk HPVs that cause about 70 percent of cervical cancers. In addition, Gardasil 9 adds protection against five additional HPV types, which cause approximately 20 percent of cervical cancers and are not covered by previously FDA-approved HPV vaccines. The FDA has approved Gardasil and Gardasil 9 for use in females ages 9 to 26 to protect against cervical cancer and prevent genital warts, and for males ages 9 to 26 to prevent genital warts. Cervarix, which does not protect against genital warts, is approved for females ages 10 to 26 to help prevent cervical cancer. Cervarix has not been approved for use in boys or men.

The CDC currently recommends using two doses—instead of the previous three—for those who start the HPV vaccine series between ages 9 and 14. Older patients (ages 15 through 26 for women, and 15 through 21 for men) and immunocompromised patients should still receive three doses—the second dose 1 to 2 months after the first and the third dose 6 months after the first.[69]

Rates of HPV vaccination remain lower than for other routinely recommended immunizations.[70] Vaccination against HPV has lagged in part because of fear that it might encourage teenagers to initiate sexual activity at earlier ages or to engage in riskier sexual behaviors.[71] However, several studies have confirmed that girls vaccinated against HPV are no more (and in some cases are less) likely than others to initiate sex or, if they are already sexually active, to have more partners or not use condoms during sex.[72]

Adverse effects, reported in about 6 percent of vaccinated patients, include:

- Fainting.
- Itchiness.
- Headache.
- Nausea.
- Blood clots.
- Allergic reactions.

Although young women under age 25 are most likely to develop HPV, older women at risk for cervical cancer can also benefit from vaccination, according to initial tests of the HPV vaccine in various age groups. If you are age 26 or older and have not been vaccinated, talk to your health-care provider about the relative risks and benefits for you.[73]

Since HPV vaccination began more than a decade ago, prevalence of the cancer-causing virus has significantly decreased in girls 14 to 19 years of age and in those 20 to 24—the age groups at highest risk for HPV. Health-insurance claims indicate lower rates of changes in cervical cells among women ages 25 to 29 years who've been vaccinated and in anogenital warts among vaccinated young women and men.[74]

HPV Vaccination on Campus Sexually active young adults are at the highest risk of HPV infection. More than half of college students—56 percent—report having been vaccinated against HPV.[75] Many of those who remain unvaccinated describe themselves as not being in a committed relationship or not living with a romantic partner. (See Consumer Alert.)

✓**check-in** Have you been vaccinated against HPV?

Signs and Symptoms HPV lives on the skin or in mucous membranes and usually causes no symptoms. Some people get visible genital warts or have precancerous changes in the cervix, vulva, anus, or penis. After contact with an infected individual, genital warts may appear within 3 weeks to 18 months, with an average period of about 3 months.

Most HPV infections are asymptomatic in men, who may unwittingly increase their partners' risk. Men who test positive for HPV typically report significantly more sex partners than those who do not. HPV may also cause genital warts in men and increase the risk of cancer of the penis.

HPV infection may invade the urethra and cause urinary obstruction and bleeding. It greatly increases a woman's risk of developing a precancerous condition called cervical *intraepithelial neoplasia*, which can lead to cervical cancer. Adolescent girls infected with HPV appear to be particularly vulnerable to developing cervical cancer.

It is not known if HPV itself causes cancer or acts in conjunction with cofactors (such as other infections, smoking, or suppressed immunity). A woman's risk of cervical cancer is strongly related to the number of her partner's current and lifetime female partners. Women are significantly more likely to get cervical cancer if their steady sex partner has had 20 or more previous partners.

Diagnosis and Treatment Most women are diagnosed with HPV after an abnormal Pap test or HPV DNA test. The results of HPV DNA testing can help health-care providers decide whether treatment is necessary to prevent or treat

HEALTH NOW!

Telling a Partner You Have an STI

Even though the conversation can be awkward and embarrassing, you need to talk honestly about any STI that you may have been exposed to or contracted. What you don't say can be hazardous to your partner's health. Here are some guidelines:

- **Talk before you become intimate.** A good way to start is simply by saying, "There is something we need to talk over first."

- **Be honest.** Don't downplay any potential risks.

- **Don't blame.** Even if you suspect that your partner was the source of your infection, focus on the need for medical attention.

- **Be sensitive to your partner's feelings.** Anger and resentment are common reactions when someone feels at risk. Try to listen without becoming defensive.

- **Seek medical attention.** Do not engage in sexual intimacies until you obtain a doctor's assurance that you are no longer contagious.

Even if you are not sexually active or have never had an STI, imagine yourself in this situation. What would be your biggest concern if you were the one with the STI? What would be your biggest concern if you were the partner of someone with an STI? What do you think is the best possible way to deal with such circumstances? Record your thoughts in your online journal.

Source: Bacchus and Gamma Peer Education Network, www.smartersex.org.

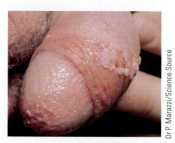

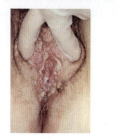

Dr. P. Marazzi/Science Source

Joe Millar/CDC

Human papillomavirus, which causes genital warts, is the most common viral STI.

cervical cancer. (See Chapter 12 for a discussion of cervical cancer.) Warning signs for cervical cancer include irregular bleeding and unusual vaginal discharge. Precancerous cervical cells can be destroyed by laser surgery or freezing during a visit to a doctor's office.

No form of therapy has been shown to completely eradicate HPV, nor has any single treatment been uniformly effective in removing warts or preventing their recurrence. CDC guidelines suggest treatments that focus on the removal of visible warts—laser therapy, cryotherapy (freezing), and topical applications of podofilox, podophyllin, or trichloroacetic acid—and then eradication of the virus. At least 20 to 30 percent of treated individuals experience recurrence.

Genital Herpes

Herpes (from the Greek word that means "to creep") collectively describes some of the most common viral infections in humans.

Characteristically, herpes simplex causes blisters on the skin or mucous membranes.

Herpes simplex exists in several varieties. *Herpes simplex virus 1 (HSV-1)* can be transmitted by kissing and generally causes cold sores and fever blisters around the mouth. *Herpes simplex virus 2 (HSV-2)* is sexually transmitted and may cause blisters on the penis, inside the vagina, on the cervix, in the pubic area, on the buttocks, on the thighs, or in the mouth and throat (transmitted via oral sex). In recent years HSV-1 infections of the genitals have increased among young adults, in part because of an increase in oral sex.[76]

About one in five women and one in nine men have genital herpes. More than 80 percent do not realize they are infected.[77] HSV transmission occurs through close contact with mucous membranes or abraded skin. Condoms help prevent infection but aren't foolproof.

In the past, physicians viewed herpes as an episodic disease with the greatest risk of transmission during a flare-up. But as newer research has documented, "classic herpes" that produces acute symptoms is not typical. For many people genital herpes is a chronic, nearly continuously active infection that may produce subtle, varied, and often-overlooked symptoms. Most cases are transmitted by sexual partners who are unaware of their infections or do not have symptoms at the time of transmission.

When herpes sores are present, the infected person is highly contagious and should avoid bringing the lesions into contact with someone else's body through touching, sexual interaction, or kissing. However, the herpes virus is present in genital secretions even when patients do not notice any signs of the disease, and people infected with genital herpes can spread it even between flare-ups, when they have no symptoms.

A newborn can be infected with genital herpes while passing through the birth canal, and the frequency of mother-to-infant transmission seems to be increasing. Most infected infants develop typical skin sores, which can be cultured to confirm a herpes diagnosis. Some physicians recommend treatment with acyclovir. Because of the risk to the infant of severe damage and possible death, caesarean delivery may be advised for a woman with active herpes lesions.

Incidence At least 50 million people in the United States have genital herpes, including 21 percent of women. Only a minority know they are affected, and many believe they could tell if a sexual partner were infected. About 40 percent of new cases of genital herpes occur in young people ages 15 to 24.

⊘ CONSUMER ALERT

Should You Get the HPV Vaccine?

Some states are considering legislation to make HPV vaccination mandatory for all girls because the vaccine is most effective when given before a girl becomes sexually active. Some religious groups oppose mandatory immunization because they feel that vaccinating girls against an STI gives them the wrong message about sexual responsibility. Consumer advocates worry about the unknown long-term effects. Others feel that the decision should be made privately by parents, in consultation with their pediatricians. Vaccination is recommended for both sexes.

Facts to Know

- The HPV vaccines have been extensively tested worldwide and are considered safe. However, the long-term effects are not known.
- No one yet knows whether a booster shot or shots will be necessary.
- Adverse effects include fainting, nausea, headache, blood clots, allergic reactions,

and death. The most common side effects are pain at the injection site and fever.

- Annually, an estimated 4,000 women in the United States and about 274,000 women internationally die from cervical cancer. The National Cancer Institute estimates 11,300 new cases of cervical cancer each year.

Steps to Take

- Talk with your doctor if you are under age 26 or at risk for cervical cancer and have not yet been vaccinated.
- Check with your insurance provider. Vaccination costs about $400. Most insurance companies cover recommended vaccines.
- Do *not* get the HPV vaccine if you
  - Are pregnant
  - Have ever had a life-threatening allergic reaction to any component of HPV vaccine
  - Are moderately to severely ill at the time of vaccination

Signs and Symptoms Most people with genital herpes have no symptoms or very mild symptoms that go unnoticed or are not recognized as a sign of infection. The most common is a cluster of blistery sores, usually on the vagina, vulva, cervix, penis, buttocks, or anus. They may last several weeks and go away. They may return in weeks, months, or years.

Other symptoms include blisters, burning feelings if urine flows over sores, inability to urinate if severe swelling of sores blocks the urethra, and itching and pain in the infected area. Severe first episodes of herpes may also cause swollen, tender lymph glands in the groin, throat, and under the arms; fever; chills; headache; and achy flulike feelings.

The virus that causes herpes never entirely goes away; it retreats to nerves near the lower spinal cord, where it remains for the life of the host. Herpes sores can return without warning weeks, months, or even years after their first occurrence, often during menstruation or times of stress, or with sudden changes in body temperature. Of those who experience HSV recurrence, 10 to 35 percent do so frequently—that is, about six or more times a year. In most people, attacks diminish in frequency and severity over time.

....
✓**check-in** Did you know that individuals can transmit genital herpes even when they don't have visible lesions?
....

Diagnosis and Treatment Testing for the herpes virus has become much more accurate. Several highly effective antiviral therapies not only reduce symptoms and heal herpes lesions but also, if taken continuously, significantly reduce the risk of transmission of the virus to sexual partners.

The three antiviral medications approved for the treatment of genital herpes are as follows:

- **Acyclovir.** The oldest antiviral medication for herpes, acyclovir is sold as a generic drug and under the brand name Zovirax. Available as an ointment and pill, acyclovir has been shown to be safe in persons who have used it continuously (every day) for as long as 10 years.

- **Valacyclovir.** Sold as Valtrex, this medication delivers acyclovir more efficiently so that the body absorbs more of the drug and medication can be taken fewer times during the day.

- **Famcyclovir.** Sold as Famvir, this drug utilizes penciclovir as its active ingredient

to stop HSV. Like valacyclovir, it is well absorbed, persists for a long time in the body, and can be taken less frequently than acyclovir.

These antiviral medications are prescribed for initial and recurrent episodes of herpes. In episodic therapy, a person begins taking medication at the first sign of recurrence and continues for several days to hasten healing or prevent a full outbreak from occurring. In suppressive therapy, people with genital herpes take antiviral medication daily to prevent symptoms. For individuals who have frequent recurrences (six or more per year), suppressive therapy can reduce the number of outbreaks by at least 75 percent. Suppressive therapy may also reduce asymptomatic shedding of HSV. They may be less effective for a first episode of genital herpes.[78]

Various treatments—compresses made with cold water, skim milk, or warm salt water; ice packs; or a mild anesthetic cream—can relieve discomfort. Herpes sufferers should avoid heat, hot baths, and nylon underwear. Some physicians have used laser therapy to vaporize the lesions. Clinical trials of an experimental vaccine to protect people from herpes infections are underway.

Chlamydia

The most widespread sexually transmitted bacterium in the United States is *Chlamydia trachomatis*, which causes more than a million cases of **chlamydia** each year, a number that continues to rise. Almost half of reported cases occur among sexually active young adults between ages 15 and 24. The use of condoms with spermicide can reduce, but not eliminate, the risk of chlamydial infection.

Incidence An estimated 1.7 million cases of chlamydia were reported in 2017.[79] Chlamydia is much more prevalent in young black adults than in young white adults. However, this may be because black and Hispanic women are much more likely to be screened. Women have three times the rate of chlamydia as men. Chlamydial infections are more common in younger than in older women, and they also occur more often in both men and women with gonorrhea.

Those at greatest risk of chlamydial infection are individuals 25 years old or younger who engage in sex with more than one new partner within a 2-month period and women who use birth control pills or other nonbarrier contraceptive methods. The USPSTF recommends regular screening for chlamydia for all sexually active women under age 25.

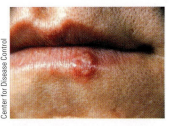

Center for Disease Control

Herpes simplex virus (HSV-1) as a mouth sore.

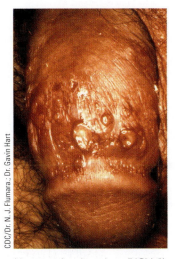

CDC/Dr. N. J. Flumara.; Dr. Gavin Hart

Herpes simplex virus (HSV-2) as a genital sore.

chlamydia A common sexually transmitted infection caused by bacteria known as *Chlamydia trachomatis*.

The incidence of chlamydia is lower in older women, and screening is recommended only for those with multiple sexual partners, a history of STIs, or inconsistent use of condoms.[80]

✓**check-in** Have you ever been screened for chlamydia?

Signs and Symptoms

As many as 75 percent of women and 50 percent of men with chlamydia have no symptoms or have symptoms so mild that they don't seek medical attention. Without treatment, up to 40 percent of cases of chlamydia can lead to pelvic inflammatory disease (PID), a serious infection of the woman's fallopian tubes that can also damage the ovaries and uterus. Also, women infected with chlamydia may have three to five times the risk of getting infected with HIV if exposed. Babies exposed to chlamydia in the birth canal during delivery can be born with pneumonia or with an eye infection called conjunctivitis, both of which can be dangerous unless treated early with antibiotics. Symptomless women who are screened and treated for chlamydial infection are almost 60 percent less likely than unscreened women to develop PID. Chlamydia may also be linked to cervical cancer.

When women have symptoms of chlamydia, they may experience:

- Abdominal pain.
- Abnormal vaginal discharge.
- Bleeding between menstrual periods.
- Cervical or rectal inflammation.
- Low-grade fever.
- Yellowish discharge from the cervix that may have a foul odor.
- Vaginal bleeding after intercourse.
- Painful intercourse.
- Painful urination.
- The urge to urinate more than usual.

When men have symptoms of chlamydia, they may experience:

- Pain or burning while urinating.
- Pus or watery or milky discharge from the penis.
- Swollen or tender testicles.
- Rectal inflammation.

Men often don't take these symptoms seriously because the symptoms may appear only early in the day and can be very mild.

Chlamydia, which can spread from a man's urethra to his testicles, can also cause a condition called epididymitis, which can cause sterility. Symptoms include fever, swelling, and extreme pain in the scrotum. Six percent of men with epididymitis develop reactive arthritis, which causes swelling and pain in the joints and can progress and become disabling.

In women and men, chlamydia may cause the rectum to itch and bleed. It can also result in a discharge and diarrhea. If it infects the eyes, it may cause redness, itching, and a discharge. If it infects the throat, it may cause soreness. Babies exposed to chlamydia during birth may develop an eye infection that causes swollen eyelids and a bloody discharge.

Diagnosis and Treatment

Various antibiotics such as *azithromycin* and doxycycline kill *Chlamydia* bacteria. Some are taken in a single dose; others over several days. Both partners must be treated to avoid reinfections.[81]

The CDC recommends that all women with chlamydia be rescreened 3 to 4 months after treatment is completed. The reason is that reinfection, which often happens because a patient's sex partners were not treated, increases the risk of PID and other complications. Immediately treating the partners of people infected with gonorrhea or chlamydia can reduce rates of recurrence of these infections.

Pelvic Inflammatory Disease

Infection of a woman's fallopian tubes or uterus, called **pelvic inflammatory disease (PID)**, is not actually an STI but a complication of STIs involving the uterus, oviducts, and/or ovaries.[82] Ten to 20 percent of initial episodes of PID lead to scarring and obstruction of the fallopian tubes severe enough to cause infertility. Other long-term complications are ectopic pregnancy and chronic pelvic pain. Smoking may also increase the likelihood of PID.

Two bacteria—*Gonococcus* (the culprit in gonorrhea) and *Chlamydia*—are responsible for one-half to one-third of all cases of PID. Other organisms are responsible for the remaining cases. Several studies have shown that women with PID are more likely to have used douches than those without the disease. Consistent condom use may decrease PID risk.

✓**check-in** Did you know that PID can cause infertility in women?

Incidence

About one in every seven women of reproductive age has PID; half of all adult women may have had it. Each year, about 1 million new cases are reported.

pelvic inflammatory disease (PID) An inflammation of the internal female genital tract, characterized by abdominal pain, fever, and tenderness of the cervix.

Most cases of PID occur among women under age 25 who are sexually active. *Gonococcus*-caused cases tend to affect poor women; those caused by *Chlamydia* range across all income levels. One-third to one-half of all cases are transmitted sexually, and others have been traced to some IUDs that are no longer on the market.

Signs and Symptoms   PID is a silent disease that in half of all cases produces no noticeable symptoms as it progresses and causes scarring of the fallopian tubes. Early symptoms include:

- Abdominal pain or tenderness.
- Fever.
- Vaginal discharge that may have a foul odor.
- Painful intercourse or urination.
- Irregular menstrual bleeding.
- Rarely, pain in the right upper abdomen.

Diagnosis and Treatment   Urine testing is a cost-effective method of detecting gonorrhea and chlamydia in young women and can prevent development of PID. For women with symptoms, a pelvic ultrasound can show whether fallopian tubes are enlarged or an abscess is present. Magnetic resonance imaging (MRI) can also establish a diagnosis of PID and detect other diseases that may be responsible for the symptoms. Treatment consists of antibiotic therapy, usually with at least two antibiotics effective against a wide range of bacteria. A woman's sex partner(s) should also be treated to decrease the risk of reinfection, even if they have no symptoms. PID causes an estimated 15 to 30 percent of all cases of infertility every year and about half of all cases of ectopic pregnancy.

Gonorrhea

Gonorrhea (sometimes called "the clap"), the second most commonly reported STI in the United States, can lead to pelvic inflammatory disease, ectopic pregnancy, and infertility.[83]

Incidence   More than 550,000 new cases of gonorrhea were reported to the CDC in 2017, an increase of 75 percent in the previous decade.[84] Gonorrhea rates have increased among both men and women and across all racial and ethnic groups.[85]

Signs and Symptoms   Most men who have gonorrhea know it. Thick, yellow-white pus oozes from the penis, and urination causes a burning sensation. These symptoms usually develop 2 to 9 days after the sexual contact that infected them. Men have a good reason to seek help: It hurts too much not to.

In men, untreated gonorrhea can spread to the prostate gland, testicles, bladder, and kidneys. Among the serious complications are urinary obstruction and sterility caused by blockage of the vas deferens (the excretory duct of the testis).

Women may also experience discharge and burning on urination. However, as many as 8 in 10 infected women have no symptoms.

Gonococcus, the bacterium that causes gonorrhea, can live in the vagina, cervix, and fallopian tubes for months, even years, and continue to infect the woman's sexual partners. Approximately 5 percent of sexually active American women have positive gonorrhea cultures but are unaware that they are silent carriers.

If left untreated in men or women, gonorrhea spreads through the urinary–genital tract. In women, the inflammation travels from the vagina and cervix, through the uterus, to the fallopian tubes and ovaries. The pain and fever are similar to those caused by stomach upset, so a woman may dismiss the symptoms. Eventually these symptoms diminish, even though the disease spreads to the entire pelvis. Pus may ooze from the fallopian tubes or ovaries into the peritoneum (the lining of the abdominal cavity), sometimes causing serious inflammation. However, this, too, can subside in a few weeks.

Gonorrhea, the leading cause of sterility in women, can cause PID. In pregnant women, gonorrhea becomes a threat to the newborn. It can infect the infant's external genitals and cause a serious form of conjunctivitis. As a preventive step, newborns may have penicillin dropped into their eyes at birth.

In both sexes, gonorrhea can develop into a serious, even fatal, bloodborne infection that can cause arthritis in the joints, attack the heart muscle and lining, cause meningitis, and attack the skin and other organs.

Diagnosis and Treatment   Although a blood test has been developed for detecting gonorrhea, the tried-and-true method of diagnosis is still a microscopic analysis of cultures from the male's urethra, the female's cervix, and the throat and anus of both sexes.

Because gonorrhea often occurs along with chlamydia, practitioners often prescribe an agent effective against both, such as ofloxacin. Fluoroquinolones are no longer advised for use in its treatment. The CDC recommends a cephalosporin antibiotic plus azithromycin or doxycyline, but recommendations for treatment are rapidly evolving. A new strain of gonorrhea resistant to available antibiotics has emerged in North America. Antibiotics taken for other reasons may not affect or cure gonorrhea because of their dosage or type. The CDC estimates that at least 2 million Americans contract

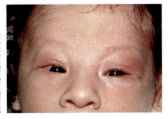

A baby exposed to chlamydial infection in the birth canal during delivery may develop an eye infection. Symptoms include a bloody discharge and swollen eyelids.

Dr. Allan Harris/Phototake

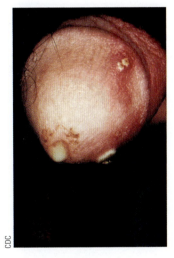

A cloudy discharge is symptomatic of gonorrhea.

CDC

gonorrhea A sexually transmitted infection caused by the bacterium Neisseria gonorrhoeae; symptoms include discharge from the penis; women are generally asymptomatic.

infections—including gonorrhea—that are resistant to at least one antibiotic.

Symptoms of the infection are often absent. Undiagnosed and untreated gonorrhea may lead to pelvic inflammatory disease, infertility, ectopic pregnancy (a pregnancy that occurs outside of the uterus), and/or chronic pelvic pain. At risk older women and all sexually active women age 24 and younger should be routinely screened for the infection.

The CDC advises medical professionals to treat gonorrhea with a combination that includes the injectable antibiotic ceftriaxone and the antibiotic pill azithromycin. However, there is concern about the growing threat of resistance to these drugs.[86]

Nongonococcal Urethritis

The term **nongonococcal urethritis (NGU)** refers to any inflammation of the urethra that is not caused by gonorrhea. NGU is the most common STI in men, accounting for 4 to 6 million visits to a physician every year. Three microorganisms—*Chlamydia trachomatis*, *Ureaplasma urealyticum*, and *Mycoplasma genitalium*—are the primary causes; the usual means of transmission is sexual intercourse. Other infectious agents, such as fungi or bacteria, allergic reactions to vaginal secretions, or irritation by soaps or contraceptive foams or gels may also lead to NGU.

In the United States, NGU is more common in men than gonococcal urethritis. The symptoms in men are similar to those of gonorrhea, including discharge from the penis (usually less than with gonorrhea) and mild burning during urination. Women frequently develop no symptoms or very mild itching, burning during urination, or discharge. Symptoms usually disappear after 2 or 3 weeks, but the infection may persist and cause cervicitis or PID in women and, in men, may spread to the prostate, epididymis, or both. Treatment usually consists of doxycycline or azithromycin and should be given to both sexual partners.

Syphilis

A corkscrew-shaped, spiral bacterium called *Treponema pallidum* causes syphilis. This frail microbe dies in seconds if dried or chilled but grows quickly in the warm, moist tissues of the body, particularly in the mucous membranes of the genital tract. Entering the body through any tiny break in the skin, the germ burrows its way into the bloodstream. Sexual contact, including oral sex or intercourse, is a primary means of transmission. Genital ulcers caused by syphilis may increase the risk of HIV infection, while individuals with HIV may be more likely to develop syphilis.

Incidence
The rates of syphilis, which was nearly eliminated more than a decade ago, have been increasing. Men account for almost 9 in 10 cases, with gay, bisexual, and other men having sex with men accounting for about two-thirds of these cases. Syphilis also has increased among injection drug users, women, and newborns infected before birth.[87]

Signs and Symptoms
Syphilis has clearly identifiable stages:

- **Primary syphilis.** The first sign of syphilis is a lesion, or *chancre* (pronounced "shanker"), an open lump or crater the size of a dime or smaller, teeming with bacteria. The incubation period before its appearance ranges from 10 to 90 days; 3 to 4 weeks is average. The chancre appears exactly where the bacteria entered the body: in the mouth, throat, vagina, rectum, or penis. Any contact with the chancre is likely to result in infection.

- **Secondary syphilis.** Anywhere from 1 to 12 months after the chancre's appearance, secondary-stage symptoms may appear. Some people have no symptoms. Others develop a skin rash or a small, flat rash in moist regions on the skin; whitish patches on the mucous membranes of the mouth or throat; temporary baldness; low-grade fever; headache; swollen glands; or large, moist sores around the mouth and genitals. These sores are loaded with bacteria; contact with them, through kissing or intercourse, may transmit the infection. Symptoms may last for several days or several months. Even without treatment, symptoms eventually disappear as the syphilis microbes go into hiding.

- **Late and latent syphilis.** Although there are no signs or symptoms and no sores or rashes at this stage, the bacteria are invading various organs inside the body, including the heart and brain. For 2 to 4 years, there may be recurring infectious and highly contagious lesions of the skin or mucous membranes. However, syphilis loses its infectiousness as it progresses: After the first 2 years, a person rarely transmits syphilis through intercourse.

- After 4 years, even congenital syphilis is rarely transmitted. Until this stage of the disease, however, a pregnant woman can pass syphilis to her unborn child. If the fetus is infected in its fourth month or earlier, it may be disfigured or even die. If infected late in pregnancy, the child may show no signs of infection for months or years after birth, but may then become disabled with the symptoms of tertiary syphilis.

- **Tertiary syphilis.** Ten to 20 years after the beginning of the latent stage, the most serious symptoms of syphilis emerge, generally in the

nongonococcal urethritis (NGU) Inflammation of the urethra caused by organisms other than the *Gonococcus* bacterium.

organs in which the bacteria settled during latency. Syphilis that has progressed to this stage has become increasingly rare. Victims of tertiary syphilis may die of a ruptured aorta or of other heart damage, or may have progressive brain or spinal cord damage, eventually leading to blindness, insanity, or paralysis. About one-third of those who are not treated during the first three stages of syphilis enter the tertiary stage later in life.

Diagnosis and Treatment   Health experts urge screening with a blood test for syphilis for everyone who seeks treatment for an STI, especially adolescents; for anyone using illegal drugs; and for the partners of those in these two groups. They also recommend that anyone diagnosed with syphilis be screened for other STIs and be counseled about voluntary testing for HIV.

Penicillin is the drug of choice for treating primary, secondary, and latent syphilis. The earlier the treatment begins, the more effective it is. Those allergic to penicillin may be treated with doxycycline, ceftriaxone, or erythromycin. An added danger of not getting treatment for syphilis is an increased risk of HIV transmission.

Chancroid

A **chancroid** is a soft, painful sore or localized infection caused by the bacterium *Haemophilus ducrevi* and is usually acquired through sexual contact. Half of the cases heal by themselves. In other cases, the infection may spread to the lymph glands near the chancroid, where large amounts of pus can accumulate and destroy much of the local tissue. The incidence of this STI, widely prevalent in Africa and tropical and semitropical regions, is rapidly increasing in the United States, with outbreaks in several states, including Louisiana, Texas, and New York. Chancroids, which may increase susceptibility to HIV infection, are believed to be a major factor in the heterosexual spread of HIV. This infection is treated with antibiotics (ceftriaxone, azithromycin, or erythromycin) and can be prevented by keeping the genitals clean and washing them with soap and water in case of possible exposure.

Pubic Lice and Scabies

These infections are sometimes, but not always, transmitted sexually. *Pubic lice* (or "crabs") are usually found in the pubic hair, although they can migrate to any hairy areas of the body. Lice lay eggs called nits that attach to the base of the hair shaft. Irritation from the lice may produce intense itching. Scratching to relieve the itching can produce sores. *Scabies* is caused by mites that burrow under the skin, where they lay eggs that hatch and undergo many changes in the course of their life cycle, producing great discomfort, including intense itching. Lice and scabies are treated with applications of permethrin cream and lindane shampoo to all the areas of the body where there are concentrations of body hair (genitals, armpits, scalp).

Trichomoniasis

An estimated 7.4 million new cases of this common curable STI appear each year in men and women. The cause is a single-celled protozoan parasite *Trichomonas vaginalis*, transmitted by vaginal intercourse or vulva-to-vulva contact with an infected partner. Women can acquire this disease from male or female partners; men usually contract it only from infected women.

Most men have no signs or symptoms; some experience irritation inside the penis, mild discharge, or slight burning on urination or ejaculation. Some women develop a frothy, yellow-green vaginal discharge with a strong odor and may experience discomfort during intercourse and urination as well as genital itching and irritation.

Diagnosis is based on a physical examination and a laboratory test. Treatment consists of a single dose of oral medication, either metronidazole or tinidazole. If untreated, an infected man, even if he has never had symptoms or if his symptoms have gone away, can continue to infect or reinfect partners.

Bacterial Vaginosis

Bacterial vaginosis (BV), the most common vaginal infection in women ages 15 to 44, is caused by an imbalance of normal bacteria in the vagina. Having a new sex partner or multiple sex partners and douching can increase a woman's risk for getting BV. Although not considered an STD, BV increases vulnerability to STIs.[88]

Women cannot get bacterial vaginosis from toilet seats, bedding, or swimming pools. The best ways to prevent BV are:

- Not having sex.
- Limiting the number of sexual partners.
- Not douching.

Many women with BV do not have symptoms. Others may notice a thin white or gray vaginal discharge and odor, pain, itching, or burning in the vagina. Some women detect a strong fishlike odor, especially after sex; burning when urinating; or itching around the outside of the vagina.

Laboratory tests of vaginal fluid can determine if BV is present. Antibiotics can treat BV, although the infection may recur. Male sex partners of women diagnosed with BV generally do not need to be treated. Antibiotic treatment for sexual partners of women with BV does not increase the

chancroid A soft, painful sore or localized infection usually acquired through sexual contact.

bacterial vaginosis (BV) A common vaginal infection caused by an imbalance of normal bacteria in the vagina.

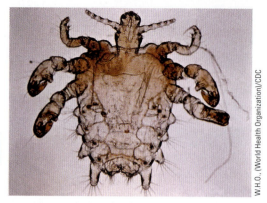

W.H.O. (World Health Organization)/CDC

Pubic lice or "crabs" usually are found in pubic hair but can migrate to other hairy parts of the body.

rate of clinical or symptomatic improvement or a lower recurrence rate.

Without treatment, BV increases the risk of various STIs, including chlamydia, gonorrhea, and HIV, and, in pregnant women, the risk of having a premature or low-birth-weight baby.

HIV and AIDS

Decades ago no one knew about **human immunodeficiency virus (HIV)** or had ever heard of **acquired immune deficiency syndrome (AIDS)**. Once seen as an epidemic affecting primarily gay men and injection drug users, AIDS has taken on very different forms. Thanks to medical advances, HIV has evolved into a chronic disease instead of a fatal one. But those who are infected must take medications for their entire lives and face higher risk of various health problems as they age.

The U.S. Department of Health and Human Services (HHS) has proposed a new initiative with the goals of reducing new HIV infections by 75 percent within 5 years and by 90 percent within 10 years. Its fundamental strategies are:

- Diagnose all individuals with HIV as early as possible after infection.
- Treat HIV infection rapidly and effectively to achieve sustained viral suppression.
- Prevent at-risk individuals from acquiring HIV infection, including the use of preexposure prophylaxis (PrEP)
- Rapidly detect and respond to emerging clusters of HIV infection to further reduce new transmissions.[89]

human immunodeficiency virus (HIV) A virus that causes a spectrum of health problems, ranging from a symptomless infection to changes in the immune system, to the development of life-threatening diseases because of impaired immunity.

acquired immune deficiency syndrome (AIDS) The final stages of HIV infection, characterized by a variety of severe illnesses and decreased levels of certain immune cells.

Incidence More than 700, 000 people in the United States have died as a result of HIV/AIDS since the disease was first recognized in 1981. An estimated 1.1 million people are currently living with HIV; about 15 percent are unaware of their HIV infection.[90] Globally, about 35 million have died, and an estimated 36.9 million to 43.9 million people are living with HIV.[91] Women comprise half of adults estimated to be living with HIV/AIDS worldwide. More than 1.1 million people in the United States are living with HIV; 1 in 7 do not realize they are infected.[92]

More than 38,000 people were diagnosed with HIV in the United States in 2017. The majority were young black/African American and Hispanic/Latino men who have sex with men (MSM). There is also a high incidence of HIV among transgender individuals, high-risk heterosexuals, and those who inject drugs. More than half of new HIV diagnoses have been reported in southern states and Washington, D.C.[93]

Who Is at Risk?

Approximately 1 in 4 new infections are transmitted by individuals who are unaware that they are HIV-positive. About 7 in 10 new infections are transmitted by individuals diagnosed with HIV infection but who are not receiving treatment.[94] At highest risk are the following:

- **Gay and bisexual men.** HIV infection rates have generally declined among gay and bisexual men, but new infections are on the rise among this group. An estimated 53 percent of new HIV infections occur in gay or bisexual men. Younger gay and bisexual men and those of color are at particularly high risk. One reason may be a misperception of risk. In a study of men engaging in behaviors such as unprotected anal sex, only 25 to 35 percent considered themselves at high risk of infection. Gay and bisexual Hispanic males—another population group at serious risk of HIV—have a one in four chance of contracting HIV, according to a CDC report. CDC researchers predict that one in six will be diagnosed with HIV in their lifetime. For gay or bisexual black males, the rate is one in two; for gay or bisexual Hispanic men, one in four; and for gay or bisexual white males, 1 in 11, according to the CDC.

- **Black Americans.** Two percent of black Americans are HIV positive, higher than any other group. The AIDS diagnosis rate for blacks is more than nine times that for whites. If current HIV rates continue, about half of gay and bisexual black men in the United States will be diagnosed with the AIDS-causing virus in their lifetime, a new government analysis says. In general, black people have the greatest lifetime HIV risk—1 in 20 for men and 1 in 48 for women, the analysis showed. The overall lifetime HIV infection rate in white men is 1 in 132, while for white women, it's 1 in 880, according to the CDC.

Blacks have had the highest age-adjusted death rate due to HIV disease throughout most of the epidemic. The reasons for this discrepancy are complex and include a higher rate of other STDs in black communities, disparities in health care, and poverty. While HIV diagnoses dropped significantly over the past decade in the United States, blacks with HIV are less likely than whites or Hispanics to receive routine, ongoing care, according to the CDC. Black women with HIV fared better than black men, the CDC noted. While 44 percent of black women benefited from routine care, just 35 percent of black men did the same. Most of the black HIV patients who received ongoing care were infected during heterosexual contact.[95]

- **Women.** In 1985, women represented 8 percent of AIDS diagnoses; now they account for 25 percent. According to CDC estimates, almost 280,000 women in the United States are living with HIV or AIDS. Black women make up about two-thirds of women diagnosed with AIDS, but the rate of new infections among black women has dropped. Latinas account for 18 percent of new infections in women.

Women are most likely to be infected through heterosexual sex, followed by injection drug use. Mother-to-child transmission of HIV has decreased dramatically because of the use of medicines that significantly reduce the risk of transmission from a woman to her baby.

At least one case of woman-to-woman infection has been documented. Although the risk is low, female sex partners can transmit HIV when bodily fluids such as menstrual blood and vaginal fluids come into contact with a cut, an abrasion, or a mucous membrane (the tissue lining the mouth and vagina).

- **Young adults.** Teens and young adults under age 30 continue to be at risk. Those between ages 13 and 20 account for 34 percent of new HIV infections, the largest share of any age group. Most are infected sexually.

- As a result of the opioid crisis, drug injection has become a more frequent cause of HIV transmission.[96]

- An estimated 50 percent of young Americans infected with the virus that causes AIDS don't know they have it. However, the HIV testing rate is lower among those ages 18 to 24 than for older people in the United States.[97] In the National College Health Assessment, 28.8 percent of students report ever being tested for HIV.[98]

✓**check-in** How would you rate your risk of HIV infection?

Reducing the Risk of HIV Transmission

HIV/AIDS can be so frightening that some people have exaggerated its dangers, whereas others understate them. The fact is that although no one is immune to HIV, you can reduce the risk if you abstain from sexual activity or remain in a monogamous relationship with an uninfected partner and if you do not inject drugs.[99]

If you're not in a long-term monogamous relationship with a partner you're sure is safe and you're not willing to abstain from sex, there are things you can do to lower your risk of HIV infection. Remember that the risk of HIV transmission depends on sexual behavior, not sexual orientation. Among young men, the prevalence and frequency of sexual risk behaviors are similar regardless of sexual orientation, ethnicity, or age. Homosexual, heterosexual, and bisexual individuals all need to know about the kinds of sexual activity that increase their risk.

Sexual Transmission

Here is what you should know about sexual transmission of HIV:

- Casual contact does *not* spread HIV infection. You cannot get HIV infection from drinking from a water fountain, contact with a toilet seat, or touching an infected person.

- Compared to other viruses, HIV is extremely difficult to get.

- HIV can live in blood, semen, vaginal fluids, and breast milk.

- Many chemicals, including household bleach, and hydrogen peroxide, can inactivate HIV.

- In studies of family members sharing dishes, food, clothing, and frequent hugs with people with HIV infection or AIDS, those who have contracted the virus have shared razor blades or toothbrushes or had other means of blood contact.

- You cannot tell visually whether a potential sexual partner has HIV. A blood test is needed to detect the antibodies that the body produces to fight HIV, thus indicating infection. As noted in Chapter 9, circumcision greatly reduces the risk for HIV infection.

- HIV can be spread in semen and vaginal fluids during a single instance of anal, vaginal, or oral sexual contact between heterosexuals, bisexuals, or homosexuals. The risk increases with the number of sexual encounters with an infected partner.

- Teenage girls may be particularly vulnerable to HIV infection because the immature cervix is easily infected.
- Anal intercourse is an extremely high-risk behavior because HIV can enter the bloodstream through tiny breaks in the lining of the rectum. HIV transmission is much more likely to occur during unprotected anal intercourse than vaginal intercourse.
- Other behaviors that increase the risk of HIV infection include having multiple sexual partners, engaging in sex without condoms or virus-killing spermicides, having sexual contact with persons known to be at high risk (e.g., prostitutes or injection drug users), and sharing injection equipment for drugs.
- Condom use significantly reduces the risk of HIV transmission (by as much as 78 percent).[100]
- Individuals are at greater risk if they have an active sexual infection. STIs—such as herpes, gonorrhea, and syphilis—facilitate transmission of HIV during vaginal or anal intercourse.
- No cases of HIV transmission by deep (French) kissing have been reported, but it could happen. Studies have found blood in the saliva of healthy people after kissing; other lab studies have found HIV in saliva. Social (dry) kissing is safe.
- Oral sex can lead to HIV transmission. The virus in any semen that enters the mouth could make its way into the bloodstream through tiny nicks or sores in the mouth. A man's risk in performing oral sex on a woman is smaller because an infected woman's genital fluids have much lower concentrations of HIV than does semen.
- HIV infection is not widespread among lesbians, although there have been documented cases of possible female-to-female HIV trans-mission. However, in each instance, one partner had had sex with a bisexual man or male injection drug user or had injected drugs herself.

Nonsexual Transmission

Efforts to prevent nonsexual forms of HIV transmission have been very effective. Screening the blood supply has reduced the rate of transfusion-associated HIV transmission by 99.9 percent. Treatment with antiretroviral drugs during pregnancy and birth has reduced transmission to newborns by about 90 percent in optimal conditions. Drug injection has become a more frequent cause of HIV transmission.[101]

Prevention and Protection

Behavioral methods, such as safer sex practices, remain the primary means of preventing transmission of HIV (see Health on a Budget). Individuals at very high risk for HIV can lower their risk of becoming infected using preexposure prophylaxis (PrEP), which consists of daily HIV medicines. PrEP, which can stop HIV from spreading throughout the body, reduces the risk of sexual transmission by more than 90 percent if taken consistently and by even more if combined with condoms.

Among people who inject drugs, PrEP reduces the risk of HIV infection by more than 70 percent. For those who have been exposed to HIV through sexual contact, sharing needles, or accidental exposure (as can happen for medical personnel), PEP (postexposure prophylaxis) consists of antiretroviral therapy (ART) to protect against infection. For use only in emergency situations, PEP must be started within 72 hours after a possible exposure to HIV.

Recognizing and Treating HIV/AIDS

HIV infection refers to a spectrum of health problems that results from immunologic abnormalities caused by the virus when it enters the bloodstream. In theory, the body may be able to resist infection by HIV. In reality, in almost all cases, HIV destroys the cell-mediated immune system, particularly the CD4+ T lymphocytes (also called *T4 helper cells*). The result is greatly increased susceptibility to various cancers and opportunistic infections (infections that take hold because of the reduced effectiveness of the immune system).

HIV triggers a state of all-out war within the immune system. Almost immediately following infection with HIV, the immune system responds aggressively by manufacturing enormous numbers of CD4+ cells. It eventually is overwhelmed, however, as the viral particles continue to replicate, or multiply. The intense war between HIV and the immune system indicates that the virus itself, not a breakdown in the immune system, is responsible for disease progression.

Without treatment, HIV infection typically progresses through three stages:

Stage 1: Acute HIV Infection
Flu-like symptoms develop within two to four weeks after infection and may last for a few weeks. During this stage, individuals often do not realize that they have been infected, yet they have high levels of virus in their blood and are extremely contagious.

Stage 2: HIV Inactivity or Latency
Individuals may not feel sick or develop any symptoms but the HIV continues to reproduce at low levels. With proper treatment, people can remain in this stage for a decade or even several decades. They

can still transmit HIV to others during this stage. However, those who receive ART and have a very low level of virus in their blood are much less likely to infect a partner.[102] As the amount of virus in the blood (the viral load) increases, individuals develop more symptoms and enter Stage 3.

Stage 3: Acquired Immunodeficiency Syndrome (AIDS)

Because their immune systems are so severely impaired, people with AIDS are susceptible to severe complications and opportunistic illnesses, with symptoms such as chills, fever, sweats, swollen lymph glands, weakness, and weight loss. Because they have such high levels of HIV in their blood, they are very infectious. Without treatment, people with AIDS may survive for about three years. Psychological problems, including depression, anxiety, and stress, occur "in epidemic proportions" in individuals with HIV, according to recent research, and can affect their behavior (such as taking steps to prevent transmitting the virus) and treatment outcome.

HIV Testing

All HIV tests measure antibodies, cells produced by the body to fight HIV infection. A negative test indicates no exposure to HIV. It can take 3 to 6 months for the body to produce the telltale antibodies, however, so a negative result may not be accurate, depending on the timing of the test. Faster tests that can detect HIV earlier are under development.[103]

HIV testing can be either confidential or anonymous. In confidential testing, a person's name is recorded along with the test results, which are made available to medical personnel and, in 32 states, the state health department. In anonymous testing, no name is associated with the test results. Anonymous testing is available in 39 states.

The only home HIV test approved by the FDA, Home Access, is available in drugstores or online for $40 to $50. An individual draws a blood sample by pricking a finger and sends it to a laboratory, along with a personal identification number. Results are given over the phone by a trained counselor, usually within several days.

Newly developed blood tests can determine how recently a person was infected with HIV and distinguish between long-standing infections and those contracted within the previous 4 to 6 months.

Diagnosing AIDS

A diagnosis of AIDS applies to anyone with HIV whose immune system is severely impaired, as indicated by a CD4+ count of fewer than 200 cells per cubic millimeter of blood, compared to normal CD4+ cell counts in healthy people not infected with HIV of 800 to 1,200 per cubic millimeter of blood. In addition, AIDS is diagnosed in persons with HIV infection who experience recurrent pneumonia, invasive cervical cancer, or pulmonary tuberculosis.

People with AIDS may also experience persistent fever, diarrhea that persists for more than a month, or involuntary weight loss of more than 10 percent of normal body weight. Neurological disease—including dementia (confusion and impaired thinking) and other problems with thinking, speaking, movement, or sensation—may occur. Secondary infectious diseases that may develop in people with AIDS include *Pneumocystis carinii* pneumonia, tuberculosis, or oral candidiasis (thrush). Secondary cancers associated with HIV infection include Kaposi's sarcoma and cancer of the cervix.

Treatment

New forms of therapy have been remarkably effective in boosting levels of protective T cells and reducing *viral load*—the amount of HIV in the bloodstream. Starting HIV treatment early, before a patient's immune system is badly weakened, can dramatically improve survival. People with high viral loads are more likely to progress rapidly to AIDS than people with low levels of the virus.

ART dramatically reduces viral load but does not eradicate the virus. This complex regimen uses 1 of 250 different combinations of three or more antiretroviral drugs, often available in a single tablet. Treatment begins much earlier than in the past, even before moderate immune suppression. This benefits the individual patient and helps prevent HIV transmission to a sexual partner.

Early ART has shown promise in treating newborns with HIV infection but also causes serious complications. HIV resistance to the antiretroviral drug tenofovir (Viread) is increasingly common, which is alarming because the drug plays a major role in treating and preventing infection with HIV, the virus that causes AIDS.

Resistance often occurs when patients don't take their drugs as directed. To prevent resistance, people need to take the drugs correctly about 85 to 90 percent of the time. Tenofovir-resistant HIV strains could be passed on to other people and become more widespread, potentially weakening global efforts to control HIV.[104] A significant number of people with HIV have strains of the AIDS-causing virus that are resistant to both older and newer drugs.

Among the 40 million people living with HIV, there is only one confirmed cure: a patient who also developed cancer and underwent intensive chemotherapy, total body radiation, and bone marrow transplantation. A key challenge is that once HIV invades an individual's genome, it is extremely difficult to remove all HIV-infected cells, which—even with treatment—persist in the body for decades.[105]

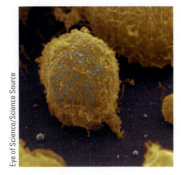
Eye of Science/Science Source

Electron micrograph of a white blood cell being attacked by HIV (light blue particles), the virus that causes AIDS.

- What are the basic hormonal and anatomical differences between men and women?

- What should college students know about hooking up?

- What are the sexual preferences and behaviors of American adults?

- What do you know about the incidence, signs, symptoms, and treatments for the most common STIs?

Reflection

In this chapter, you learned about the diversity of sexual identities, orientations, and behaviors. Has this perspective affected your perceptions of your own sexuality? You also learned about the sexually transmitted infections that can threaten your health. How would a diagnosis of an STI affect your attitudes and behaviors?

TAKING CHARGE OF YOUR HEALTH

Protecting Your Sexual Health

As with other aspects of your well-being, your sexual health depends on your choices and behaviors. Here are some basic guidelines:

_____ **Talk first.** Get to know your partner. Before having sex, establish a committed relationship that allows trust and open communication. You should be able to discuss past sexual histories and any previous STIs or IV drug use. You should not feel coerced or forced into having sex.

_____ **Stay sober.** Alcohol and drugs impair your judgment, make it harder to communicate clearly, and can lead to forgetting or failing to use condoms properly.

_____ **Practice safe sex.** Avoid risky sex practices that can tear or break the skin, such as anal intercourse. Use latex condoms. Limit sexual partners.

_____ **Be honest.** If you have an STI, like HPV or herpes, advise any prospective sexual partner. Allow him or her to decide what to do. If you mutually agree on engaging in sexual activity, use latex condoms and other protective measures.

_____ **Don't feel you have to have sex** for fear of hurting someone's feelings or fear of being the "only one" who isn't doing it.

If you don't want to have sex, be honest, discuss the reasons behind your decision with your partner, and stay true to you.

_____ **Respect everyone's right to make his or her own personal decision—including yours.** There is no perfect point in a relationship where sex has to happen. If your partner tells you that he or she is not ready to have sex, respect this decision, discuss the reasons behind it, and be supportive.

_____ **Be prepared for a sex emergency.** Consider carrying two condoms with you just in case one breaks or tears. Men and women are equally responsible for preventing STIs, and both should carry condoms.

_____ **Abstinence doesn't mean less affection.** Practicing abstinence—the most effective way to protect against STIs—doesn't mean you can't have an intimate relationship with someone. It just means you don't have vaginal or anal intercourse or oral sex.

_____ **Make your sexual health a priority.** Whether you are having sex or not, both men and women need regular checkups to make sure they are sexually healthy. Get immunized against HPV.

SELF-SURVEY

Assessing Your STI Risk

This self-survey looks at your risk of acquiring or transmitting any sexually transmitted infection.

STI Quiz

1. **True** or **False**: A person can have an STI and not know it.

2. **True** or **False**: It is normal for women to have some vaginal discharge.

3. **True** or **False**: Once you have had an STI and have been cured, you can't get it again.

4. **True** or **False**: HIV is mainly present in semen, blood, vaginal secretions, and breast milk.

5. **True** or **False**: Chlamydia and gonorrhea can cause pelvic inflammatory disease.

6. **True** or **False**: A pregnant woman who has an STI can pass the disease on to her baby.

7. **True** or **False**: Most STIs go away without treatment, if people wait long enough.

8. **True** or **False**: STIs that aren't cured early can cause sterility.

9. **True** or **False**: Birth control pills offer excellent protection from STIs.

10. **True** or **False**: Condoms can help prevent the spread of STIs.

11. **True** or **False**: If you know your partner, you can't get an STI.

12. **True** or **False**: Chlamydia is the most common bacterial STI.

13. **True** or **False**: A sexually active woman should get an annual Pap test from her doctor.

Scoring

1. **True** Some of the most common symptoms of an STI infection include abnormal discharge, painful urination, burning, and itching or tingling in the genital area, but it is important to remember that many women and men who have an STI often do not experience any symptoms at all. Chlamydia, for example, often has no symptoms.

2. **True** Normal vaginal discharge has several purposes: cleaning and moistening the vagina and helping to prevent and fight infections. Although it's normal for the color, texture, and amount of vaginal fluids to vary throughout a woman's menstrual cycle, some changes in discharge may indicate a problem.

   If you think you may have a problem, you should see a doctor as soon as possible. First, though, it helps to learn some of the differences between what is normal and abnormal vaginal discharge for you.

3. **False** Having an STI and being cured from it does not mean that your body now has a built-in immunity to the bacteria that causes the infection. You must protect yourself from becoming infected again by using a condom. Remember, it is your body!

4. **True** Although small traces of HIV can be found in tears, saliva, urine, and perspiration, extensive studies have shown that there is not enough of the virus or the virus is not strong enough to be transmitted. Only blood, semen, vaginal secretions, and breast milk have been proven to transmit HIV and hepatitis B. HIV cannot be passed on by casual contact.

5. **True** Many different organisms can cause PID, but most cases are associated with gonorrhea and genital chlamydial infections, two very common STIs. Scientists have found that bacteria normally present in small numbers in the vagina and cervix also may play a role.

6. **True** STIs can be passed from a pregnant woman to the baby before, during, or after the baby's birth. Some STIs (e.g., syphilis) cross the placenta and infect the baby while it is in the uterus (womb). Other STIs (e.g., gonorrhea, chlamydia, hepatitis B, and genital herpes) can be transmitted from the mother to the baby during delivery as the baby passes through the birth canal. HIV can cross the placenta during pregnancy, infect the baby during the birth process, and unlike most other STIs, can infect the baby through breastfeeding.

7. **False** Even if symptoms appear to go away, the infected person will still have the infection and is able to pass the infection on to others until he or she gets treatment. STIs that aren't cured early can cause sterility.

8. **True** If the fallopian tubes are blocked at one or both ends, the egg can't travel through the tubes into the uterus. Blocked tubes may result from pelvic inflammatory disease, which is often caused by untreated STIs.

9. **False** The birth control pill does not protect against sexually transmitted infections. For those having sex, condoms must always be used along with birth control pills to protect against STIs. Abstinence (the decision to not have sex) is the only method that always prevents pregnancy and sexually transmitted infections.

10. **True** Most condoms are made of latex. Those made of lambskin may offer less protection against some sexually transmitted infections, including HIV, so use of latex condoms is recommended. For people who may have an allergic skin reaction to latex, both male and female condoms made of polyurethane are available.

    When properly used, latex and plastic condoms are effective against most STIs. Condoms do not protect against infections spread from sores on the skin not covered by a condom (such as the base of the penis or scrotum).

11. **False** As stated in question 1, a person can have an STI and not know it. If they can't tell, how can you?

12. **True** The U.S. Centers for Disease Control and Prevention estimates that more than 4 million new cases of chlamydia occur each year. The highest rates of chlamydial infection are in 15- to 19-year-old adolescents regardless of demographics or location.

13. **True** The Pap test is a way to find cell changes on the cervix. Abnormal cells may lead to cancer, so having a Pap test can find and treat them early, before they have time to progress to cancer.

    Although Pap tests do not test for STIs, some STIs, such as HPV (human papillomavirus infection), can cause abnormal Pap test results. Certain types of HPV are linked to cancer in both women and men.

Source: Material from The Bacchus Network™ Website, smartersex.org.

REVIEW QUESTIONS

(LO 8.1)   1. At its deepest and most fulfilling level, when sexuality uplifts the soul of an individual by allowing her or him to connect to something greater than oneself, the _____ aspect of sexuality is the focus.
     a. spiritual   c. emotional
     b. intellectual   d. environmental

(LO 8.1)   2. Awareness of the impact of one's decisions on others is part of the _____ dimension of sexuality.
     a. social   c. emotional
     b. intellectual   d. environmental

(LO 8.1)   3. The uterine walls of human females are lined by a layer of tissue called the _____.
     a. endometrium   c. cervix
     b. perineum   d. labia

(LO 8.1)   4. The condition in which women may stop menstruating for a variety of reasons, including a hormonal disorder, drastic weight loss, strenuous exercise, or change in the environment, is known as _____.
     a. premenstrual syndrome   c. dysmenorrhea
     b. amenorrhea   d. toxic shock syndrome

(LO 8.1)   5. The collection of coiled tubes adjacent to each testis where immature sperm are stored is known as the _____.
     a. ejaculatory ducts   c. prostate glands
     b. scrotum   d. epididymis

(LO 8.1)   6. Which of the following statements is true of circumcision?
     a. It increases the risk of HIV infection.
     b. It increases the risk of cancer of the penis.
     c. It may decrease the risk of prostate cancer.
     d. It leads to foreskin infections and retraction.

(LO 8.2)   7. Which of the following is a characteristic of sexually healthy relationships, according to the Sexuality Information and Education Council of the United States?
     a. It is open ended.
     b. It is procreational.
     c. It is pleasurable to at least one of the sexual partners.
     d. It is protected against unintended pregnancy.

(LO 8.2)   8. Which of the following statements is true of communication about sex?
     a. It is important to prioritize the partner's feelings over one's own feelings and values.
     b. Men impute more sexual meaning to gestures than women.
     c. When declining sex, suggestive gestures are preferred over direct communication.
     d. Saying no to sex means the same for men and women.

(LO 8.3)   9. Which of the following is true of the sexual behavior of young adults in college?
     a. Studies have reported that very few college students hook up.
     b. Young adults who graduated from college report more lifetime sexual partners than those without a high school degree.
     c. Men are likely to judge attractive women as more risky sexual partners.
     d. About a third of students who've reported hooking up have described the experience as "traumatic" or "very difficult to handle."

(LO 8.3)   10. Which of the following is one of the strongest predictors of hooking up?
     a. Feeling sad or lonely
     b. Knowing a wide variety of people
     c. More frequent viewing of pornography
     d. Being unattractive

(LO 8.4)   11. Which of the following statements is true about sexual behaviors among young adults?
     a. An individual's sexual identity remains constant throughout his or her life.
     b. The average American teenager reports having sex at least once a week.
     c. College students, in general, prefer hookups over romantic relationships.
     d. The context of sexual activity affects sexual enjoyment in both sexes.

(LO 8.4)   12. Which of the following is true of bisexuality?
     a. Bisexuality usually begins to manifest itself early in life.
     b. Bisexual behavior is the lowest among married men.
     c. Individuals may identify themselves as bisexual even if they don't behave bisexually.
     d. Bisexuality raises no special concerns about HIV infection.

(LO 8.4)   13. _____ is associated with greater homophobia.
     a. White ethnicity
     b. Masculine gender identity
     c. Having spiritual meaning in life
     d. Having had homosexual experiences

(LO 8.5)   14. _____ means that a person doesn't masturbate or engage in sexual activity with a partner.
     a. Celibacy   c. Fantasy
     b. Abstinence   d. Outercourse

(LO 8.5)   15. One of the potentially negative impacts of pornography is _____.
     a. greater acceptance of rape
     b. confusion about sexual identity

c. excessive spending of money
d. decreased number of sexual partners

(LO 8.6) 16. The process of discharge of semen by a male is known as _____.
a. masturbation   c. ejaculation
b. menstruation   d. circumcision

(LO 8.6) 17. The second stage of sexual response is _____.
a. orgasm   c. excitement
b. plateau   d. stimulation

(LO 8.6) 18. After orgasm, men typically enter a(n) _____, during which they are incapable of another orgasm.
a. abstinence period   c. excitement stage
b. refractory period   d. plateau stage

(LO 8.7) 19. 19. Besides sexual contact, sexually transmitted infections (STIs) can also be transmitted by _____.
a. cohabitation
b. sharing clothes
c. a mother to a fetus
d. drinking from the same container

(LO 8.7) 20. Which of the following statements about the risk factors of sexually transmitted infections is true?
a. A person is safe as long as the partner shows no symptoms of a sexually transmitted infection.
b. Multiple partners reduce the risk of a sexually transmitted infection.
c. Failure to use condoms increases the risk of an infection.
d. Substance abuse has a negligible contribution toward the risk associated with an infection.

(LO 8.7) 21. Which of the following statements about STIs is true?
a. Symptoms of STIs tend to be more pronounced in women than in men.
b. Women's risk of getting an infection is greater than that of men.
c. Spermicides containing nonoxynol-9 protect from gonorrhea, chlamydia, and HIV.
d. Pregnancy and fertility are unaffected by sexually transmitted infections.

(LO 8.8) 22. _____ are the only contraceptives that help prevent both pregnancy and STIs when used properly and consistently.
a. Condoms
b. Birth control pills
c. Intrauterine devices
d. Surgical sterilization methods

(LO 8.8) 23. College students are at high risk for contracting STIs primarily because _____.
a. protective measures are unavailable
b. they typically know their partners well
c. their immune systems are not yet at full strength
d. they have opportunities to engage in sex with different partners

(LO 8.7) 24. Young people 15–24 years of age _____.
a. acquire one-fifth of all new sexually transmitted infections
b. make up 40 percent of new cases of genital herpes.
c. are less likely to contract sexually transmitted infections
d. have a lower risk of chlamydia than other age groups

(LO 8.8) 25. Gardasil and Cervarix are vaccines available to prevent _____ in girls and young women.
a. cervical cancer
b. nongonococcal urethritis
c. genital herpes
d. pubic lice

(LO 8.7) 26. Which of the following is true of the incidence of HIV and AIDS?
a. HIV infections are negligible in gay and bisexual men.
b. The rate of HIV infections among black Americans is less than that of whites.
c. Women are most likely to be affected through heterosexual sex.
d. Young adults are least likely to contract an HIV infection.

Answers to these questions can be found on page 531.

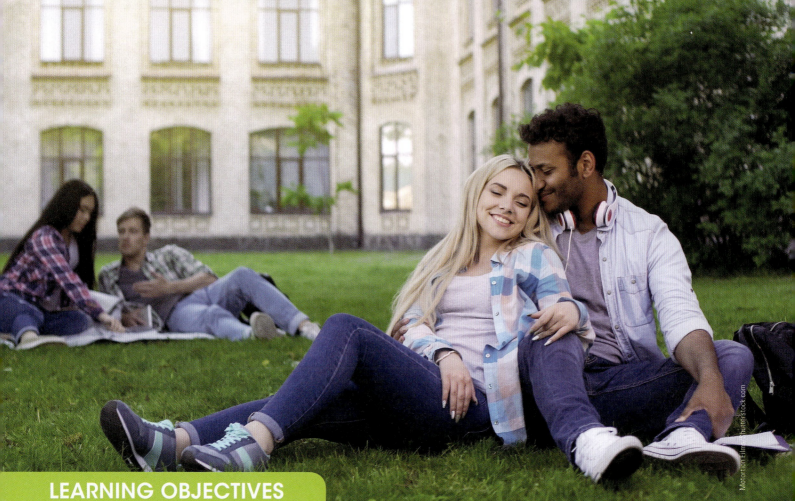

Motortion Films/Shutterstock.com

LEARNING OBJECTIVES

After reading this chapter, you should be able to:

9.1 Describe the process of conception, from spermatogenesis to implantation.

9.2 Review the reasons for practicing abstinence and nonpenetrative sexual activity.

9.3 Summarize the methods, benefits, risks, and use of contraception on campuses.

9.4 Explain the advantages and disadvantages of the major types of barrier contraceptives.

9.5 Review the types of hormonal contraceptives, their advantages, and their disadvantages.

9.6 Describe the fertility awareness methods, as well as their advantages and disadvantages.

9.7 Discuss the incidence and use of emergency contraception.

9.8 Explain male and female sterilization.

9.9 Outline several reasons some individuals and couples choose not to have children.

9.10 Discuss the options available when women are faced with an unwanted pregnancy.

9.11 Compare medical and surgical abortion.

9.12 Summarize preconception care, home pregnancy tests, prenatal care, and complications of pregnancy.

9.13 Identify the stages of childbirth.

9.14 Discuss the causes of infertility and the options available to infertile couples.

WHAT DO YOU THINK?

• What do college students need to know about contraception?

• How do you decide on the best birth control method for you and your partner?

• How can you prevent pregnancy after unprotected intercourse or failed birth control?

• What changes do a mother-to-be and her unborn child undergo during pregnancy?

9

Reproductive Options

Justin and Katie, second-year students at the same community college, can't remember a time when abortion was illegal, when AIDS wasn't a deadly threat, and when safe sex wasn't a concern of every sexually active individual. Yet even though they were aware of the risks and the realities involved, neither used contraception during every single sexual encounter. Then one of Justin's partners had a pregnancy scare. He decided never again to engage in unprotected sex. Katie had a different reality check: At her regular physical, she learned that she had contracted chlamydia, the most common sexually transmitted infection (STI) in the United States.

"When we started dating," Katie recalls, "both of us felt that something was special about our relationship." Despite their mutual attraction, they decided to take every step toward intimacy slowly. Both considered and talked about their personal priorities and concerns. Even though it was awkward, they also discussed their own sexual histories and underwent tests for STIs.

Looking toward a continuing committed relationship, they decided on a long-acting reversible contraceptive (LARC). In the future, they realized that they might switch to other forms of birth control or consider different options, including both marriage and parenthood.

As human beings, we have a unique power: the ability to choose to conceive or not to conceive. No other species on Earth can separate sexual activity and pleasure from reproduction. However, simply not wanting to get pregnant is never enough to prevent conception, nor is wanting to have a child always enough to get pregnant. Both desires require individual decisions and actions.

This chapter provides information on conception, birth control, abortion, infertility, adoption, and the processes by which a new human life develops and enters the world. <

Reproductive Responsibility

Anyone who engages in vaginal intercourse must be willing to accept the consequences of this activity, including the possibility of conceiving a child, or take action to avoid an unintended pregnancy. Across the world, including the United States, an estimated 40 to 45 percent of pregnancies are unintended.[1] If a woman did not want to become pregnant at the time a pregnancy occurred but wants to do so in the future, an unintended pregnancy is considered "mistimed" (this occurs in 27 percent of pregnancies). If the woman did not want to become pregnant then or at any time in the future, an unintended pregnancy is considered "unwanted." This occurs in 18 percent of pregnancies.[2] Almost half of all unintended pregnancies occur among women who reported no or inconsistent use of of birth control. About 4 in 10 unintended pregnancies end in abortion.[3]

Reproductive responsibility involves more than protection against pregnancy. Even on a woman's most fertile day of the month, her risk of becoming pregnant is less than half her risk of acquiring an STI (see Chapter 11). The risk of an STI occurs only with an infected partner; the risk of pregnancy occurs with virtually all partners who have not undergone sterilization.

Since it takes two people to conceive a child, two people should be involved in deciding *not* to conceive a baby. In the process, they can also enhance their skills in communication, critical thinking, and negotiating.

✓check-in How do you take responsibility for your reproductive ability?

Conception

The equation for making a baby is quite simple: One sperm plus one egg equals one fertilized egg, which can develop into an fetus. But the processes that affect or permit **conception** are quite complicated.

- The creation of sperm, or **spermatogenesis**, starts in the male at puberty, and the production of sperm is regulated by hormones.

- Sperm cells form in the seminiferous tubules of the testes and are passed into the epididymis, where they are stored until ejaculation.

- A single male ejaculation may contain 500 million sperm. Each sperm released into the vagina during intercourse moves on its own, propelling itself toward its target, an ovum.

- To reach its goal, the sperm must move through the acidic secretions of the vagina, enter the uterus, travel up the fallopian tube containing the ovum, then fuse with the nucleus of the egg (**fertilization**). Almost every sperm produced by a man in his lifetime fails to accomplish its mission.

- There are far fewer human egg cells than there are sperm cells. Each woman is born with her lifetime supply of ova, and between 300 and 500 eggs eventually mature and leave her ovaries during ovulation.

- As discussed in Chapter 9, every month, one of the woman's ovaries releases an ovum to the nearby fallopian tube. It travels through the fallopian tube until it reaches the uterus, a journey that takes 3 to 4 days.

- An unfertilized egg lives for about 24 to 36 hours, disintegrates, and during menstruation is expelled along with the uterine lining.

- Even if a sperm, which can survive in the female reproductive tract for 2 to 5 days, meets a ripe egg in a fallopian tube, its

conception The merging of a sperm and an ovum.

spermatogenesis The process by which sperm cells are produced.

fertilization The fusion of sperm and egg nucleus.

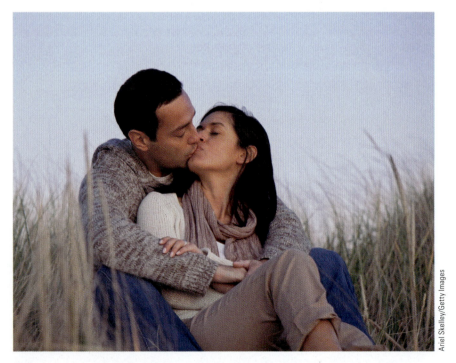

Some couples refrain from intercourse by engaging in outercourse, or intimacy that includes kissing and hugging.

Ariel Skelley/Getty Images

success is not ensured. A mature ovum releases the chemical allurin, which attracts the sperm. A sperm is able to penetrate the ovum's outer membrane because of a protein called fertilin. The egg then pulls the sperm inside toward its nucleus (Figure 9.1).

- The fertilized egg, called the **zygote**, travels down the fallopian tube, dividing to form a tiny clump of cells called a **blastocyst**. When it reaches the uterus, about a week after fertilization, it burrows into the endometrium, the lining of the uterus. This process is called **implantation**.

What are the chances that a single act of intercourse will result in pregnancy? It depends on a woman's menstrual cycle. If intercourse occurs within her fertile window (menstrual days 12–22), the odds of pregnancy can be as high as 25 percent.[4]

Abstinence and Nonpenetrative Sexual Activity

The contraceptive methods discussed in this chapter are designed to prevent pregnancy resulting from vaginal intercourse. Couples who choose abstinence make a very different decision—to abstain from vaginal intercourse and forms of nonpenetrative sexual activity that could result in conception (any in which ejaculation occurs near the vaginal opening). People choose abstinence for various reasons, including:

- Waiting until they are ready for a sexual relationship.
- Waiting until they find the "right" partner.
- Respecting religious or moral values.
- Enjoying friendships without sexual involvement.
- Recovering from a breakup.
- Preventing pregnancy and STI.

✓**check-in** What do you think are good reasons for choosing abstinence?

Practicing abstinence is the only form of birth control that is 100 percent effective and risk- and cost-free. It can also be a valid and valued lifestyle choice. A growing number of individuals,

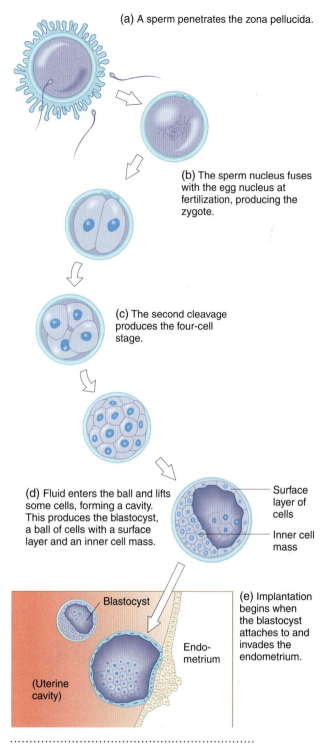

(a) A sperm penetrates the zona pellucida.

(b) The sperm nucleus fuses with the egg nucleus at fertilization, producing the zygote.

(c) The second cleavage produces the four-cell stage.

(d) Fluid enters the ball and lifts some cells, forming a cavity. This produces the blastocyst, a ball of cells with a surface layer and an inner cell mass.

Surface layer of cells

Inner cell mass

Blastocyst

(Uterine cavity)

Endo-metrium

(e) Implantation begins when the blastocyst attaches to and invades the endometrium.

FIGURE 9.1 Fertilization

(a) The efforts of hundreds of sperm may allow one to penetrate the ovum's corona radiate, an outer layer of cells, and then the zona pellucida, a thick inner membrane. (b) The nuclei of the sperm and the egg cells merge, and the male and female chromosomes in the nuclei come together, forming a zygote. (c) The zygote divides into two cells, then four cells, and so on. (d) As fluid enters the ball, cells form a ball of cells called a blastocyst. (e) The blastocyst implants itself in the endometrium.

zygote A fertilized egg.

blastocyst In embryonic development, a ball of cells with a surface layer and an inner cell mass.

implantation The embedding of the fertilized ovum in the uterine lining.

including some who have been sexually active in the past, are choosing abstinence until they establish a relationship with a long-term partner.

Abstinence offers special health benefits for women. Those who abstain until their 20s and engage in sex with fewer partners during their lifetime are less likely to get STIs, suffer infertility, or develop cervical cancer. However, there is a risk that people will abruptly end their abstinence without being prepared to protect themselves against pregnancy or infection.

Individuals who choose abstinence from vaginal intercourse often engage in activities sometimes called *outercourse*, such as kissing, hugging, sensual touching, and mutual masturbation. Pregnancy is possible if the man ejaculates near the vaginal opening because sperm can swim up the vagina and fallopian tubes to fertilize an egg. Outercourse may lower the risk of contracting STIs but does not eliminate the danger of transmission via a parasite or skin-to-skin contact.

Contraception

The average woman in the United States spends about 5 years pregnant, postpartum (the time immediately after giving birth), or trying to become pregnant, and three decades—more than three-quarters of her reproductive life—trying to avoid an unintended pregnancy. **Contraception**, also referred to as birth control or family planning, includes methods that prevent ovulation or implantation or block the sperm from reaching the egg. Some forms of contraception are temporary; others permanently alter one's fertility.[5]

Contraception has an enormous impact on women's lives. According to the World Health Organization (WHO), 87 million women experience an unintended pregnancy every year. Many, particularly in low-income developing countries, face the risks of lower educational and job opportunities, disability, disease, and even death.[6] The use of modern methods of contraception—condoms, intrauterine devices, oral and injectable contraceptives, implants, and sterilization—could prevent as many as four in five unwanted pregnancies every year[7]. However, despite the advances that have been made, the rate of unintended pregnancies remains high, and many myths persist among young adults.[8]

Some couples, for instance, use withdrawal, or **coitus interruptus** (removal of the penis from the vagina before ejaculation), to prevent pregnancy, even though this is not a reliable form of birth control. About half the men who have tried coitus interruptus find it unsatisfactory, either because they cannot anticipate when they're going to ejaculate or because they cannot withdraw quickly enough. Also, the Cowper's glands, two pea-size structures located on each side of the urethra, often produce a fluid that appears as drops at the tip of the penis any time from arousal and erection to orgasm. This fluid can contain active sperm and, in infected men, human immunodeficiency virus (HIV).

Good decisions about birth control are based on sound information. Consult a physician or family-planning counselor if you have questions or want to know how certain methods might affect medical conditions such as high blood pressure or diabetes.

✓**check-in** How well informed are you about contraceptive options?

Table 9.1 presents your contraceptive choices. When you evaluate any contraceptive, always consider its effectiveness (the likelihood that it will indeed prevent pregnancy). The failure rate refers to the number of pregnancies that occur per year for every 100 women using a particular method of birth control (Figure 9.2).

Women or their partners may not use contraception consistently or correctly and thereby become pregnant without intending to do so. This is why researchers distinguish between "perfect" and "typical" use. The average probability of unintended pregnancy in 1 year of typical use is about 12 percent. Women under age 25 have higher rates of contraceptive failures during the first year of use than older women.

Hormonal methods (the pill, patch, ring, and injectable and implantable contraceptives) and the intrauterine device (IUD) are more effective than other alternatives in preventing pregnancy. A woman has a 1 in 15 chance of becoming pregnant within a year of typical use of a hormonal implant, for instance, compared with a 1 in 4 likelihood if she uses fertility awareness.

Over the course of their reproductive years, women switch to different contraceptive methods for a variety of reasons, including changes in their life circumstances. In a common pattern, young women initially use condoms, begin a hormonal contraceptive in addition to condoms, and eventually discontinue condoms, often because of their partners' negative attitude toward their use. (See Health Now in this chapter for some criteria for choosing a form of contraceptive that works best for you.)

There have been attempts to develop male contraceptives, and in international surveys 44 to 83 percent of men express willingness to use

contraception The prevention of conception; birth control.

coitus interruptus The removal of the penis from the vagina before ejaculation.

TABLE 9.1 Birth Control Guide

Methods	MD Visit Needed	How to Use It	Some Risks	Noncontraceptive Benefits
Sterilization surgery for women	yes	One-time procedure; nothing to do or remember	• Pain • Bleeding • Infection or other complications after surgery • Ectopic (tubal) pregnancy	Reduces risk of ovarian cancer
Surgical sterilization implant for women	yes	One-time procedure; nothing to do or remember	• Mild to moderate pain after insertion • Ectopic (tubal) pregnancy	Reduces risk of ovarian cancer
Sterilization surgery for men	yes	One-time procedure; nothing to do or remember	• Pain • Bleeding • Infection	Possible reduction in risk for prostate cancer
Implantable rod	yes	One-time procedure; nothing to do or remember	• Acne • Hair loss • Weight gain • Headache • Cysts of the ovaries • Upset stomach • Mood changes • Dizziness • Depression • Sore breasts	Can use while breastfeeding; reduced menstrual flow and cramping
IUD	yes	One-time procedure; nothing to do or remember	• Cramps • Lower interest in sexual activity • Bleeding • Pelvic inflammatory disease • Changes in your periods • Infertility • Tear or hole in the uterus	Decreased menstrual flow and cramping; can use while breastfeeding; reduced risk of endometrial cancer
Shot/injection	yes	Need a shot every 3 months	• Bone loss • Bleeding between periods • Weight gain • Breast tenderness • Headaches	
Oral contraceptives (combined pill): "the pill"	yes (some states are making oral contraceptives available at pharmacies without a doctor's prescription)	Must swallow a pill every day	• Dizziness • High blood pressure • Nausea • Blood clots • Changes in your cycle (period) • Heart attack • Changes in your mood • Strokes • Weight gain	Decreases menstrual flow, cramping, PMS, acne, risk of ovarian and endometrial cancers, and the development of ovarian cysts
Oral contraceptives (progestin-only): "the pill"	yes	Must swallow a pill every day	• Irregular bleeding • Weight gain • Breast tenderness	May have similar noncontraceptive benefits as combined pills; reduction of uterine and ovarian cancer risk

(continues)

TABLE 9.1 (continued)

Methods	MD Visit Needed	How to Use It	Some Risks	Noncontraceptive Benefits
Oral contraceptives (extended/continued use): "the pill"	yes	Must swallow a pill every day	• Risks are similar to other oral contraceptives • Bleeding • Spotting between periods	Four periods per year and fewer menstrual-related problems; may reduce uterine fibroids and endometriosis symptoms
Patch	yes	Must wear a patch every day	• Exposure to higher-than-average levels of estrogen than most oral contraceptives	Decreases menstrual flow and cramping, PMS, acne, risk of ovarian and endometrial cancers, and the development of ovarian cysts
Vaginal contraceptive ring	yes	Must leave the ring in every day for 3 weeks	• Vaginal discharge • Swelling of the vagina • Irritation • Similar to oral contraceptives	Decreases menstrual flow and cramping, PMS, acne, risk of ovarian and endometrial cancers, and the development of ovarian cysts
Male condom	no	Must use every time you have sex; requires partner's cooperation	• Allergic reactions	Protects against STIs; delays premature ejaculation Except for abstinence, latex condoms are the best protection against HIV/AIDS and other STIs
Diaphragm with spermicide	yes	Must use every time you have sex	• Irritation • Urinary tract infection • Allergic reactions • Toxic shock	
Sponge with spermicide	no	Must use every time you have sex	• Irritation • Allergic reactions • Hard time removing • Toxic shock	Possible STI protection
Cervical cap with spermicide	yes	Must use every time you have sex	• Irritation • Allergic reactions • Abnormal Pap test • Toxic shock	
Female condom	no	Must use every time you have sex	• Irritation • Allergic reactions	Possible STI protection
Spermicide	no	Must use every time you have sex	• Irritation • Allergic reactions • Urinary tract infection	
Emergency Contraception (If your primary method of birth control fails)				
Emergency contraceptives "the morning-after pill"	no	Must be used within 72 hours of unprotected sex should not be used as a regular form of birth control	• Nausea • Vomiting • Abdominal pain • Fatigue • Headache	

Effectiveness of Family Planning Methods

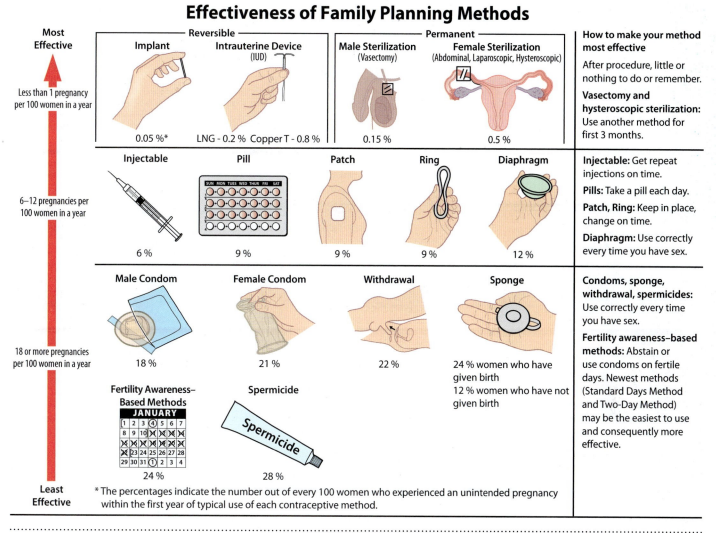

Most Effective

Less than 1 pregnancy per 100 women in a year

Reversible

Implant
0.05 %*

Intrauterine Device (IUD)
LNG - 0.2 % Copper T - 0.8 %

Permanent

Male Sterilization (Vasectomy)
0.15 %

Female Sterilization (Abdominal, Laparoscopic, Hysteroscopic)
0.5 %

How to make your method most effective

After procedure, little or nothing to do or remember.

Vasectomy and hysteroscopic sterilization: Use another method for first 3 months.

6–12 pregnancies per 100 women in a year

Injectable
6 %

Pill
9 %

Patch
9 %

Ring
9 %

Diaphragm
12 %

Injectable: Get repeat injections on time.

Pills: Take a pill each day.

Patch, Ring: Keep in place, change on time.

Diaphragm: Use correctly every time you have sex.

18 or more pregnancies per 100 women in a year

Male Condom
18 %

Female Condom
21 %

Withdrawal
22 %

Sponge
24 % women who have given birth
12 % women who have not given birth

Condoms, sponge, withdrawal, spermicides: Use correctly every time you have sex.

Fertility awareness–based methods: Abstain or use condoms on fertile days. Newest methods (Standard Days Method and Two-Day Method) may be the easiest to use and consequently more effective.

Fertility Awareness–Based Methods
JANUARY
24 %

Spermicide
28 %

Least Effective

* The percentages indicate the number out of every 100 women who experienced an unintended pregnancy within the first year of typical use of each contraceptive method.

FIGURE 9.2 Comparing Effectiveness of Birth Control Methods

LNG = levonorgestrel.
Source: Centers for Disease Control and Prevention.

them. Promising methods under development include a birth control "shot," or injection, that would suppress sperm production.[9]

✓**check-in** What forms of contraception have you used or would you consider using?

The Benefits and Risks of Contraceptives

Using birth control is safer and healthier than not using it (Table 9.2). According to the Population Reference Bureau, the use of contraceptives, including oral contraceptives, saves millions of lives each year. The Affordable Care Act (ACA) requires health insurance coverage for specific contraceptive methods specified by the Food and Drug Administration (FDA), including counseling, prescribed drugs and devices, and methods

available with a prescription from a health-care professional. Churches, religiously affiliated elementary and secondary schools, and, potentially, some religious charities and universities—but not hospitals—are allowed to refuse to provide coverage for birth control. States vary in their required coverage for contraception, including which types of institutions are exempt. Some require coverage of sterilization (for women more often than for men); some prohibit restrictions or delays by insurers. You can check the details of your state's provisions online.[10]

If you have one of the following conditions, you should talk with your doctor about which types of contraceptive may increase your health risks[11]:

- **High blood pressure (180/110 mmHg or higher).** Avoid birth control pills or injections containing estrogen, which may increase your risk of a heart attack or stroke.[12]

HEALTH NOW!

Choosing a Contraceptive

You may choose different types of birth control at different stages of your life, or you may switch contraceptives for various reasons. (See Self-Survey: Which Contraceptive Method Is Best for You?) You and your partner should always consider and discuss these factors:

- **Effectiveness:** Keep in mind that your own conscientiousness will play an important role. (See Figure 9.2.)

- **Suitability:** If you don't have sex very often, a contraceptive with many risks and side effects, such as the pill, may be a bad match for you.

- **Side effects:** Some complications related to contraceptives are serious health threats. Be sure to ask questions and gather information.

- **Safety:** The risks of certain contraceptives, such as the pill, may be too great to allow their use if, for example, you have high blood pressure.

- **Future fertility:** Some women don't return to regular menstrual cycles for 6 months to a year after discontinuing oral contraceptives.

- **Reduced risk of sexually transmitted infections:** Some forms of contraception, in particular barrier contraceptives and spermicides, help reduce the risk of transmission of some STIs. However, none provides complete protection.

What is your top priority for any form of birth control? Why? What is your top concern or source of hesitation? Record your reflections in your online journal.

TABLE 9.2 Noncontraceptive Benefits of Birth Control

Method	Benefits
Male sterilization	Possible reduction in prostate risk
Female sterilization	Reduces risk for ovarian cancer
Implanon	Reduced menstrual flow and cramping; can be used while breastfeeding
Mirena IUD	Decreases menstrual flow and cramping; reduced risk for endometrial cancer
ParaGard IUD	Reduced risk for endometrial cancer
Depo-Provera	Reduced menstrual flow and cramping; decreased risk for pelvic inflammatory disease (PID) and ovarian and endometrial cancers; can be used while breastfeeding
NuvaRing	Decreases menstrual flow and cramping, premenstrual syndrome (PMS), acne, ovarian and endometrial cancers, the development of ovarian cysts, uterine and breast fibroids, and PID
Ortho Evra Patch	Decreases menstrual flow and cramping, PMS, acne, ovarian and endometrial cancers, the development of ovarian cysts, uterine and breast fibroids, and PID
Combination birth control pill	Decreases menstrual flow and cramping, PMS, acne, ovarian and endometrial cancers, the development of ovarian cysts, uterine and breast fibroids, and PID
Progestin-only birth control pill	May have similar contraceptive benefits as combination pills
Extended-use birth control pill	Four periods or less per year and fewer menstrual-related problems; may reduce uterine fibroids and endometriosis symptoms
Male condom	Protects against sexually transmitted infections (STIs); delays premature ejaculation
Female condom	Protects against STIs
Cervical barrier	Diaphragm may protect from cervical dysplasia
Contraceptive sponge	None
Fertility awareness methods	Can help a woman learn her cycle and eventually help in getting pregnant
Withdrawal	None
Spermicide	Provides lubrication
No method	n/a

Source: Carroll J, *Sexuality Now*, 6th ed. San Francisco, CA: Cengage Learning, 2019.

- **Episodes of depression.** Avoid products that contain progestin, such as Depo-Provera, the contraceptive implant, and the minipill. In some women with depression, progestin may worsen depressive symptoms. Also, check with your doctor if you are taking an antidepressant medication; it may affect or be affected by oral contraceptives and you may require a different dose.

- **Seizure disorder.** Avoid low-dose birth control pills. Some antiseizure medications, such as Dilantin, accelerate liver metabolism of all substances, including oral contraceptives, and make them less effective.

- **Ectopic pregnancy.** Avoid IUDs. Although IUDs do not cause ectopic pregnancies, if your fallopian tubes have been scarred by a previous ectopic gestation, you're more likely to have another ectopic pregnancy if you use an IUD.

- **Hepatitis.** Avoid birth control pills or injections containing estrogen, which is metabolized in the liver—an organ damaged by hepatitis.

You also have to recognize the specific risks associated with various methods of contraception. If you are a woman, the risks are chiefly yours. Various methods of birth control have side effects, although pregnancy and childbirth account for much higher rates of medical complications and deaths than any contraceptive. Most women never experience any serious complications, but it's important to be aware of potential problems.

Reproductive Coercion

Reproductive coercion refers to "behaviors intended to maintain power and control in a relationship" by someone who is, was, or wishes to be involved in an intimate or dating relationship.

In a study of almost 1,000 female undergraduates at a large public university, nearly 8 percent reported reproductive coercion, including the following:

- Being told not to use any birth control.
- Being forced or pressured to become pregnant.
- Having her partner say he would have a baby with someone else or leave if they did not get pregnant.
- Being hurt physically because they did not agree to get pregnant.
- Having her partner refuse to pay for contraceptives.
- Having her partner break, puncture, remove, or refuse to use a condom so that she would get pregnant.
- Having birth control pills taken away.

As part of their regular screening exams, obstetrician-gynecologists now ask women if they have been the victims of reproductive coercion or any other form of intimate partner violence (discussed in Chapter 18).

Contraception Choices

Culture, religion, sex roles, and tradition can affect birth control options and decisions. In countries that are predominantly Catholic, such as Ireland, Italy, and the Philippines, the Church promotes fertility awareness and the rhythm method and condemns other contraceptive methods. Because Jewish law teaches men not to "spill their seed," methods that can cause damage to sperm, such as vasectomy, condoms, or spermicides, are less acceptable in Israel than oral contraceptives. According to the United Nations, about 6 in 10 women who are married or in a union use contraception. People around the world use sterilization more than any other birth control method; and the IUD is the most commonly used reversible form of contraception. The most popular methods of birth control among women using contraception in the United States are pills (28 percent) and female sterilization (27 percent).[13]

Birth Control on Campus

In the ACHA's *National College Health Assessment*, 54 percent of students—50 percent of men and 56 percent of women—reported using contraception the last time they had vaginal intercourse. (See Snapshot: On Campus Now.) Among students who had vaginal intercourse in the past 12 months, 15.6 percent reported that they or their partner had used emergency contraception (the morning-after pill), discussed later in this chapter; 1 percent reported an unintended pregnancy.[14]

Even students who know and understand the risks associated with unprotected sex often do not take steps to prevent pregnancy or STIs. One reason is that many believe that "a known partner is a safe partner" and that sex with someone they know as a friend or have been dating for a while is safe.

In a study at a community college, women who were not using birth control or who were relying on less-effective methods expressed a desire to try hormonal contraceptives, such as the birth control pills, injectable contraceptives, or long-acting reversible contraceptives. However, various factors, including cost, limited their access to more effective contraceptives.[15]

✓**check-in** If you are sexually active, do you use condoms every time you engage in sex? Are you less likely to do so with a partner you know well?

Hormonal Contraceptives

In recent years, birth control methods made with synthetic hormones have become available in a variety of forms. Oral contraceptives, in widespread use for decades, are among the most well researched of all medications.

Other options for hormonal birth control include a skin patch, a vaginal ring, a 3-month injection, and a 3-year implant. All are extremely

Birth Control Choices of College Students

Contraceptive use reported by students or their partners the last time they had vaginal intercourse:

	Percent (%)		
	Male	Female	Total
Yes, used a method of contraception	50.1	56.4	54.2
Not applicable/Didn't use a method/Don't know	49.9	43.6	45.8

If YES to contraceptive use the last time student had vaginal intercourse, reported means of birth control used among college students or their partners to prevent pregnancy:

	Percent (%)		
	Male	Female	Total
Birth control pills (monthly or extended cycle)	56.3	52.9	53.5
Birth control shots	4.2	3.3	3.6
Birth control implants	9.7	8.9	9.1
Birth control patch	1.6	0.8	1.0
Vaginal ring	3.0	2.7	2.8
Intrauterine device	13.4	14.2	14.1
Male condom	65.5	56.2	58.8
Female condom	0.9	0.6	0.7
Diaphragm or cervical cap	0.5	0.2	0.3
Contraceptive sponge	0.4	0.1	0.2
Spermicide (foam, jelly, cream)	4.6	2.2	2.9
Fertility awareness (calendar, mucus, basal body temperature)	6.3	8.0	7.6
Withdrawal	27.7	32.5	31.1
Sterilization (hysterectomy, tubes tied, vasectomy)	2.1	2.3	2.3
Other method	2.4	1.7	1.9
Male condom use plus another method	50.3	45.4	46.7
Any two or more methods (excluding male condoms)	32.8	33.9	33.6

✓**check-in** If you engage in heterosexual intercourse, do you always use a form of birth control? If not, why not? If so, which type? How did you choose it? Did you discuss contraception with your sexual partner? Did you find this difficult? Write down your reflections in your online journal.

Source: American College Health Association. American College Health Association-National College Health Assessment II: Reference Group Executive Summary Spring 2018. Silver Spring, MD: American College Health Association, 2018.

effective when used consistently and conscientiously (Table 9.3).

Hormonal contraceptives can provide benefits beyond birth control, including:

- Regular menstrual cycles.

- Reduction of menstrual pain and excess bleeding.

- Treatment of premenstrual syndrome, polycystic ovarian syndrome, uterine fibroids, and endometriosis.

- Prevention of menstrual migraines.

- Decreased risk of endometrial cancer, ovarian cancer, and colorectal cancer.

- Treatment of acne and excess facial hair.

- Improved bone mineral density.

Hormonal contraceptives do not protect against HIV infection and other STIs, so condoms and spermicides should also be used unless or until both partners have been tested for possible infections.

Oral Contraceptives

The *pill*—the popular term for **oral contraceptives**—is the method of birth control preferred by unmarried women and by those under age 30, including college students. About one in five American women of childbearing age uses the pill.

Oral contraceptives come in two forms:

- *Monophasic pills* release a constant dose of estrogen and progestin throughout a woman's menstrual cycle.

- *Multiphasic pills* mimic normal hormonal fluctuations of the natural menstrual cycle by providing different levels of estrogen and progesterone at different times of the month. Multiphasic pills reduce total hormonal dose and side effects.

Both monophasic and multiphasic pills block the release of hormones that would stimulate the process leading to ovulation. They also thicken and alter the cervical mucus, making it more hostile to sperm, and they make implantation of a fertilized egg in the uterine lining more difficult.

Combination Oral Contraceptives

Consisting of two hormones, synthetic estrogen and progestin, **combination oral contraceptives (COCs)** play important roles in controlling ovulation and the menstrual cycle.[16]

The doses in today's oral contraceptives are much lower—less than one-fourth the amount of estrogen and one-twentieth the progestin—than in the original pill. However, they may still increase the risk of cardiovascular problems in some women.[17] Obese women who take oral contraceptives may have a higher risk for a rare type of stroke known as cerebral venous thrombosis (CVT), compared with women of normal weight who don't take birth control pills.[18] Researchers are just beginning to investigate the ways in which oral contraceptives may affect emotions, social behavior, and the brain itself.[19]

Newer birth control pills appear to be less effective than those approved decades ago, with twice the failure rate of previous products. The reason seems to be the lower doses of hormones that stop ovulation. Women on low-dose oral contraceptives should take their pills at the same time every day and follow their doctor's advice if they miss a dose.

One combination pill, Yasmin, contains a unique progestin that works like a mild diuretic and prevents fluid retention. YAZ, a lower-dose 24-day version, can ease emotional and physical premenstrual symptoms (discussed in Chapter 8). Women who are taking potassium supplements, daily anti-inflammatory drugs, or heparin (a blood thinner) should talk with their doctor because of potentially dangerous drug interactions. Other pills offer different benefits, such as clearer skin and reduced facial hair, and less spotting.

Progestin-Only Pills

Also called **minipills**, the **progestin-only pills** contain a smaller amount of progestin and no estrogen. They work somewhat differently than combination pills. Women taking minipills probably ovulate, at least occasionally. In those cycles, the pills prevent pregnancy by thickening cervical mucus, making it hard for sperm to penetrate, and by interfering with implantation of a fertilized egg. Their typical effectiveness is slightly less than that for combination oral contraceptives, and there may be more breakthrough bleeding but fewer serious adverse effects.[20] Researchers have found a slightly elevated risk with continuous rather than cyclic use of combination oral contraceptives, but the absolute difference in risk is small.[21]

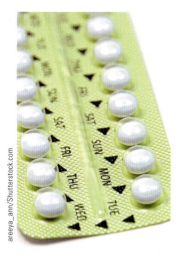

Various types of birth control pills contain different hormones and combinations of hormones.

oral contraceptives Preparations of synthetic hormones that inhibit ovulation; also referred to as *birth control pills* or simply *the pill.*

combination oral contraceptives (COCs) Combination oral contraceptives are birth control pills that consist of two hormones, synthetic estrogen and progestin, which play important roles in controlling ovulation and the menstrual cycle.

minipills Oral contraceptives containing a small amount of progestin and no estrogen, which prevent contraception by making the mucus in the cervix so thick that sperm cannot enter the uterus.

progestin-only pills Oral contraceptives containing a small amount of progestin and no estrogen, which prevent contraception by making the mucus in the cervix so thick that sperm cannot enter the uterus.

TABLE 9.3 How Effective Are Hormonal Contraceptives?

The number of women out of 100 who will become pregnant during the first year of typical use (when a method is used by the average person who does not always use the method correctly or consistently) of each of these methods is as follows:

- Implant—The odds are lower than 1 in 100 women.
- Injection—3 in 100 women will become pregnant.
- Vaginal ring—8 in 100 women will become pregnant.
- Skin patch—8 in 100 women will become pregnant.
- Birth control pill—8 in 100 women will become pregnant.

Source: American College of Obstetricians and Gynecologists.

The risk of heart disease and stroke is lower with progestin-only pills than with any combination pill. For this reason, they are a good choice for women over age 35 and others who cannot take estrogen-containing pills because of high blood pressure, diabetes, or clotting disorders. Because they do not affect the quality or quantity of breast milk, progestin-only pills often are recommended for nursing mothers; and they are recommended for smokers. Because progestin can affect mood and worsen the symptoms of depression, progestin-only pills are not recommended for women with a history of depression. Antiseizure medications, such as Dilantin, which accelerate liver metabolism, may make the mini-pill less effective.

Users of progestin-only pills have to be conscientious about taking these pills—not just every day, but at the same time every day. If you take a progestin-only pill 3 or more hours later than usual, use a backup method of contraception, such as a condom, for 2 days after you resume taking the pill.

....
✓**check-in** If you are a woman, how do you view the benefits and potential risks of using the pill?
....

Although some people incorrectly think that the risks of the pill are greater than those of pregnancy and childbirth, long-term studies show that oral contraceptive use does not increase mortality rates or disease risks. The pill significantly cuts women's risk of dying from colon cancer and the risk of developing ovarian and endometrial cancer. It also does not increase rates of diabetes, multiple sclerosis, rheumatoid arthritis, or liver disease.[22]

Before Using Oral Contraceptives Before starting the pill, a woman should undergo a physical examination that includes a blood pressure test, a breast exam, blood tests, and a urine sample. Let your doctor know about any personal or family incidence of high blood pressure or heart disease; diabetes; liver dysfunction; hepatitis; unusual menstrual history; severe depression; sickle cell anemia; cancer of the breast, ovaries, or uterus; high cholesterol levels; or migraine headaches.

How They Work Oral contraceptives usually come in 28-day packets: 21 of the pills contain the hormones, and 7 are "blanks," included so that the woman can take a pill every day, even during her menstrual period. If a woman forgets to take one pill, she should take it as soon as she remembers. However, if she forgets during the first week of her cycle or misses more than one pill, she should rely on another form of birth control until her next menstrual period.

Even if she experiences no discomfort or side effects while on the pill, a woman should see a physician at least once a year for an examination, which should include a blood pressure test, a pelvic exam, and a breast exam. She should notify her doctor at once if she develops severe abdominal pain, chest pain, coughing, shortness of breath, pain or tenderness in the calf or thigh, severe headaches, dizziness, faintness, muscle weakness or numbness, speech disturbance, blurred vision, a sensation of flashing lights, a breast lump, severe depression, or yellowing of the skin.

Generally, when a woman stops taking the pill, her menstrual cycle resumes the next month, but it may be irregular for the next couple of months. However, 2 to 4 percent of pill users experience prolonged delays. Women who become pregnant during the first or second cycle after discontinuing use of the pill may be at greater risk of miscarriage; they are also more likely to conceive twins.

A Special Caution Common antibiotics, including many prescribed for dental procedures or skin conditions, may lower the effectiveness of oral contraceptives, particularly low-dose birth control pills. Always ask a dentist or doctor who prescribes an antibiotic about its potential effect on your oral contraceptive, and check with your gynecologist or primary physician about using an additional nonhormonal means of contraception (such as a condom) to ensure protection against an unwanted pregnancy.

Other medicines and supplements that may make hormonal contraceptives less effective include St. John's wort, certain pills prescribed for yeast infections, some HIV medications, and specific antiseizure medication. Body weight does not generally affect efficacy.

Advantages

- Extremely effective when taken consistently.
- Convenient.
- Moderately priced.
- Does not interrupt sexual activity.
- Reversible within 3 months of stopping the pill.
- Reduces the risk of benign breast lumps, ovarian cysts, iron-deficiency anemia, pelvic inflammatory disease, and endometrial and ovarian cancer.
- May relieve painful menstruation.

Disadvantages

- In real life, rates of unintended pregnancies among pill users are as high as 2.8 percent in the first year of use and 5.7 percent after 3 years.

- Usually requires a prescription. Oregon was the first state to make birth control pills available to women directly from a pharmacist without a doctor's prescription. The American College of Obstetricians and Gynecologists (ACOG) is supporting similar legislation in other states.

- Increases risk of cardiovascular problems such as blood clotting, primarily for women over age 35 who smoke and those with high blood pressure or other health problems.[23]

- Side effects vary with different brands but include spotting between periods, weight gain or loss, nausea and vomiting, breast tenderness, and decreased sex drive. Progestin-only pills may cause acne, body hair growth, and weight gain.

- Must be taken at the same time every day (especially critical with low-dose estrogen and progestin-only pills).

- No protection against STIs.

- Must use a secondary form of birth control for the initial 7 days of use.

For years, physicians have prescribed prolonged use of birth control pills to lessen the number of menstrual cycles for women with asthma, migraines, rashes, or other conditions that flare up during their periods. Eliminating periods eliminates symptoms, and having fewer cycles may also lower a woman's long-term risk of ovarian cancer. However, some women are wary of long-term hormone use or consider a lack of menstrual cycles unnatural.

Long-Acting Oral Contraceptives

Seasonale and Seasonique As prescription forms of oral contraception, Seasonale and Seasonique prevent pregnancy as effectively as other birth control pills but produce only four menstrual periods a year.

How They Work Unlike traditional birth control pills, women take "active" pills continuously for 3 months, or 84 days. During this time, Seasonale prevents the uterine lining from thickening enough to produce a full menstrual period. Every 3 months, a woman takes 7 days of inactive pills to produce a "pill period," which may be lighter than a regular period. With Seasonique, women take a very low dose of estrogen for 7 days to eliminate any symptoms of complete hormone withdrawal.

The chance of getting pregnant ranges from 5 percent with typical use to 1 percent with perfect use. For maximum effectiveness, each pill should be taken at the same time of day.

Advantages

- Fewer periods.

- Trimonthly periods are usually lighter, with less blood flow.

Disadvantages

- Similar to those of other oral contraceptives in terms of health risks, costs, and side effects. Cigarette smoking increases these risks.

- No protection from STIs.

- More spotting and breakthrough bleeding than with a 28-day pill.

- Determining pregnancy is difficult without a monthly period.

Lybrel, the "No-Period" Pill Lybrel, described as a continuous contraceptive, works the same way as other combination hormonal birth control pills; however, women take the "365-day" pill every single day without interruption.

How They Work Like other oral contraceptives, Lybrel stops the body's monthly preparation for pregnancy by lowering the production of hormones that make pregnancy possible; however, it does not include the "week off" of placebo pills that leads to vaginal bleeding. Most women resume menstruation within 90 days of stopping Lybrel. Medical experts see no long-term risk in doing away with regular monthly periods, but the long-term safety of menstrual suppression is unknown.

Advantages

- No menstrual periods, cramps, or other symptoms.

- No need to stop taking pills or to switch to dummy pills for a week.

- Relief from menstruation-linked conditions such as endometriosis and menstrual migraine.

Disadvantages

- Spotting, which generally tapers off over the first year of use.

- Health risks similar to those of other combination pills.

- Determining pregnancy is difficult without a monthly period.

- Some women feel that eliminating periods is unnatural.

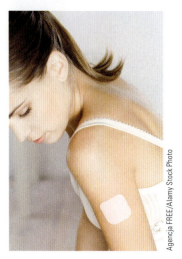

Contraceptive hormones can be delivered through the skin with the patch.

Contraceptive Patch

The Ortho Evra birth control patch, the first transdermal (through the skin) contraceptive, works like a combination pill but looks like a Band-Aid. Embedded in its adhesive layer are two hormones, a low-dose estrogen and a progestin. The contraceptive patch prevents pregnancy by delivering continuous levels of estrogen and progestin through the skin directly into the bloodstream so women are exposed to higher overall levels of estrogen, which may increase their risk of blood clots. The patch is waterproof and stays on in the shower, swimming pool, or hot tub.

How It Works A woman applies the 1.75-inch square to her back, upper arm, lower abdomen, or buttocks and changes it every 7 days for 3 weeks. During the patch-free week, she experiences menstrual bleeding. A user should check every day to make sure the patch is still in place. If you don't replace a detached patch within 24 hours, use a backup method of contraception until your next period.

Advantages

- Good alternative for women who can't remember, don't like, or have problems swallowing daily pills.
- Highly effective when used correctly.
- Does not interrupt sexual activity.
- Fewer side effects, such as nausea, breakthrough bleeding, and mood swings, than pills.
- Fertility returns quickly after you stop using it.

Disadvantages

- Must apply a new patch every week.
- Requires a prescription.
- No protection against STIs.
- Increases risk of blood clots, heart attack, and stroke, particularly for women who smoke or have certain health conditions. The risk of dying or suffering a survivable blood clot while using the patch is estimated to be about two times higher than with birth control pills. However, an FDA panel has concluded that the patch can be especially useful for younger women and those who have trouble taking a daily pill.
- Less effective in women who weigh more than 198 pounds.
- Some women report breast tenderness, headaches, bleeding between periods, upper respiratory infections, or self-consciousness wearing the patch.

- Contact lens wearers may experience vision changes.
- Five percent of women report that at least one patch slipped off; 2 percent report skin irritation.
- Must use another form of birth control for the initial 7 days of use.

Contraceptive Vaginal Ring

A contraceptive vaginal ring (CVR), NuvaRing, is a 1-month combination hormonal ring that is as effective as combined contraceptive pills with similar side effects. Progering, tested and approved in South America, is a 3-month progesterone-releasing ring. Other longer-acting rings are under development.[24]

The silver-dollar-size NuvaRing, a 2-inch ring made of flexible, transparent plastic, slowly emits the same hormones as oral contraceptives through the vaginal tissues (Figure 9.3). Smaller than the smallest diaphragm, it contains less estrogen than any pill. NuvaRing is not associated with weight gain and may have many noncontraceptive benefits, including a positive effect on sexual function, dysmenorrhea, premenstrual syndrome, and heavy menstrual bleeding. Contraindications are the same as for combined oral contraceptives, and serious complications are rare. The risk of venous thromboembolism with the ring is comparable with that of combined oral contraceptives.[25]

How It Works Unlike a diaphragm, the NuvaRing does not have to be exactly positioned within the vagina or used with a spermicide. The flexible, plastic 2-inch ring compresses so a woman can easily insert it. Each ring stays in place for 3 weeks and then is removed for the fourth week of the menstrual cycle.

If a NuvaRing pops out (uncommon but possible), it should be washed, dried, and replaced within 3 hours. If a longer time passes, users should rely on a backup form of birth control until the ring has been reinserted for a week and the medications have risen to protective levels again.

Advantages

- Under medical supervision, may be safer than birth control pills for women with mild hypertension or diabetes.
- Less likelihood of pill-related side effects, such as nausea, mood swings, spotting, and cramping.
- No need to remember a daily pill or weekly patch.
- Fertility returns quickly when ring is removed.
- Reduced pain during menstrual periods.

Agencja FREE/Alamy Stock Photo

- May improve acne and reduce excess body hair.
- Can help prevent menstrual migraines.

Disadvantages

- Slightly increased risk of blood clots, heart attack, and stroke in women older than 35 who smoke 15 or more cigarettes a day or who have other cardiovascular risk factors.

- Some women do not feel comfortable placing and removing something inside their vagina.

- Possible side effects include vaginal discharge, irritation, infection, headaches, weight gain, and nausea.

- Cannot use oil-based vaginal medications for yeast infections while ring is in place.

- No protection against STIs.

Long-Acting Reversible Contraceptives

Long-acting reversible contraceptives (LARCs), which provide protection from pregnancy for an extended period without any action by users, include intrauterine devices (IUDs), injections, and implants. Their use has jumped fivefold in the last decade, particularly among women who have had at least one child and those between ages 25 and 34. After oral contraceptives and sterilization, long-acting reversible contraceptives (LARCs), including intrauterine contraceptives (IUCs) and implants, are the most effective methods of birth control. In a study of nearly 1,000 women, LARC methods have an unintended pregnancy rate of 0.27 per hundred. However, some women are hesitant to try LARCs because of a lack of information about them or misinformation in the form of negative stories about their side-effects or complications.[26]

The primary disadvantage of LARCS is that they do not protect against STIs. Their advantages include the following:

- No need to remember to take a pill every day or insert a cap or diaphragm prior to sex.

- Long-lasting, quickly reversible, and 20 times more effective than oral contraceptive pills, patches, and rings.

- Cost effective; can save thousands of dollars for users over a 5-year period compared to the cost of oral contraceptives and other birth control methods.

- Better control of menstrual bleeding and spotting.

- Can be inserted immediately after delivery or abortion.

- Rapid restoration of fertility following removal.[27]

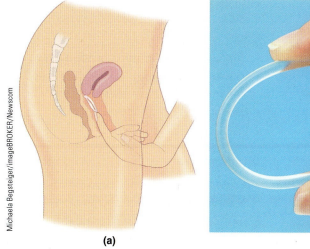

Michaela Begsteiger/imageBROKER/Newscom

(a)   **(b)**

FIGURE 9.3 NuvaRing

The NuvaRing releases estrogen and progestin, preventing ovulation. The exact position of the NuvaRing in the vagina is not critical.

Intrauterine Device

An **intrauterine device (IUD)** is a small piece of molded plastic, with a nylon string attached, that is inserted into the uterus through the cervix. It prevents pregnancy by interfering with implantation. Once widely used, IUDs became less popular after most brands were removed from the market because of serious complications such as pelvic infection and infertility. However, the use of intrauterine contraception, particularly of devices that remain effective for 7 to 12 years, is rising in the United States.[28] According to a recent meta-analysis of more than 3,000 studies, young women are not at greater risk of complications, including pregnancy, perforation, infection, or heavy bleeding, than older IUD users.[29]

How It Works A physician must insert the IUD in a woman's uterus. In a 5-year clinical trial, about 5 in every 100 women reported that an IUD had slipped out of the uterus.[30] Users should check for the string that extends from the device through the vagina at least once a month. Varying brands of hormonal IUDs protect from pregnancy for different amounts of time: Skyla and Liletta for 3 years, Kyleena for 5 years, and Mirena for 6 years. The copper IUD prevents pregnancy for up to 10 years.

Advantages

- Highly effective at preventing pregnancy.

- No need to think about contraception for several years.

long-acting reversible contraceptives (LARCs) Contraceptive devices that provide protection from pregnancy for an extended period without any action by users. Examples include intrauterine devices, injections, and implants.

intrauterine device (IUD) A device inserted into the uterus through the cervix to prevent pregnancy by interfering with implantation.

- Allows sexual spontaneity; neither partner can feel it.
- Starts working immediately.
- New mothers can breastfeed while using it.
- Periods become shorter and lighter or stop altogether.
- Low incidence of side effects.
- Can be removed at any time.

Disadvantages

- Available sizes may be too large for some women, which can cause pain or embedment.
- Spotting or breakthrough bleeding in first 3 to 6 months.
- No protection against STIs.
- Potential side effects include acne, headaches, nausea, breast tenderness, and mood changes.
- Increased risk of benign ovarian cysts.
- May take up to a year for fertility to return after discontinuation.

Contraceptive Injection

A progestin-only contraceptive is available in the form of a birth control "shot" or injection. Depo-Provera or its newer form, Depo-subQ Provera, must be given every 12 weeks. Contraceptive injections provide no protection against HIV and other STIs.

Because of the risk of significant bone mineral loss, the FDA has recommended that women not use Depo-Provera for longer than 2 years. Although mineral loss is common and greater in the first year of use, most individuals regain bone density after discontinuing its use.

How It Works One injection of this synthetic version of the natural hormone progesterone provides 3 months of contraceptive protection. This long-acting hormonal contraceptive raises levels of progesterone, thereby simulating pregnancy. The pituitary gland doesn't produce FSH and LH, which normally cause egg ripening and release. The endometrial lining of the uterus thins, preventing implantation of a fertilized egg. Self-administered injectables also have proven effective.[31]

Advantages

- Because it contains only progestin, it is safe for women who cannot take combination birth control pills.
- No risk of user error.
- No worry about buying, storing, or using contraceptives.

- No need to think about contraception for 3 months at a time.
- Possible protection against endometrial and ovarian cancer.
- Can be used by women who are breastfeeding.
- May decrease menstrual migraines.

Disadvantages

- Must visit a doctor or clinic every 3 months for injection.
- Menstrual cycles become irregular. After a year, 50 percent of women stop having periods.
- Potential side effects include decreased sex drive, depression, headaches, nervousness, dizziness, frequent urination, allergic reactions, hair loss, or increased hair growth.
- Increased weight gain, especially for obese women and teenage girls.
- No protection against STIs.
- May increase the risk of acquiring chlamydia and gonorrhea compared with women not using a hormonal contraceptive.
- Delayed return of fertility.
- Long-term use may significantly reduce bone density, particularly for women who smoke, don't get enough calcium, and have never been pregnant.

Contraceptive Implant

This thin, flexible, plastic implant—about the size of a matchstick—is inserted under the skin of the upper arm to provide birth control that is 99 percent effective for up to 3 years. Easier to insert and remove than earlier implants (Norplant and Jadelle), Implanon has been used in other countries for years and is now available throughout the United States. Nexplanon is a newer version designed for easier insertion and removal.

How It Works Contraceptive implants work primarily by releasing progestin and suppressing ovulation. They also thicken cervical mucus, which inhibits sperm movement, inhibit the development and growth of the uterine lining, and limit secretion of progesterone during the second half of the menstrual cycle.

Advantages

- Can be used while breastfeeding.
- Can be used by women who cannot take estrogen.

- Provides continuous long-lasting birth control without sterilization.

- No medicine to take every day.

- Does not interfere with sexual foreplay.

- Ability to become pregnant returns quickly once implant is removed.

Disadvantages

- Irregular bleeding, especially in the first 6 to 12 months of use. Periods stop completely in one of three women after a year of use.

- Side effects include dizziness, acne, hair loss, headache, nausea, nervousness, pain at the insertion site, and weight gain.

- No protection against STIs.

- Change in appetite.

- Change in sex drive.

- Cysts on the ovaries.

- Depression and mood changes.

- Discoloring or scarring of the skin over the implant.

If implanted during the first 5 days of a woman's period, a contraceptive implant protects against pregnancy immediately. Otherwise, a woman needs to use some form of backup birth control for the first week after getting the implant.

Barrier Contraceptives

As their name implies, **barrier contraceptives** block the meeting of egg and sperm by means of a physical barrier (condom, sponge, diaphragm, cervical cap, or FemCap) or a chemical one (vaginal spermicide in jellies, foams, creams, suppositories, or film). As shown in Table 9.4, they vary in effectiveness.

The nonprescription barrier contraceptives include the male and female condom, the contraceptive sponge, and vaginal spermicides.

Condoms

Unlike other barrier contraceptives, **condoms** provide some protection against HIV infection and other STIs; spermicides, sponges, and films do not.

✓**check-in** Do you think condoms have a negative effect on sexual pleasure?

Advantages

- Effective when used correctly.

- Lowers a woman's risk of pelvic inflammatory disease (PID) and may protect against some urinary tract and genital infections.

TABLE 9.4 How Effective Are Barrier Contraceptives?

Method	Number of women out of 100 who will become pregnant during the first year of typical use (when a method is used by the average person who does not always use the method correctly or consistently)
Diaphragm	12
Sponge	
Women who have not given birth	12
Women who have given birth	24
Cervical cap	
Women who have not given birth	13
Women who have given birth	23
Male condom	18
Female condom	21
Spermicide	28

Source: American Congress of Obstetricians and Gynecologists.

barrier contraceptives Birth control devices that block the meeting of egg and sperm, either by physical barriers, such as condoms, diaphragms, or cervical caps, or by chemical barriers, such as spermicide, or both.

condoms Latex or polyurethane sheaths worn over the penis during sexual acts to prevent conception and/or the transmission of disease; the female condom lines the walls of the vagina.

- No side effects.

- No prescription required.

- Can be carried in a pocket or purse.

- Inexpensive.

- No effect on a woman's natural hormones or fertility.

- The female condom can be inserted up to 8 hours before sex.

- The female condom gives women more control in reducing their risk of pregnancy and STIs and does not require a prescription or medical appointment.

Disadvantages

- Requires consistent and diligent use.

- Not 100 percent effective in preventing pregnancy or STIs.

- Risk of manufacturing defects, such as pin-size holes, and breaking or slipping off during intercourse.

- May inhibit sexual spontaneity.

- Users or partners may complain about odor, lubrication (too much or too little), feel, taste, difficulty opening the packages, and disposal.

- Some men complain of reduced penile sensitivity or cannot sustain an erection while putting on a condom.

- Some women complain that the female condom is difficult to use, squeaks, and looks odd.

Male Condom Worldwide, more than 25 percent of contraception relies on the male partner.[32] Currently the only reliable birth control option for men is the condom, which covers the erect penis and catches the ejaculate in order to avoid fertilization of an egg. The male condom also prevents the exchange of bodily fluids during oral and anal sex in same- and opposite-sex partners (Figure 9.4).

How It Works Most condoms are made of thin surgical latex or polyurethane. The polyurethane condom has proven to be less effective than the latex condom for pregnancy prevention. However, polyurethane condoms may be a good option for those allergic to latex. Membrane condoms ("natural" or "sheepskin") are not recommended. Avoid use of condoms with non-oxynol-9, which may increase rather than lower the risk of sexual infections (see Chapter 11).

Here are some additional guidelines for condom use:

- Before using a condom, check the expiration date and make sure it's soft and pliable.

- Do not tear open a packet with your teeth; you could puncture the condom.

- If it's yellow or sticky, throw the condom out.

- Don't check for leaks by blowing up a condom before using it; you may weaken or tear it.

- Put the condom on at the beginning of sexual activity, before genital contact occurs.

- Leave a little space at the top of the condom to catch the semen (see Figure 9.4).

- If a female partner is using a vaginal lubricant, it should be water-based. Petroleum-based

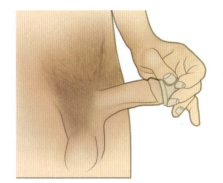
Pinch or twist the tip of the condom, leaving one-half inch at the tip to catch the semen.

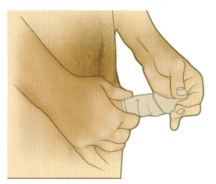
Holding the tip, unroll the condom.

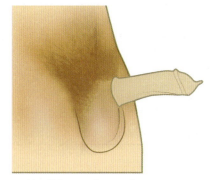
Unroll the condom until it reaches the pubic hairs.

FIGURE 9.4 Male Condom

Condoms effectively reduce the risk of pregnancy as well as STIs if used consistently and correctly.

creams or jellies (such as petroleum jelly, baby oil, massage oil, vegetable oils, or oil-based hand lotions) can deteriorate latex.

- After ejaculation, hold the condom firmly against the penis so that it doesn't slip off or leak during withdrawal.

- Couples engaging in anal intercourse should use a water-based lubricant as well as a condom but should never assume that the condom will provide 100 percent protection from HIV infection or other STIs.

Effectiveness. Although the theoretical effectiveness rate for condoms is 97 percent, the actual rate is only 80 to 85 percent. The condom can be torn during the manufacturing process or during use. Careless removal can also decrease the effectiveness of condoms. Users who have little experience with condoms—who are young, single, or childless, or who engage in risky behaviors—are more likely to have condoms break. However, the major reason that condoms have such a low actual effectiveness rate is that couples don't use them each and every time they have sex.

Condoms are second only to the pill in popularity among college-age adults. Half of sexually active students report using condoms the last time they had vaginal intercourse (Table 9.5).[33] Men give multiple reasons for using condoms, including fear of transmitting HIV or another STI; protecting themselves from a STI; protecting a partner from a STI or pregnancy; complying with a partner's request and showing that they care; and concern about whether a partner might be engaging in sex with someone else.[34]

The reasons college men give for *not* using a condom include:

- **Concerns about diminished pleasure or performance.** Research disputes this common misconception. Investigators have found that, whether heterosexual or homosexual, most men and women describe their most recent sexual experiences as highly arousing and pleasurable, regardless of whether they used condoms or engaged in oral, vaginal, or anal intercourse. The men in the study reported that condom use had no significant impact on the ease of their erections or their sexual pleasure.[35]

- **Condom fit or feel.** The most common complaints from condom users include decreased sensation, lack of naturalness, condom size, decreased pleasure, and pain and discomfort.[36]

- **Familiarity with a partner.** In a study of young adults ages 18 to 29, 55 percent of the men and 36 percent of the women reported condom use the first time a couple had

TABLE 9.5 Condoms on Campus

Using a condom or other protective barrier within the past 30 days (mostly or always):			
	Percent (%)		
	Male	**Female**	**Average**
Sexually active students reported*			
Oral sex	5.6	5.2	5.4
Vaginal intercourse	52.6	46.0	47.8
Anal intercourse	36.8	21.3	27.5

*Students responding "Never did this sexual activity" or "Have not done this during the past 30 days" were excluded from the analysis.

Source: American College Health Association. American College Health Association-National College Health Assessment II: Reference Group Executive Summary Spring 2018. Silver Spring, MD: American College Health Association, 2018.

intercourse. Only 16 percent of the men and 8 percent of the women reported using condoms after nine "coital events."[37]

- **Norms and beliefs about masculinity.** More traditional views of masculinity, such as toughness, correlates with negative attitudes toward condom use.[38]

- **Availability.** Among colleges and universities with health centers, about half provide free condoms.[39] At other schools, students may have limited access to condoms and may need to leave campus to buy condoms at convenience stores, pharmacies, or grocery stores.[40]

Female Condom The second-generation female condom, known as FC2, is a strong, thin, flexible nitrile sheath or pouch about 6.5 inches long, the same length as a male condom. It consists of a flexible polyurethane ring at the closed end of the pouch, the end that is inserted into the vagina, and a soft nitrite ring at the end that remains outside the vagina. There is a silicone-based lubricant on the inside of the condom; additional lubrication can be used.

How It Works As shown in Figure 9.5, a woman removes the condom and applicator from the wrapper and inserts the condom slowly by gently pushing the applicator toward the small of the back. When properly inserted, the outer ring should rest on the folds of skin around the vaginal opening, and the inner ring (the closed end) should fit against the cervix. The female condom may be placed up to 8 hours before intercourse.

Effectiveness. The female condom is about 75 to 82 percent effective with normal use; if it were used correctly during every occasion of

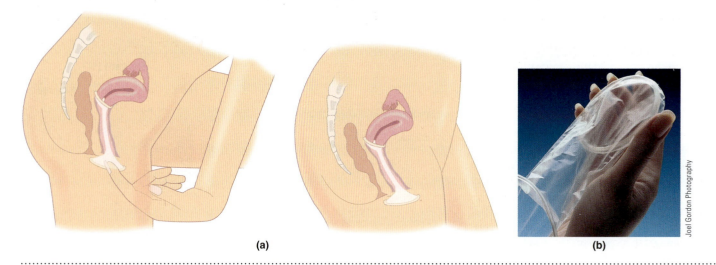

(a)　**(b)**

Joel Gordon Photography

FIGURE 9.5 Female Condom

No spermicide is used with the female condom. Like the male condom, this method does not require a prescription.

intercourse, it is about 95 percent effective in preventing pregnancy. Female condoms can fail for the same reasons as male condoms, such as having a tear, not being put in place before the penis touches the vagina, and spilling the contents as the condom is being removed.

Friction of the female condom may reduce clitoral stimulation and lubrication, which may make intercourse less enjoyable, although lubricants may help. Some users have reported irritation and allergic reactions. A couple should not use a male and female condom together because friction between them can cause them to tear or bunch and should avoid petroleum-based lubricants such as Vaseline, which can break down latex.

Properly used, the female condom is considered as good as or better than the male condom for preventing infections, including HIV, because it is stronger and covers a slightly larger area. Female condoms may be more prone to slipping and other mechanical problems but are as effective as male condoms in blocking semen. The efficacy of female condoms increases with a woman's experience in using them.

Contraceptive Sponge

The contraceptive sponge, which is made of soft polyurethane foam laced with spermicide, is available at retail and online stores as well as family planning centers. It may prevent about 88 in 100 pregnancies in women who have never had children but is less effective in those who have given birth.

How It Works　The contraceptive sponge acts as a barrier by blocking the entrance to the uterus and absorbing and deactivating sperm. Prior to

inserting it in the vagina, moisten the sponge with water to activate the spermicide. Then fold it in half and insert deep into the vagina. Check to make sure it is covering the cervix. Intercourse can occur immediately or at any time during the next 24 hours. However, the sponge must remain in place for 6 hours after intercourse. To remove, gently pull the cloth loop or the tabs on the outside.

Advantages

- Does not require a prescription.
- Easy to carry and use.
- Can be inserted up to 24 hours before intercourse.
- Effective immediately if used correctly.
- No effect on fertility or a woman's natural hormones.
- Generally cannot be felt by a woman or her partner.
- Can be used by women who are breastfeeding for 6 weeks after childbirth.

Disadvantages

- May be difficult to remove.
- May be less effective in women who have had children.
- Does not provide reliable protection against STIs.
- Requires advance planning to place the sponge.
- Side effects include vaginal irritation and allergic reactions.

- Should not be used during menstruation.

- Slightly increased risk of toxic shock syndrome if left in place longer than 24 to 30 hours.

Vaginal Spermicides and Film

The various forms of **vaginal spermicide** include chemical foams, creams, jellies, vaginal suppositories, gels, and film. Some creams and jellies are made for use with a diaphragm; others can be used alone. Several vaginal suppositories claim high effectiveness, but no American studies have confirmed these claims. In general, failure rates for vaginal suppositories are as high as 10 to 25 percent.

Frequent use of spermicides can increase the risk of getting HIV from an infected partner. They should be used only by those at low risk of HIV infection. One widely used spermicide, nonoxynol-9, has proven to be less effective than once believed. It does not protect against many STIs, including HIV, chlamydia, and gonorrhea. Nonoxynol-9 may also increase the risk of infection with human papillomavirus (HPV) and with HIV. The Centers for Disease Control and Prevention has concluded that it is ineffective against HIV, and the WHO describes it as only "moderately effective" for pregnancy prevention.

Vaginal contraceptive film (VCF), a thin 2-inch-square film laced with spermicide, is folded and inserted into the vagina, where it dissolves into a stay-in-place gel (Figure 9.6). VCF, which can be used by people allergic to foams and jellies, is as effective as most spermicides.

Spermicides consist of a chemical that kills sperm and potential pathogens and an inert base, such as jelly, cream, foam, or film, that holds the spermicide close to the cervix. The jelly, cream, or foam spermicide is inserted into the vagina with an applicator or finger. Vaginal suppositories take about 20 minutes to dissolve and cover the vaginal walls. Follow package directions precisely.

You must apply additional spermicide or insert another VCF film before each additional intercourse. After sex, women should shower rather than bathe to prevent the spermicide from being rinsed out of the vagina, and they should not douche for at least 6 hours.

Advantages

- Easy to use.

- Effective if used with another form of contraception.

- Reduces the risk of some vaginal infections, PID, and STIs.

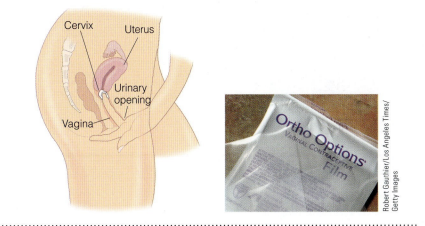

FIGURE 9.6 Vaginal Contraceptive Film
The effectiveness of this thin film, laced with spermicide, is similar to that for other spermicides.

Robert Gauthier/Los Angeles Times/Getty Images

- No effect on a woman's natural hormones or fertility.

Disadvantages

- When used alone, does not protect against STIs.

- Frequent use can increase risk of HIV from an infected partner.

- Insertion interrupts sexual spontaneity.

- May cause irritation.

- Some people cannot use foams or jellies because of an allergic reaction.

- Some users complain that spermicides are messy or interfere with oral–genital contact.

- Spermicidal suppositories that do not dissolve completely can feel gritty.

The prescription barrier contraceptives—the diaphragm, cervical cap, and FemCap, all used by women—are placed in the vagina with a spermicide. They do not protect against HIV infection and most STIs.

Diaphragm

The **diaphragm** is a bowl-like rubber cup with a flexible rim that is inserted into the vagina to cover the cervix and prevent the passage of sperm into the uterus during sexual intercourse (Figure 9.7).

When used with a spermicide, the diaphragm is both a physical and a chemical barrier to sperm. The effectiveness of the diaphragm in preventing pregnancy depends on strong motivation (to use it faithfully) and a precise understanding of its use. Without spermicide, the diaphragm is not effective.

vaginal spermicide A substance that kills or neutralizes sperm, inserted into the vagina in the form of a foam, cream, jelly, suppository, or film.

vaginal contraceptive film (VCF) A small dissolvable sheet saturated with spermicide that can be inserted into the vagina and placed over the cervix.

diaphragm A bowl-like rubber cup with a flexible rim that is inserted into the vagina to cover the cervix and prevent the passage of sperm into the uterus during sexual intercourse; used with a spermicidal foam or jelly, it serves as both a chemical and a physical barrier to sperm.

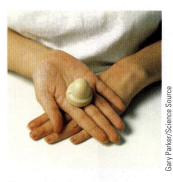

The cervical cap, preferred by some women, is about as effective as a diaphragm if used with a spermicide and inserted correctly.

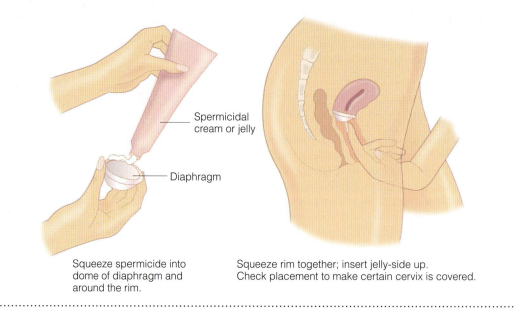

Squeeze spermicide into dome of diaphragm and around the rim.

Squeeze rim together; insert jelly-side up. Check placement to make certain cervix is covered.

FIGURE 9.7 Diaphragm

When used correctly and consistently with a spermicide, the diaphragm is effective in preventing pregnancy. It must be fitted by a health-care professional.

How It Works Diaphragms are fitted and prescribed by a qualified health-care professional in diameter sizes ranging from 2 to 4 inches (50 to 105 millimeters). The diaphragm's main function is to serve as a container for a spermicidal (sperm-killing) foam or jelly, which is available at pharmacies without a prescription. A diaphragm should remain in the vagina for at least 6 hours after intercourse to ensure that all sperm are killed. If intercourse occurs again during this period, additional spermicide must be inserted with an applicator tube.

A sexually active woman should keep her diaphragm in the most accessible place—her purse, bedroom, or bathroom. Before every use, a diaphragm should be checked for tiny leaks (to do so, hold up to the light or place water in the dome). A health-care provider should check its fit and condition every year. Oil-based lubricants will deteriorate the latex of the diaphragm and should not be used.

Cervical Cap

Like the diaphragm, the **cervical cap** combined with spermicide serves as both a chemical and physical barrier blocking the path of the sperm to the uterus. The rubber or plastic cap is smaller and thicker than a diaphragm. It resembles a large thimble that fits snugly around the cervix and may work better for some women than others. It is about as effective as a diaphragm.

How It Works The cervical cap is fitted by a qualified health-care professional. For use, a woman

fills it one-third to two-thirds full with spermicide and inserts it by holding its edges together and sliding it into the vagina. The cup is then pressed onto the cervix. (Most women find it easiest to do so while squatting or in an upright sitting position.) The cap can be inserted up to 6 hours prior to intercourse and should not be removed for at least 6 hours afterward. It can be left in place up to 24 hours. Pulling on one side of the rim breaks the suction and allows easy removal. Oil-based lubricants should not be used with the cap because they can deteriorate the latex.

FemCap

The FemCap is a nonhormonal, latex-free barrier contraceptive that works with a spermicide (Figure 9.8). The FemCap, designed to conform to the anatomy of the cervix and vagina, comes in three sizes. The smallest usually best suits women who have never been pregnant; the medium size, for women who have been pregnant but have not had a vaginal delivery; the largest, for those who have delivered a full-term baby vaginally.

How It Works A prescription is required to purchase FemCap, and the woman selects the appropriate size. To use, a woman applies spermicide to the bowl of the FemCap (which goes over the cervix), to the outer brim, and to the groove that will face into the vagina. She inserts the squeezed, flattened cap into the vagina with the bowl facing upward. The FemCap must be pushed all the way in to cover the cervix completely and left in place at least 6 hours after intercourse.

cervical cap A thimble-size rubber or plastic cap that is inserted into the vagina to fit over the cervix and prevent the passage of sperm into the uterus during sexual intercourse; used with a spermicidal foam or jelly, it serves as both a chemical and a physical barrier to sperm.

Advantages

- Can be inserted up to 6 hours before sex so it doesn't interrupt sexual activity.
- Usually not felt by either partner.
- Can easily be carried in pocket or purse.
- No effect on a woman's natural hormones or fertility.
- Cervical caps are an alternative for women who cannot use diaphragms or find them too messy.

Disadvantages

- Less effective than hormonal contraceptives.
- Available by prescription only.
- Requires advance planning or interruption of sexual activity to position the device before intercourse.
- May slip out of place during intercourse.
- May be uncomfortable for some women and their partners.
- Spermicidal foams, creams, and jellies may be messy, cause irritation, and detract from oral–genital sex.
- Some diaphragm users report bladder discomfort, urethral irritation, or recurrent cystitis.
- Some cap users find it difficult to insert and remove and is uncomfortable to wear.
- Slightly increased risk of toxic shock syndrome.

Fertility Awareness and Digital Birth Control

Awareness of a woman's cyclic fertility can help in both contraception and conception. The different methods of birth control based on a woman's menstrual cycle are sometimes referred to as *natural family planning* or *fertility awareness methods (FAMs)*. New fertility monitors that use saliva to determine time of ovulation can improve the accuracy of these methods. There is no difference in the use of periodic abstinence by religious affiliation, importance of religion, or frequency of attendance at religious services.

Women's menstrual cycles vary greatly. To use one of the fertility awareness methods, a woman must know and understand her cycle. She should track her cycle for at least 8 months—marking day 1 (the day bleeding begins) on a calendar and counting the length of each cycle. Figure 9.9 shows the days in a 28-day cycle when abstinence or other contraceptive methods would be necessary.

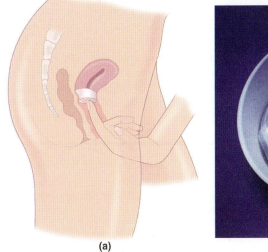
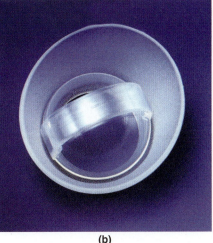

(a)   **(b)**

Joel Gordon Photography

FIGURE 9.8 FemCap

The FemCap must be used with spermicide and correctly positioned to cover the cervix completely.

Source: Reproduced with permission from FemCap, Inc., and Alfred Shihata, MD.

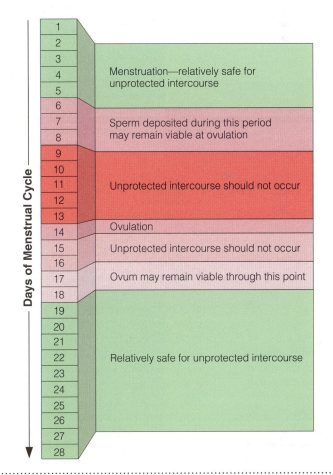

Days of Menstrual Cycle

Day	
1–5	Menstruation—relatively safe for unprotected intercourse
6–8	Sperm deposited during this period may remain viable at ovulation
9–13	Unprotected intercourse should not occur
14	Ovulation
15–16	Unprotected intercourse should not occur
17–18	Ovum may remain viable through this point
19–28	Relatively safe for unprotected intercourse

FIGURE 9.9 Safe and Unsafe Days

Events in the menstrual cycle determine the relatively safe days for avoiding pregnancy in unprotected intercourse.

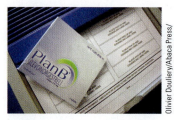

Emergency contraception can prevent unintended pregnancy after unprotected intercourse or when another form of contraception fails.

How It Works The calendar method, often called the **rhythm method**, is based on counting the woman's safe days based on her individual menstrual cycle. The basal-body-temperature method determines the safe days based on the woman's *basal body temperature*, which rises after ovulation. The cervical mucus method, also called the *ovulation method*, is based on observation of changes in the consistency of the woman's vaginal mucus throughout her menstrual cycle. The period of maximum fertility occurs when the mucus is smooth and slippery.

Advantages

- No expense.
- No side effects.
- No need for a prescription, medical visit, or fittings.
- Nothing to insert, swallow, or check.
- No effect on fertility.
- Complies with the teachings of the Roman Catholic Church.

Disadvantages

- Less reliable than other forms of birth control.
- Couples must abstain from vaginal intercourse 8 to 11 days a month or use some form of contraception.
- Conscientious planning and scheduling are essential.
- May not work for women with irregular menstrual cycles.
- Some women find the mucus or temperature methods difficult to use.

Digital Birth Control

Technology has brought a new twist to fertility awareness: mobile apps that make family planning more user-friendly. Fertility trackers use different methods to monitor a woman's menstrual cycle and identify nonfertile days (often marked green) and fertile days (marked red). A woman enters her body temperature into the app every morning (taken with a precise basal body thermometer), and the app, identifying the spike in temperature that signals ovulation, calculates the five or six days when she might become pregnant. The longer a woman continues to input her daily temperature, the more accurately the app can forecast fertility—either to abstain from sex or use a barrier contraceptive to lower the odds of conception or to engage in sex to improve the likelihood of conceiving.

Birth control app designers estimate that, with typical use, they have an effectiveness rate of 93 percent—which means that 7 of every 100 women relying on the app will get pregnant in the course of a year. The failure rate is higher in women with irregular cycles, fluctuating sleep hours, or conditions that might affect their body temperature.

The benefits of digital birth control include:

- No side effects.
- No hormones or surgical procedures required.
- No prescription needed.
- No risk to a woman's health.

The disadvantages include the need for a daily commitment to taking and recording body temperature, the lack of protection against STIs, and the need to abstain or use protection on fertile days.

Emergency Contraception

Emergency contraception (EC) is the use of a method of contraception to prevent unintended pregnancy after unprotected intercourse or the failure of another form of contraception, such as a condom breaking or slipping off. EC is available without a prescription. EC has proved extremely safe in almost all women.

The use of emergency contraception has more than doubled in recent years, particularly among women in their early 20s:

- Nearly one in four women between ages 20 and 24 who have ever had sex has used the morning-after pill.
- Among sexually active college women, 14.9 percent report having used emergency contraception in the past year.[41]
- Overall, one in nine sexually experienced women has used emergency contraception, including one in five never-married women, one in seven cohabiting women, and one in twenty currently or formerly married women.
- The most common reasons for using EC are unprotected sex and fear of contraceptive failure.

✓**check-in** Have you or your partner ever used emergency contraception?

Emergency contraception provides a second chance to prevent pregnancy following unprotected sexual intercourse or contraceptive failure. The copper IUD is the most effective method for emergency contraception, but hormonal methods are often considered more convenient and acceptable.

rhythm method A birth control method in which sexual intercourse is avoided during those days of the menstrual cycle in which fertilization is most likely to occur.

emergency contraception (EC) Types of oral contraceptive pills, usually taken after unprotected intercourse or failed birth control, that can prevent pregnancy.

An IUD can safely be inserted on the same day it is prescribed without increasing the risk of infection.

The progestin-only pill levonorgestrel, marketed as Plan B, Preven, One Step, or Next Choice, has proved more effective with fewer side effects than combination pills.[42] Plan B morning-after pills, which are available without a prescription, should be taken within 5 days (120 hours) of unprotected sex. They can reduce the risk of pregnancy up to 89 percent.

Most women can safely use emergency contraception pills (ECPs), even if they cannot use birth control pills as their regular method of birth control. (Although ECPs use the same hormones as birth control pills, not all brands of birth control pills can be used for emergency contraception.) Some women may experience spotting or a full menstrual period a few days after taking ECPs, depending on where they were in their cycle when they began therapy. Most women have their next period at the expected time.

As multiple studies have shown, increased access to EC does not increase sexual risk taking or lead couples to abandon use of contraceptives. However, awareness of EC remains limited among both consumers and health-care providers. In a recent study of young men, most of whom were sexually active, only about 4 in 10 had heard of EC.[43] Although most physicians knew of the "morning-after pill," those who were not reproductive specialists knew little of and rarely provided alternative and more effective methods, such as a copper IUD.[44]

How It Works EC methods stop pregnancy in the same way as other hormonal contraceptives: They delay or inhibit ovulation, inhibit fertilization, or block implantation of a fertilized egg, depending on a woman's phase of the menstrual cycle. They have no effect once a pregnancy has been established. EC pills may be moderately effective even if started between the third and fifth days (up to 120 hours) after unprotected sexual intercourse or contraceptive failure.

The morning-after pill may also be safe for use as a regular birth control method and may appeal to women who do not have sex regularly and who could use it before or after sex. However, it is not as effective as regular birth control pills, patches, or rings. The most common side effect is irregular bleeding. Pregnancy rates after use of EC are less than 3 percent but slightly higher among obese women.[45]

Sterilization

The most popular method of birth control among married couples in the United States is **sterilization** (surgery to end a person's reproductive capability). Each year an estimated 1 million men and women

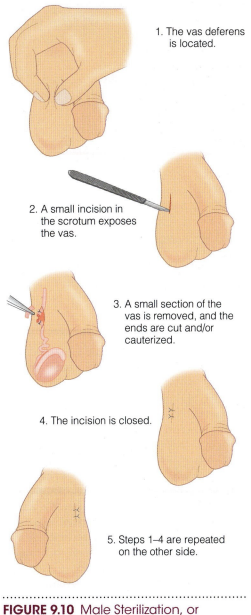

1. The vas deferens is located.

2. A small incision in the scrotum exposes the vas.

3. A small section of the vas is removed, and the ends are cut and/or cauterized.

4. The incision is closed.

5. Steps 1–4 are repeated on the other side.

FIGURE 9.10 Male Sterilization, or Vasectomy

in the United States undergo sterilization procedures. Fewer than 25 percent ever seek reversal.

✓**check-in** Would you consider sterilization as a contraceptive option?

Male Sterilization In men, the cutting of the vas deferens, the tube that carries sperm from one of the testes into the urethra for ejaculation, is called **vasectomy**. During the 15- or 20-minute office procedure, done under a local anesthetic, the doctor makes small incisions in the scrotum, lifts up each vas deferens, cuts it, and ties off the ends to block the flow of sperm (Figure 9.10). Sperm continue to form, but they are broken down and absorbed by the body.

sterilization A surgical procedure to end a person's reproductive capability.

vasectomy A surgical sterilization procedure in which each vas deferens is cut and tied shut to stop the passage of sperm to the urethra for ejaculation.

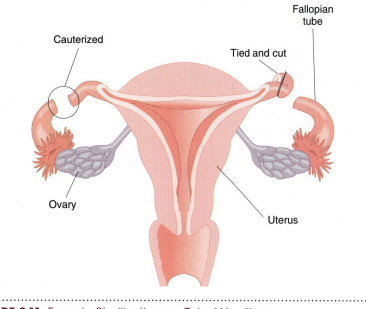

Fallopian tube

Cauterized

Tied and cut

Ovary

Uterus

FIGURE 9.11 Female Sterilization, or Tubal Ligation

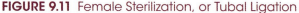

The man usually experiences some local pain, swelling, and discoloration for about a week after the procedure. More serious complications, including the formation of a blood clot in the scrotum (which usually disappears without treatment), infection, and an inflammatory reaction, occur in a small percentage of cases.

Sometimes men want to reverse their vasectomies, usually because they want to have children with a new spouse. Although anyone who chooses to have a vasectomy should consider it permanent, surgical reversal (*vasovasostomy*), thanks to new microsurgical techniques, can restore fertility in more than 90 percent of vasectomized men, but it may take up to 2 years for fertility to return after vasectomy reversal.

Female Sterilization Eleven million U.S. women ages 15 to 44 rely on tubal sterilization for contraception. An estimated 750,000 tubal sterilization procedures are performed each year in the United States. The average age of sterilization is about 30. Female sterilization procedures modify the fallopian tubes, which each month normally carry an egg from the ovaries to the uterus.

The two terms used to describe female sterilization are **tubal ligation** (the cutting or tying of the fallopian tubes) and **tubal occlusion** (the blocking of the tubes). The tubes may be cut or sealed with thread, a clamp, or a clip, or by electrical coagulation to prevent the passage of eggs from the ovaries (Figure 9.11). They can also be blocked with bands of silicone.

One of the common methods of tubal ligation or occlusion uses **laparoscopy**, commonly called *belly-button surgery* or *band-aid surgery*. This procedure is done on an outpatient basis and takes 15 to 30 minutes. A lighted tube called a laparoscope is inserted through a 0.5-inch incision made right below the navel, giving the doctor a view of the fallopian tubes. Using surgical instruments that may be inserted through the laparoscope or through other tiny incisions, the doctor then cuts or seals the tubes, most commonly by electrical coagulation.

The cumulative failure rate of tubal sterilization is about 1.85 percent during a 10-year period. Complications include problems with anesthesia, hemorrhage, organ damage, and mortality.

Essure. Essure involves placement of small, flexible microcoils into the fallopian tubes via the vagina by a physician. Unlike other methods, it does not require the risks of general anesthesia and surgery. The procedure itself does not require incisions and takes approximately 35 minutes. Recovery occurs quickly; most women resume normal activities within 24 hours. For the first 3 months after insertion, women should use another form of contraception. An X-ray called a hysterosalpingogram must confirm that the inserts are correctly placed and the fallopian tubes are completely blocked.

Advantages

- Offers permanent protection against unwanted pregnancy.

- No effect on sex drive in men or women. Many couples report greater sexual activity and pleasure because they no longer have to worry about pregnancy or deal with contraceptives.

- Vasectomy and tubal ligation are performed as outpatient procedures, with a quick recovery time.

- Use of Essure requires no incision, so there's less discomfort and very rapid recovery. Essure may be an option for women with chronic health conditions, such as obesity, diabetes, or heart disease.

Disadvantages

- All procedures should be considered permanent and used only if both partners are certain they want no more children.

- No protection against STIs.

- Must use another form of birth control for first 3 months.

- Many long-term risks remain unknown, but there is no evidence of any link between vasectomy and prostate cancer.

tubal ligation The suturing or tying shut of the fallopian tubes to prevent pregnancy.

tubal occlusion The blocking of the fallopian tubes to prevent pregnanc

laparoscopy A surgical sterilization procedure in which the fallopian tubes are observed with a laparoscope inserted through a small incision, and then cut or blocked.

When Pregnancy Occurs

Unintended Pregnancy

A woman faced with an unintended pregnancy—often alone, unwed, and desperate—can find it extremely difficult to decide what to do. The political debate over the right to life almost always is secondary to practical and emotional matters, such as her relationship with the baby's father, their capacity to provide for the child, the impact on any children she already has, her age and health, and other important life issues.

Giving up the child for adoption is an option for women who do not feel abortion is right for them. Because the number of would-be adoptive parents greatly exceeds the number of available newborns, some women considering adoption may feel pressured by offers of money from couples eager to adopt. Others, particularly minority women, may feel cultural pressures to keep a child—regardless of their age, economic situation, or ability to care for an infant.

Advocates of adoption reform are pressing for mandatory counseling for all pregnant women considering adoption (available now in agency-arranged, but not private, adoptions) and for extending the period of time during which a new mother can change her mind about giving up her child for adoption. (See the discussion of adoption on page 293.)

✓**check-in** Which alternatives would you consider if faced with an unplanned pregnancy?

Abortion

An *abortion* is a procedure that uses medicine or surgery to end a pregnancy. The number and rates of elective abortions have been declining since 2002 to all-time lows. According to the Centers for Disease Control and Prevention, about 730,000 elective abortions are performed every year—13.9 per 1,000 women ages 15 to 44.

Women in their 20s account for the majority of abortions. Most take place early in gestation: 9 in 10 at less than 13 weeks' gestation and just 1 percent at 21 weeks' gestation. The complication rate for abortions is 2.1 percent, ranging from 1.3 percent for first-trimester aspiration abortions to 5.2 percent for medical abortions.[46]

Claims that abortion increases the risk of breast cancer, based on retrospective studies that are less accurate because they rely on individuals' recall, have proved false. Research has found no correlation between the termination of a pregnancy, whether induced or spontaneous, and increased risk of breast cancer.

The term **medical abortion** describes the use of drugs, also called *abortifacients*, to terminate a pregnancy. Medical abortion accounts for about one in five abortions.

The abortion pill mifepristone (Mifeprex), formerly known as RU-486, is 97 percent effective in inducing abortion by blocking progesterone, the hormone that prepares the uterine lining for pregnancy. According to FDA guidelines updated in 2016, mifepristone, used in combination with misoprostol to induce abortion, may now be taken as late as 70 days after the start of a woman's last menstrual period and in lower doses than previously prescribed.[47] On day 1, a woman wishing to terminate a pregnancy takes 200 mg (instead of the previously prescribed dose of 600 mg) of mifepristone. Within 24 to 48 hours, she places 800 mg misoprostol in the pouch of her cheek for 30 minutes (instead of swallowing the pills, as previously recommended, which causes more gastrointestinal upset).

Two days after taking this compound, a woman takes a prostaglandin to increase uterine contractions. The uterine lining is expelled, along with the fertilized egg (Figure 9.12). Sometime within the next 7 to 14 days, the woman returns to the clinic to confirm termination.

Women have compared the discomfort of medical abortion to severe menstrual cramps. Common side effects include excessive bleeding, nausea, fatigue, abdominal pain, and dizziness. About 1 woman in 100 requires a

medical abortion Method of ending a pregnancy within 9 weeks of conception using hormonal medications that cause expulsion of the fertilized egg.

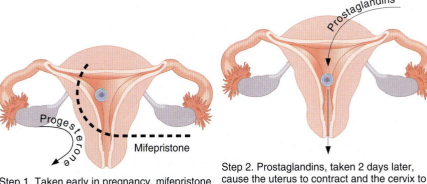

Step 1. Taken early in pregnancy, mifepristone blocks the action of progesterone and makes the body react as if it weren't pregnant.

Step 2. Prostaglandins, taken 2 days later, cause the uterus to contract and the cervix to soften and dilate. As a result, the fertilized egg is expelled in 97 percent of cases.

FIGURE 9.12 Medical Abortion

Mifepristone works by blocking the action of progesterone, a hormone produced by the ovaries that is necessary for the implantation and development of a fertilized egg.

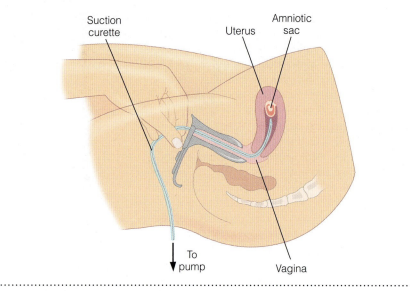

FIGURE 9.13 Suction Curettage

The contents of the uterus are extracted through the cervix with a vacuum apparatus.

blood transfusion. The FDA has warned doctors about rare but deadly bloodstream infections in women using mifepristone. The rate of infection is about 1 in 100,000 uses, comparable to infection risks with surgical abortions and childbirth.

Medical abortion does not require anesthesia and can be performed very early in pregnancy. However, women experience more cramping and bleeding during medical abortion than during surgical abortion, and bleeding lasts for a longer period.

About three-fourths of abortions performed in the United States today are surgical. **Suction curettage**, usually done from 7 to 13 weeks after the last menstrual period, involves the gradual dilation (opening) of the cervix. If this in itself does not bring on a miscarriage, dilators are used to further enlarge the cervical opening. The physician inserts a suction tip into the cervix, and the uterine contents are drawn out via a vacuum system (Figure 9.13). A *curette* (a spoon-shaped surgical instrument used for scraping) is used to check for complete removal of the contents of the uterus. With suction curettage, the risks of complication are low. Major complications, such as perforation of the uterus, occur in fewer than 1 in 100 cases.

The Psychological Impact of Abortion
Abortion can have various psychological effects. As decades of research have shown, the primary emotion of women who have just had an abortion is relief. Although many women also express feelings of guilt or sadness, usually their anxiety

suction curettage A procedure in which the contents of the uterus are removed by means of suction and scraping.

levels drop to lower levels than immediately before the abortion.

Women who experienced violence, including rape, or high anxiety levels prior to becoming pregnant have more anxiety symptoms following an abortion. The best predictor of psychological well-being after abortion is a woman's emotional well-being prior to pregnancy. At highest risk are women who have had a psychiatric illness, such as an anxiety disorder or clinical depression, prior to an abortion, and those whose abortions occurred among complicated circumstances (such as a rape, or coercion by parents or a partner). The vast majority of women manage to put the abortion into perspective as one of many life events.

In a 2-year follow-up, women who underwent abortions had similar or lower levels of depression and anxiety than those who sought but were denied abortion. This finding, according to the researchers, refutes "the notion that abortion is a cause of mental health problems."[48] Women who have had abortions are at no higher risk of post-traumatic stress than those who did not, nor are they more likely to develop depression, anxiety, or substance use disorders.[49]

The Politics of Abortion Abortion is one of the most controversial political, religious, and ethical issues of our time. The issues of when life begins, a woman's right to choose, and an unborn child's right to survival are among the most divisive Americans face. Here is some background:

- Abortions were legal in the United States until the 1860s.

- For decades after that, women who decided to terminate unwanted pregnancies did so by attempting to abort on their own or by obtaining illegal abortions—often performed by untrained individuals using unsanitary and unsafe procedures.

- In the late 1960s, some states changed their laws to make abortions legal.

- In 1973, the U.S. Supreme Court, following a 1970 ruling on the case of *Roe v. Wade* by the New York Supreme Court, said that an abortion in the first trimester of pregnancy was a decision between a woman and her physician and was protected by privacy laws.

- The court further ruled that abortion during the second trimester could be performed on the basis of health risks and that abortion during the final trimester could be performed only for the sake of the mother's health.

- The controversy over abortion has at times become violent: Physicians who perform abortions have been shot and killed; abortion clinics have been bombed, wounding and killing patients and staff members.

- The Supreme Court has upheld a federal law banning "partial-birth" abortions, a late-term procedure involving the removal of a fetus from the uterus and the collapsing of its skull. Pro-life groups hailed this ruling as a step toward the overthrow of *Roe v. Wade*.

- The number of abortions has declined in recent years to 14.5 abortions per 1,000 women ages 15 to 44, while the number of clinics providing abortions has decreased.[50]

- The debate over abortion continues to stir passionate emotions, with pro-life supporters arguing that life begins at conception and that abortion is therefore immoral, and pro-choice advocates countering that an individual woman should have the right to make decisions about her body and health. In 2017, a total of 19 states adopted 63 new restrictions on abortion rights, service provision, and patient access. Increasingly, geography—the county and state where a woman lives and her ability to travel to a different location—can influence whether she can obtain an abortion.[51]

Although the majority of Americans continue to support abortion, many feel that it should be more restricted and difficult to obtain. Some states have required women to view ultrasounds, imposed waiting periods, cut funding for clinics, or banned abortions after 20 weeks. As a result, the number of medical centers providing abortions has decreased, making it particularly difficult for low-income women to obtain abortions. Health-care professionals have united to support the need for "access to comprehensive reproductive health care, including abortion" for all women in the United States.[52]

✓**check-in** How do you view the politics of abortion?

Pregnancy

Pregnancy and birth rates in the United States have declined to the lowest rate ever recorded: 62.5 births per 1,000 women. According to the most recent statistics, total annual births number 3,932,181.[53] Mothers' mean age at first birth is 26.3 years, a significant increase from a decade ago.[54] Pregnancy rates have fallen for women in their teens and 20s, while they have increased for women in their 30s. Despite a decline, the United States continues to have the highest teenage pregnancy rate in the developed world.[55]

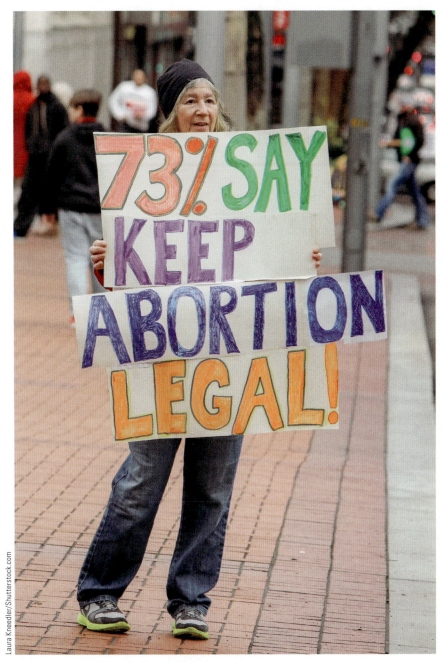

Laura Kneedler/Shutterstock.com

The controversy over abortion has triggered countless demonstrations and encounters between pro-choice and pro-life supporters.

Preconception Care

The time *before* a child is conceived can be crucial in ensuring that an infant is born healthy, full size, and full term. The best chance for lowering the infant mortality rate and preventing birth defects is before pregnancy. Preconception care—the enhancement of a woman's health and well-being prior to conception in order to

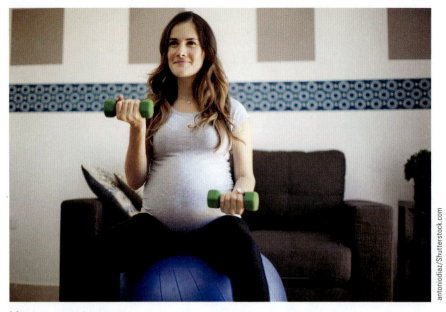

Most pregnant women benefit from mind–body practices and regular moderate exercise.

ensure a healthy pregnancy and baby—includes the following:

- Risk assessment (evaluation of medical, genetic, and lifestyle risks).
- Health promotion (such as teaching good nutrition).
- Interventions to reduce risk (such as treatment of infections and other diseases, assistance in quitting smoking or drug use, and taking folic acid supplements to prevent pregnancy).

Home Pregnancy Tests

Home pregnancy tests detect the presence of human chorionic gonadotropin (hCG), which is secreted as the fertilized egg implants in the uterus. If the concentration of hCG is high enough, a woman will test positive for pregnancy. If the test is done too early, the result will be a false negative. A follow-up test a week later can usually confirm a pregnancy. Although home pregnancy tests are 85 to 95 percent accurate, medical laboratory tests provide definitive confirmation of a pregnancy.

Prenatal Care

From the moment she learns she is pregnant, a woman must assume responsibility for the new life growing inside her. Fortunately, the same habits that maintain her good health also enhance her baby's well-being. These include a healthy diet, exercise, and avoidance of smoking and alcohol.

A Healthy Diet Doctors have long recommended a well-balanced diet that provides a complete variety of key nutrients. In addition, pregnant women should:

- Make sure they are getting an adequate level of folic acid in order to prevent neural tube defects.
- Avoid soft unpasteurized cheeses to prevent *Listeria* infections, which can be harmful to a fetus.
- Eat a diet rich in fruits and vegetables, which provides an additional benefit: a lower risk of premature birth.[56]
- If overweight or obese, increase their caloric intake to ensure adequate nutrition for the fetus but not put on so much weight that it increases the risks to their own health and their baby's.[57]
- Not avoid any specific foods unless they are allergic to them. Recent research suggests that eating nuts during pregnancy lowers a child's risk of having a nut allergy—as long as the mother is not allergic.[58]

Exercise The proven benefits of light to moderate exercise during pregnancy include a greater sense of well-being, enhanced mood, shorter labor, fewer obstetric complications, and healthier infant birth weights.[59] However, women should not exercise more strenuously than they did before pregnancy and should consult their doctors about any precautions they should take, particularly if working out on hot or smoggy days. They should also avoid certain high-risk activities, such as water-skiing, scuba-diving, or contact sports.

Avoid Smoking and Smoke As discussed in Chapter 17, smoking during pregnancy can put a growing fetus in jeopardy.[60] Quitting has been proven to lower the risk of low birth weight and other pregnancy complications.[61] Exposure to secondhand smoke puts a woman and her unborn child in jeopardy; the risk increases with the duration of her exposure.[62]

Don't Use Alcohol or Drugs Alcohol (see Chapter 16) and illegal drugs (see Chapter 15) are well-documented threats to an unborn child.[63] However, even some common prescription drugs, such as acetaminophen and antidepressants, can pose short- and long-term risks.[64] A pregnant woman should discuss any medication with her doctor to weigh the risks and benefits.

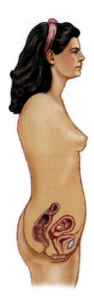

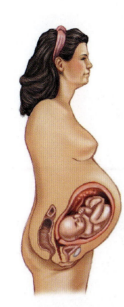

First Trimester

Increased urination because of hormonal changes and the pressure of the enlarging uterus on the bladder.
Enlarged breasts as milk glands develop.
Darkening of the nipples and the area around them.
Nausea or vomiting, particularly in the morning, may occur.
Fatigue.
Increased vaginal secretions.
Pinching of the sciatic nerve, which runs from the buttocks down through the back of the legs, may occur as the pelvic bones widen and begin to separate.

Second Trimester

Thickening of the waist as the uterus grows.
Weight gain.
Increase in total blood volume.
Slight increase in size and change in position of the heart.
Darkening of the pigment around the nipple and from the navel to the pubic region.
Darkening of the face.
Increased salivation and perspiration.
Secretion of colostrum from the breasts.

Third Trimester

Increased urination because of pressure from the uterus.
Tightening of the uterine muscles (called Braxton–Hicks contractions).
Shortness of breath because of increased pressure by the uterus on the lungs and diaphragm.
Interrupted sleep because of the baby's movements or the need to urinate.
Descending ("dropping") of the baby's head into the pelvis about 2–4 weeks before birth.
Navel pushed out.

FIGURE 9.14 Physiological Changes of Pregnancy

A Woman's Bodily Changes During Pregnancy

The 40 weeks of pregnancy, divided into 3-month periods called trimesters, transform a woman's body:

- At the beginning of pregnancy, the woman's uterus becomes slightly larger, and the cervix becomes softer and bluish owing to increased blood flow.

- Progesterone and estrogen trigger changes in the milk glands and ducts in the breasts, which increase in size and feel somewhat tender.

- The pressure of the growing uterus against the bladder causes a more frequent need to urinate.

- As the pregnancy progresses, the woman's skin stretches as her body shape changes, her center of gravity changes as her abdomen protrudes, and her internal organs shift as the baby grows (Figure 9.14).

Neonatal Development

Silently and invisibly, over a 9-month period, a fertilized egg develops into a human being:

- When the zygote reaches the uterus, it's still smaller than the head of a pin.

- Once nestled into the spongy uterine lining, it becomes an **embryo**.

- The embryo takes on an elongated shape, rounded at one end. A sac called the **amnion** envelops it.

embryo An organism in its early stage of development; in humans, the embryonic period lasts from the second to the eighth week of pregnancy.

amnion The innermost membrane of the sac enclosing the embryo or fetus.

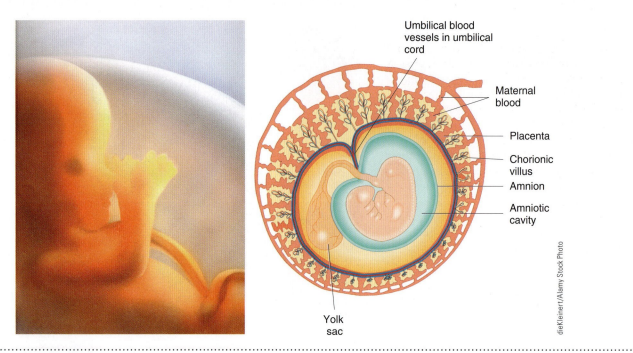

Umbilical blood
vessels in umbilical
cord

Maternal
blood

Placenta

Chorionic
villus

Amnion

Amniotic
cavity

Yolk
sac

dieKleinert/Alamy Stock Photo

FIGURE 9.15 The Placenta

The placenta supplies the growing embryo with fluid and nutrients from the maternal bloodstream and carries waste back for disposal.

- As water and other small molecules cross the amniotic membrane, the embryo floats freely in the absorbed fluid, cushioned from shocks and bumps.

- At 9 weeks the embryo is called a **fetus**.

- A special organ, the **placenta**, forms (Figure 9.15). Attached to the embryo by the umbilical cord, it supplies the growing baby with fluid and nutrients from the maternal bloodstream and carries waste back to the mother's body for disposal.

Complications of Pregnancy

In about 10 to 15 percent of all pregnancies, there is increased risk of some problem, such as a baby's failure to grow normally. The mother-to-be can also be at risk. Pregnancy-related mortality rates have risen in recent years to 16 deaths per 100,000 live births. The danger increases with age and varies with race, with Hispanic black women at the greatest risk.[65] *Perinatology*, or maternal-fetal medicine, focuses on the special needs of high-risk mothers and their unborn babies, including the following potential complications.

Ectopic Pregnancy
Any woman who is of childbearing age, has had intercourse, and feels abdominal pain with no reasonable cause may have an **ectopic pregnancy**, in which the fertilized egg remains in the fallopian tube instead of traveling to the uterus. Ectopic, or tubal, pregnancies have increased dramatically in recent years, now accounting for 2 percent of all reported pregnancies.[66] Risk factors include chlamydia (Chapter 11); previous pelvic surgery, particularly involving the fallopian tubes; pelvic inflammatory disease; infertility; and use of an IUD.

Miscarriage
About 10 to 20 percent of pregnancies end in **miscarriage**, or spontaneous abortion, before the twentieth week of gestation. Major genetic disorders may be responsible for 33 to 50 percent of pregnancy losses. The most common cause is an abnormal number of chromosomes. An estimated 70 to 90 percent of women who miscarry eventually become pregnant again.[67]

Infections
The infectious disease most clearly linked to birth defects is **rubella** (German measles). All women should be vaccinated against this disease at least 3 months prior to conception to protect themselves and any children they may bear. The most common prenatal infection today is *cytomegalovirus*, which produces mild flulike symptoms in adults but can cause brain damage, retardation, liver disease, cerebral palsy, hearing problems, and other malformations in unborn babies. STIs, such as syphilis, gonorrhea, and genital herpes, can be particularly dangerous during pregnancy if not recognized and treated.

fetus The human organism developing in the uterus from the ninth week until birth.

placenta An organ that develops after implantation and to which the embryo attaches, via the umbilical cord, for nourishment and waste removal.

ectopic pregnancy A pregnancy in which the fertilized egg has implanted itself outside the uterine cavity, usually in the fallopian tube.

miscarriage A pregnancy that terminates before the 20th week of gestation; also called spontaneous abortion.

rubella An infectious disease that may cause birth defects if contracted by a pregnant woman; also called German measles.

Zika Virus The Zika virus, discussed in Chapter 13, poses a special danger to pregnant women. Health officials are recommending at least 8 weeks of abstinence or contraception for women who or whose partners may have been exposed to the Zika virus (discussed in Chapter 13), regardless of whether they developed any symptoms. This recommendation is based on the length of the time that Zika has been found in blood or semen after infection and the risk of serious birth defects, including microencephaly, a condition characterized by abnormally small head size caused by impaired brain development, prematurity, stillbirths, and blindness.[68]

Genetic Disorders Every individual has an estimated four to six defective genes, but the chances of passing them on to a child are slim. Almost all are recessive, which means they are "masked" by a more influential dominant gene. The likelihood of a child inheriting the same faulty recessive gene from both parents is remote—unless the parents are so closely related that they have very similar genetic makeup.

The child of a parent with an abnormal dominant gene has a 50 percent likelihood of inheriting it. The most common of such defects are minor, such as the growth of an extra finger or toe. However, some single-gene defects can be fatal. Huntington's chorea, for example, is a degenerative disease that in the past was usually not diagnosed until midlife.

A mother's age has long been associated with increased risk of chromosomal disorders such as Down syndrome. More recent research has linked a father's age of 45 or older to several neuropsychiatric disorders, including autism spectrum disorder, attention-deficit/hyperactivity disorder, psychosis, bipolar disorders, and substance use problems.

Preterm Labor Approximately 8 percent of all babies are born too soon (before 37 weeks of pregnancy). The increasing rates of preterm birth worldwide have been linked to hypertension and low levels of maternal education.[69] Prematurity is the main underlying cause of stillbirth and infant deaths within the first few weeks after birth. Bedrest, close monitoring, and, if necessary, medications for at-risk women can buy more time in the womb for their baby. The warning signs of **preterm labor** include a dull, low backache; a feeling of tightness or pressure on the lower abdomen; and intestinal cramps, sometimes with diarrhea.

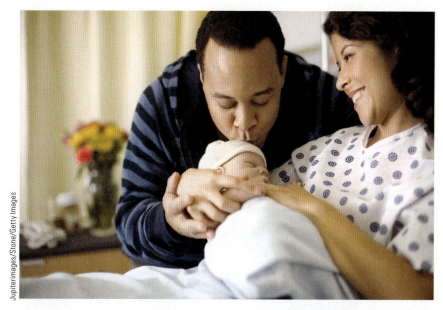

Jupiterimages/Stone/Getty Images

The birth of a child marks a new chapter in the life of a family.

Childbirth

Today, parents can choose from many birthing options, including a birth attendant, who can be a physician or a nurse-midwife, and a birthing center, hospital, or home birth.

Preparing for Childbirth Women who attend prenatal classes are less likely than others to undergo cesarean deliveries and more likely than others to breast feed. They also tend to have fewer complications and require fewer medications. However, painkillers or anesthesia are always an option if labor is longer or more painful than expected. The lower body can be numbed with an *epidural block*, which involves injecting an anesthetic into the membrane around the spinal cord, or a spinal block, in which the injection goes directly into the spinal canal. General anesthesia is often used only for emergency cesarean births.

The American College of Obstetricians and Gynecologists recommends minimal interventions for healthy women in labor, who may not need constant fetal monitoring or continuous intravenous (IV) fluids. They encourage healthcare providers to involve the parents in decisions that may increase a woman's comfort and do not compromise the health of her unborn baby.[70]

Labor and Delivery There are three stages of **labor**. The first starts with *effacement* (thinning) and *dilation* (opening up) of the cervix:

• Effacement is measured in percentages, and dilation in centimeters or finger-widths. Around this time, the amniotic sac of fluids usually breaks, a sign that the woman should call her doctor or midwife.

preterm labor Labor that occurs after the 20th week but before the 37th week of pregnancy.

labor The process leading up to birth: effacement and dilation of the cervix; the movement of the baby into and through the birth canal, accompanied by strong contractions; and contraction of the uterus and expulsion of the placenta after the birth.

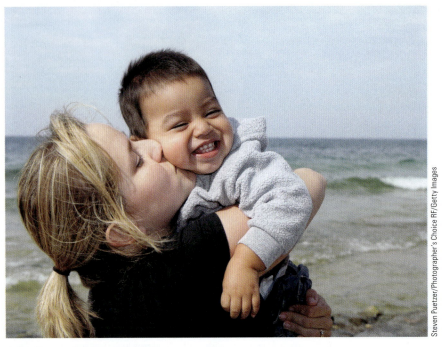

Adoption matches would-be parents yearning for youngsters to love with infants or children who need loving homes.

- The first contractions of the early, or *latent*, phase of labor are usually not uncomfortable; they last 15 to 30 seconds, occur every 15 to 30 minutes, and gradually increase in intensity and frequency.

- The most difficult contractions come after the cervix is dilated to about 8 centimeters, as the woman feels greater pressure from the fetus. The first stage ends when the cervix is completely dilated to a diameter of 10 centimeters (or five finger-widths) and the baby is ready to come down the birth canal. For women having their first baby, this first stage of labor averages 12 to 13 hours. Women having another child often experience shorter first-stage labor.

When the cervix is completely dilated, the second stage of labor occurs:

- The baby moves into the vagina, or birth canal, and out of the mother's body.

- As this stage begins, women who have gone through childbirth preparation training often feel a sense of relief from the acute pain of the transition phase and at the prospect of giving birth.

This second stage can take up to an hour or more. Strong contractions may last 60 to 90 seconds and occur every 2 to 3 minutes. As the baby's head descends, the mother feels an urge to push. By bearing down, she helps the baby complete its passage to the outside:

- As the baby's head appears, or *crowns*, the doctor may perform an *episiotomy*—an incision from the lower end of the vagina toward the anus to enlarge the vaginal opening. The purpose of the episiotomy is to prevent the baby's head from causing an irregular tear in the vagina, but routine episiotomies have been criticized as unnecessary.

- Usually the baby's head emerges first, then its shoulders, then its body. With each contraction, a new part is born. However, the baby can be in a more difficult position, facing up rather than down, or with the feet or buttocks first (a *breech birth*), and a cesarean birth may then be necessary.

In the third stage of labor, the uterus contracts firmly after the birth of the baby:

- Within about 5 minutes, the placenta separates from the uterine wall.

- The woman may bear down to help expel the placenta, or the doctor may exert gentle external pressure.

- If an episiotomy has been performed, the doctor sews up the incision. To help the uterus contract and return to its normal size, it may be massaged manually, or the baby may be put to the mother's breast to stimulate contraction of the uterus.

Cesarean Birth In a **cesarean delivery** (also referred to as a *cesarean section*, or *C-section*), the doctor lifts the baby out of the woman's body through an incision made in the lower abdomen and uterus. The most common reason for cesarean birth is *failure to progress*, a vague term indicating that labor has gone on too long and may put the baby or mother at risk. Other reasons include the baby's position (if feet or buttocks are first) and signs that the fetus is in danger.

Nearly one in three babies is delivered by this method, many in women who had a previous C-section. More than 95 percent are performed because of risk factors complicating labor or delivery.

Infertility

The WHO defines **infertility** as the failure to conceive after 1 year of unprotected intercourse. Infertility affects one in six couples in the United States. Women between ages 35 and 44 are about twice as likely to have fertility problems as women ages 30 to 34. An estimated 12 percent of women between ages 15 and 44 may have impaired fertility; 6.7 percent of married women in this age group are infertile; 12 percent of women have used infertility services.[71]

cesarean delivery A surgical procedure in which an infant is delivered through an incision made in the abdominal wall and uterus.

infertility The inability to conceive a child.

Steven Puetzer/Photographer's Choice RF/Getty Images

Infertility is a problem of the couple, not of the individual man or woman. Male factors are estimated to be involved, at least partially, in half of the cases.[72] In women, the most common causes of subfertility or infertility are age, untreated sexual transmitted diseases, abnormal menstrual patterns, suppression of ovulation, and blocked fallopian tubes.[73] A woman's fertility peaks between ages 20 and 30 and then drops quickly—by 20 percent after 30, by 50 percent after 35, and by 95 percent after 40.

Male subfertility or infertility is usually linked to either the quantity or the quality of sperm, which may be inactive, misshapen, or insufficient (fewer than 20 million sperm per milliliter of semen in an ejaculation of 3 to 5 milliliters).[74] Sometimes the problem is hormonal or a blockage of a sperm duct. Some men suffer from the inability to ejaculate normally, or from retrograde ejaculation, in which some of the semen travels in the wrong direction, back into the body of the male. Lifestyle factors, such as smoking, may also impair fertility.[75]

Infertility can have an enormous emotional impact. Many women yearn to experience pregnancy and childbirth and feel great loss if they cannot conceive. Women in their 30s and 40s fear that their biological clock is running out of time. Men may be confused and surprised by the intensity of their partner's emotions.

Options for Infertile Couples

The odds of successful pregnancy range from 30 to 70 percent, depending on the specific cause of infertility. One result of successful infertility treatments has been a boom in multiple births, including quintuplets and sextuplets.

Artificial Insemination The introduction of viable sperm into the vagina by artificial means, called **artificial insemination**, is used primarily by couples in which the husband is infertile.

Assisted Reproductive Technology An estimated 500,000 babies have been born in the United States through assisted reproductive technology (ART) since 1985. The most common ART procedure is *in vitro fertilization (IVF)*, which removes the ova from a woman's ovary and places the woman's egg and her mate's sperm in a laboratory dish for fertilization. If the fertilized egg cell shows signs of development, within several days it is returned to the woman's uterus,

the egg cell implants itself in the lining of the uterus, and the pregnancy continues as normal. ART accounts for slightly more than 1 percent of total U.S. births. One of the most common complications of ART is the birth of multiples.

✓**check-in** Under what circumstances, if any, might you consider ART?

Transgender Individuals

As discussed in Chapter 8, transgender individuals who do not identify with their biological sex may undergo hormonal and surgical treatment that can affect their fertility. Health-care providers are encouraged to ask individuals considering gender transition about their hopes and plans for children and their options for "fertility preservation." However, the medical community generally has limited knowledge and experience in fertility preservation for transgender men and women.

In some cases, individuals whose biological sex is male continue to manufacture sperm after receiving gender-affirming hormones. Conception and pregnancy also may occur in transgender individuals whose biological sex is female despite testosterone treatments. However, there are few data on these possibilities and their outcomes. Another option for transgender individuals undergoing gender transition is freezing of sperm or eggs for possible use in the future, but cost is often an obstacle.[76]

Adoption

Adoption matches would-be parents yearning for youngsters to love with infants or children who need loving homes. Couples interested in adoption can work with either public agencies or private counselors who contact obstetricians directly. Or they can contact organizations that arrange adoptions of children in need from other countries.

There are no reliable statistics on the annual number of adoptions in the United States, but census records indicate there are currently 1.6 million adopted children in the United States. Each year some 50,000 U.S. children become available for adoption—far fewer than the number of would-be parents looking for youngsters to adopt. An estimated 13 percent of adopted children are foreign born.

artificial insemination The introduction of viable sperm into the vagina by artificial means for the purpose of inducing conception.

adoption The legal process for becoming the parent to a child of other biological parents.

- What do college students need to know about contraception?

- How do you decide on the best birth control method for you and your partner?

- How can you prevent pregnancy after unprotected intercourse or failed birth control?

- What changes do a mother-to-be and her unborn child undergo during pregnancy?

Reflection

Your perspective on fertility—the ability to conceive new life—depends on many factors, including your age, sex, sexual orientation, beliefs, and values. Reflect on what fertility means to you and what impact it may have on your future.

TAKING CHARGE OF YOUR HEALTH

Protecting Your Reproductive Health

The decisions you make about birth control can affect your reproductive health—and your partner's. Here are guidelines that can help prevent pregnancy and protect your reproductive well-being. Check those that you have used or think you will use in the future.

_____ **Abstinence.** The only 100 percent safe and effective way to avoid unwanted pregnancy is not to engage in heterosexual intercourse.

_____ **Limiting sexual activity to outercourse or oral sex.** You can engage in many sexual activities—kissing, hugging, touching, massage, oral–genital sex—without risking pregnancy.

_____ **Talking about birth control with any potential sex partner.** If you are considering sexual intimacy with a person, you should feel comfortable enough to talk about contraception.

_____ **Knowing what doesn't work—and not relying on it.** There are many misconceptions about ways to avoid getting pregnant, such as having sex in a standing position or during menstruation. Only the methods described in this chapter are reliable forms of birth control.

_____ **Talking with a health-care professional.** A great deal of information and advice is available—in writing, from family planning counselors, and from physicians on the Internet. Check it out.

_____ **Choosing a contraceptive method that matches your personal habits and preferences.** If you can't remember to take a pill every day, oral contraceptives aren't for you. If you're constantly forgetting where you put things, a diaphragm might not be a good choice.

_____ **Considering long-term implications.** Since you may well wish to have children in the future, find out about the reversibility of various methods and possible effects on future fertility.

_____ **Resisting having sex without contraceptive protection "just this once."** It only takes once—even the very first time—to get pregnant. Be wary of drugs and alcohol. They can impair your judgment and make you less conscientious about using birth control—or using it properly.

_____ **Using backup methods.** If there's a possibility that a contraceptive method might not offer adequate protection (for instance, if it's been almost 3 months since your last injection of Depo-Provera), use an additional form of birth control.

_____ **Informing yourself about emergency contraception.** Just in case a condom breaks or a diaphragm slips, find out about the availability of forms of after-intercourse contraception.

SELF-SURVEY

Which Contraceptive Method Is Best for You?

Answer Yes or No to each statement as it applies to you and, if appropriate, your partner.

1. You have high blood pressure or cardiovascular disease.

2. You smoke cigarettes.

3. You have a new sexual partner.

4. An unwanted pregnancy would be devastating to you.

5. You have a good memory.

6. You or your partner have multiple sexual partners.

7. You prefer a method with little or no bother.

8. You have heavy, crampy periods.

9. You need protection against STIs.

10. You are concerned about endometrial and ovarian cancer.

11. You are forgetful.

12. You need a method right away.

13. You're comfortable touching your own and your partner's genitals.

14. You have a cooperative partner.

15. You like a little extra vaginal lubrication.

16. You have sex at unpredictable times and places.

17. You are in a monogamous relationship and have at least one child.

Scoring:

Recommendations are based on Yes answers to the following numbered statements:

The combination pill: 4, 5, 6, 8, 10, 16

The progestin-only pill: 1, 2, 5, 7, 16

The patch: 4, 7, 8, 11, 16

The NuvaRing: 4, 7, 8, 11, 13, 16

Condoms: 1, 2, 3, 6, 9, 12, 13, 14

Depo-Provera: 1, 2, 4, 7, 11, 16

Diaphragm, cervical cap, or FemCap: 1, 2, 13, 14

Mirena IUD: 1, 2, 7, 8, 11, 13, 16, 17

Spermicides: 1, 2, 12, 13, 14, 15

Sponge: 1, 2, 12, 13

REVIEW QUESTIONS

(LO 9.1) 1. Fusion of a sperm with the nucleus of an egg is known as _____.
a. ejaculation
b. fertilization
c. ovulation
d. implantation

(LO 9.1) 2. A fertilized egg is called a(n) _____.
a. zygote
b. blastocyst
c. fetus
d. ovary

(LO 9.2) 3. Which of the following is a common reason that people choose abstinence?
a. Avoiding having to break up with their partner.
b. Messages from the media.
c. Conformity with their peers.
d. Fear of contracting an STI.

(LO 9.3) 4. Which of the following is true about the use of contraceptives?
a. Progestin checks depression in women.
b. Birth control pills may increase the risk of heart attacks.
c. Antiseizure medications slow down the liver metabolism of birth control pills.
d. Birth control injections prevent the occurrence of strokes.

(LO 9.4) 5. Which of the following is an advantage of using a condom?
a. It allows for sexual spontaneity.
b. It is 100 percent effective in preventing STIs and pregnancies.

c. It increases penile sensitivity.
d. It is inexpensive.

(LO 9.5) 6. The most effective contraceptives for preventing pregnancy are _____.
a. digital birth control/fertility awareness method
b. condoms
c. sponges
d. hormonal methods

(LO 9.5) 7. Which of the following is one of the benefits of hormonal contraceptives beyond birth control?
a. Weight loss
b. Decreased depression
c. Improved bone density
d. Increased sex drive

(LO 9.6) 8. What is a disadvantage to digital birth control?
a. The rhythm method is more effective than using an app.
b. They have difficult side effects.
c. They use hormones.
d. Seven out of every 100 women relying on the temperature monitoring app will get pregnant in the course of a year.

(LO 9.7) 9. Which of the following is true of the use of emergency contraception (EC)?
a. Awareness of EC methods remains limited.
b. Access to EC has been shown to increase sexual risk-taking.
c. EC pills contain different hormones from regular birth control.
d. Only women who can safely use hormonal contraceptives can use EC.

10. Which of the following is one of the disadvantages of sterilization?
a. It can affect sex drive.
b. It does not protect against STIs.
c. The effects are often not permanent.
d. It sometimes leads to hormonal imbalances.

(LO 9.10) 11. Which of the following is true of the circumstances of unwanted pregnancies?
a. Women faced with an unwanted pregnancy are often happily married.
b. Minority women generally feel less cultural pressure to keep the child.
c. Women faced with an unwanted pregnancy are often alone.
d. The number of would-be adoptive parents is less than the number of children available for adoption, so adoption is an unfavorable option.

(LO 9.11) 12. In the context of the psychological impact of abortion, which of the following statements is true?
a. The primary emotion of women following an abortion is stress.
b. Women generally do not express feelings of guilt following an abortion.
c. Women who were raped tend to have high anxiety levels following an abortion.
d. Research has documented no link between abortion and long-term depression or anxiety.

(LO 9.12) 13. _____ is defined as the failure to conceive after one year of unprotected intercourse
a. Sterilization
b. Infertility
c. Miscarriage
d. Abortion

(LO 9.12) 14. In vitro fertilization refers to _____.
a. a surgical technique to prevent conception
b. an assisted reproductive technology
c. natural conception
d. a procedure to overcome male infertility

Answers to these questions can be found on page 531.

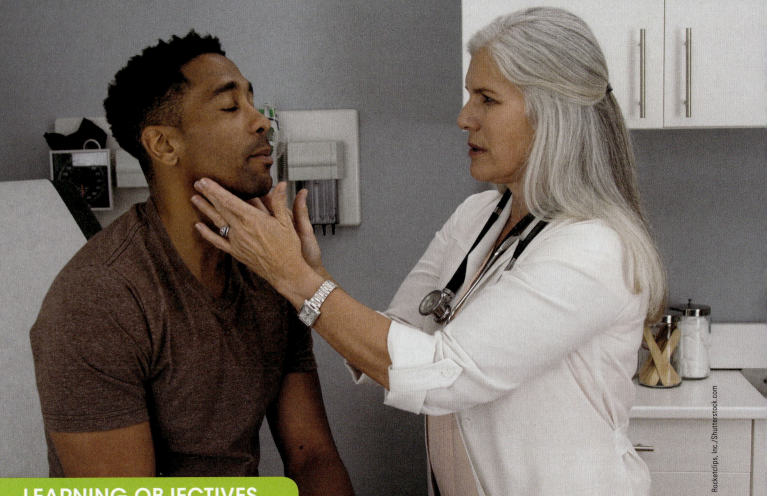

Rocketclips, Inc./Shutterstock.com

After reading this chapter, you should be able to:

10.1 List the risk factors for cardiovascular diseases.

10.2 Summarize the risks and signs of metabolic syndrome and diabetes.

10.3 Discuss the risk factors and management of hypertension and high blood cholesterol.

10.4 Explain the patterns and consequences of cardiovascular diseases.

10.5 Identify the risk factors and common causes of strokes.

10.6 Outline the risk factors for cancer.

10.7 Review the signs, causes, and treatments of common types of cancer.

10.8 Describe the agents of infection and their effects on human health.

WHAT DO YOU THINK?

- Do college students need to think about their risk for major diseases?
- What behaviors can you change to protect your cardiometabolic health?
- What steps are you taking to prevent cancer?
- What do you see as the greatest infectious threats to your health?

10

Diseases and Disorders

"**W**hat did your great-great-grandparents die of?"

Like many of the other students in her Personal Health class, Serena didn't know the answer to her teacher's question.

"Probably an infectious disease," she guessed—with good reason. At the turn of the twentieth century, the major killers of Americans were two deadly infections: tuberculosis and pneumonia.

By 1925, diseases of the heart had become the number one cause of death in the United States, followed by pneumonia and influenza. By the 1940s, cancer had edged out

pneumonia for the dubious distinction of being the nation's second most lethal disease. Today, heart disease and cancer account for nearly half of all deaths in the United States.[1]

Serena's family followed this pattern. Heart disease killed her great-grandfather; a series of strokes led to her great-grandmother's death. Her grandparents are still alive, but Serena worries about their health. Her grandfather has undergone bypass surgery for blocked arteries in his heart. Her grandmother is a breast cancer survivor. <

✓**check-in** Which of the American Heart Association's recommended steps are you taking to safeguard your well-being?

____ Get moving. As research has confirmed, being sedentary may be twice as deadly as being obese.[2] The good news: Increased physical activity, especially vigorous exercise, reduces cardiovascular risks in the young, starting in adolescence.[3] (See Chapter 6.)

____ Eat healthfully. Diets lower in saturated and trans fats, sugar-sweetened drinks, and red or processed meats and

higher in fiber, nuts, coffee, and polyunsaturated fats (all discussed in Chapter 5) significantly reduce the risk of type 2 diabetes as well as heart disease and stroke.[4]

____ Maintain a healthy weight. General obesity increases the risk of cardiovascular disease and diabetes, while abdominal obesity increases the danger of dying of all causes, including cardiovascular illness and cancer.[5]

____ Control blood sugar. As long-term follow-up studies have shown, diabetics who intensively control their blood glucose early in their disease live longer than those who do not.[6]

____ Control cholesterol. The sooner that blood fat levels rise and the longer they remain elevated, the greater the danger to your health.[7]

____ Stop smoking. Death rates among current smokers are two to three times as high as those of people who never smoked. (See Chapter 13.)

Men and women who adopt these healthy habits early in life enjoy longer lives, higher quality of life, and greater mobility and functioning as they age.[8]

Your Cardiometabolic Health

Medical science has increasingly focused on the complex connections between various risk factors, symptoms, and diseases. Physical inactivity, for instance, increases the likelihood of obesity, which in turn leads to greater risk of many diseases. This awareness has led to a focus on **cardiometabolic** health. "Cardio" refers to the heart and blood vessels of the cardiovascular system; "metabolic" refers to the biochemical processes involved in the body's functioning.

Every day more than 2,200 Americans die of cardiovascular diseases—an average of one death every 39 seconds. Cardiovascular diseases (all diseases of the heart and blood vessels) account for one of every three deaths, including an increasing number among younger adults ages 35 to 54. Medical scientists fear that the obesity epidemic and the rise in metabolic disorders may be responsible.

Only about half of young Americans get passing grades for heart-healthy behaviors. Fewer than 1 percent eat "ideal" diets; about one-third have high body mass indexes (BMIs) (discussed in Chapter 5), and one-third have unfavorable cholesterol readings.[9] Unhealthy habits in youth, such as drinking sugary beverages, not only increase the odds of disease in

old age but also lower the likelihood of surviving to age 55.[10]

The opposite is also true: For individuals who reach age 55 with low blood pressure and cholesterol levels, do not smoke, and are not diabetic, the risk for heart disease or a heart attack is significantly lower than for those with two or more risk factors.

Cardiometabolic Risk Factors

Specific risk factors determine your cardiometabolic health. Once you understand your risk, you can start making changes to lower your odds of developing metabolic syndrome, diabetes, and heart disease (see Health on a Budget).

✓check-in Are you "metabolically unhealthy"? You are if you have two or more of the following risk factors:

____ High cholesterol

____ High blood pressure

____ High blood sugar levels

____ Elevated triglycerides

____ Insulin resistance

____ High C-reactive protein

Risk Factors You Can Control

The choices you make and the habits you follow can have a significant impact on whether you remain healthy. For the sake of your cardiometabolic health, avoid the following potential risks.

Overweight/Obesity Excess weight, an increasingly common and dangerous cardiometabolic risk factor in both men and women, undermines good health:

- The higher your body mass index (BMI) during adolescence, the greater your risk of type 2 diabetes and heart disease in the future. Even teens with a BMI in the high "normal" range face an increased likelihood of health problems.

- Overweight and obese individuals are more likely to have additional risk factors for cardiovascular disease, including physical inactivity, hypertension, high cholesterol, and diabetes mellitus.

- Overweight teens who lose weight and keep their BMI within a healthy range as adults can eliminate the danger of diabetes, but being obese at any age endangers cardiovascular health.

cardiometabolic Referring to the heart and to the biochemical processes involved in the body's functioning.

$ HEALTH ON A BUDGET

Lowering Your Cardiometabolic Risks

Yes, advances in treatment can help if you eventually develop a cardiometabolic condition. But changes in lifestyle can do even more. To make healthy changes, consider these behavioral modifications that require little or no expense.

Changes You Can Make Today

- Eat a good breakfast: whole-grain cereal, juice, yogurt, and so forth.
- Take a walk after lunch.
- Skip dessert at dinner.
- Eat one more serving of vegetables.
- Eat one more piece of fruit.
- Drink one more glass of water.
- Take the stairs for one or two flights rather than ride the elevator in your dorm or classroom building.
- Get 7 to 8 hours of sleep tonight.
- Don't smoke.

Changes You Can Make This Term

- **Block out time for exercise on your calendar.** Try for at least 30 minutes of physical activity most days.
- **If you haven't had your lipoproteins checked within the past year, schedule a test.**
- **If you don't know your blood pressure, find out what it is.**
- **Make a list of stress-reducing activities, such as meditation or listening to music.** Select two or three to try every week.
- **Learn your family history.** If you've inherited a predisposition to high blood pressure, diabetes, or heart disease, you need extra preventive care.
- **Develop and use a support system of friends and family members.** Identify individuals you can talk to, work out with, or call.

✓**check-in** Is your weight increasing your risk of cardiometabolic disorders?

Body Fat Apple-shaped people who carry most of their excess weight around their waists are at greater risk of cardiometabolic conditions than are pear-shaped individuals who carry most of their excess weight below their waist. The more visceral (abdominal) fat that you have, the more resistant your body's cells become to the effects of your own insulin. However, as newer research suggests, fat alone, regardless of where it is stored, boosts the likelihood of heart attack or stroke. Subcutaneous fat (located under the skin) as well as visceral fat can pose dangers to cardiometabolic health.[11]

Waist Circumference A measurement of more than 40 inches in men and more than 35 inches in women indicates increased health risks.[12] A "pot belly" raises risk even when a person's weight is normal. Rather than waist circumference alone, the ratio of waist to height may be a more precise indicator of risk (see Chapter 5). Among college students, the ratio of muscle mass to visceral fat is a significant predictor of metabolic syndrome. The lower an individual's muscle mass and physical fitness, the greater the risk.[13]

✓**check-in** Do you know your waist measurement? Does it indicate increased risk?

Physical Inactivity As discussed in Chapter 6, about one-quarter of U.S. adults are sedentary and another third are not active enough to reach a healthy level of fitness. Among young people, physical activity—or inactivity—is the most influential factor in cardiometabolic health.[14] One significant culprit: smartphones. In a study of adults between the ages of 18 and 89, cell phone use (an average of 239 minutes a day) contributed to sedentary behavior and physical inactivity.[15] Simply replacing sedentary time with physical activity, whether light, moderate, or vigorous, has been shown to improve cardiometabolic health 10 years later.[16]

The greater the exercise "dose," the more benefits it yields. In studies that compare individuals of different fitness levels, the least fit are at much greater risk of dying than the fittest. In men, more rigorous exercise, such as jogging, produces greater protection against heart disease and boosts longevity. High-intensity interval training improves metabolic control and provides significant cardiovascular benefits.[17]

✓**check-in** Did you know that the World Health Organization estimates that 3.2 million people around the globe die each year because they are not active enough?

Too Much Sitting, Not Enough Sleep

Defined as being seated from 8 to 12 hours a

day, prolonged sitting significantly increases the odds of heart disease, diabetes, cancer, and death, according to an analysis of about four dozen studies of the impact of inactivity.[18] To prevent these problems, take a 3-minute break every 30 minutes to stand, lift, or extend your legs, stretch your arms overhead, twist your torso side to side, lunge to the back or side, or walk in place.

The quantity and quality of your time in bed also matters. In a study of healthy young adults, ages 21 to 35, sleep disturbances—including getting less than 6 hours of total sleep time and waking for more than 60 minutes after sleep onset—increased the risk factors for metabolic syndrome.[19]

Healthy Diet

As research has consistently confirmed, closely following the Mediterranean diet—high in fresh fruits and vegetables, whole grains, beans, nuts, fish, and olive oil—can reduce the risk of heart disease by almost half. Additional benefits include weight loss, lower blood pressure and cholesterol levels, and a lower risk of diabetes.[20] Even a single meal can trigger metabolic changes that lower the risk of cardiometabolic diseases.[21]

"Problematic" eating behaviors and attitudes, such as binge-eating, among young adults (ages 27–41) increase the risk of metabolic syndrome and diabetes.[22] According to the most recent research, vitamin D supplements do not prevent or lower the risk of cardiovascular disease or cancer.[23] Fish oil supplements also do not protect against these diseases.[24]

Tobacco Use

Chapter 13 provides compressive coverage of smoking's harmful effects, but here are some key facts to keep in mind

- Each year smoking causes more than 250,000 deaths from cardiovascular disease—far more than it causes from cancer and lung disease.

- Smokers who have heart attacks are more likely to die from them than are nonsmokers.

- Smoking is the major risk factor for peripheral arterial disease, in which the vessels that carry blood to the leg and arm muscles become hardened and clogged.

- Both active and passive smoking accelerate the process by which arteries become clogged and increase the risk of heart attack and stroke.

✓**check-in** Is active or passive smoking putting you at risk?

systolic blood pressure
Highest blood pressure, which occurs when the heart contracts.

diastolic blood pressure
Lowest blood pressure, which occurs between contractions of the heart.

hypertension High blood pressure that occurs when the blood exerts excessive pressure against the arterial walls.

High Blood Glucose

Your stomach and digestive system break down the food you eat into glucose, a type of sugar. The hormone insulin acts like a key, letting glucose into cells and providing energy. "Insulin-resistant" cells no longer respond well to insulin, and so glucose, unable to enter the cells, builds up in the bloodstream.

Frequent thirst, blurry vision, weakness, unexplained weight loss, and unusual hunger can be signs of high blood glucose. A simple blood test will tell you if your glucose levels are too high. Here is what the readings mean:

Healthy blood glucose	Under 100
Prediabetes	100–125
Diabetes	More than 125

✓**check-in** Have you ever had your blood glucose level tested? If so, what was it?

High Blood Pressure (Hypertension)

Blood pressure is a result of the contractions of the heart muscle, which pumps blood through your body, and the resistance of the walls of the vessels through which the blood flows. Each time your heart beats, your blood pressure goes up and down within a certain range:

- It is highest when the heart contracts; this is called **systolic blood pressure**.

- It is lowest between contractions; this is called **diastolic blood pressure**.

- A blood pressure reading consists of the systolic measurement "over" the diastolic measurement, recorded in millimeters of mercury (mmHg).

- High blood pressure, or **hypertension**, occurs when the artery walls become constricted so that the force exerted as the blood flows through them is greater than it should be. Physicians see blood pressure as a continuum: The higher the reading, the greater the risk of stroke and heart disease.

- In studies of young adults ages 18 to 40, elevated blood pressure predicted hypertension and other metabolic abnormalities later in life.[25]

As a result of increased effort in pumping blood, the heart muscle of a person with hypertension can become stiffer. This stiffness increases resistance to filling up with blood between beats, which can cause the following:

- Shortness of breath with exertion.

- Damage to the arteries in the kidneys, which can lead to kidney failure.

- Accelerated development of plaque buildup in the arteries.

✓**check-in** What's your blood pressure reading?

Lipoprotein Levels   **Cholesterol** is a fatty substance found in certain foods and is also manufactured by the body. Figure 10.1 shows food sources of cholesterol. The measurement of cholesterol in the blood is one of the most reliable indicators of the formation of plaque, the sludge-like substance that builds up on the inner walls of arteries. You can lower blood cholesterol levels by cutting back on high-fat foods and exercising more, thereby reducing the risk of a heart attack.

Lipoproteins are compounds in the blood that are made up of proteins and fat. The different types are classified by their size or density. The heaviest are *high-density lipoproteins*, or HDLs, which have the highest proportion of protein. These "good guys," as some cardiologists refer to them, pick up excess cholesterol in the blood and carry it back to the liver for removal from the body. An HDL level of 40 mg/dL or lower substantially increases the risk of heart disease. (Cholesterol levels are measured in milligrams of cholesterol per deciliter of blood [mg/dL].) The average HDL for men is about 45 mg/dL; for women, it is about 55 mg/dL.

Low-density lipoproteins (LDLs), and very low-density lipoproteins (VLDLs) carry more cholesterol than HDLs and deposit it on the walls of arteries—they're the "bad guys." The higher your LDL cholesterol, the greater your risk for heart disease. If you are at high risk of heart disease, any level of LDL higher than 100 mg/dL may increase your danger.

Triglycerides are fats that flow through the blood after meals and have been linked to increased risk of coronary artery disease, especially in women.[26] Triglyceride levels tend to be highest in those whose diets are high in calories, sugar, alcohol, and refined starches. High levels of these fats may increase the risk of obesity, and cutting back on these foods can reduce high triglyceride levels. In assessing an individual's risks, cardiologists consider not just the levels of various blood fats, but also their ratios and associations.[27]

✓**Check-in** Have you ever had your lipoproteins measured?

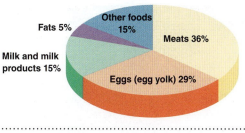

FIGURE 10.1 Cholesterol in Our Food

Percentages indicate the proportion of cholesterol each type of food contributes to the diet.

Risk Factors You Can't Control

Family History   Certain cardiometabolic risk factors, such as abnormally high blood levels of lipids, can be passed down from generation to generation. Individuals with an inherited vulnerability can lower the danger by changing the risk factors within their control, such as body weight and fat.

Race and Ethnicity   Cardiometabolic risk factors occur at increased rates and increase mortality rates among ethnic minority populations such as African Americans, Hispanic Americans, and Native Americans.[28] Here are some examples:

- Blacks and Hispanics have double the rates of diabetes as whites.

- The incidence of diabetes is even higher among American Indians. Among the Pima Indians of Arizona, half of all adults have type 2 diabetes, one of the highest rates of diabetes in the world.

- Mexican Americans are likely to have heart-damaging risk factors such as high blood pressure and high blood sugar levels, even if they are not obese.[29]

- Nearly 4 in every 10 black adults have cardiovascular disease.

- Among Hispanic Americans, nearly 3 in 10 have cardiovascular disease.

- African Americans are twice as likely to develop high blood pressure as whites and suffer strokes at an earlier age and of greater severity.

- Black women are twice as likely as white women to suffer heart attacks and to die from heart disease. They are also less likely to receive common medications, such as cholesterol-lowering drugs, to lower their risk.

Socioeconomic Status   Poverty in childhood and young adulthood can contribute to

cholesterol An organic substance found in animal fats; it is linked to cardiovascular disease, particularly atherosclerosis.

lipoproteins Compounds in blood that are made up of proteins and fat; high-density lipoproteins (HDL) pick up excess cholesterol in the blood; low-density lipoproteins (LDL) carry more cholesterol and deposit it on the walls of arteries.

triglycerides Fats that flow through the blood after meals and are linked to increased risk of coronary artery disease.

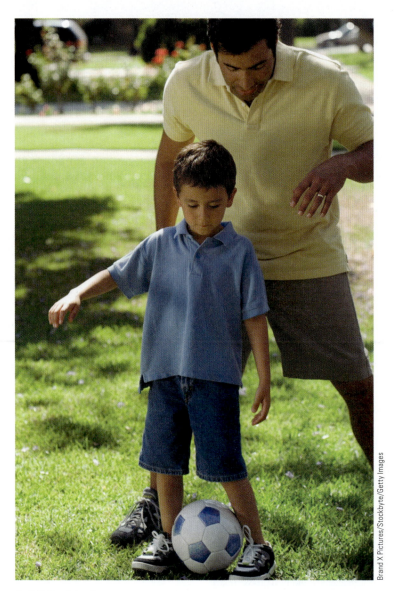
Brand X Pictures/Stockbyte/Getty Images

A child's risk of developing heart disease later in life depends on many factors, including family history, diet, and physical activity.

metabolic syndrome A cluster of disorders of the body's metabolism that make diabetes, heart disease, or stroke more likely.

increased cardiometabolic risk, in part because families with low incomes are less likely to receive medical treatments or undergo corrective surgery.[30]

Age Cardiometabolic risk factors increase as people get older, especially past age 45. This may be because many individuals tend to exercise less, lose muscle mass, and gain weight as they age.

Height Shorter men are more likely to develop cardiovascular disease, regardless of their smoking status, blood pressure, body mass index, blood fats, alcohol consumption, education level, or occupation. Every extra 2.5 inches of height brings a 13.5 percent reduction in heart disease risk Researchers theorize that the same gene variations that

determine height may also affect the likelihood of atherosclerosis.

Metabolic Syndrome

Metabolic syndrome, once called Syndrome X, or insulin-resistance syndrome, is not a disease but a cluster of disorders of the body's metabolism—including high blood pressure, high insulin levels, abdominal obesity, and abnormal cholesterol levels—that make a person more likely to develop diabetes, heart disease, or stroke. Each of these conditions is by itself a risk factor for other diseases. In combination, they dramatically boost the chances of potentially life-threatening illnesses.

Who Is at Risk?

The national prevalence of metabolic syndrome has fallen, particularly among teenagers who have lower levels of triglycerides (blood fats are discussed on page 312) and higher levels of "good" HDL cholesterol. However, teen obesity has risen.[31] Researchers have targeted sugary beverages as contributors to weight and metabolic problems by leading to unhealthy waist circumference, blood glucose, and dietary patterns.[32]

What Are the Signs?

Three or more of the following characteristics indicate metabolic syndrome:

- **A larger-than-normal waist measurement:** 40 inches or more in men and 35 inches or more in women (for Asians and individuals with a genetic predisposition to diabetes, 37 to 39 inches in men and 31 to 35 inches in women).

- **A higher-than-normal triglyceride level:** 150 mg/dL or more.

- **A lower-than-normal high-density lipoprotein (HDL) level:** Less than 40 mg/dL in men or 50 mg/dL in women.

- **A higher-than-normal blood pressure:** 130 mmHg systole over 85 mmHg diastole (130/85) or higher.

- **A higher-than-normal fasting blood sugar:** 110 mg/dL or higher.

Compared with people with no factors of metabolic syndrome, those with three factors are nearly twice as likely to have a heart attack or stroke and more than three times likely to develop heart disease. Men with four or five characteristics of the syndrome have nearly four times the risk of heart attack or stroke and more than 24 times the risk of diabetes. Young adults with metabolic syndrome are more likely than others their age to have thicker neck arteries, an indicator of atherosclerosis, the buildup of fatty plaques in arteries.

✓**check-in** Do you have any risk factors for metabolic syndrome?

College-age men and women who maintain their weights as they get older are much less likely to develop metabolic syndrome. Among those who are obese, losing 7 to 10 percent of their body weight may reverse the symptoms of metabolic syndrome.

Diabetes

Glucose is the primary form of sugar that body cells use for energy. When a person without diabetes eats a meal, the level of glucose in the blood rises, triggering the production and release of insulin by special cell clusters in the pancreas.

Insulin enhances the movement of glucose into various body cells, bringing down the level of glucose in the blood.

In those who have diabetes, however, insulin secretion is either nonexistent or deficient. Without sufficient insulin, the glucose in the blood is unable to enter most body cells, so the energy needs of the cells aren't met. The levels of glucose in the blood rise higher and higher after each meal. This unused glucose eventually passes through the kidneys, which are unable to process the excessive glucose, and out of the body in urine.

Deprived of the fuel it needs, the body begins to break down stored fat as a source of energy. This process produces weak acids, called ketones. A buildup of ketones leads to ketoacidosis, an upheaval in the body's chemical balance that brings on nausea, vomiting, abdominal pain, lethargy, and drowsiness. Severe ketoacidosis can lead to coma and, eventually, death (see Figure 10.2).

An estimated 29 million Americans—almost 1 in 10—have diabetes. The Centers for Disease Control and Prevention (CDC) projects that up to one-third of Americans could have diabetes by 2050 if they continue to gain weight and avoid exercise.

The rate of diabetes is much higher in 15 states, mostly in the South. People living in this so-called diabetes belt are more likely to be obese, sedentary, and less educated than in the country as a whole. Certain racial and ethnic minorities—American Indians/Alaska Natives, African Americans, and

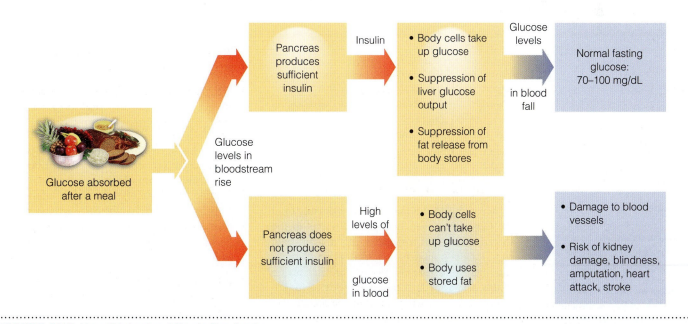

FIGURE 10.2 How Diabetes Affects the Body
Diabetes affects almost every organ system of the body in complex and often subtle ways.

Hispanic American—around the country also have higher rates of diabetes.

Before the development of insulin injections, diabetes was a fatal illness. Today, diabetics can have normal lifespans. However, diabetes still can lead to devastating complications. Uncontrolled glucose levels slowly damage blood vessels throughout the body; thus, individuals who become diabetic early in life may face major complications even before they reach middle age. Diabetes is the number one cause of blindness, nontraumatic amputations, and kidney failure, and diabetes increases by two or three times the risk of heart attack or stroke.

Insulin Resistance

In a healthy body, the digestive system breaks down food into glucose, which then travels in the bloodstream to cells throughout the body. As blood glucose rises after a meal, the pancreas releases insulin to help cells take in the glucose. As noted earlier, **insulin resistance** is a condition in which the body produces insulin but does not use it properly.

When muscle, fat, and liver cells do not respond properly to insulin, the pancreas tries to keep up with the increased demand for insulin by producing more, but eventually it cannot. Excess glucose builds up in the bloodstream, setting the stage for diabetes. Many people with insulin resistance have high levels of both glucose and insulin circulating in their blood at the same time. Excess weight, particularly in men, and lack of physical activity, along with genetic factors, contribute to insulin resistance.

Prediabetes

Sometimes called impaired fasting glucose, impaired glucose tolerance, or intermediate hyperglycemia, **prediabetes** is a condition in which blood glucose levels are higher than normal but not high enough for a diagnosis of diabetes.[33] There is no standard definition of prediabetes, and many individuals told that they are prediabetic do not develop diabetes over time.[34]

According to the most recent estimates from the CDC, more than one-third of adults in the United States—an estimated 79 million men and women—could be assessed as prediabetic, although more than 90 percent are not aware of this risk. They face increased odds of cardiovascular events, such as heart attack and stroke, although regular exercise (Chapter 6) and the Mediterranean diet (Chapter 5) can lower the likelihood of developing diabetes.

One way to reduce this risk is by walking. Adding 2,000 steps more per day could lower the risk for heart disease in subsequent years by 10 percent.

✓**check-in** Have you ever had your blood glucose tested?

Diabetes Mellitus

In those with **diabetes mellitus**, the pancreas, which produces insulin (the hormone that regulates carbohydrate and fat metabolism), doesn't function as it should. When the pancreas either stops producing insulin or doesn't produce sufficient insulin to meet the body's needs, almost every body system can be damaged (see Figure 10.2).

✓**check-in** Does anyone in your family have diabetes?

Diabetes mellitus, the seventh-leading cause of death in the United States, can shorten life expectancy by a decade or more. The risk of premature death among people with diabetes is about twice that of people without the disease. Obesity, diabetes, and heart disease can also work together to speed dementia and other brain disorders, such as cognitive impairment.

Who Is at Risk?

Several factors—some of which you can control—increase your risk for prediabetes and diabetes.

- Being overweight or obese is the strongest predictor of undiagnosed type 2 diabetes.[35]

- Age 60 or older.

- Physically inactive.

- Parent or sibling with diabetes.

- Family background that is African American, Alaska Native, American Indian, Asian American, Hispanic/Latino, or Pacific Islander. Asian Americans start developing diabetes at lower weights. The reason may be that Asian Americans tend to deposit "visceral" fat around their internal organs, which increases the risk of insulin resistance, a precursor to type 2 diabetes. The American Diabetes Association recommends that Asian Americans with a body mass index (BMI) of 23 or higher, rather than the 25 used for other races, undergo screening for type 2 diabetes.

insulin resistance A condition in which the body produces insulin but does not use it properly.

prediabetes A condition in which blood glucose levels are higher than normal but not high enough for a diagnosis of diabetes.

diabetes mellitus A disease in which the inadequate production of insulin leads to failure of the body tissues to break down carbohydrates at a normal rate.

- Sitting—the more time that individuals spend on a chair or sofa, the greater their odds of developing high blood sugar.

- Exercising fewer than three times a week.

- Giving birth to a baby weighing more than 9 pounds or being diagnosed with diabetes during pregnancy.

- High blood pressure—140/90 mmHg or above—or being treated for high blood pressure.

- HDL, or "good," cholesterol level below 35 mg/dL or a triglyceride level above 250 mg/dL.

- Impaired fasting glucose (IFG) or impaired glucose tolerance (IGT) on previous testing.

- Other conditions associated with insulin resistance, such as severe obesity.

- History of cardiovascular disease.

- Sugary drinks—even a single can of sugary soda a day can increase the risk of prediabetes and diabetes.

- Certain common medications, including antibiotics such as penicillin and cholesterol-lowering statin drugs, may increase the risk of type 2 diabetes.

Types of Diabetes

Diabetes includes several conditions in which the body has difficulty controlling levels of glucose in the bloodstream. After an overnight fast, most people have blood glucose levels between 70 and 100 mg/dL. This is considered normal. If your fasting blood glucose level is between 101 and 125 mg/dL, you have prediabetes. If your fasting blood glucose is consistently 126 mg/dL or higher, you have diabetes. There are three types of diabetes: type 1 diabetes, type 2 diabetes, and gestational diabetes.[36]

Type 1 Diabetes In this form of diabetes (once called juvenile-onset or insulin-dependent diabetes), the body's immune system attacks the insulin-producing beta cells in the pancreas and destroys them. The pancreas then produces little or no insulin, and therefore blood glucose cannot enter the cells to be used for energy.

Type 1 diabetes develops most often in young people but can appear in adults. People with type 1 diabetes lose an average of 11 years for men and 13 years for women to the chronic disease, compared to those without diabetes. The largest single cause of lost years is the impact diabetes has on the heart. However, type 1 diabetics under age 50 also die because of conditions related to management of their disease, such as a diabetic coma triggered by low blood sugar.[37] Women with type 1 diabetes have a nearly 40 percent greater risk of dying from any cause and more than double the risk of dying from heart disease than men with type 1 diabetes. The reason may be that high levels of blood sugar may cause more damage to women's blood vessels than to men's.

Individuals with type 1 diabetes require insulin therapy because their own bodies no longer supply this vital hormone. As long-term follow-up studies have shown, people with type 1 diabetes who intensively control their blood glucose early in their disease are likely to live longer than those who do not.

Type 2 Diabetes In type 2 diabetes (once called adult-onset or non-insulin-dependent diabetes), either the pancreas does not make enough insulin or the body is unable to use insulin correctly. Type 2 diabetes, which affects 90 to 95 percent of diabetics, is becoming more common in children and teenagers because of the increase in obesity in the young.

Although type 1 and type 2 diabetes have different causes, two factors are important in both: an inherited predisposition to the disease and something in the environment that triggers diabetes. Genes alone are not enough. In most cases of type 1 diabetes, people need to inherit risk factors from both parents and to experience some environmental trigger, which might involve prenatal nutrition, a virus, or an unknown agent.

In type 2 diabetes, family history is one of the strongest risk factors for getting the disease, but only in Westernized countries. African Americans, Mexican Americans, and Native Americans have the highest rates, but people who live in less developed nations tend not to get type 2 diabetes, no matter how high their genetic risk.

Excess weight, especially around the waistline, is the major and most controllable risk factor for type 2 diabetes. Losing weight greatly reduces this risk and, in individuals with the disease, can help get blood sugar under control.[38]

Gestational Diabetes Women who get diabetes while they are pregnant are more likely to have a family history of diabetes, especially on their mothers' side; they are at increased risk of developing diabetes later in life. Children of mothers who develop gestational diabetes early in pregnancy may be at increased risk for autism spectrum disorders (discussed in Chapter 3). Early screening and good control of glucose levels during pregnancy may reduce this risk.

Detecting Diabetes To identify individuals with this disease as early as possible, the American Diabetes Association recommends screening every 3 years for all men and women beginning at age 45. The American College of Endocrinology recommends screening at age 30 for individuals at risk, including those who are overweight, are sedentary, have a family history of diabetes, or have high blood pressure or heart disease.

Tests that can detect diabetes include:

- **Random blood sugar test.** Because you don't necessarily fast for this test, your blood glucose may be high because you've just eaten. Even so, it shouldn't be higher than 200 mg/dL.

- **Fasting blood glucose test.** In general, glucose is lowest after an overnight fast. That's why the preferred way to test your blood sugar is after you've fasted overnight or for at least 8 hours.

- **Glucose challenge test.** Often used to screen pregnant women for gestational diabetes, this test measures glucose before drinking 8 ounces of an extremely sweet liquid after fasting for 6 hours, then every hour for a 3-hour period. If your blood sugar rises more than expected and doesn't return to normal by the third hour, you likely have diabetes.

Diabetes Signs and Symptoms About one-third of individuals with type 2 diabetes do not realize they have the illness. If you have risk factors for the disease, watch for the following warning signs:

- **Increased thirst and frequent urination.** Excess glucose circulating in your body draws water from your tissues, making you feel dehydrated. Drinking water and other beverages to quench thirst leads to more frequent urination.

- **Flulike symptoms.** Type 2 diabetes can sometimes feel like a viral illness, with such symptoms as extreme fatigue and weakness. When glucose, your body's main fuel, doesn't reach cells, you may feel tired and weak.

- **Weight loss or weight gain.** Because your body is trying to compensate for lost fluids and glucose, you may eat more than usual and gain weight, or the opposite may occur. Although eating more than normal, you may lose weight because your muscle tissues don't get enough glucose to generate growth and energy.

- **Blurred vision.** High levels of blood glucose pull fluid from body tissues, including the lenses of the eyes, which affects ability to focus. Vision should improve with treatment of diabetes.

- **Slow-healing sores or frequent infections.** Diabetes affects the body's ability to heal and fight infection. Bladder and vaginal infections can be a particular problem for women.

- **Nerve damage (neuropathy).** Excess blood glucose can damage the small blood vessels to your nerves, leading to symptoms such as tingling and loss of sensation in hands and feet.

- **Red, swollen, tender gums.** Diabetes increases the risk of infection in your gums and in the bones that hold your teeth in place.

Diabetes Management

Before the development of insulin injections, diabetes was a fatal illness. Today, diabetics can have normal lifespans. However, uncontrolled glucose levels slowly damage blood vessels throughout the body. Diabetes is the number one cause of blindness, nontraumatic amputations, and kidney failure, and diabetes increases by two or three times the risk of heart attack or stroke.

Unlike many other medical conditions, patients must take charge of their diabetes and monitor their blood glucose regularly to prevent or delay the serious complications of the disease. Diabetes educators teach patients a new set of ABCs:

- **A** is for the *A1c* test. This test measures the amount of glucose attached to hemoglobin molecules, the iron-rich molecules in red blood cells that deliver oxygen to the body. The higher your blood glucose levels, the more hemoglobin molecules you will have with glucose attached—and the greater the risk of damage to eyes, kidneys, and feet. In general, the life cycle of a red blood cell is 75 to 90 days, which is why the A1c test shows average blood glucose levels for the past 2 to 3 months. The American Diabetes Association recommends a goal for A1c of less than 7 percent. The American College of Endocrinology recommends a goal of 6.5 percent. (Normal A1c levels are below 6.) Individuals with diabetes should have their A1c levels checked at least twice a year.

- **B** is for *blood pressure*. High blood pressure can cause heart attack, stroke, and kidney disease.

- **C** is for *cholesterol*. The LDL goal for most people is less than 160 mg/dL (see Table 10.2). Bad cholesterol, or LDL, can build up and clog your blood vessels.

✓**check-in** If you have been diagnosed with diabetes, how vigilant are you in controlling your blood sugar levels?

Regular exercise and healthy eating are critical to diabetes management. In its most recent recommendations, the American Diabetes Associations advises individuals with diabetes to engage in mild to moderate physical activity—such as walking, standing in place, torso twists, and lunges—for 3 minutes at 30-minute intervals.[39]

Treatment   The goal for diabetics is to keep blood sugar levels as stable as possible to prevent complications, such as kidney damage. Home glucose monitoring, including new continuous glucose monitors, allows diabetics to check their blood sugar levels as many times a day as necessary and to adjust their diet or insulin doses as appropriate.

Types of insulin differ in how long they take to start working after injection (onset), when they work hardest (peak), and how long they last in the body (duration). Individuals with diabetes may use different types in various combinations, depending on time of day and timing of meals. New insulin inhalers offer an alternative to injections for those with type 2 diabetes.

Those with type 1 diabetes require daily doses of insulin via injections, an insulin infusion pump, or oral medication. Those with type 2 diabetes can often control their disease through a well-balanced diet, exercise, and weight management. However, insulin therapy may be needed to keep blood glucose levels normal or near normal, thereby reducing the risk of damage to the eyes, nerves, and kidneys. New medications help control weight and lower blood pressure and cholesterol.

In most cases, diabetes requires lifelong management and treatment. However, a cure for some patients no longer seems impossible. About 400 to 500 pancreas transplants are performed in the United States every year; when successful they normalize glucose levels, thereby curing diabetes. However, only about half of these transplants continue to function for 10 years.

Gastric bypass surgery (which limits the amount of food a person can ingest) for extremely obese individuals has led to lasting remission of diabetes, sometimes even before a patient loses weight. (See Chapter 6.) Scientists believe that bypass surgery "cures" diabetes by changing the hormones and amino acids produced during digestion. Some surgeons are advocating this approach for all diabetics with body mass indexes (BMIs) over 50; others, as an option for those with BMIs over 35.

Among other promising approaches are, the use of stem cells to "rejuvenate" the pancreas, antibodies to block the autoimmune response of type 1 diabetes, and a more sophisticated artificial pancreas to monitor and manage glucose levels.

✓**check-in** Could the future be pinch-free for diabetics?

High-tech alternatives to the dreaded fingerstick may include smartphone apps, a contact lens to monitor blood sugar in tears, a breathalyzer, a saliva test, and a tattoo that would refract infrared light back through the skin to a monitor that could translate the readings into blood sugar levels.

Hypertension

Blood pressure refers to the force of blood against the walls of arteries. When blood pressure remains elevated over time—a condition called *hypertension*—the heart must pump harder than is healthy. Because the heart must force blood into arteries that are offering increased resistance to blood flow, the left side of the heart becomes enlarged. If untreated, high blood pressure can cause a variety of cardiovascular complications, including heart attack and stroke—as well as blindness and kidney disease (Figure 10.3).[40]

The "silent killer" continues to live up to its nickname. Since 2000, the overall death rate from hypertension has increased 23 percent for both men and women, with the greatest spike in those ages 45 to 64.[41] People living in low-income states are more likely to have high blood pressure than the residents of more affluent states.[42] Globally blood pressure in less developed countries has increased significantly over the past four decades.[43]

Regulating blood pressure for all Americans could prevent 56,000 heart attacks and strokes and 13,000 deaths each year. However, 44 percent of adults with elevated blood pressure do not have it under control. Globally, treating half of people with uncontrolled high blood pressure could prevent 10 million heart attacks and strokes over 10 years.[44]

✓**check-in** Are you too young to worry about blood pressure? Read the following section, and think again.

Hypertension in the Young

In a young person, even mild hypertension can cause organs such as the heart, brain, and kidneys to start to deteriorate. High blood pressure can damage the structure of the brain in people as young as age 40. In individuals at genetic risk,

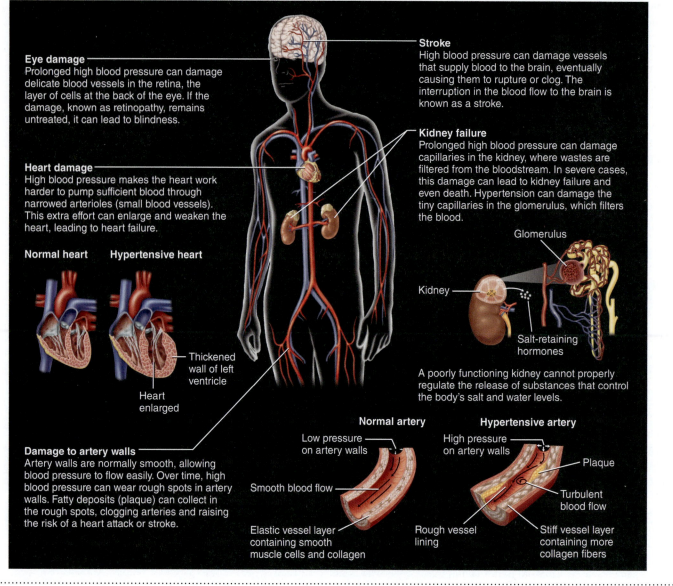

FIGURE 10.3 Consequences of High Blood Pressure

If left untreated, elevated blood pressure can damage blood vessels in several areas of the body and lead to serious health problems.

high blood pressure may spur development of the brain plaques characteristic of Alzheimer's disease.

Especially when combined with obesity, smoking, high cholesterol levels, or diabetes, hypertension greatly increases the risks of cardiovascular problems. Young adults in their 20s with even mildly elevated blood pressure may face an increased risk of clogged arteries by middle age, according to a 25-year study of nearly 4,700 people.[45] Among college students, binge drinking has been linked with an increased short- and long-term risk of hypertension.[46]

✓**check-in** Do you know your systolic blood pressure?

For young adults, high systolic blood pressure—the top number in a reading—may herald increased risk for heart disease. A systolic reading of 120 mmHg or higher may signal a significantly greater risk of dying from heart disease over time, particularly for women.

Who Is at Risk?

According to the CDC, about 3 in 10 adults ages 18 or older in the United States—some 65 million men and women—have high blood pressure.

- Blood pressure has increased among children and adolescents as well as adults, with the highest rates among African American and

Mexican American children. The primary culprit is the increase in obesity in the young.

- Binge drinking, discussed in Chapter 16, can raise systolic blood pressure (the top number in a blood pressure reading) among young adults and increase their risk of hypertension later in life.

- An African American with the same elevated blood pressure reading as a Caucasian faces a greater likelihood of hospitalization and risk of stroke, heart disease, and kidney problems.[47] Even small increases in blood pressure can be dangerous for black people. A rise of as little as 10 mmHg in systolic blood pressure in blacks raises the risk of dying and is even greater for black people under age 60.[48]

- Family history increases the risk. If one or both of your parents have high blood pressure, have yours checked regularly.

- Men and women are equally likely to develop hypertension. Women who develop high blood pressure during pregnancy may face an increased risk of heart and kidney disease. Blood pressure also tends to rise around the time of menopause.

- People with chronic insomnia who take longer than 14 minutes to fall asleep may have a 300 percent higher risk of high blood pressure. The longer before sleep onset, the greater their risk.[49]

- Lowering blood pressure is a key to preventing stroke, discussed on page 321.[50]

✓**check-in** Do you know if your parents have high blood pressure?

What Your Blood Pressure Reading Means

Based on the most recent federal guidelines, nearly half of Americans (46 percent) have high blood pressure. The blood pressure categories in the guidelines are:

- Normal: Less than 120/80 mmHg.

- Elevated: Systolic between 120 and 129 *and* diastolic less than 80.

- Stage 1: Systolic between 130 and 139 *or* diastolic between 80 and 89.

- Stage 2: Systolic at least 140 *or* diastolic at least 90 mmHg.

- Hypertensive crisis: Systolic over 180 *and*/or diastolic over 120, with patients needing prompt changes in medication if there are no other

YOUR STRATEGIES FOR PREVENTION

Checking Your Blood Pressure at Home

Monitors can range from $40 to $100 on average, but insurance may cover part or all of the cost.

- Select a monitor that goes around your upper arm. Wrist and finger monitors are not as precise.

- Choose an automated monitor with a self-inflating cuff.

- Opt for a large, bright digital readout that you can see clearly.

- If possible, choose a monitor that can transfer readings to an app on your smartphone and create a graph.

- Don't drink caffeinated or alcoholic beverages 30 minutes before testing.

- Sit quietly for five minutes with your back supported. Do not cross your legs. Rest your arm in a position where your elbow is at or near heart level.

- Wrap the cuff over bare skin.

- Don't talk.

- Leave the deflated cuff in place, wait a minute, then take a second reading. If the readings are close, average them. If not, repeat again and average the three readings.

- Record your blood pressure readings, including the time of day.

TABLE 10.1 What Your Blood Pressure Reading Means

Normal Results
In adults, the systolic pressure should be less than 120 mmHg and the diastolic pressure should be less than 80 mmHg.
What Abnormal Results Mean
Prehypertension
The top number is consistently 120–139 or the bottom number reads 80–89.
Stage 1: Mild hypertension
The top number is consistently 140–159 or the bottom number reads 90–99.
Stage 2: Moderate to severe hypertension
The top number is consistently 160 or over or the bottom number reads 100 or over.
Low blood pressure (hypotension)
The top number reads lower than 90 mmHg, or pressure 25 mmHg lower than usual.
Blood pressure readings may be affected by many different conditions, including cardiovascular disorders; neurological conditions; kidney and urological disorders; psychological factors such as stress, anger, or fear; various medications; and "white coat hypertension," which may occur if the medical visit itself produces extreme anxiety.

Source: National Institute of Medicine, National Institutes of Health.

indications of problems or immediate hospitalization if there are signs of organ damage.

Unlike previous recommendations, the new guidelines do not differentiate on the basis of age.

How to Lower Your Blood Pressure

- **Get moving.** Regular exercise can lower blood pressure by 10 points, prevent the onset of high blood pressure, or enable you to reduce your dosage of blood pressure medications.

- **Eat your way to better blood pressure.** Choose more fruits, vegetables, low-fat dairy products, whole grains, poultry, fish, and nuts. Cut down on red meat, sweets, sugar-containing beverages, and saturated fat and cholesterol.

- **Lose 10.** Shedding 10 percent of your current weight—or even 10 pounds—can make a big difference.

- **Don't smoke.** A single cigarette can cause a 20-point spike in systolic blood pressure. Don't light up. (See Chapter 13 for tips on quitting.)

- **Hold the salt.** If you're salt sensitive, you may be spiking your blood pressure as you season your food.

- **Stick with your medications.** If your doctor has prescribed medication to lower your blood pressure, take it conscientiously. Your future health may depend on it.

- **Avoid caffeinated energy drinks,** which can increase blood pressure and disrupt your heart rhythm.

Medications are recommended to lower blood pressure in stage 1 hypertension only if individuals have already had a heart attack or stroke. For others with stage 1 hypertension, lifestyle changes alone are recommended.[51]

Monitoring Your Blood Pressure

In healthy adults, blood pressure screening should begin at age 21, with repeat evaluations at least every 2 years, or more often, depending on a person's current health, medical history, and risk factors for cardiovascular disease. According to the National College Health Assessment survey, 3.2 percent of undergraduates have been diagnosed or treated for high blood pressure.[52]

Lowering High Blood Pressure

Lifestyle changes are a first-line weapon in the fight against high blood pressure. Rather than make a single change, a combination of behavioral changes, including losing weight, eating heart-healthy foods, reducing sodium, and exercising more, yields the best results.

Reducing Sodium Medical scientists continue to debate the risks of sodium consumption.[53] Low sodium intake (less than 3 grams a day) has been linked with cardiovascular problems and greater risk of dying regardless of an individual's blood pressure. High sodium intake (of 71 grams daily) increases the risks—but only

for those with hypertension.[54] Talk with your health-care providers about how much sodium may be too much for you.

✓check-in Do you monitor your salt intake?

The DASH Eating Pattern The National Heart, Lung, and Blood Institute (NHLBI) has developed the DASH (Dietary Approaches to Stop Hypertension) eating pattern, which has proved as effective as drug therapy in lowering blood pressure. An additional benefit: DASH also lowers harmful blood fats, including cholesterol and LDL, and the amino acid homocysteine (one of the new suspects in heart disease risk).

Exercise Regular exercise, both aerobic workouts and resistance training, can lower blood pressure. Walking has proven as beneficial as running in lowering blood pressure and other cardiovascular risk factors.[55] See Your Strategies for Change for ways to lower your blood pressure.

Medications Making healthy lifestyle modifications can help reduce Stage 1 hypertension, but most people also require a medication. Drugs for lowering blood pressure come in a range of regimens (once a day to several times a day) with a range of effects on other conditions, interactions with other drugs, and potential side effects. They have been shown to lower the risk of stroke and add years to life expectancy. Treatment with a combination of medications may lead to a faster reduction in blood pressure and earlier protection for individuals at high cardiovascular risk.[56]

✓check-in Did you know that only one-third of people with hypertension have it effectively controlled? Reducing blood pressure to healthy levels could prevent 1 death in every 11 people treated for hypertension.

Your Lipoprotein Profile

Medical science has changed the way it views and targets the blood fats that endanger a healthy heart. In the past, the focus was primarily on total cholesterol in the blood. The higher this number was, the greater the risk of heart disease. The NHLBI's National Cholesterol Education Program has recommended more comprehensive testing, called a *lipoprotein profile*, for all individuals age 20 or older.

This blood test, which should be performed after a 9- to 12-hour fast and repeated at least once every 5 years, provides readings of:

- **Total cholesterol.**
- **LDL (bad) cholesterol**, the main culprit in the buildup of plaque within the arteries.
- **HDL (good** or **healthy) cholesterol**, which helps prevent cholesterol buildup.
- **Triglycerides**, the blood fats released into the bloodstream after a meal.

✓**check-in** Are you too young to have to pay attention to how much fatty food you eat? Even if you are still in your teens, the answer is "no."

Long-term exposure to higher cholesterol levels can damage a person's future heart health. Individuals who live for more than a decade with high cholesterol have four times the risk of heart disease than those with shorter exposure. The longer your cholesterol remains high, the more likely you are to develop heart problems.

What Is a Healthy Cholesterol Reading?

Total cholesterol is the sum of all the cholesterol in your blood. Less than 200 mg/dL total cholesterol is ideal, and 200 to 239 mg/dL is borderline high. Total cholesterol above 240 mg/dL is high and doubles your risk of heart disease. However, total cholesterol is not the only crucial number you should know. Because LDL increases your risk for heart disease, you should always find out your LDL level. Even if your total cholesterol is higher than 200, you may not be at high risk for a heart attack. Some people—such as women before menopause and young, active men who have no other risk factors—may have high HDL cholesterol and desirable LDL levels. Ask your doctor to interpret your results so you both know your numbers and understand what they mean (Table 10.2).

HDL, good cholesterol, is important in everyone, but particularly in women. Federal guidelines define an HDL reading of less than 40 mg/dL as a major risk factor for developing heart disease. HDL levels of 60 mg/dL or more are protective and lower the risk of heart disease.

Triglycerides, the free-floating molecules that transport fats in the bloodstream, should ideally be below 150 mg/dL. Individuals with readings of 150 to 199 mg/dL, considered borderline, as well as those with higher readings, may benefit from weight control, physical activity, and, if necessary, medication.

Lowering Cholesterol

According to federal guidelines, about one in five Americans may require treatment to lower his or her cholesterol level. However, nearly half of people who need cholesterol treatment, which can reduce the risk of heart disease by 30 percent over 5 years, don't get it. Depending on your lipoprotein profile and an assessment of other risk factors, your physician may recommend that you take steps to lower your LDL cholesterol.

Lifestyle Changes

Some individuals with elevated cholesterol can improve their lipoprotein profile with lifestyle changes:

- **Dietary changes.** In the past, dietary changes produced relatively modest improvements compared to the effects of medications, which can cut cholesterol by as much as 35 percent. However, a diet consisting of cholesterol-lowering foods, including nuts, soy, oats, and plant sterols (in margarine and green leafy vegetables), reduced LDL cholesterol by about 30 percent. Researchers are recommending this diet as an effective first treatment for individuals with high cholesterol levels, particularly coupled with exercise and weight loss.

- **Weight management.** For individuals who are overweight, losing weight can help lower LDL. This is especially true for those with high triglyceride levels and/or low HDL levels and those who have a large waist measurement (more than 40 inches for a man and more than 35 inches for a woman).

- **Physical activity.** Regular activity can help lower LDL, lower blood pressure, reduce triglycerides, and, particularly important, raise HDL. Again, these benefits are especially important for those with high triglyceride levels or large waist measurements.

✓**check-in** Which lifestyle changes would you make to improve your cholesterol profile?

Lifestyle changes can lower harmful LDL levels by 5 to 10 percent. Alternative therapies, such as

TABLE 10.2 How to Interpret Your Lipoprotein Profile

Total Cholesterol Level	Category
Less than 200 mg/dL	Desirable level that puts you at lower risk for coronary heart disease. A cholesterol level of 200 mg/dL or higher raises your risk.
200–239 mg/dL	Borderline high
240 mg/dL and above	High blood cholesterol. A person with this level has more than twice the risk of coronary heart disease as someone whose cholesterol is below 200 mg/dL.

HDL Cholesterol Level	Category
Less than 40 mg/dL (for men)	Low HDL cholesterol—a major risk factor for heart disease.
Less than 50 mg/dL (for women)	
60 mg/dL and above	High HDL cholesterol. An HDL of 60 mg/dL and above is considered protective against heart disease.

LDL Cholesterol Level	Category
Less than 100 mg/dL	Optimal
100–129 mg/dL	Near or above optimal
130–159 mg/dL	Borderline high
160–189 mg/dL	High
190 mg/dL and above	Very high

Your LDL cholesterol goal depends on how many other risk factors you have.

- If you don't have coronary heart disease or diabetes and have one or no risk factors, your LDL goal is less than 160 mg/dL.

- If you don't have coronary heart disease or diabetes and have two or more risk factors, your LDL goal is less than 130 mg/dL.

- If you do have coronary heart disease or diabetes, your LDL goal is less than 100 mg/dL.

Triglyceride Level	Category
Less than 150 mg/dL	Normal
150–199 mg/dL	Borderline high
200–499 mg/dL	High
500 mg/dL or above	Very high

Source: National Cholesterol Education Program (NCEP) and American Heart Association. Adapted from www.americanheart.org/presenter.jhtml?identifier54500.

garlic, may have some limited benefit but remain unproven. A greater reduction of 30 to 40 percent requires either intensive lifestyle changes, including an extremely low-fat diet or the addition of cholesterol-lowering medication.

Medications

Drugs called statins—best known by brand names such as Lipitor, Mevacor, Pravachol, and Zocor—can cut the risk of dying of a heart attack by as much as 40 percent. Initially tested in men, statins have proved equally beneficial for women, including those whose cholesterol levels rise after menopause.

Statins work in the liver to block production of cholesterol. When the liver can't make cholesterol, it draws LDL cholesterol from the blood to use as raw material. This means that less LDL is available to trigger or promote the artery-clogging process known as *atherosclerosis*. Statins also appear to stabilize cholesterol-filled deposits in artery walls and to cool down inflammation. The combination of statins with moderate exercise, such as 30 minutes a day of brisk walking, has the most dramatic effect on cholesterol levels and reduced risk of dying.

Statins also protect patients who have not had a heart attack but are at high risk for developing cardiovascular disease because of high cholesterol or other risk factors. Large-scale studies indicate that statins protect against heart attacks and strokes even in older adults without known cardiovascular disease or diabetes and with low cholesterol—if these patients also have high levels of CRP or C-reactive protein.

Cardiovascular (Heart) Disease

Heart disease, stroke, and other cardiovascular diseases cause about one of every three deaths in the United States, killing about 787,000 Americans annually. Globally, cardiovascular disease is the leading cause of death, claiming more lives than all cancers combined. An American dies of a heart-related disease every 40 seconds.[57]

✓**check-in** Fewer than 20 percent of adults meet at least five of the following American Heart Association criteria for ideal heart health. Do you?

• Never smoked or quit more than a year ago

• Body mass index (BMI) less than 25

• Physical exercise—at least 150 minutes of moderate intensity or 75 minutes of vigorous intensity a week

• At least four components of a healthful diet, such as fewer calories and more fruits and vegetables (see Chapter 4)

• Total cholesterol lower than 200 mg/dL

• Blood pressure below 120/80 mmHg

• Fasting blood sugar below 100 mg/dL

How the Heart Works

The heart is a hollow, muscular organ with four chambers that serve as two pumps (Figure 10.4). Its key characteristics include:

• A human heart is about the size of a clenched fist.

• Each pump consists of a pair of chambers formed of muscles. The upper two—each

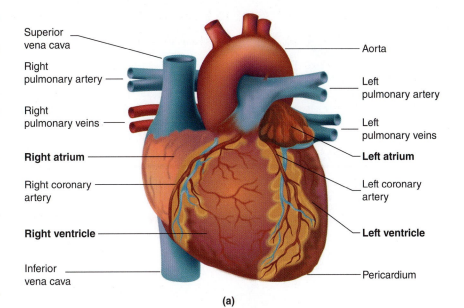

(a)

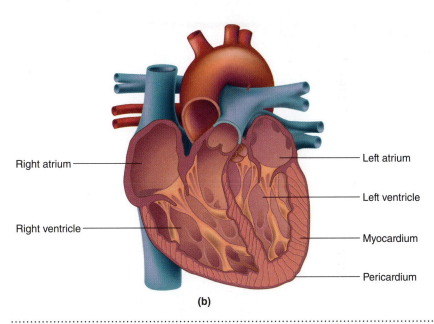

(b)

FIGURE 10.4 The Healthy Heart

(a) The heart muscle is nourished by blood from the coronary arteries, which arise from the aorta. (b) The cross section shows the four chambers and the myocardium, the muscle that does the heart's work. The pericardium is the outer covering of the heart.

called an **atrium**—receive blood, which then flows through valves into the lower two chambers, the **ventricles**, which contract to pump blood out into the arteries through a second set of valves.

• A thick wall divides the right side of the heart from the left side; even though the two sides are separated, they contract at almost the same time. Contraction of the ventricles is

atrium Either of the two upper chambers of the heart, which receive blood from the veins.

ventricles The two lower chambers of the heart, which pump blood out of the heart and into the arteries.

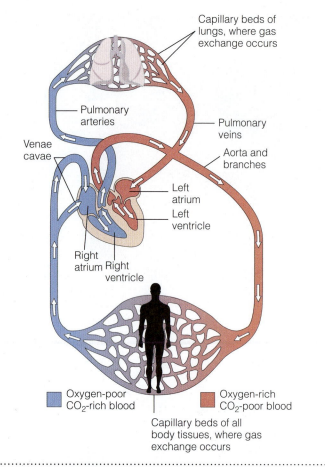

Capillary beds of lungs, where gas exchange occurs

Pulmonary arteries

Pulmonary veins

Venae cavae

Aorta and branches

Left atrium

Left ventricle

Right atrium

Right ventricle

■ Oxygen-poor CO₂-rich blood

■ Oxygen-rich CO₂-poor blood

Capillary beds of all body tissues, where gas exchange occurs

FIGURE 10.5 The Path of Blood Flow

Blood is pumped from the right ventricle into the pulmonary arteries, which lead to the lungs, where gas exchange (oxygen for carbon dioxide) occurs. Oxygenated blood returning from the lungs drains into the left atrium and is then pumped into the left ventricle, which sends the blood into the aorta and its branches. The oxygenated blood flows through the arteries, which extend to all parts of the body. Again gas exchange occurs in the body tissues; this time oxygen is "dropped off" and carbon dioxide "picked up"

systole The contraction phase of the cardiac cycle.

diastole The period between contractions in the cardiac cycle, during which the heart relaxes and dilates as it fills with blood.

aorta The main artery of the body, arising from the left ventricle of the heart.

capillaries Minute blood vessels that connect arteries to veins.

called **systole**; the period of relaxation between contractions is called **diastole**.

• The heart valves, located at the entrance and exit of the ventricular chambers, have flaps that open and close to allow blood to flow through the chambers of the heart.

• The *myocardium* (heart muscle) consists of branching fibers that enable the heart to contract, or beat, between 60 and 80 times per minute, or about 100,000 times a day. With each beat, the heart pumps about 2 ounces of blood. This may not sound like much, but it adds up to nearly 5 quarts of blood pumped by the heart in 1 minute, or about 75 gallons per hour.

• The heart is surrounded by the *pericardium*, which consists of two layers of a tough membrane. The space between the two contains a

lubricating fluid that allows the heart muscle to move freely. The *endocardium* is a smooth membrane lining the inside of the heart and its valves.

• Blood circulates through the body by means of the pumping action of the heart, as shown in Figure 10.5. The right ventricle (on your own right side) pumps blood, via the *pulmonary arteries*, to the lungs, where it picks up oxygen (a gas essential to the body's cells) and gives off carbon dioxide (a waste product of metabolism). The blood returns from the lungs via the *pulmonary veins* to the left side of the heart, which pumps it, via the **aorta**, to the arteries in the rest of the body.

• The arteries divide into smaller and smaller branches and finally into **capillaries**, the smallest blood vessels of all (only slightly larger in diameter than a single red blood cell). The blood within the capillaries supplies oxygen and nutrients to the cells of the tissues and takes up various waste products.

• Blood returns to the heart via the veins: The blood from the upper body (except the lungs) drains into the heart through the *superior vena cava*, while blood from the lower body returns via the *inferior vena cava*.

The workings of this remarkable pump affect your entire body. If the flow of blood to or through the heart or to the rest of the body is reduced, or if a disturbance occurs in the small bundle of highly specialized cells in the heart that generate electrical impulses to control heartbeats, the result may at first be too subtle to notice. However, without diagnosis and treatment, these changes could develop into a life-threatening problem.

Heart Risks on Campus

Many people, including college students and other young adults, are unaware of habits and conditions that put their hearts at risk. Many undergraduates view heart disease as mainly a problem for white men and underestimate the risks for women and ethnic groups. Students rate their own knowledge of heart disease as lower than that of sexually transmitted infections and psychological disorders.

✓**check-in** How would you rate your knowledge of heart disease?

Here are some crucial facts:

• Heart disease is the third leading cause of death among adults ages 25 to 44. Diabetes, family history, and other risk factors increase the likelihood of heart disease.

- It's never too soon to start protecting your heart. High aerobic fitness in the college-age years has been linked with a lower risk of heart attack later in life.

- Among the behaviors that put students' hearts at risk is binge drinking, which may hinder the function of the blood vessels and increase the likelihood of stroke, sudden cardiac death, and heart attack.

- Young athletes face special risks. Each year, seemingly healthy teens or young adults die suddenly on playing fields and courts. The culprit in one of every three cases of sudden cardiac death in young athletes is a silent condition called hypertrophic cardiomyopathy (HCM), an excessive thickness of the heart muscle. Because of HCM, the heart is more prone to dangerous heart irregularities. Some medical groups have recommended routine electrocardiograms to reduce risk of sudden cardiac death in competitive collegiate sports; others believe that a simpler physical exam-based screening is sufficient.

Psychosocial Risk Factors

Researchers classify psychological risk factors for heart disease into three categories:

- **Chronic factors**, such as job strain or lack of social support, play an important role in the buildup of artery-clogging plaque and may increase blood pressure. Even feeling that life has treated you unfairly boosts your chance of having a heart attack.

- **Episodic factors**, such as depression, can last from several weeks to 2 years and may lead to the creation of "unstable" plaque, which is more likely to break off and block a blood vessel within the heart.

- **Short-term, or acute, factors**, such as an angry outburst, can directly trigger a heart attack in people with underlying heart disease.

These factors may act alone or combine and exert different effects at different ages and stages of life. They may influence behaviors such as smoking, diet, alcohol consumption, and physical activity, as well as directly cause changes in physiology.

Stress How you respond to stress (discussed in Chapter 3) can affect your heart as well as your overall health. Even stressed teenagers may be at risk. In a longitudinal analysis that followed teens into middle age, those who

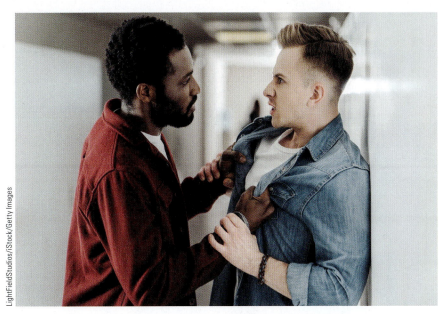

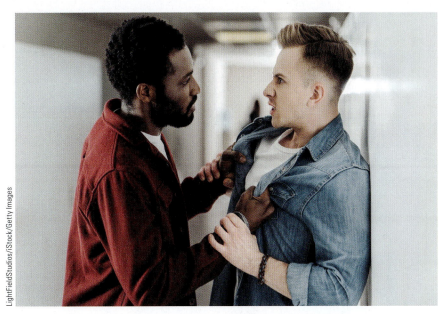

scored high in stress early in life were more likely to develop atherosclerosis by their mid-40s.[58] Although you may not be able to control the sources of stress, you can change how you habitually respond to it.

✓**check-in** Do you think the way you respond to stress increases or decreases your cardiovascular risk?

Depression Depression and heart disease often occur together. People with heart disease are more likely than others to be depressed, and some seemingly healthy people with depression are at greater risk of heart problems. Depressed women younger than age 60 are more likely to suffer a heart attack than those who do not suffer from depression.

The combination of stress, depression, and heart disease can be so deadly that researchers have dubbed the combination a "psychosocial perfect storm" that increases the risk of heart attack or death among men and women with heart disease.[59]

Anger and Hostility Anger and hostility have both short- and long-term consequences for the heart, particularly for men. In general, the angriest men are three times more likely to develop heart disease than the most placid ones. Hostility more than doubles the risk of recurrent heart attacks in men (but not women). Research has linked hostility to increased cardiac risk factors, to decreased survival in men with coronary artery disease below the age of 61, to an increased risk of heart attack in men with

Hostility in men of any age can increase their risk of heart attacks and heart disease.

LightFieldStudios/iStock/Getty Images

metabolic syndrome, and to an increased risk of abnormal heart rhythms. The risk of a heart attack or other cardiovascular "event" is highest in the 2 hours following an angry outburst. The more frequent the outbursts, the greater the danger to heart health.

Angry young men may be putting their future heart health in jeopardy. In longitudinal studies the angriest young men were more likely to suffer heart attacks by age 55 and, more significantly, to develop any form of cardiovascular disease.

✓**check-in** If you are male, do you think anger may be putting your heart health at risk?

How does hostility harm the heart? Anger triggers a surge in stress hormones that can provoke abnormal and potentially lethal heart rhythms and activates platelets, the tiny blood cells that trigger blood clotting. High levels of anger can also trigger a spasm in a coronary artery, which results in the additional narrowing of a partially blocked blood vessel.

In women, anger and hostility do not always lead to heart troubles. However, women who outwardly express anger may be at increased risk if they also have other risk factors for heart disease, such as diabetes or unhealthy levels of lipoproteins.

Personality Types In addition to stress, anger, and depression, other psychological traits can increase the risk of heart disease. Based on more than a decade of research, Dutch scientists have identified a "Type D" (for distressed) personality type. Type D people tend to be anxious, self-conscious, irritable, insecure, and negative, and they go to great lengths not to say or do anything that others might not like. In the Dutch study, almost four times as many Type D individuals as others in cardiac rehabilitation programs died within an 8-year period.

In the past, other personality types were linked to disease—for example, hard-charging, hostile Type A persons were associated with heart disease, and conflict-avoiding, emotion-suppressing Type C persons with cancer; However, these traits have not proved to be significant risk factors for these illnesses.

The Power of Positive Emotions Our psychological and social health affects not just our minds but our bodies, including the heart. While problems such as depression and stress may increase cardiovascular risk, happiness may help keep our hearts healthy. In a study that followed men and women for 10 years, those who showed more "positive" emotions—such as enthusiasm, joy, and contentment—were less likely to develop heart disease than less happy individuals. The happier people were, the lower their risk of heart disease became.

An optimistic outlook may also boost heart health. When socioeconomic factors such as education and income are taken into account, optimistic people are more likely to be in ideal cardiovascular health, with lower blood sugar, cholesterol, blood pressure, and BMIs, compared with pessimists.

A sense of purpose affects your heart as well as your mindset. Individuals who feel motivated by a sense of meaning and direction in life and view life as worth living are at lower risk of cardiovascular disease, stroke, and death from any cause.

The Heart of a Woman

Many people still think of heart disease as a "guy problem." Men do have a higher incidence of cardiovascular problems than women before age 45, but young women who have heart attacks are more likely to die as a result.[60]

- Every year 35,000 women under age 65 experience a heart attack.

- More than 15,000 women younger than age 55 die from heart disease in the United States each year.

- High blood pressure is a stronger risk factor for women than for men. Diabetes raises a young woman's heart disease risk up to five times higher compared to young men.[61]

- Black women of any age have a higher incidence of heart attack than white women; and black and Hispanic women have more risk factors such as obesity, diabetes, and high blood pressure at the time of heart attack compared to white women.

For men and women, chest pain or discomfort is the most common heart attack symptom, but women are more likely to report:

- Shortness of breath, back or jaw pain, and nausea and vomiting.

- Tiredness, even after getting adequate sleep.

- Trouble breathing.

- Trouble sleeping.

- Feeling sick to the stomach.

- Feeling scared or nervous.

- New or worse headaches.

- An ache in the chest.

- "Heaviness" or "tightness" in the chest.

- A burning feeling in the chest.

- Pain in the back, between the shoulders.

- Pain or tightness in the chest that spreads to the jaw, neck, shoulders, ear, or the inside of the arms.

- Pain in the belly, above the belly button.

Unhealthy lifestyles may be responsible for almost 75 percent of heart disease cases in young and middle-aged women. Healthful habits can reduce the danger. Even a few bouts of moderate exercise each week can cut a middle-aged woman's odds for heart disease, blood clots, and stroke. More frequent exercise, at least in this study of more than 1.1 million middle-aged women with no history of heart disease, did not yield more benefits than walking, gardening, cycling, or engaging in other activities that caused sweating or increased heart rate 2 or 3 days a week.[62]

✓**check-in** Would you like to cut your odds of heart disease by 90 percent over the next 20 years?

Here are six behaviors proven to do so:

_____ Not smoking.

_____ Exercising at least 2.5 hours a week.

_____ Maintaining a healthy weight.

_____ Watching fewer than 7 hours of television a week.

_____ Following a healthy diet.

_____ Drinking no more than one glass of alcohol a day. Moderate alcohol consumption has been linked with biochemical indicators of reduced cardiovascular risk.[63] However, heavier drinking increases the risk of heart-related problems.

Coronary Artery Disease

The general term for any impairment of blood flow through the blood vessels, often referred to as "hardening of the arteries," is **arteriosclerosis**. The most common form is **atherosclerosis**, a disease of the lining of the arteries in which **plaque**—deposits of fat, fibrin (a clotting material), cholesterol, other cell parts, and calcium— narrows the artery channels. Inflammation also plays a crucial role.

Atherosclerosis

This process begins when LDL cholesterol penetrates the wall of an artery. Ideally, HDL cholesterol carries the cholesterol out of the artery wall to the liver for disposal. However, if LDL accumulates, the artery responds by releasing chemical messengers called cytokines, which trigger active inflammation in the artery wall.

Elevated levels of LDL cholesterol and apolipoprotein B (apoB), the main structural protein of LDL, are directly associated with the risk of atherosclerosis.[64] T lymphocytes and macrophages, specialized white blood cells that are part of the body's defensive immune system, move from the bloodstream into the artery and engulf the LDL. As they ingest the LDL, the macrophages enlarge and become foam cells, which rupture, releasing cholesterol into the artery wall, where the cycle of damage begins again. In response, the smooth muscle cells in the artery wall create a fibrous cap over the inflamed area (Figure 10.6).

arteriosclerosis Any of a number of chronic diseases characterized by degeneration of the arteries and hardening and thickening of arterial walls.

atherosclerosis A form of arteriosclerosis in which fatty substances (plaque) are deposited on the inner walls of arteries.

plaque A sludgelike substance that builds up on the inner walls of arteries.

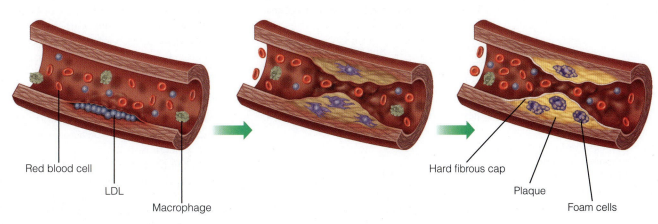

Red blood cell

LDL

Macrophage

Hard fibrous cap

Plaque

Foam cells

FIGURE 10.6 How Atherosclerosis Happens

LDL cholesterol penetrates an artery wall, and the accumulation of LDL cholesterol triggers an inflammation. Macrophages engulf the LDL and become foam cells. The artery wall creates a fibrous cap over this plaque, and the artery is narrowed. If the plaque ruptures, blood clots can block flow to the heart or to the brain.

These hard-capped plaques are dangerous: They narrow arteries, reduce the flow of blood, and produce **angina** (chest pain). However, the usual culprits in heart attacks are smaller, softer plaques that can rupture. As the body responds with clotting factors, platelets, and blood cells, a blood clot, or thrombus, forms on the disrupted plaque's surface. The clot ultimately blocks the artery and kills heart muscle cells. Similar clots can block blood flow to the brain and lead to other complications, including kidney failure and circulation problems in the legs and feet.

Heart Attack (Myocardial Infarction)

The medical name for a heart attack, or coronary, is **myocardial infarction (MI)**. The *myocardium* is the cardiac muscle layer of the wall of the heart. It receives its blood supply, and thus its oxygen and other nutrients, from the coronary arteries. If an artery is blocked by a clot or plaque, or by a spasm, the myocardial cells do not get sufficient oxygen, and the portion of the myocardium deprived of its blood supply begins to die.

Although such an attack may seem sudden, usually it has been building up for years, particularly if the person has ignored risk factors and early warning signs. According to research, 80 to 90 percent of those who develop heart disease and 95 percent of those who suffer a fatal heart attack have at least one major risk factor.

Is It a Heart Attack?
If they experience the following symptoms, individuals should seek immediate medical care and take an aspirin (325 mg) to keep the blood clot in a coronary artery from getting any bigger:

- A tight ache; heavy, squeezing pain; or discomfort in the center of the chest, which may last for 30 minutes or more and is not relieved by rest.

- Chest pain that radiates to the shoulder, arm, neck, back, or jaw.

- Anxiety.

- Sweating or cold, clammy skin.

- Nausea and vomiting.

- Shortness of breath.

- Dizziness, fainting, or loss of consciousness.

Women often experience heart attacks differently than men. In the month before an attack, many report unusual fatigue and disturbed sleep.

Far fewer women than men experience chest pain. More common symptoms are shortness of breath, weakness and fatigue, a clammy sweat, dizziness, and nausea.[65]

✓**check-in** Would you recognize the symptoms of a heart attack?

Many everyday activities—eating, drinking coffee, having sex, even breathing—can spur a heart attack. Air pollution from traffic poses the greatest risk. Other triggers include drinking alcohol, physical exertion, and eating a heavy meal.

If you are with someone who's exhibiting the classic signs of a heart attack and if these signs last for 2 minutes or more, act at once. Expect the person to deny the possibility of anything as serious as a heart attack, but insist on taking prompt action.

Time is of the essence when a heart attack occurs. Call 911 immediately. The sooner emergency personnel get to a heart attack victim and administer cardiac life support, the greater the odds of survival. Yet according to the American Heart Association, most patients wait 3 hours after the initial symptoms begin before seeking help. By that time, half of the affected heart muscle may already be lost.

Cardiac Arrest Cardiac arrest occurs when the heart stops beating. If circulation is not restored within 4 or 5 minutes, the brain shuts down completely, and the person dies.

Cardiopulmonary resuscitation (CPR) is an emergency procedure for a person whose heart has stopped or who is no longer breathing. CPR can maintain circulation and breathing until emergency medical help arrives.

The combination of mouth-to-mouth "rescue" breathing and chest compressions performed by individuals trained in CPR is the most effective method. However, according to the most recent research, chest compressions or "hands-only" CPR, which does not require extensive training, can also keep blood circulating until emergency help arrives.

Automated external defibrillators (AEDs), portable computerized devices, can actually restart a heart with a lethal rhythm (ventricular fibrillation) or that is not beating at all. The machines, widely available on airplanes and in public places like stadiums and terminals, can also be purchased by individuals. Written and voice instructions allow laypeople as well as trained professionals to use them in case of emergency. A combination of CPR and defibrillation boosts the survival rate much higher than from CPR alone.

angina Chest pain.

myocardial infarction (MI)
A condition characterized by the dying of tissue areas in the myocardium, caused by interruption of the blood supply to those areas; the medical name for a heart attack.

cardiopulmonary resuscitation (CPR) Emergency treatment to maintain circulation in a person whose heart has stopped or who is no longer breathing.

Stroke

When the blood supply to a portion of the brain is blocked, a cerebrovascular accident, or **stroke**, occurs. The proportion of strokes among young adults between ages 20 and 45 has been rising, perhaps as a consequence of the higher incidence of obesity, hypertension, and diabetes.[66] Young adults who suffer strokes are at higher risk of diabetes and further "vascular events."[67]

✓**check-in** Did you know that 10 percent of strokes occur in 18- to 50-year-olds?

Although the number and mortality rate have declined, strokes rank third, after heart disease and cancer, as a cause of death in this country.

Worldwide, stroke is second only to heart disease as a cause of death. An estimated 20 percent of stroke victims die within 3 months; 50 to 60 percent are disabled.

Among those who survive a stroke before age 50, one-third are unable to live independently or require assistance with daily activities 10 years later.[68] (See Your Strategies for Prevention: How to Recognize a Stroke.)

As many as 80 percent of strokes are preventable, primarily through lifestyle modification. The most important steps are as follows:

- Treating hypertension.
- Not smoking.
- Managing diabetes.
- Lowering cholesterol.
- Taking aspirin, which reduces stroke risk in women but not in men.

✓**check-in** Which of these steps are you taking?

Quick treatment with a clot-busting drug at a hospital can reduce the chance of disability after a stroke, but few people recognize the signs of a stroke and seek medical care within 3 hours of the first symptoms.

Who Is at Risk?

Risk factors for stroke, like those for heart disease, include some that cannot be changed (such as gender, race, and age) and some that can be modified:

- **Sex.** Up to age 85, men have a greater risk of stroke than women. However, women are at increased risk at times of marked hormonal changes, particularly pregnancy and childbirth. Although older oral contraceptives had been linked with stroke, particularly in women over age 35 who smoke, the newer low-dose oral contraceptives have not shown an increased stroke risk among women ages 18 to 44. Early menopause (before age 42) may double a woman's stroke risk.

- **Race.** The incidence of strokes is two to three times greater in blacks than in whites in the same communities. Hispanics are also more likely to develop hemorrhagic strokes than whites.

- **Age.** A person's risk of stroke more than doubles every decade after age 55.

- **Obesity.** The more overweight individuals are, the more likely they are to have a stroke. Obesity may increase stroke risk by contributing to high blood pressure and diabetes.

- **Hypertension.** Detection and treatment of high blood pressure are the best means of stroke prevention.

- **High red blood cell count.** A moderate to marked increase in the number of a person's red blood cells increases the risk of stroke.

- **Heart disease.** Heart problems can interfere with the flow of blood to the brain; clots that form in the heart can travel to the brain, where they may clog an artery. Atrial fibrillation, the most common abnormal heart rhythm, also may increase the risk of stroke.

- **Blood fats.** Although the standard advice from cardiologists is to lower harmful LDL levels, what may be more important to lower stroke risk is an increase in the levels of protective HDL.

YOUR STRATEGIES FOR PREVENTION

How to Recognize a Stroke

Researchers have found that the following steps can identify facial weakness, arm weakness, and speech problems, all signs of stroke:

- **Ask the individual to smile.**
- **Ask him or her to raise both arms.**
- **Ask the person to speak a simple sentence, such as "It is sunny out today."**

If he or she has trouble with any of these tasks, call 911 immediately and describe the symptoms to the dispatcher.

stroke A cerebrovascular event in which the blood supply to a portion of the brain is blocked.

- **Diabetes mellitus.** Diabetics have a higher incidence of stroke than nondiabetics.

- **Estrogen therapy.** In the Women's Health Initiative—a series of clinical trials of hormone therapy for postmenopausal women—estrogen-only therapy significantly increased the risk of stroke.

- **A diet high in fat and sodium.** Individuals consuming the largest amounts of fatty foods and sodium are at much greater risk than those eating low-fat, low-salt diets.

- **Marijuana.** According to current research, smoking marijuana (discussed in Chapter 15) may double the risk of stroke in young adults.

✓**check-in** Do you have any risk factors for stroke?

Types of Stroke

There are two types of strokes:

- *Ischemic stroke* results from a blockage that disrupts blood flow to the brain. One of the most common causes is the blockage of a brain artery by a thrombus, or blood clot—a *cerebral thrombosis*. Clots generally form around deposits sticking out from the arterial wall. Sometimes a wandering blood clot (embolus), carried in the bloodstream, becomes wedged in one of the cerebral arteries. This is called a *cerebral embolism*, and it can completely plug up a cerebral artery.

- *Hemorrhagic stroke* occurs when a diseased artery in the brain floods the surrounding tissue with blood. The cells nourished by the artery are deprived of blood and can't function, and the blood from the artery forms a clot that may interfere with brain function. This is most likely to occur if the patient suffers from a combination of hypertension and atherosclerosis. Hemorrhage (bleeding) may also be caused by a head injury or by the bursting of an aneurysm, a blood-filled pouch that balloons out from a weak spot in the wall of an artery.

Why Quick Treatment Matters Brain tissue, like heart muscle, begins to die if deprived of oxygen, which may then cause difficulty speaking and walking, as well as loss of memory. These effects may be slight or severe, temporary or permanent, depending on how widespread the damage and whether other areas of the brain can take over the function of the damaged area (Figure 10.7).

For patients who suffer a thrombotic stroke, thrombolytic drugs such as tissue-type plasminogen activator (tPa) can restore brain blood flow and save blood cells. Other medications called heparinoids can reduce the blood's tendency to clot. For thrombolytic drugs to be effective, they must be administered within 3 hours after the stroke; heparinoids must be given within 24 hours. People who get to a hospital within an hour of having the first symptoms of a stroke are twice as likely to receive tPa. However, more than one-third of people having a stroke do not call 911, and an equally large percentage live more than an hour away from a stroke center.[69]

✓**check-in** Would you recognize the signs of a stroke in time to get quick treatment?

📷 SNAPSHOT: ON CAMPUS NOW
Cancer Prevention Strategies

Percentage of students who	%
Used sunscreen regularly when outdoors	52.4
If male, performed a testicular self-exam in the past 30 days	33.3
If female, performed a breast self-exam in the past 30 days	35.6
If female, had a gynecological exam in the past 12 months	40.5

Source: American College Health Association. American College Health Association-National College Health Assessment II: Reference Group Executive Summary Spring 2018. Silver Spring, MD: American College Health Association, 2018.

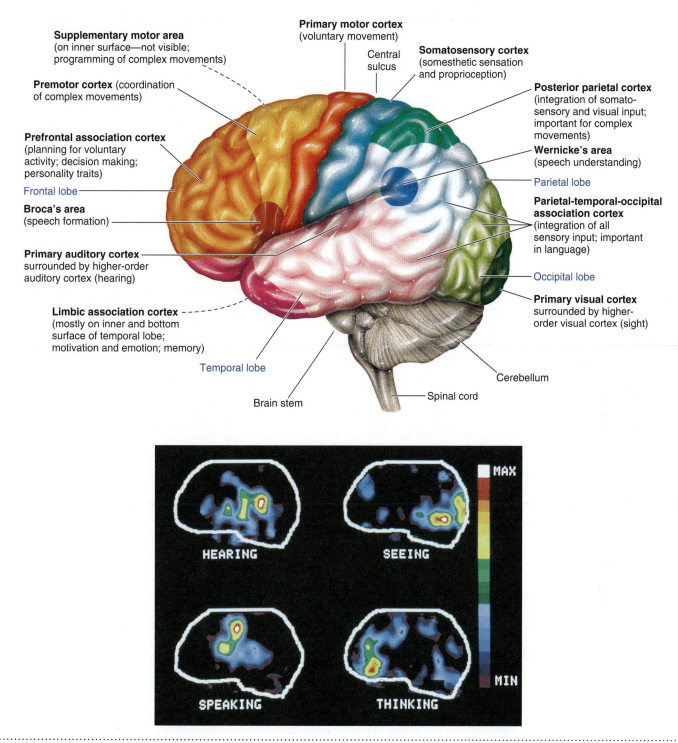

FIGURE 10.7 The Effects of Stroke on the Brain

Cancer

Cancer refers to a group of diseases characterized by the uncontrolled growth and spread of abnormal cells. Cancer is the second leading cause of death worldwide; 8.7 million die from the disease. The lifetime risk of developing cancer is one in three for men and one in four for women.[70]

In the United States, about 1.7 million new cancers are diagnosed every year and about 607,000 Americans die of cancer every year.[71] The gap in cancer deaths among blacks and whites has narrowed for most cancers, but disparities remain.

An estimated 42 percent of cancers are preventable, including those caused by the following:

- Tobacco smoking.
- Heavy alcohol consumption.
- Overweight and obesity.
- Physical inactivity.
- Poor nutrition.
- Excessive sun exposure and indoor tanning.
- Infections that could be avoided by behavioral changes or vaccination.
- Cancers such as colorectal and cervical cancers in which screening can detect precancerous lesions that can be removed.[72]

✓check-in Which of the following preventive steps are you taking to reduce your risk of cancer?

____ Higher fruit and vegetable intake

____ Lower red meat intake

____ Lower fat intake

____ Lower BMI

____ More physical activity

Prevention, early detection, and improved treatment have lowered the death rates for cancers of the lungs, colon, breast, and prostate. Since 1991 cancer death rates have declined by 27 percent.[73]

Understanding Cancer

The uncontrolled growth and spread of abnormal cells cause cancer. Normal cells follow the code of instructions embedded in DNA (the body's genetic material); cancer cells do not. Think of the DNA within the nucleus of a cell as a computer program that controls the cell's functioning, including its ability to grow and reproduce itself. If this program or its operation is altered, the cell goes out of control. The nucleus no longer regulates growth. The abnormal cell divides to create other abnormal cells, which again divide, eventually forming *neoplasms* (new formations), or tumors.

Tumors can be either benign (slightly abnormal, not considered life threatening) or malignant (cancerous). The only way to determine whether a tumor is benign is by microscopic examination of its cells. Cancer cells have larger nuclei than the cells in benign tumors; they vary more in shape and size; and they divide more often. In general, 1 billion cancer cells need to have formed before a cancer can be detected. This is the number of cells in a tumor that measures 1 centimeter (about 0.3 inch).

✓check-in Do you know your lifetime risk of developing cancer?

If you're male: slightly less than one in two.

If you're female: a little more than one in three.

Without treatment, cancer cells continue to grow, crowding out and replacing healthy cells. This process is called **infiltration**, or invasion. Cancer cells may also **metastasize**, or spread to other parts of the body via the bloodstream or lymphatic system (Figure 10.8). For many cancers, as many as 60 percent of patients may have metastases (which may be too small to be felt or seen without a microscope) at the time of diagnosis. Early detection and treatment result in the highest rate of cure.

Who Is at Risk?

Cancer strikes individuals at all social, economic, and educational levels (Table 10.4).

Heredity An estimated 13 million to 14 million Americans may be at risk of a hereditary cancer. In hereditary cancers, such as retinoblastoma (an eye cancer that strikes young children) or certain colon cancers, a specific cancer-causing gene is passed down from generation to generation. The odds of any child with one affected parent inheriting this gene and developing the cancer are 50–50.

Other people are born with genes that make them susceptible to having certain cells grow and divide uncontrollably, which may contribute to cancer development. The most well known are mutations of the BRCA gene, linked with increased risk of breast, colon, and ovarian cancer.

Genetic tests can identify some individuals who are born with an increased susceptibility to cancer. Spotting a mutated gene in an individual may alert doctors to increase screening and possibly detect cancer years earlier than they otherwise would have. The most likely sites for inherited cancers to develop are the breast, brain, blood, muscles, bones, and adrenal glands. A growing number of women who develop breast cancer before age 40 are being tested for the BRCA gene mutations that substantially raise the risks of breast and ovarian tumors.[74]

✓check-in If you had a family history of cancer, would you undergo genetic tests to find out if you are at risk? Why or why not?

infiltration A gradual penetration or invasion.

metastasize To spread to other parts of the body via the bloodstream or lymphatic system.

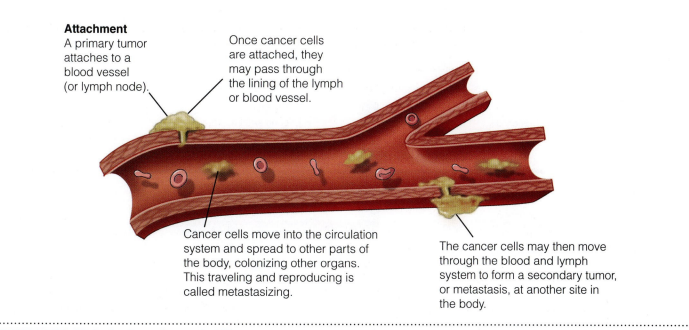

Attachment
A primary tumor attaches to a blood vessel (or lymph node).

Once cancer cells are attached, they may pass through the lining of the lymph or blood vessel.

Cancer cells move into the circulation system and spread to other parts of the body, colonizing other organs. This traveling and reproducing is called metastasizing.

The cancer cells may then move through the blood and lymph system to form a secondary tumor, or metastasis, at another site in the body.

FIGURE 10.8 Metastasis, or Spread of Cancer

Cancer cells can travel through the blood vessels to spread to other organs or through the lymphatic system to form secondary tumors.

Racial and Ethnic Groups Although cancer death rates have fallen in the United States, they vary in different racial and ethnic groups[75]:

- Biological, racial, and ethnic differences can affect whether a cancer is aggressive and will spread beyond its initial site. In breast cancer, for instance, black women had a higher risk of dying compared with white women, even when both were diagnosed with small tumors.

- African Americans have the highest rates of fatal cancers. Black women have the highest incidence of colorectal and lung cancers of any ethnic group, while black men have the highest rates of prostate, colorectal, and lung cancers. African Americans also have higher rates of incidence and deaths from other cancers, including those of the mouth, throat, esophagus, stomach, pancreas, and larynx. Cancer death rates have been declining annually since the 1990s for black men and women.

- Hispanics have a six times lower risk of developing melanoma than Caucasians yet tend to have a worse prognosis than Caucasians when they do develop this skin cancer.

- The incidence of female breast cancer is highest among white women and lowest among Native American women.

- Cervical cancer is most common in Hispanic women.

- Vietnamese men have much higher rates of liver cancer than whites, while Korean men and women are much more likely to develop stomach cancer.

- Compared with other Asian Americans, Chinese and Vietnamese women have higher rates of lung cancer.

- Asian Americans who have lived in the United States the longest are likely to develop the cancers that are most common here, such as breast and colon cancer, although at lower rates than whites.[76]

Obesity Long recognized as threats to cardiovascular health, overweight and obesity may play a role in an estimated 90,000 cancer deaths each year.

The higher an individual's BMI, the greater the likelihood of dying of cancer. An unhealthy body weight increases the risk of many types of cancer, including non-Hodgkin's lymphoma, multiple myeloma, and cancers of the following:

- Breast (in postmenopausal women).
- Colon and rectum.
- Kidney.
- Cervix.
- Ovary.
- Uterus.
- Esophagus.
- Gallbladder.
- Stomach (in men).

TABLE 10.3 Leading New Cancer Cases and Deaths, 2019 Estimates

Estimated new cases

		Males		Females		
Prostate	174,650	20%		Breast	268,600	30%
Lung and bronchus	116,440	13%		Lung and bronchus	111,710	13%
Colon and rectum	78,500	9%		Colon and rectum	67,100	8%
Urinary bladder	61,700	7%		Uterine corpus	61,880	7%
Melanoma of the skin	57,220	7%		Melanoma of the skin	39,260	4%
Kidney and renal pelvis	44,120	5%		Thyroid	37,810	4%
Non-Hodgkin lymphoma	41,090	5%		Non-Hodgkin lymphoma	33,110	4%
Oral cavity and pharynx	38,140	4%		Kidney and renal pelvis	29,700	3%
Leukemia	35,920	4%		Pancreas	26,830	3%
Pancreas	29,940	3%		Leukemia	25,860	3%
All sites	**870,970**	**100%**		**All sites**	**891,480**	**100%**

Estimated deaths

		Males		Females		
Lung and bronchus	76,650	24%		Lung and bronchus	66,020	23%
Prostate	31,620	10%		Breast	41,760	15%
Colon and rectum	27,640	9%		Colon and rectum	23,380	8%
Pancreas	23,800	7%		Pancreas	21,950	8%
Liver and intrahepatic bile duct	21,600	7%		Ovary	13,980	5%
Leukemia	13,150	4%		Uterine corpus	12,160	4%
Esophagus	13,020	4%		Liver and intrahepatic bile duct	10,180	4%
Urinary bladder	12,870	4%		Leukemia	9,690	3%
Non-Hodgkin lymphoma	11,510	4%		Non-Hodgkin lymphoma	8,460	3%
Brain and other nervous system	9,910	3%		Brain and other nervous system	7,850	3%
All sites	**321,670**	**100%**		**All sites**	**285,210**	**100%**

American Cancer Society. Cancer Facts & Figures 2019. Atlanta: American Cancer Society; 2019.

- Liver.

- Pancreas.

- Prostate.

The degree to which extra pounds affect cancer risk varies by the site of the cancer. Obesity elevates the risk of esophageal cancer fivefold; increases the risk of breast or uterine cancer by two to four times; and boosts the risk for colon cancer by 35 to 50 percent.

Carcinogens

The federal government has identified 248 specific substances implicated in cancer, including metals, chemicals, physical agents such as X-rays and ultraviolet radiation, and infectious agents.[77] Each represents a cancer hazard, but does not by itself mean that a substance or a virus will cause cancer. Many factors, including an individual's susceptibility to a substance, and the amount and duration of exposure, can affect whether a person will develop cancer. In the case of viruses, a weakened immune system may also be a contributing factor. Of all known carcinogens, tobacco takes the biggest toll. Smoking is linked to almost one-third of fatal cancers in people 35 or older.[78]

Infectious agents. An estimated 12 percent of cancers in the United States can be attributed to infection, including the following:

- Human papillomavirus (HPV) with cancer of the cervix, mouth and throat, vulva, and anus.

- *Helicobacter pylori* with stomach cancer.

- Epstein-Barr virus (EBV), a herpesvirus, transmitted primarily through saliva infecting more than 90 percent of adults worldwide. Although most people infected with EBV

THE SEVEN WARNING SIGNS OF CANCER

The American Cancer Society uses the word

C-A-U-T-I-O-N

to help recognize the seven early signs of cancer:

- Change in bowel or bladder habits
- A sore that does not heal
- Unusual bleeding or discharge
- Thickening or lump in the breast, testicles, or elsewhere
- Indigestion or difficulty swallowing
- Obvious change in the size, color, shape, or thickness of a wart, mole, or mouth sore
- Nagging cough or hoarseness

trentemoller/Shutterstock.com

remain healthy, EBV can lead to certain types of lymphomas and stomach cancers as well as nasopharyngeal cancer.

- Human immunodeficiency virus (HIV) with certain lymphomas and leukemias and a type of cancer called Kaposi's sarcoma.[79]

Generally, the presence of a bacterium or a virus per se is not enough to cause cancer. A predisposing environment and other cofactors—most still unknown—are needed for cancer development and growth.

Common Types of Cancer

Cancer refers to a group of more than a hundred diseases characterized by abnormal cell growth. Although all cancers have similar characteristics, each is distinct. Some cancers are relatively simple to cure, whereas others are more threatening and mysterious (see Table 10.3). The earlier any cancer is found, the easier it is to treat and the better the patient's chances of survival.

Cancers are classified according to the type of cell and the organ in which they originate, such as the following:

- **Carcinoma,** the most common kind, which starts in the epithelium, the layers of cells that cover the body's surface or line internal organs and glands.
- **Sarcoma,** which forms in the supporting, or connective, tissues of the body: bones, muscles, and blood vessels.
- **Leukemia,** which begins in the blood-forming tissues: bone marrow, lymph nodes, and the spleen.
- **Lymphoma,** which arises in the cells of the lymph system, the network that filters out impurities.

Skin Cancer One of every five Americans can expect to develop skin cancer in his or her lifetime. Once scientists thought exposure to the B range of ultraviolet light (UVB), the wavelength of light responsible for sunburn, posed the greatest danger. However, longer-wavelength UVA, which penetrates deeper into the skin, also plays a major role in skin cancers. UV light can damage DNA in melanocytes, cells in the skin that make the substance called melanin, which gives skin its color. Damage to melanocytes can continue long after UV exposure, even in the dark.

Exposure to tanning salons and sunlamps also increase the risk of skin cancer because they produce UV radiation. A 30-minute dose of radiation from a sunlamp can be equivalent to the amount you'd get from an entire day in the sun. Often skin damage is invisible to the naked eye but shows up under special diagnostic lights.

According to a recent analysis of data on more than 400,000 people, more than one-third of all Americans—and nearly 6 of 10 U.S. university students—have used indoor tanning.[80] Even when they perceive the seriousness of skin cancer, college students—particularly women—describe suntanned skin as attractive, healthy, and athletic looking and view the benefits of getting a suntan as outweighing the risks of skin cancer or premature aging. (See Consumer Alert.) However, a CDC report concluded that indoor tanning is "simply not safe" and causes sunburn, infection, eye damage, and increased risk of skin cancer.

In Canada, where more than 10 percent of adults (particularly young women) report using an indoor tanning device, this exposure contributes to 7 percent of melanomas, as well as 5 percent of basal cell carcinomas and 8 percent of squamous cell carcinomas.[81]

Using tanning beds at a young age significantly raises a woman's risk of developing melanoma

Are You Addicted to Tanning?

You know that exposure to UV rays increases your risk of developing skin cancer, but maybe you still can't stay out of the sun or a tanning booth. Why?

Facts to Know

- Researchers theorize that repetitive tanning behavior may be the result of a kind of addiction.
- College students who have symptoms of mental or substance abuse disorders may be more susceptible to developing dependency.

Steps to Take

- Test your risk of "ultraviolet light (UVL) dependency" by taking the CAGE screening test for addictive behavior. Ask yourself the following questions:

  - **Cut:** Ever felt you ought to cut down on your behavior?

  - **Annoyed:** Have people annoyed you by criticizing your behavior?

  - **Guilt:** Ever felt bad or guilty about your behavior?

  - **Eye opener:** Ever engaged in your behavior to steady your nerves in the morning?

Answering yes to two of the CAGE questions is a strong indication for an addictive behavior; answering yes to three confirms it.

---

before the age of 50. Among adults ages 25 to 49, the risk for the deadly skin cancer increased two to six times for women who tanned indoors, with the greatest odds seen for those who used tanning beds in their teens and 20s. Younger women with melanoma also reported more tanning sessions than older women—an average of 100 tanning sessions compared with 40 sessions for women diagnosed at 40 to 49.[82]

In a recent study, some college women reported that indoor tanning eased negative feelings such as being upset, nervous, irritable, jittery, or afraid and increased positive mood states. Frequent tanners who report relatively high rates of psychiatric and substance abuse symptoms may be especially vulnerable to dependence.[83] One novel approach being tried to alert people to the potential dangers is text messaging.[84]

✓**check-in** Have you ever gone to indoor tanning salons? If so, how often?

The most common skin cancers are *basal cell* (involving the base of the epidermis, the top level of the skin) and *squamous cell* (involving cells in the epidermis). Their incidence is increasing among men and women under age 40. Long-term exposure to the sun is the biggest risk factor for these cancers.

Young men and women who use tanning beds are significantly more likely than nonusers to develop early-onset basal cell skin cancers before age 40. The more extensive their use, the greater their risk of skin cancers, particularly on the extremities and the torso. Researchers

estimate that avoiding tanning beds could cut the percentages of early-onset skin cancer by 27 percent overall and by 43 percent among women.

Every year more than 5 million Americans develop skin lesions known as actinic keratoses (AKs), rough red or brown scaly patches that develop in the upper layer of the skin, usually on the face, lower lip, bald scalp, neck, back of the hands, and forearms. Forty percent of squamous cell carcinomas, the second leading cause of skin cancer deaths, begin as AKs. Treatments include surgical removal, cryosurgery (freezing the skin), electrodesiccation (heat generated by an electric current), topical chemotherapy, and removal with lasers, chemical peels, or dermabrasion.

Malignant *melanoma*, the deadliest type of skin cancer, causes 1 to 2 percent of all cancer deaths. Melanoma has become the most common cancer among young adults between ages 25 and 29 and the second most common cancer among 15- to 24-year-olds. During the 1930s, the lifetime risk of melanoma was about 1 in 1,500. Today it is 1 in 75. This increase in risk is due mostly to overexposure to UV radiation. Although melanoma occurs more often among people over age 40, its incidence is increasing in younger people, particularly those who had severe sunburns in childhood.

Individuals with any of the following characteristics are at increased risk:

- Fair skin, light eyes, or fair hair.

- A tendency to develop freckles and to burn instead of tan.

- A history of childhood sunburn or intermittent, intense sun exposure.

- A personal or family history of melanoma.

Detection. Although a large number of nevi or moles (200 or more, or 50 or more if under age 20) or dysplastic (atypical) moles was long considered a risk factor, a recent study found that patients with melanoma skin cancer often had few moles and no abnormal ones. The most common predictor for melanoma is a change in an existing mole or development of a new and changing pigmented mole. The most important early indicators are change in color, an increase in diameter, and changes in the borders of a mole (Figure 10.9). Thickness or an increase in height signals a corresponding growth in depth under the skin.[85] Itching in a new or long-standing mole also should not be ignored.

Treatment. If caught early, melanoma is highly curable, usually with surgery alone. Once it has spread, chemotherapy with a single drug or a combination can temporarily shrink tumors in some people. Melanomas that have penetrated deep into the body or spread to lymph nodes may be treated with surgery, immunotherapy, chemotherapy, and/or radiation. The five-year survival rate for melanoma is 92 percent.[86] (See Your Strategies for Prevention.)

Breast Cancer
About one in eight women in the United States (12 percent) develops invasive breast cancer in her lifetime.[87] Every 3 minutes, a woman in the United States learns that she has breast cancer. Although death rates for breast cancer have declined, every 12 minutes a woman dies of it. Many women misjudge their own likelihood of developing breast cancer, either overestimating or underestimating their susceptibility. In a national poll, 1 in every 10 surveyed considered herself at no risk at all. This is never the case. Every woman is at risk for breast cancer simply because she's female.

Risk Factors. The most common risk factors include the following:

- **Age.** As shown in Table 10.4, at age 25, a woman's chance of developing breast cancer is 1 in 19,608; by age 45, it has increased to 1 in 93; by 65, it is 1 in 17. The mean age at which women are diagnosed is 63. However, more young women are being diagnosed with advanced metastatic breast cancer.

- **Family history.** The overwhelming majority of breast cancers—90 to 95 percent—are not

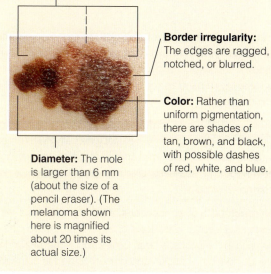

Asymmetry: One half doesn't match the other half.

Border irregularity: The edges are ragged, notched, or blurred.

Color: Rather than uniform pigmentation, there are shades of tan, brown, and black, with possible dashes of red, white, and blue.

Diameter: The mole is larger than 6 mm (about the size of a pencil eraser). (The melanoma shown here is magnified about 20 times its actual size.)

Callista Images/Alamy Stock Photo

FIGURE 10.9 ABCD: The Warning Signs of Melanoma

An estimated 95 percent of cases of melanoma arise from an existing mole. A normal mole is usually round or oval, less than 6 mm (about ¼ inch) in diameter, and evenly colored (black, brown, or tan). Seek prompt evaluation of any moles that change in ways shown in the photo.

due to strong genetic factors. However, having a first-degree relative—mother, sister, or daughter—with breast cancer does increase risk, and if the relative developed breast cancer before menopause, the cancer is more likely to be hereditary.

- **Long menstrual history.** Women who had their first period before age 12 are at greater risk than women who began menstruating later. The reason is that the more menstrual cycles a woman has, the longer her exposure to estrogen, a hormone known to increase breast cancer danger. For similar reasons, childless women, who menstruate continuously for several decades, are also at greater risk. Neither miscarriage nor induced abortion increases the risk of breast cancer.

- **Age at birth of first child.** An early pregnancy—in a woman's teens or 20s—changes the actual maturation of breast cells and decreases risk. But if a woman has her first child in her 40s, precancerous cells may actually flourish with the high hormone levels of the pregnancy.

- **Breast biopsies.** Even if laboratory analysis finds no precancerous abnormalities, women who require such tests are more likely to develop breast cancer. Fibrocystic breast disease, a term often used for "lumpy" breasts, is not a risk factor.

TABLE 10.4 A Woman's Risk of Developing Breast Cancer

By age 25	1 in 19,608
By age 30	1 in 2,525
By age 35	1 in 622
By age 40	1 in 217
By age 45	1 in 93
By age 50	1 in 50
By age 55	1 in 33
By age 60	1 in 24
By age 65	1 in 17
By age 70	1 in 14
By age 75	1 in 11
By age 80	1 in 10
By age 85	1 in 9
Ever	1 in 8

Source: Surveillance Program, National Cancer Institute.

YOUR STRATEGIES FOR PREVENTION

Save Your Skin

- **Once a month, stand in front of a full-length mirror to examine your front and back, as well as your left and right sides with your arms raised.** Check the backs of your legs, the tops and soles of your feet, and the surfaces between your toes. Use a hand mirror to check the back of your neck, behind your ears, and your scalp.

- **Watch for changes in the size, color, number, and thickness of moles.** Suspicious moles are likely to be asymmetrical (one half doesn't match the other), with ragged, notched, or blurred edges. Also look for any signs of darkly pigmented growth, oozing, scaliness, bleeding, or a change in sensation, itchiness, tenderness, or pain.

- **Don't put too much faith in sunscreens.** Wearing sunscreen (with a sun protection factor, or SPF, of at least 15) is good, but protective clothing is better—and staying in the shade is best. Check your shadow. One simple guideline for reducing the risk of skin cancer is avoiding the sun anytime your shadow is shorter than you are. According to the National Cancer Institute (NCI), this shadow method—based on the principle that the closer the sun comes to being directly overhead, the stronger its ultraviolet rays—works for any location and at any time of year.

- **Check for photosensitivity.** If you are taking any drugs, ask your doctor or pharmacist to see if the medication could make you more sensitive to sun damage. Be especially cautious about sun exposure if you have been using a synthetic preparation derived from vitamin A (Retin A) as an acne or antiwrinkle treatment; it can increase your susceptibility.

- **Use extra caution near water, snow, and sand since they reflect the damaging rays of the sun and increase the risk of sunburn.** Wear protective clothing, such as a wide-brimmed cap or hat, whenever possible.

- **Race and ethnicity.** Breast cancer rates are lower in Hispanic and Asian American populations than in white and African American women. Caucasian women over age 40 have the highest incidence rate for breast cancer in this country, but African American women at every age have a greater likelihood of dying from breast cancer.[88] One reason may be that minority women wait longer for treatment, whether surgery or chemotherapy. Hispanic women, particularly those of Mexican descent, are more likely than white or black women to have hereditary forms of cancer.

- **Occupation.** Based on two decades of following more than a million women, Swedish researchers have developed a list of jobs linked with a high risk of breast cancer. These include pharmacists, certain types of teachers, schoolmasters, systems analysts and programmers, telephone operators, telegraph and radio operators, metal platers and coaters, and salon workers. Shift work, particularly at night, may be associated with an increased risk of breast cancer.

- **Alcohol.** Women's risk of breast cancer increases with the amount of alcohol they drink. Those who have two or more drinks per day are 40 percent more likely to develop breast cancer than women who don't drink at all. For a nondrinking woman, the lifetime risk of breast cancer by age 80 is 1 in 11. For heavy drinkers it's about 1 in 7, regardless of race, education, family history, use of hormone therapy, or other risk factors.

- **Smoking.** Cigarette smoking, with or without alcohol use, increases the risk of breast cancer, especially when women start smoking early in life.

- **Hormone therapy (HT).** Several studies confirm an increased risk with a combination of estrogen and progestin, particularly in women who use combination HT for 5 years or longer. With the decreasing use of hormone therapy, breast cancer rates have declined by 40 percent from their peak in 1989.[89]

- **Obesity.** Excess weight, particularly after menopause, increases the risk of getting breast cancer. Overweight women, both pre- and postmenopausal, with breast cancer are more likely to die of their disease.

- **Sedentary lifestyle.** According to the World Health Organization, regular physical activity may cut the risk of developing breast cancer by 20 to 40 percent, regardless of a woman's menopausal status or the type or intensity of the activity. The reason may be that exercise lowers levels of circulating ovarian hormones.

✓**check-in** Do you know which factors may lower a woman's risk of breast cancer?
- Breastfeeding for at least 1 year.
- Regular, moderate, or vigorous exercise.
- Maintaining a healthy body weight.
The answer: All of the above.

Screening for Breast Cancer. Early detection of breast cancer can help save thousands of lives each year by improving the odds that breast cancer can be found early and be treated successfully. According to the American Cancer Society's most recent guidelines:

- **Women ages 40 to 44** at average risk who do not have a personal or family history of breast cancer, a genetic mutation known to increase risk of breast cancer (such as BRCA), or radiation therapy to the chest before the age of 30, should have the choice to start annual breast cancer screening with mammograms if they wish to do so.

- **Women ages 45 to 54** should get mammograms every year.
- **Women ages 55 or older** should switch to mammograms every 2 years, or have the choice to continue yearly screening.

The primary downside of more frequent mammograms is a false-positive diagnosis—when breast cancer is first suspected but then ruled out with further testing—which can be extremely upsetting.

✓**check-in** If you are a woman, have you ever had a mammogram or breast biopsy?

Medical organizations disagree as to the value of breast self-examination to check for changes in the appearance and feel of the breast for women starting in their 20s. Talk to your doctor about the benefits and limitations of examining your breasts on a regular basis. (Figure 10.10 provides step-by-step instructions.)

Treatment. Because breast cancer is a heterogeneous disease, treatment must be targeted to the individual, depending on factors such as tumor size, extent of spread, and certain key receptors. In general, options include:

- Breast-conserving surgery (surgical removal of the tumor and surrounding tissue).
- **Mastectomy** (surgical removal of the breast). Women treated with breast-conserving surgery plus radiation and those who undergo mastectomy have similar long-term survival rates.[90] Surgeons usually remove underarm lymph nodes to determine if a tumor has spread beyond the breast.

Breast cancer treatment may also involve:

- Radiation.
- Chemotherapy (before or after surgery).
- Hormone therapy (with agents such as estrogen receptor modifiers or aromatase inhibitors).

More women diagnosed with cancer in one breast are opting to have their other, healthy breast removed. However, recent analysis of nearly 500,000 women with breast cancer has found no survival benefits in doing so.[91]

Survival. About 6 in 10 diagnosed breast cancers are localized and have not spread to lymph

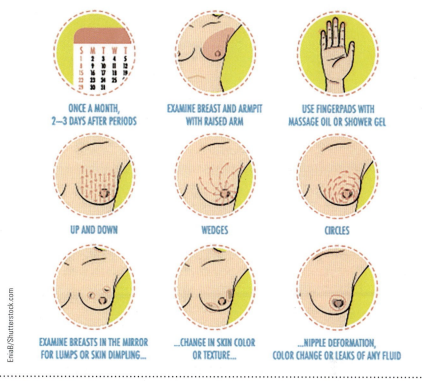

BREAST SELF-EXAMINATION

ONCE A MONTH, 2–3 DAYS AFTER PERIODS

EXAMINE BREAST AND ARMPIT WITH RAISED ARM

USE FINGERPADS WITH MASSAGE OIL OR SHOWER GEL

UP AND DOWN

WEDGES

CIRCLES

EXAMINE BREASTS IN THE MIRROR FOR LUMPS OR SKIN DIMPLING...

...CHANGE IN SKIN COLOR OR TEXTURE...

...NIPPLE DEFORMATION, COLOR CHANGE OR LEAKS OF ANY FLUID

EniaB/Shutterstock.com

FIGURE 10.10 Women should check their breasts regularly for changes in the way they look or feel.

nodes or other locations outside the breast. The 5-year survival rate for women with these cancers is 99 percent. If the cancer has spread to tissues or lymph nodes under the arm, the survival rate is 85 percent. If the cancer has spread to lymph nodes around the collarbone or more distant nodes or an organ, the survival rate falls to 25 percent. Survival rates are lower for black women, who may be diagnosed and seek treatment later.[92] Increased physical activity after breast cancer diagnosis has been associated with lower risk of dying, either of cancer or other causes.[93]

Male breast cancer accounts for 1 percent of all breast cancers and less than 1 percent of all malignancies in men. Stage for stage, men have similar outcomes to those for female breast cancer patients, but they tend to be diagnosed at a more advanced stage, waiting an average of 10 months after the onset of symptoms.[94]

Cervical Cancer Cervical cancer, the second most common cancer in women worldwide, claims 250,000 lives every year. An estimated 11,000 cases of invasive cervical cancer are diagnosed in the United States every year. The highest incidence rate occurs among Vietnamese, Alaska Native, Korean, and Hispanic women.

mastectomy The surgical removal of an entire breast.

Human papillomavirus (HPV) infection is the primary risk factor for cervical cancer. Women are at higher risk for cervical cancer if they:

- Engaged in sexual activity before age 16.

- Have had multiple sexual partners (more than five in a lifetime).

- Have genital herpes.

- Smoke.

- Have been exposed to secondhand smoke.

Screening. Two types of tests are used for cervical cancer screening:

- The Pap test, which can find early cell changes and cancerous growths and treat them (Table 10.5).

- The HPV test, which detects infections that can lead to cell changes and cancer. The HPV test may be used along with a Pap test or to help doctors decide how to treat women with an abnormal Pap test.

The American Cancer Society's latest screening recommendations are:

- All women should begin cervical cancer screening at age 21.

- Women between the ages of 21 and 29 should have a Pap test every 3 years but should not be tested for HPV unless they have an abnormal Pap test result.

- Women between the ages of 30 and 65 should have both a Pap test and an HPV test every 5 years. Recent evidence suggests that the screening interval can be extended beyond 5 years for women over age 40.[95]

- Women over age 65 who have had regular screenings with normal results should not be screened for cervical cancer. Women who have been diagnosed with cervical precancer should continue to be screened.

- Women who have had their uterus and cervix removed in a hysterectomy and have no history of cervical cancer or precancer should not be screened.

- Women who have had the HPV vaccine should still follow the screening recommendations for their age group.

- Women who are at high risk for cervical cancer—for example, those with HIV infection, organ transplant, or exposure to the drug DES—should talk with their doctor or nurse about more frequent screening.

Doctors no longer recommend annual Pap tests because it generally takes 10 to 20 years for cervical cancer to develop and overly frequent screening could lead to unneeded medical and surgical procedures.

✓**check-in** If you're a woman, have you had any screening test for cervical cancer?

TABLE 10.5 What Your Pap Test Results Mean

A Pap test may come back as "normal," "unclear," or "abnormal."	
Normal 	A normal (or "negative") result means that no cell changes were found on the cervix.
Unclear	It is common for test results to come back unclear. Doctors may use other words to describe this result, such as inconclusive, or ASC-US. These mean the same thing: that some cervical cells could be abnormal, perhaps because of an infection. An HPV test will indicate whether the changes are related to HPV.
Abnormal	An abnormal result means that cell changes were found on the cervix. This usually does not indicate cervical cancer.

Abnormal changes on your cervix are likely caused by HPV. The changes may be minor (low grade) or serious (high grade). Most of the time, minor changes go back to normal on their own. But more serious changes can turn into cancer if the cells are not removed. The more serious changes are often called "precancer" because they are not yet cancer but could turn into cancer over time.

Ovarian Cancer Ovarian cancer is the leading cause of death from gynecological cancers. Each year, more than 21,000 women in the United States are diagnosed with ovarian cancer; more than 14,000 women die from the disease each year. Ovarian cancer isn't a single disease, according to an expert panel, but a number of different malignancies involving the ovaries. Many ovarian cancers begin in other tissues, such as the fallopian tubes, and eventually spread to the ovaries.[96]

Risk factors include:

- Family history of ovarian cancer

- Smoking

- Testing positive for inherited mutations in BRCA1 and BRCA2 genes. (Preventive surgery to remove the ovaries and fallopian tubes decreases the risk for these women.)

Ovarian cancer may be diagnosed through pelvic examination, ultrasound, MRI, computed tomography, or positron emission tomography (PET) scan. Women with ovarian cancer are more likely to report abdominal pain, feeling full quickly after eating, and urinary urgency, but these symptoms are so common that they are often overlooked or dismissed.

Treatment involves surgery and usually chemotherapy. Survival rates depend on whether the cancer has spread to distant sites.

Testicular Cancer In the past 20 years the incidence of testicular cancer has risen by about 50 percent in the United States, to 5.44 per 100,000. It is not clear why testicular cancer is on the rise, although researchers speculate that changing environmental or socioeconomic risk factors could have a role. Chronic use of marijuana increases the risk of an especially aggressive form of testicular cancer. Testicular cancer occurs mostly among young men between the ages of 18 and 35, who are not normally at risk of cancer.

Risk factors for testicular cancer include:

- An undescended testicle
- Family history of testicular cancer
- HIV infection
- Cancer in the other testicle
- Caucasian race (white men have a four to five times greater risk than black or Asian American men)

To detect possibly cancerous growths, men should perform monthly testicular self-exams (Figure 10.11).

✓**check-in** If you're a man, do you examine your testicles regularly?

Often the first sign of this cancer is a slight enlargement of one testicle. There may also be a change in the way it feels when touched. Sometimes men with testicular cancer report a dull ache in the lower abdomen or groin, along with a sense of heaviness or sluggishness. Lumps on the testicles may also indicate cancer.

A man who notices any abnormality should consult a physician. If a lump is indeed present, a surgical biopsy is necessary to find out if it is cancerous. If the biopsy is positive, a series of tests is generally needed to determine whether the disease has spread.

Treatment for testicular cancer generally involves surgical removal of the diseased testis, sometimes along with radiation therapy, chemotherapy, and the removal of nearby lymph nodes. The remaining testicle is capable of maintaining a man's sexual potency and fertility. Only in rare cases is removal of both testicles necessary. Testosterone injections following such surgery can maintain potency. The chance for a cure is very high if testicular cancer is spotted early.

Colon and Rectal Cancer Colon and rectal, or colorectal, cancer is the third most common cancer and accounts for 10 percent of cancer deaths. Long considered a disease of older men and women, colon cancer is rising

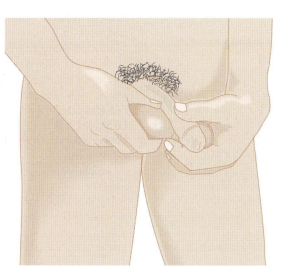

FIGURE 10.11 Testicular Self-Exam

The best time to examine your testicles is after a hot bath or shower, when the scrotum is most relaxed. Place your index and middle fingers under each testicle and the thumb on top, and roll the testicle between the thumb and fingers. If you feel a small, hard, usually painless lump or swelling, or anything unusual, consult a urologist.

among men and women under 55, who now account for one in seven colon cancer patients. Younger patients are more likely to have advanced-stage cancer, but they live slightly longer without a cancer recurrence because they are treated aggressively.[97] In a recent epidemiological study, African Americans and American Indian/Alaska Natives had a significantly greater risk of dying from colorectal cancer as compared with whites.[98]

Several factors may lower your odds of developing colon cancer. Men who are physically fit in middle age are less likely to develop colon cancer later in life.[99] A healthy vegetarian diet that features fruits, vegetables, whole grains, beans, and nuts may cut the risk by as much as 20 percent.[100] A federal task force has recommended daily low-dose aspirin to provide a "modest" preventive effect in certain adults over age 55.[101]

....
✓**check-in** Do you have any of the risk factors for colon cancer?
....

Risk factors include:

- Personal or family history of colon and rectal cancer.

- Polyps in the colon or rectum.

- Ulcerative colitis.

- Smoking.

- Alcohol consumption.

- Prolonged high consumption of red and processed meat.

- High-fat or low-fiber diet.

- Inadequate intake of fruits and vegetables.

- Low calcium intake.

- Obesity.

- Physical inactivity.

Long-term constipation does not raise the risk of colorectal cancer. Low doses of aspirin or other nonsteroidal anti-inflammatory drugs (NSAIDs) appear to reduce the risk of precancerous polyps that can lead to colon and rectal cancer. Smokers have a worse prognosis than nonsmokers.

Under the Affordable Care Act (discussed in Chapter 14), insurance companies must pay the full cost of colon cancer screening, Current guidelines recommend that clinicians screen for colorectal cancer in average-risk adults starting at age 50 and in high-risk adults starting at age 40, or 10 years younger than the age at which the youngest affected relative was diagnosed with colorectal cancer. The screening options include a stool-based test, flexible sigmoidoscopy, and optical colonoscopy in patients who are at average risk.

Tests for blood in the stool—known as fecal immunochemical tests—can consistently detect colon cancer when used on an annual basis. According to one study, stool testing can be a reasonable screening alternative to colonoscopy.[102] This invasive procedure, in which a tiny camera is inserted into a person's colon, requires sedation and powerful laxatives to "prep" the bowels for examination. By comparison, a fecal blood test is less intrusive and unpleasant. However, a colonoscopy provides the opportunity to detect and remove dangerous polyps, which has proven to reduce deaths from colon and rectal cancer by 70 percent. If 80 percent of older adults underwent colon cancer screening, 21,000 fewer Americans would die of the cancer every year.[103]

Early signs of colorectal cancer are bleeding from the rectum, blood in the stool, and a change in bowel habits. Treatment may involve surgery, radiation therapy, and/or chemotherapy.

Prostate Cancer After skin cancer, prostate cancer is the most common form of cancer in American men. The risk of prostate cancer is 1 in 6; the risk of death due to metastatic prostate cancer is 1 in 30. More than one-quarter of men diagnosed with cancer have prostate cancer. The incidence of prostate cancer is about 60 percent higher in blacks than in whites; the reasons for this difference are not known.[104]

The risk of prostate cancer increases with age, family history, exposure to the heavy metal cadmium, high number of sexual partners, and history of frequent sexually transmitted infections. A diet high in saturated fat may be a risk factor. An inherited predisposition may account for 5 to 10 percent of cases. A purported link between vasectomy and prostate cancer has been disproved. Statin drugs, commonly prescribed to lower cholesterol, may also lower the risk of prostate cancer.

Annual screening with a test that measures levels of a protein called prostate-specific antigen (PSA) in the blood is no longer recommended. Annual prostate cancer screening does not reduce deaths from the disease, regardless of the man's age or overall health.

Some prostate cancers never progress. Treatment options include a conservative, wait-and-watch approach, various forms of radiation and ablative technologies, and different surgical approaches.[105] The 10-year survival rate for all stages combined is 98 percent.[106]

Infectious Diseases

Infection is a complex process, triggered by various pathogens (disease-causing organisms) and countered by the body's own defenders. Physicians explain infection in terms of a host (either a person or a population) that contacts one or more agents in an environment. A vector—a biological or physical vehicle that carries the agent to the host—provides the means of transmission.

Agents of Infection

The types of microbes that can cause infection are viruses, bacteria, fungi, protozoa, and helminths (parasitic worms) (Figure 10.12).

Viruses   The tiniest pathogens—viruses—are also the toughest; they consist of a bit of nucleic acid (DNA or RNA, but never both) within a protein coat. Unable to reproduce on its own, a virus takes over a body cell's reproductive machinery and instructs it to produce new viral particles, which are then released to enter other cells. The common cold, the flu, herpes, hepatitis, and AIDS are viral diseases.

The most common viruses are as follows:

- **Rhinoviruses and adenoviruses,** which get into the mucous membranes and cause upper respiratory tract infections and colds.

- **Coronaviruses,** named for their corona, or halolike appearance, are second only to rhinoviruses in causing the common cold and other respiratory infections. Coronaviruses have recently been implicated in outbreaks of deadly diseases such as severe acute respiratory syndrome (SARS).[107] A deadly new strain was identified in the Middle East and Great Britain several years ago.

- **Influenza viruses,** which can change their outer protein coats so dramatically that individuals resistant to one strain cannot fight off a new one.

- **Herpes viruses,** which take up permanent residence in the cells and periodically flare up.

- **Papillomaviruses,** which cause few symptoms in women and almost none in men but may be responsible, at least in part, for a rise in the incidence of cervical cancer among younger women.

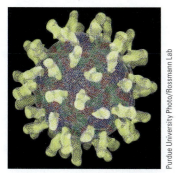

(a)

Purdue University Photo/Rossmann Lab

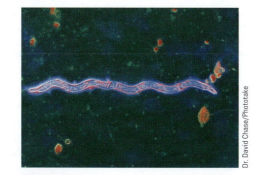

(b)

Dr. David Chase/Phototake

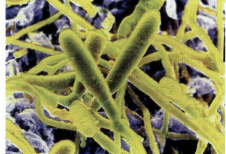

(c)

E. Gueho/Science Source

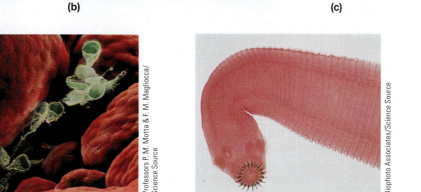

(d)

Professors P. M. Motta & F. M. Magliocca/Science Source

(e)

Biophoto Associates/Science Source

FIGURE 10.12 Examples of Major Categories of Organisms That Cause Disease in Humans.

Except for the helminths (parasitic worms), pathogens are microorganisms that can be seen only with the aid of a microscope. (a) Viruses: common cold; (b) Bacteria: syphilis; (c) Fungi: athlete's foot fungus; (d) Protozoa: *Giardia lamblia;* (e) Helminths: tapeworm.

- **Hepatitis viruses,** which cause several forms of liver infection, ranging from mild to life threatening.

- **Slow viruses,** which give no early indication of their presence but can produce fatal illnesses within a few years.

- **Retroviruses,** which are named for their backward (retro) sequence of genetic replication compared to other viruses. One retrovirus, human immunodeficiency virus (HIV), causes acquired immune deficiency syndrome (AIDS) (discussed in Chapter 12).

- **Filoviruses,** which resemble threads and are extremely lethal.

The problem in fighting viruses is that it's difficult to find drugs that harm the virus and not the cell it has commandeered. Antibiotics (drugs that inhibit or kill bacteria) have no effect on viruses. Antiviral drugs don't completely eradicate a viral infection, although they can decrease its severity and duration. Because viruses multiply very quickly, antiviral drugs are most effective when taken before an infection develops or in its early stages.

Bacteria   Simple one-celled organisms, bacteria are the most plentiful microorganisms as well as the most pathogenic. Most kinds of bacteria don't cause disease; some, like certain strains of *Escherichia coli* that aid in digestion, play important roles within the body. Even friendly bacteria, however, can get out of hand and cause acne, urinary tract infections, vaginal infections, and other problems.

Bacteria harm the body by releasing either enzymes that digest body cells or toxins that produce the specific effects of diseases such as diphtheria or toxic shock syndrome. In self-defense, the body produces specific proteins (called *antibodies*) that attack and inactivate the invaders. Tuberculosis, tetanus, gonorrhea, scarlet fever, and diphtheria are examples of bacterial diseases.

Because bacteria are sufficiently different from the cells that make up the body, antibiotics can kill them without harming the cells. Antibiotics work only against specific types of bacteria. If your doctor thinks you have a bacterial infection, tests of your blood, pus, sputum, urine, or stool can identify the particular bacterial strain.

Fungi   Single-celled or multicelled organisms, fungi consist of threadlike fibers and reproductive spores. Fungi lack chlorophyll and must obtain their food from organic material, which may include human tissue. Fungi release enzymes that digest cells and are most likely to attack hair-covered areas of the body, including the scalp, beard, groin, and external ear canals. They also cause athlete's foot. Treatment consists of antifungal drugs.

Researchers have identified a new "superbug": *Candida auris*, a potentially deadly fungal infection that has been reported in health-care facilities in the United States and Europe. Most strains of this fungus are resistant to current drug treatment.[108]

Protozoa   These single-celled, microscopic animals release enzymes and toxins that destroy cells or interfere with their function. Diseases caused by protozoa are not a major health problem in this country, primarily because of public health measures. Around the world, however, some 2.24 billion people (more than 40 percent of the world's population) are at risk for acquiring malaria—a protozoan-caused disease. Up to 3 million die from this disease annually. Many more come down with amoebic dysentery. Treatment for protozoa-caused diseases consists of general medical care to relieve the symptoms, replacement of lost blood or fluids, and drugs that kill the specific protozoan.

The most common disease caused by protozoa in the United States is *giardiasis*, an intestinal infection caused by microorganisms in human and animal feces. It has become a threat at day-care centers, as well as among campers and hikers who drink contaminated water. Symptoms include nausea, lack of appetite, gas, diarrhea, fatigue, abdominal cramps, and bloating. Treatment usually consists of antibiotics.

Helminths (Parasitic Worms)   Small parasitic worms that attack specific tissues or organs and compete with the host for nutrients are called helminths. One major worldwide health problem is *schistosomiasis*, a disease caused by a parasitic worm, the fluke, that burrows through the skin and enters the circulatory system. Infection with another helminth, the tapeworm, may be contracted from eating undercooked beef, pork, or fish containing larval forms of the tapeworm. Helminthic diseases are treated with appropriate medications.

✓**check-in** Which of these agents do you see as the greatest threat to your health?

How Infections Spread

The major *vectors*, or means of transmission, for infectious disease are animals and insects, people, food, and water.

Animals and Insects Disease can be transmitted by house pets, livestock, birds, and wild animals. Insects also spread a variety of diseases. The housefly may spread dysentery, diarrhea, typhoid fever, or trachoma (an eye disease rare in the United States but common in other parts of the world). Other insects—including mosquitoes, ticks, mites, fleas, and lice—can transmit such diseases as malaria, yellow fever, encephalitis, dengue fever (a growing threat in Mexico), and Lyme disease. West Nile virus (WNV) can be spread to humans by mosquitoes that bite infected birds; monkeypox virus is carried by various animals, including prairie dogs. Concern has grown about avian influenza, or bird flu, which has spread to wild and domestic birds around the world. The Zika virus, discussed on page 347, is spread primarily through the bite of an infected *Aedes* species mosquito.

The CDC has identified a new tickborne pathogen: the "Bourbon virus," named for the Kansas county in which it was first discovered.[109] The newfound virus belongs to a family of germs called Thogotoviruses, which have been linked to transmission by ticks and mosquitoes in parts of Europe, Asia, and Africa. Another tickborne virus, the Heartland virus, was identified in Missouri in recent years.

People The people you're closest to can transmit pathogens through the air, by touch, or from sexual contact. To avoid infection, stay out of range of anyone who's coughing, sniffling, or sneezing; and don't share food or dishes. Carefully wash your dishes, utensils, and hands, and abstain from sex or make self-protective decisions about sexual partners.

✓**check-in** What precautions do you take to avoid being infected by others?

Food Every year foodborne illnesses strike millions of Americans, sometimes with fatal consequences. Bacteria account for two-thirds of foodborne infections, and thousands of suspected cases of infection with *Escherichia coli* bacteria in undercooked or inadequately washed food have been reported.

Every year as many as 4 million Americans have a bout with *Salmonella* bacteria, which have been found in about one-third of all poultry sold in the United States. These infections can be serious enough to require hospitalization and can lead to arthritis, neurological problems, and even death. Consumers can greatly reduce the number of salmonella infections through proper handling, cooking, and refrigeration of poultry (see Chapter 5).

Water Waterborne diseases, such as typhoid fever and cholera, are still widespread in less developed areas of the world. They have been rare in the United States, although outbreaks caused by inadequate water purification have occurred.

The Process of Infection

If someone infected with the flu sits next to you on a bus and coughs or sneezes, tiny viral particles may travel into your nose and mouth. Immediately, the virus finds or creates an opening in the wall of a cell, and the process of infection begins. During the incubation period, the time between invasion and the first symptom, you're unaware of the pathogen multiplying inside you. In some diseases, incubation may go on for months or even years; for most, it lasts several days or weeks.

The early stage of the battle between your body and the invaders is called the *prodromal period*. As infected cells die, they release chemicals that help block the invasion. Other chemicals, such as *histamines*, cause blood vessels to dilate, thus allowing more blood to reach the battleground. During all this, you feel mild, generalized symptoms, such as headache, irritability, and discomfort. You're also highly contagious. At the height of the battle—the typical illness period—you cough, sneeze, sniffle, ache, feel feverish, and lose your appetite.

Recovery begins when the body's forces gain the advantage. With time, the body destroys the last of the invaders and heals itself. However, the body is not able to develop long-lasting immunity to certain viruses, such as colds, flu, or HIV.

Who Develops Infections?

Among the most vulnerable populations are the following groups:

- **Children and their families.** Youngsters get up to a dozen colds annually; adults average two a year. When a flu epidemic hits a community, about 40 percent of school-age boys and girls get sick, compared with only 5 to 10 percent of adults. Parents of young children get up to six times as many colds as do other adults.

- **Older adults.** Statistically, fewer older men and women are likely to catch a cold or flu, but when they do, they face greater danger than the rest of the population. People over age 65 who get the flu have a 1 in 10 chance of being hospitalized for pneumonia or other respiratory problems and a 1 in 50 chance of dying from the disease.

- **The chronically ill.** Lifelong diseases, such as diabetes, kidney disease, or sickle cell anemia, decrease an individual's ability to fend off infections. Individuals taking

Infection Protection

Here are some basic principles of self-defense:

- Eat a balanced diet.
- Avoid fatty foods.
- Get enough sleep.
- Exercise regularly.
- Don't smoke.
- Control your alcohol intake.
- Wash your hands frequently with hot water and soap.
- Don't share food, drinks, silverware, or glasses.
- Spend as little time as possible in crowds during cold and flu season.
- Don't touch your eyes, mouth, and nose.
- Use tissues.
- Avoid irritating air pollutants.

In your online journal, write your own goals and top strategies for preventing infection.

medications that suppress the immune system, such as steroids, are more vulnerable to infections, as are those with medical conditions that impair immunity, such as infection with HIV.

- **Smokers and those with respiratory problems.** Smokers are a high-risk group for respiratory infections and serious complications, such as pneumonia. Chronic breathing disorders, such as asthma and emphysema, also greatly increase the risk of respiratory infections.

- **Those who live or work in close contact with someone sick.** Health-care workers who treat high-risk patients, nursing home residents, and others living in close quarters—such as students in dormitories—face greater risk of catching others' colds and flus.

- **Residents or workers in poorly ventilated buildings.** Building technology has helped spread certain airborne illnesses, such as tuberculosis, via recirculated air. Indoor air quality can be closely linked with disease transmission in winter, when people spend a great deal of time in tightly sealed rooms.

✓**check-in** How would you rate your risk of infection?

How Your Body Protects Itself

Various parts of your body safeguard you against infectious diseases by providing immunity, or protection, from these health threats. Your skin, when unbroken, keeps out most potential invaders. Your tears, sweat, skin oils, saliva, and mucus contain chemicals that can kill bacteria. Cilia, the tiny hairs lining your respiratory passages, move mucus, which traps inhaled bacteria, viruses, dust, and foreign matter, to the back of the throat, where it is swallowed; the digestive system then destroys the invaders.

When these protective mechanisms can't keep you infection-free, your body's immune system, which is on constant alert for foreign substances that might threaten the body, swings into action (see Health Now!).

The immune system includes structures of the lymphatic system—the spleen, thymus gland, lymph nodes, and lymph vessels—that help filter impurities from the body (Figure 10.13). The lymph nodes, or glands, are small tissue masses in which some protective cells are stored. If pathogens invade your body, many of them are carried to the lymph nodes to be destroyed. This is why your lymph nodes often feel swollen when you have a cold or the flu.

More than a dozen different types of white blood cells (lymphocytes) are concentrated in the organs of the lymphatic system or patrol the entire body by way of the blood and lymph vessels. Some of these white blood cells are generalists and some are specialists. The generalists include *macrophages*, which are large scavenger cells with insatiable appetites for foreign cells, diseased and rundown red blood cells, and other biological debris (Figure 10.14). The specialists are the *B cells* and *T cells*, which respond to specific invaders.

An *antigen* is any substance that the white blood cells recognize as foreign. B cells create antibodies, which are proteins that bind to antigens and mark them for destruction by other white blood cells. Antigens are specific to the pathogen, and the antibody to a particular antigen binds only to that antigen (see Figure 10.14). Once the human body produces antibodies against a specific antigen—the mumps virus, for instance—you're protected against that antigen for life. If you're again exposed to mumps, the antibodies previously produced prevent another episode of the disease.

But you don't have to suffer through an illness to acquire immunity. Inoculation with a vaccine containing synthetic or weakened antigens can give you the same protection. The type of long-lasting immunity in which the body makes its own antibodies to a pathogen is called *active immunity*. Immunity produced by the injection of gamma globulin, the antibody-containing part of the blood from another person or animal that has developed antibodies to a disease, is called *passive immunity*.

Immune Response

Attacked by pathogens, the body musters its forces and fights. Sometimes the invasion is handled like a minor border skirmish; other times a full-scale battle is waged throughout the body. Together, the immune cells work like an internal police force:

- When an antigen enters the body, the T cells aided by macrophages engage in combat with the invader. Certain T cells (cytotoxic T cells) can destroy infected body cells or tumor cells by "touch-killing."

- Meanwhile, the B cells churn out antibodies, which rush to the scene and join in the fray.

- Also busy at surveillance are natural killer cells that, like the elite forces of a SWAT team, seek out and destroy viruses and cancer cells (see Figure 10.14).

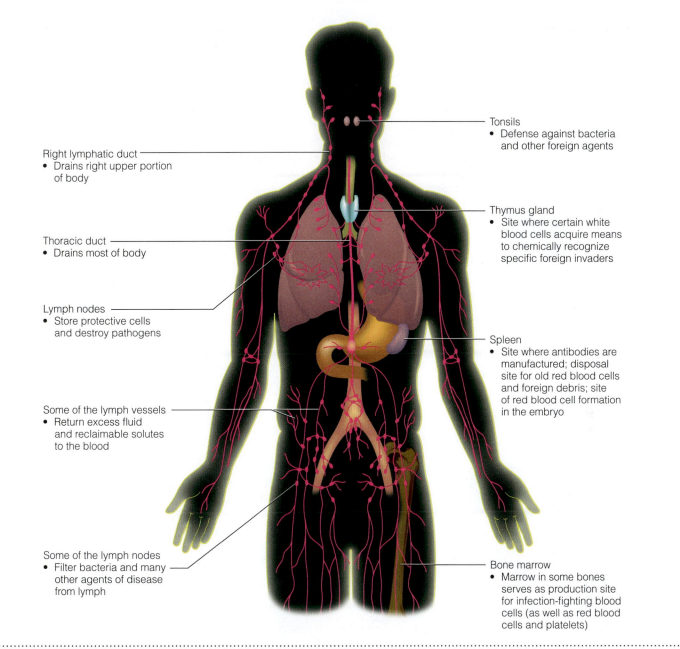

Right lymphatic duct
• Drains right upper portion of body

Thoracic duct
• Drains most of body

Lymph nodes
• Store protective cells and destroy pathogens

Some of the lymph vessels
• Return excess fluid and reclaimable solutes to the blood

Some of the lymph nodes
• Filter bacteria and many other agents of disease from lymph

Tonsils
• Defense against bacteria and other foreign agents

Thymus gland
• Site where certain white blood cells acquire means to chemically recognize specific foreign invaders

Spleen
• Site where antibodies are manufactured; disposal site for old red blood cells and foreign debris; site of red blood cell formation in the embryo

Bone marrow
• Marrow in some bones serves as production site for infection-fighting blood cells (as well as red blood cells and platelets)

FIGURE 10.13 The Human Lymphatic System and Its Functions

The lymphatic system helps filter impurities from the body.

If the microbes establish a foothold, the blood supply to the area increases, bringing oxygen and nutrients to the fighting cells. Tissue fluids, as well as antibacterial and antitoxic proteins, accumulate. You may develop redness, swelling, local warmth, and pain—the signs of inflammation.

Chronic low-grade inflammation increases by twofold to fourfold the levels of cytokines, substances secreted by certain immune cells, in the bloodstream. These elevated levels serve as inflammatory markers that have emerged as major players in the development of several major diseases, including atherosclerosis, hypertension and other cardiovascular disorders, insulin resistance, metabolic syndrome, type 2 diabetes, and cancer.

As more tissue is destroyed, a cavity, or abscess, forms and fills with fluid, battling cells and dead white blood cells (pus). If the invaders aren't killed or inactivated, the pathogens are able to spread into the bloodstream and cause systemic disease.

Some people have an immune deficiency—either inborn or acquired. A very few children are born without an effective immune system; their lives can be endangered by any infection. Although still experimental, therapy to implant a missing or healthy gene may offer new hope for a normal life.

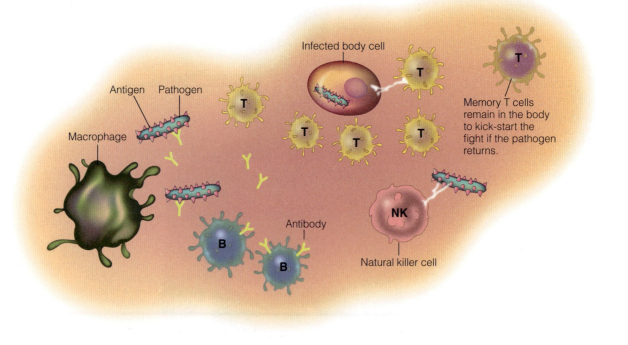

··

FIGURE 10.14 The Immune Response

Some T cells can kill infected body cells. B cells churn out antibodies to tag pathogens for destruction by macrophages and other white blood cells.

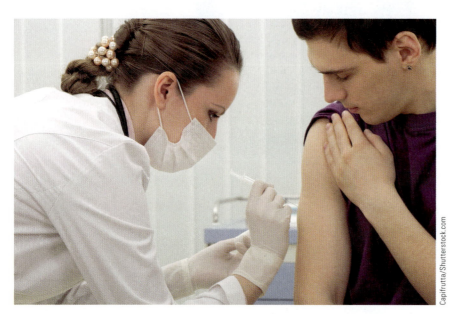

Capifrutta/Shutterstock.com

Vaccinations are as crucial for protecting adults from infectious illnesses as they are for children.

Immunity and Stress

Whenever we confront a crisis, large or small, our bodies produce powerful hormones that provide extra energy. However, this stress response dampens immunity, reducing the number of some key immune cells and the responsiveness of others.

Stress affects the body's immune system in different ways, depending on two factors: the controllability or uncontrollability of the stressor and the mental effort required to cope with the stress. An uncontrollable stressor that lasts longer than 15 minutes may interfere with cytokine interleukin-6, which plays an essential role in activating the immune defenses.

Uncontrollable stressors also produce high levels of the hormone cortisol, which suppresses immune system functioning. The mental efforts required to cope with high-level stressors produce only brief immune changes that appear to have little consequence for health. However, stress has been shown to slow proinflammatory cytokine production, which is essential for healing.

Adult Vaccinations

Although many people associate vaccination with children's health, the vast majority of vaccine-preventable deaths occur among adults. An estimated 40,000 to 50,000 American adults die every year from diseases that vaccines could have prevented. Only about 40 percent of adults get an annual flu shot. A drop in immunization with the MMR vaccine, which protects against mumps, measles and rubella, has led to an increase in cases of mumps, a contagious disease that is especially common on college campuses. Symptoms include enlarged salivary glands—which cause puffy cheeks and a swollen jaw—along with fever, fatigue, and head and muscle aches. Serious complications of mumps can occur, including meningitis and infection of the testicles, which can cause pain but also sterility.

Table 10.6 lists the vaccines recommended for college students, and Figure 10.15 shows the recommended adult immunization schedule (see Snapshot: On Campus Now).[110]

✓**check-in** Have you received all the recommended vaccinations?

Upper Respiratory Infections

Every year, about 25 million cold sufferers in the United States visit their family doctors with uncomplicated upper respiratory infections. The common cold results in about 20 million days of absence from work and 22 million days of absence from school.

College and university students are at high risk for colds and influenza-like illnesses. In one study that followed more than 3,000 students from fall to spring, 9 in 10 had at least one cold or flulike illness.

Common Cold

There are more than 200 distinct cold viruses. Although in a single season you may develop a temporary immunity to one or two, you may then be hit by a third. Americans come down with 1 billion colds annually.

TABLE 10.6 Vaccines Recommended for College Students

Tetanus–diphtheria–pertussis (Tdap) vaccine*
Meningococcal vaccine
HPV vaccine series
Hepatitis A vaccine series
Hepatitis B vaccine series
Polio vaccine series
Measles–mumps–rubella (MMR) vaccine series
Varicella (chickenpox) vaccine series
Influenza vaccine
Pneumococcal polysaccharide (PPV) vaccine

*Recommended for previously unvaccinated college freshmen living in dormitories.
*Covered by the Vaccine Injury Compensation Program.

Colds can strike in any season, but different cold viruses are more common at different times of the year:

- Rhinoviruses cause most spring, summer, and early fall colds and tend to cause more symptoms above the neck (stuffy nose, headache, runny eyes).

- Adenoviruses, para-influenza viruses, coronaviruses, influenza viruses, and others that strike in the winter are more likely to get into the trachea and bronchi (the breathing passages) and cause more fever and bronchitis.

Cold viruses spread by coughs, sneezes, and touch. Cold sufferers who sneeze and then touch a doorknob or countertop leave a trail of

📷 SNAPSHOT: ON CAMPUS NOW

Vaccinations

Vaccinated against	Percentage of students	Vaccinated against	Percentage of students
Hepatitis B	68.4	Varicella (chickenpox)	65.6
Measles-mumps-rubella	73.3	Influenza (within past 12 months)	46.4
Meningococcal meningitis	65.1		

Vaccinations are your first line of defense against potentially serious infectious diseases. Do you know your vaccination history? Do you keep track of recommendations for new or booster shots? Do you get a flu vaccination every year? Jot down what you see as the pros and cons of up-to-date vaccinations in your online journal.

Source: American College Health Association. American College Health Association-National College Health Assessment II: Reference Group Executive Summary Spring 2018. Silver Spring, MD: American College Health Association, 2018.

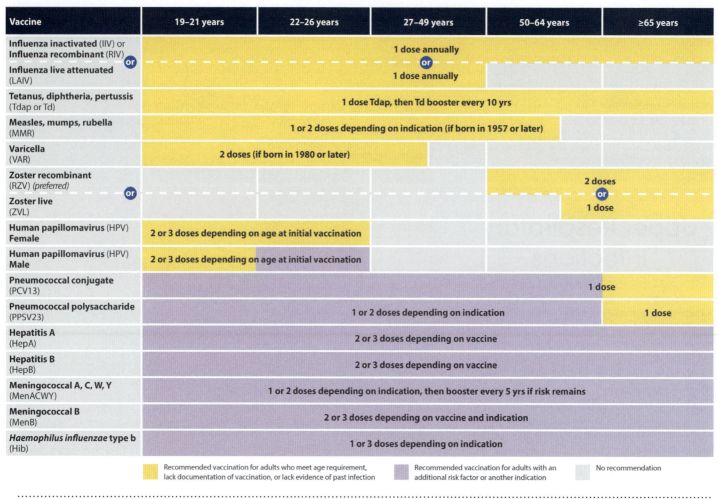

Vaccine	19–21 years	22–26 years	27–49 years	50–64 years	≥65 years
Influenza inactivated (IIV) or Influenza recombinant (RIV) or	1 dose annually				
Influenza live attenuated (LAIV)	1 dose annually				
Tetanus, diphtheria, pertussis (Tdap or Td)	1 dose Tdap, then Td booster every 10 yrs				
Measles, mumps, rubella (MMR)	1 or 2 doses depending on indication (if born in 1957 or later)				
Varicella (VAR)	2 doses (if born in 1980 or later)				
Zoster recombinant (RZV) *(preferred)* or				2 doses	
Zoster live (ZVL)				1 dose	
Human papillomavirus (HPV) Female	2 or 3 doses depending on age at initial vaccination				
Human papillomavirus (HPV) Male	2 or 3 doses depending on age at initial vaccination				
Pneumococcal conjugate (PCV13)					1 dose
Pneumococcal polysaccharide (PPSV23)	1 or 2 doses depending on indication				1 dose
Hepatitis A (HepA)	2 or 3 doses depending on vaccine				
Hepatitis B (HepB)	2 or 3 doses depending on vaccine				
Meningococcal A, C, W, Y (MenACWY)	1 or 2 doses depending on indication, then booster every 5 yrs if risk remains				
Meningococcal B (MenB)	2 or 3 doses depending on vaccine and indication				
Haemophilus influenzae type b (Hib)	1 or 3 doses depending on indication				

Recommended vaccination for adults who meet age requirement, lack documentation of vaccination, or lack evidence of past infection

Recommended vaccination for adults with an additional risk factor or another indication

No recommendation

FIGURE 10.15 Recommended Adult Immunization Schedule, by Vaccine and Age Group—the United States, 2019

https://www.cdc.gov/vaccines/schedules/downloads/adult/adult-combined-schedule.pdf

highly contagious viruses behind them. A lack of sleep can increase your odds of getting a cold. People who get less than 7 hours of sleep a night are three times more likely to catch a cold. Those who sleep poorly are five times more susceptible.

High levels of stress increase the risk of becoming infected by respiratory viruses and developing cold symptoms. People who feel unable to deal with everyday stresses have an exaggerated immune reaction that may intensify cold or flu symptoms once they've contracted a virus. Those with a positive emotional outlook are less vulnerable.

✓**check-in** When was the last time you had a cold? Do you feel that stress made you more susceptible?

Preventing Colds High-dose zinc acetate lozenges can substantially shorten the duration of various common cold symptoms. However, many zinc lozenges on the U.S. market either have too low a dose of zinc or contain ingredients that limit their effectiveness.[111] Daily Vitamin C does not ward off the common cold or significantly shorten its length or severity. (See Health on a Budget.)

In a recent review of herbal, complementary, and alternative approaches, probiotics were found better than placebo in reducing the number and rate of episodes of acute upper respiratory tract infections. Other herbal remedies that require further study include maoto, licorice roots, antiwei, North American ginseng, berries, Echinacea, plant-extracted carnosic acid, pomegranate, guava tea, and Bai Shao.[112] (See Chapter 14 for more on complementary and alternative medicine.)

$ HEALTH ON A BUDGET

Caring for Your Cold

Fortunately, the most effective treatments for a cold are inexpensive—or even free:

- **Drink plenty of fluids, particularly warm ones.** Warmth is important because the aptly named "cold" viruses replicate at lower temperatures. Hot soups and drinks (particularly those with a touch of something pungent, like lemon or ginger) raise body temperature and help clear the nose. Tea may enhance the immune system.

- **Get plenty of rest.** Taking it easy reduces demands on the body, which helps speed recovery.

- **Do not take antibiotics.** They are ineffective against colds and flu.

- **Do not take aspirin or acetaminophen (Tylenol), which may suppress the antibodies the body produces to fight cold viruses and increase symptoms such as stuffiness.** Children, teenagers, and young adults should never take aspirin for a cold or flu because of the danger of Reye's syndrome, a potentially deadly disorder that can cause convulsions, coma, swelling of the brain, and kidney damage. A better alternative for achiness is ibuprofen (brand names include Motrin, Advil, and Nuprin), which doesn't seem to affect immune response.

- **Choose the right medicines for your symptoms.**

If you want to:	Choose medicine with:
Unclog a stuffy nose	Nasal decongestant
Quiet a cough	Cough suppressant
Loosen mucus so that you can cough it up	Expectorant
Stop runny nose and sneezing	Antihistamine
Ease fever, headaches, minor aches and pains	Pain reliever (analgesic)

- **Know when to call your doctor.** You usually do not have to call a doctor right away if you have signs of a cold or flu. But be sure to call in these situations:

  - Your symptoms get worse.

  - Your symptoms last a long time.

  - After feeling a little better, you show signs of a more serious problem. Some of these signs are a sick-to-your-stomach feeling, vomiting, high fever, shaking, chills, chest pain, or coughing with thick, yellow-green mucus.

✓**check-in** Which of the following steps do you take to prevent colds?

____ Frequent handwashing.

____ Replacing toothbrushes often.

____ Exercising regularly.

____ Avoiding stress overload.

Antibiotics Although colds and sore throats—a frequent cold symptom—are caused by viruses, many people seek treatment with antibiotics, which are effective only against bacteria. Unless you're coughing up green or foul yellow mucus (signs of a secondary bacterial infection), antibiotics won't help. They also may make your body more resistant to such medications when you develop a bacterial infection in the future.[113] For effective treatments, see Health on Budget.

As many as one in four people taking antibiotics inappropriately suffers adverse effects, ranging from mild (such as a rash or diarrhea) to potentially life threatening. The American College of Physicians has issued high-value care guidelines advising against their use for uncomplicated bronchitis (infection of upper airway), pharyngitis (sore throat), rhinosinusitis (sinus infection), and the common cold.[114] Antibiotics can foster the growth of one or more strains of antibiotic-resistant

bacteria for at least 2 to 6 months inside the person taking the pills—who can pass on this drug-resistant bug to family, roommates, and others.

Influenza

Although similar to a cold, influenza—or the flu—often causes fever, achiness, cough, and other more intense and persistent symptoms.[115] Viral load, the quantity of viral particles in the body, can determine their severity.[116] Seasonal outbreaks of influenza vary in their impact, but cause an estimated 291,000 to 645,800 respiratory deaths worldwide each year, with approximately 12,000 to 56,000 deaths in the United States.[117]

Flu viruses, transmitted by coughs, sneezes, laughs, and even normal conversation, are extraordinarily contagious, particularly in the first 3 days of the disease. The usual incubation period is 2 days, but symptoms can hit hard and fast. Two varieties of viruses—influenza A and influenza B—cause most flus.

The CDC recommends an annual flu shot for everyone over the age of 6 months, except for those with certain medical conditions. Vaccination with the live, nasal-spray flu vaccine (Flu-Mist®) is an option for healthy people ages 5 to 49 years who are not pregnant. The spray provides a particular advantage for children since

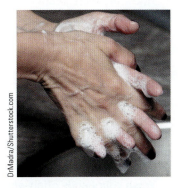

DrMadra/Shutterstock.com

Washing your hands often with soap and hot water for 15 to 20 seconds will help protect you from germs. When soap and water are not available, you can use alcohol-based disposable hand wipes or gel sanitizers. If using gel, rub your hands until the gel is dry; the alcohol in the gel kills the germs.

more than 30 percent of youngsters get the flu but most don't receive a flu shot.

✓**check-in** Do you get a flu shot every year?

For those who don't get vaccinated, antiviral drugs, which must be taken within 36 to 48 hours of the first flu symptom, have provided the next best line of defense. Two of the oldest of these medications, amantadine and rimantadine, which work only against the type A flu virus, are no longer effective, possibly because the flu virus has mutated and become resistant. According to a review of clinical trials, Tamiflu (oseltamivir) shortens the length of flu symptoms by about a day and reduces the risk of flu-related complications such as pneumonia. However, it is linked with more nausea and vomiting. (See Your Strategies for Prevention for ways to protect yourself and others from influenza.)

Although regular exercise bolsters immunity, people with flu symptoms, such as fever, fatigue, muscle aches, and swollen lymph glands, should avoid exercise while sick and for 2 weeks after recovery, according to the American Council on Exercise.

YOUR STRATEGIES FOR PREVENTION

How to Protect Yourself and Others from Influenza

If You Live

- **Get vaccinated.**

- **Do not share cups, glasses, bottles, dishes, or silverware.**

- **Frequently wash your hands with soap and water, especially after close contact with other people (on buses, in stores, at the gym, etc.).** Alcohol-based hand sanitizers are also effective.

- **Avoid touching your eyes, nose, or mouth.**

- **Try to avoid close contact with sick people.**

- **Reduce the time you spend in crowded settings.**

- **Stay in good general health: get plenty of sleep, be physically active, manage daily stress, drink plenty of fluids, and eat nutritious food.**

- **Follow public health advice regarding school closures, avoiding crowds, and other social distancing measures.**

- **Improve airflow in your living space by opening windows as much as possible.**

- **Know the facts about wearing a face mask.** There is no evidence that wearing a face mask in open areas (as opposed to enclosed spaces while in close contact with a person with flulike symptoms) reduces the risk. If you do choose to wear one, place it carefully so it covers the mouth and nose, with minimal gaps between the face and mask. Once it's on, avoid touching the mask. Wash your hands immediately after removing it. Replace a mask with a new clean, dry one as soon as it becomes damp. Do not reuse single-use masks.

If You Have Symptoms

- **Cover your nose and mouth with a tissue when you cough or sneeze.** Throw the tissue in the trash after you use it.

- **Wash your hands often with soap and water, especially after you cough or sneeze.**

- **Be prepared to stay home, in your room, or in a designated quarantine area for a week or until you have been fever-free for at least a day.** Get a supply of over-the-counter medicines, alcohol-based hand rubs, tissues, and other related items to avoid the need to go out in public while you are sick and contagious.

- **To prevent the spread of influenza virus among family members or roommates, keep surfaces (especially bedside tables, bathroom sinks, and kitchen counters) clean by wiping them down with a household disinfectant.** Wash linens, eating utensils, and dishes before sharing them.

Meningitis

Meningitis, or invasive meningococcal disease, attacks the membranes around the brain and spinal cord and can result in hearing loss, kidney failure, and permanent brain damage. One of the most common types is caused by the bacterium *Neisseria meningitidis*. Viral meningitis is typically less severe.

Most common in the first year of life, the incidence of bacterial meningitis rises in young people between ages 15 and 24. Adolescents and young adults account for nearly 30 percent of all cases of meningitis in the United States.[118]

If not treated early, meningitis can lead to death or permanent disabilities. One in five of those who survive suffers from long-term side effects, such as brain damage, hearing loss, seizures, or limb amputation. Fatality rates are five times higher among 15- to 24-year-olds.

Each year, 100 to 125 cases of meningitis occur on college campuses; an estimated 5 to 15 students die as a result. One in five survivors suffers long-term side effects.

Meningitis spreads through the exchange of respiratory droplets, which can come from sharing a drink, cigarette, or silverware; kissing; coughing; or sneezing. Even inhaling second-hand smoke can infect you with the disease.

Preventing Meningitis

Vaccination is recommended for all American adolescents, with initial immunization at age 11 or 12 and a booster at age 16. As vaccines against more meningitis pathogens have become available, they have been recommended for individuals ages 10 years or older who are at increased risk.[119] As with other immunizations, minor reactions may occur. These include pain and swelling at the injection site, headache, fatigue, or a vague sense of discomfort. The incidence of life-threatening meningitis has declined substantially since the vaccine was developed.[120]

The CDC and other major health organizations, such as the American College Health Association, recommend routine vaccination for college students because of the risk of an outbreak on campus.[121]

✓**check-in** Have you been vaccinated against meningitis? If not, why not?

Recognizing Meningitis

The early symptoms of meningitis may be mild and resemble symptoms of flu or other less severe infections. Bacterial meningitis symptoms may develop within hours; viral meningitis symptoms may develop quickly or over several days. Fever, headache, and neck stiffness are the hallmark symptoms of meningitis. Not all symptoms may appear, but they can progress very quickly, killing an otherwise healthy person in 48 hours or less, so it is critical to seek medical attention quickly.

The most common symptoms of meningitis are:

- Sudden high fever.
- Severe, persistent headache.
- Neck stiffness and pain that makes it difficult to touch the chin to the chest.
- Nausea and vomiting, sometimes along with diarrhea.
- Confusion and disorientation (acting "goofy").
- Drowsiness or sluggishness.
- Eye pain or sensitivity to bright light.
- Pain or weakness in the muscles or joints.

Other possible signs and symptoms include:

- Abnormal skin color.
- Stomach cramps.
- Ice-cold hands and feet.
- Dizziness.
- Reddish or brownish skin rash or purple spots.
- Numbness and tingling.
- Seizures.

When to Seek Medical Care

If two or more of the symptoms of meningitis appear at the same time or if the symptoms are very severe or appear suddenly, seek medical care right away. If a red rash appears along with fever, see if the rash disappears when a glass is pressed against it. If it does not, this could be a sign of blood infection, which is a medical emergency. Other symptoms that might require emergency treatment include loss of consciousness, seizures, muscle weakness, or sudden severe dementia.

About 1 in 10 people who get meningitis dies from it. Of those who survive, another 11 to 19 percent lose fingers, arms, or legs; become deaf; have problems with their nervous systems; or suffer seizures, strokes, or brain damage. Thus it is critical to seek medical care for this infection. A new concern is the emergence of the first U.S. cases of bacterial meningitis resistant to a widely used antibiotic.

Hepatitis

An estimated 500,000 Americans contract hepatitis each year, and the number of hepatitis-related deaths has been rising in the past decade. At least five different viruses, referred to as hepatitis A, B, C, Delta, and E, can cause this inflammation of the liver. Newly identified viruses also may be responsible for some cases of what is called "non-A, non-B" hepatitis.

Thanks largely to effective vaccines, rates of hepatitis A and hepatitis B infections have declined to their lowest rates in decades. Although there is no vaccine for hepatitis C, its incidence has also declined significantly. Nonetheless, hepatitis has surpassed HIV as a cause of death in the United States.

All forms of hepatitis target the liver, the body's largest internal organ. Symptoms include headaches, fever, fatigue, stiff or aching joints, nausea, vomiting, and diarrhea. The liver becomes enlarged and tender to the touch; sometimes the yellowish tinge of jaundice develops. Treatment consists of rest, a high-protein diet, and the avoidance of alcohol and drugs that may stress the liver. Alpha interferon, a protein that boosts immunity and prevents viruses from replicating, may be used for some forms.

Most people begin to feel better after 2 or 3 weeks of rest, although fatigue and other symptoms can linger. As many as 10 percent of those infected with hepatitis B and up to two-thirds of those with hepatitis C become carriers of the virus for several years or even life. Some have persistent inflammation of the liver, which may cause mild or severe symptoms and increase the risk of liver cancer.

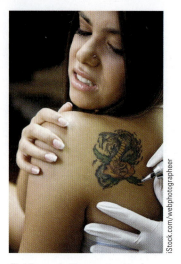

Getting a tattoo or a piercing can pose health risks, including bacterial infection and hepatitis.

Hepatitis A

Hepatitis A, a less serious form, is generally transmitted by poor sanitation, primarily fecal contamination of food or water, and is less common in industrialized nations than in developing countries. As many as 30 percent of individuals in the United States show evidence of past infection with the virus. Among those at highest risk in the United States are children and staff at day-care centers, residents of institutions for the mentally handicapped, sanitation workers, and workers who handle primates such as monkeys.

Gamma globulin can provide short-term immunity; vaccines against hepatitis A have proven effective in lowering the incidence of infection in both children and susceptible adults.[122] The CDC recommends routine immunization against hepatitis A in states with high rates, as well as for travelers to countries where hepatitis A is common, men who have sex with men, and persons who use illegal drugs.

Hepatitis B

Hepatitis B, a potentially fatal disease transmitted through the blood and other bodily fluids, infects an estimated 300 million people around the world.[123] Once spread mainly by contaminated tattoo needles, needles shared by drug users, or transfusions of contaminated blood, hepatitis B is now transmitted mostly through sexual contact. Many cases resolve on their own, but hepatitis B can cause chronic liver infection, cirrhosis, and liver cancer. Medications for hepatitis B often must be taken long term, or the disease comes back even stronger.

Who Develops Hepatitis B?
At highest risk of developing hepatitis B are:

- Young people, as 75 percent of new cases are diagnosed in those between ages 15 and 39. They usually contract hepatitis B through high-risk behaviors such as multiple sex partners and use of injected drugs.
- Athletes in contact sports, such as wrestling and football, who may transmit the hepatitis B virus (HBV) in sweat. With the discovery that HBV is more common in athletes than had been suspected, health experts are calling for mandatory HBV testing and vaccination against hepatitis B for all athletes.
- Male homosexuals.
- Heterosexuals with multiple sex partners.
- Health-care workers with frequent contact with blood.
- Injection drug users.
- Infants born to infected mothers.

Vaccination can prevent hepatitis B and is recommended for all newborns and, if not already vaccinated, for travelers to certain regions, health-care workers, dialysis patients, and anyone engaging in unprotected sexual activity (homosexual or heterosexual).

Individuals who have tattoos or body piercings may also be at risk of hepatitis B and C as well as other infections transmitted by unsterile tattooing or piercing practices.

If you choose to have a body piercing, avoid piercing guns and make certain that the piercing equipment has been sterilized. Tattoos from nonprofessionals pose two to four times greater risk than those done by professionals.

✓**check-in** Do you have a tattoo or piercing?

Hepatitis C

About 3.2 million people in the United States are infected with hepatitis C virus (HCV), but most do not realize it because the virus causes so few symptoms.[124] The most common are jaundice (a condition that causes yellow eyes and skin as well as dark urine), stomach pain, loss of appetite, nausea, and fatigue.

Hepatitis C has been increasing annually since 2010. The most common risk factors are intravenous drug use and occupational exposure from needlesticks.[125] There is controversy about whether HCV can be transmitted sexually.

Major advancements in treatment, including targeted antiviral drugs, have proven highly effective in more than 95 percent of patients with chronic HCV.[126] Medical scientists predict that, as a result, HCV may be eradicated worldwide, even without a vaccine.[127]

✓**check-in** Should you have a blood test for hepatitis C? The CDC recommends one if any of the following are true:
- You received blood from a donor who later was found to have the disease.
- You have ever injected drugs.
- You got a blood transfusion or an organ transplant before July 1992.
- You received a blood product used to treat clotting problems before 1987.
- You were born between 1945 and 1965.
- You've had long-term kidney dialysis.
- You have HIV.
- You were born to a mother with hepatitis C.

iStock.com/webphotographeer

Insect- and Animal-Borne Infections

Common insects and animals, including ticks and mosquitoes, can transmit dangerous infections, among them Lyme disease and West Nile virus. Of all emerging infections, 75 percent originate in animals; of these, 61 percent can be transmitted to humans.

Lyme Disease

Lyme disease, the most commonly reported vector-borne infectious disease in the United States, affects about 20,000 to 30,000 Americans a year. This bacterial infection is spread by ixodid ticks that carry a particular bacterium—the spirochete *Borrelia burgdorferi*.

Ticks are responsible for the spread of Lyme disease. If you spot a tick, remove it as soon as possible with tweezers or small forceps. Put it in a plastic bag or sealed bottle and save it. If you develop a rash or other symptoms, take it with you to the doctor.

Here is what you need to know:

- Symptoms include joint inflammation, heart arrhythmias, blinding headaches, and memory lapses. The disease can also cause miscarriages and birth defects.

- You are not likely to get Lyme disease if a tick is attached to your skin for less than 48 hours.

- About 70 to 80 percent of infected individuals develop a red rash at the site of the tick bite. Over a period of days to weeks, the rash grows larger. A ring of skin just beyond the bite site may fade, creating a ring or "bull's-eye" appearance. Rarely, the rash may burn or itch.

- Once diagnosed, Lyme disease is treated with antibiotics. Nonsteroidal antiinflammatory drugs, such as aspirin or ibuprofen, can relieve fever and pain.

- Without treatment, Lyme disease can cause debilitating symptoms that require extensive and expensive care.[128]

West Nile Virus

West Nile virus (WNV), transmitted by a mosquito that feeds on an infected bird and then bites a human, flares up in the summer. WNV can also be spread through blood transfusions, organ transplants, and breastfeeding, as well as from mother to fetus during pregnancy. Things to remember about WNV include the following:

- WNV interferes with normal central nervous system functioning and causes inflammation of brain tissue.

- The risk of catching WNV is low. Relatively few mosquitoes carry WNV, and fewer than 1 percent of people who are bitten by mosquitoes experience any symptoms.

- Repellents that contain an EPA-registered insect repellent can protect against these mosquitoes.

- There is no specific treatment for WNV infection. People with more severe cases usually require hospitalization and supportive treatment, including intravenous fluids and help with breathing.[129]

Zika Virus

First discovered in 1947, the Zika virus often causes no symptoms or mild ones similar to those of other infections. Cases of Zika virus disease have been reported in the United States as well as Africa, Southeast Asia, the Pacific Islands, and South America.

Infection prior to or during pregnancy is associated with serious threats, including prematurity, blindness, and congenital microcephaly (a birth defect characterized by small head size and abnormal brain development).[130] Among pregnant women in the United States possibly exposed to Zika at any time during pregnancy, 6 percent of their fetuses or infants had signs of Zika-associated birth defects, primarily brain abnormalities and microcephaly. Among women infected during their first trimester, 11 percent of fetuses or infants had evidence of Zika-associated birth defects.[131]

In adults, Zika can cause brain inflammation and Guillain-Barré syndrome, an autoimmune disorder characterized by weakness and abnormal sensation in the legs and arms.

Researchers have reported progress on promising vaccines to prevent Zika transmission; no medications are currently available to treat Zika.[132]

Transmission Zika virus can be transmitted in the following ways:

- **Through a mosquito bite.** The species that carries Zika virus typically live near standing water in such places as buckets, bowls, or flower pots (*Aedes aegypti* and *A. albopictus*). They become infected when they feed on a person already infected with the virus and spread the virus to other people through bites.

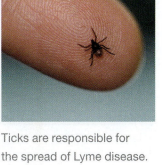

Ticks are responsible for the spread of Lyme disease. If you spot a tick, remove it as soon as possible with tweezers or small forceps. Put it in a plastic bag or sealed bottle and save it. If you develop a rash or other symptoms, take it with you to the doctor.

Lauree Feldman/Photolibrary/Getty Images

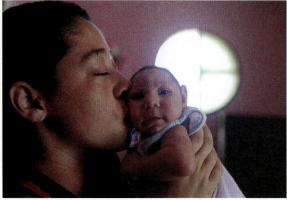

Infection with the Zika virus before or during pregnancy can lead to serious birth defects, including abnormal brain development and small head size.

Xinhua/Photoshot

- **From mother to child.** A pregnant woman can pass Zika virus to her fetus during pregnancy or childbirth. There have not been reports of infants getting Zika virus through breastfeeding.

- **Through sexual contact.** A man infected with Zika can transmit the virus to his sex partners via semen before symptoms start, when they develop, and after they resolve. Transmission of Zika virus has occurred with anal intercourse.

- **Through blood transfusion.** Cases have been traced to blood transfusions in Brazil and other countries. To protect its blood supply, the United States is not accepting donations from individuals who have travelled to areas where Zika infection has occurred.[133]

Symptoms   Most people infected with Zika virus don't have symptoms. Others may develop fever, rash, joint pain, conjunctivitis (red eyes), muscle pain, and headache a few days to a week after being bitten and may last for several days to a week. Zika virus can remain in the blood of an infected person for a week or longer.

Diagnosis and Treatment   If you develop the symptoms described and have visited an area where Zika is found, see your health-care provider for a blood test to detect Zika and similar viruses. If you are infected, health officials recommend rest, fluids to prevent dehydration, and acetaminophen (Tylenol) or paracetamol to reduce fever and pain.

Prevention   To find out where Zika has been identified, visit the CDC's traveler's health website at wwwnc.cdc.gov/travel/page/zika-travel-information.

If you are a man or a sex partner of a man who lives in or has traveled to an area with Zika and your partner is pregnant, do not have sex during pregnancy or use condoms every time you have sex, whether it's vaginal, anal, and oral (mouth-to-penis) sex. Consistent and correct use of latex condoms reduces sexual transmission of many infections, including those caused by other viruses.

To avoid mosquito bites, wear long-sleeved shirts and long pants and use insect repellents as directed.

✓**check-in** What do you think is your risk of Zika virus infection?

Avian Influenza

Avian influenza, or bird flu, is caused by viruses that occur naturally among wild birds and usually does not infect humans. However, influenza viruses jumped from birds to humans three times in the 20th century. In each case, a mutation in the genes of the virus allowed it to infect humans. Then a further change allowed the virus to pass easily from one human to another, and it spread rapidly around the world.

- Do college students need to think about their risk for major diseases?

- What behaviors can you change to protect your cardiometabolic health?

- What steps are you taking to prevent cancer?

- What do you see as the greatest infectious threats to your health?

Reflection

As you learned in this chapter, everyone is at risk for serious illness—if only because of sex, genes, or age. However, simple steps can help you stay as healthy as possible as long as possible. Are you conscientious about these protective practices? Are you better at some than at others? If you are not conscientious, why—are you too busy? Do you have other priorities? Is money an issue? Think through these issues and develop a personalized health maintenance plan.

TAKING CHARGE OF YOUR HEALTH

Defend Yourself from Disease

You may not be able to control every risk factor in your life or environment, but you can protect yourself from the obvious ones.

____ Getting your blood pressure checked regularly. Knowing your numbers can alert you to a potential problem long before you develop any symptoms.

____ Avoiding excessive exposure to ultraviolet light. If you spend a lot of time outside, protect your skin by using sunscreen and wearing long-sleeved shirts and a hat.

____ Controlling your alcohol intake. The risk of several major diseases increases with intake of more than two drinks per day for men and one drink for women.

____ Paying attention. Changes in bowel habits, skin changes, unusual lumps or discharges—anything out of the ordinary—may be clues that require further medical investigation.

____ Getting your "shots." Keep track of the vaccinations you've received and the dates you received them.

____ Washing/sanitizing your hands frequently during the cold and flu season.

____ Wiping down exercise equipment handles before using it.

____ Avoiding people who are sneezing or coughing.

____ Applying an insect spray containing an EPA-registered repellent when outdoors and wearing long-sleeved clothing and long pants when hiking.

____ Checking yourself for ticks after a walk or hike.

SELF-SURVEY

Diabetes Risk Test

Height	Weight (lbs.)		
4′ 10″	119–142	143–190	191
4′ 11″	124–147	148–197	198
5′ 0″	128–152	153–203	204
5′ 1″	132–157	158–210	211
5′ 2″	136–163	164–217	218
5′ 3″	141–168	169–224	225
5′ 4″	145–173	174–231	232
5′ 5″	150–179	180–239	240
5′ 6″	155–185	186–246	247
5′ 7″	159–190	191–254	255
5′ 8″	164–196	197–261	262
5′ 9″	169–202	203–269	270
5′ 10″	174–208	209–277	278
5′ 11″	179–214	215–285	286
6′ 0″	184–220	221–293	294
6′ 1″	189–226	227–301	3021
6′ 2″	194–232	233–310	3111
6′ 3″	200–239	240–318	319
6′ 4″	205–245	246–327	328
	(1 Point)	(2 Points)	(3 Points)

You weigh less than the amount in the left column (0 points)

Adapted from Bang et al., Ann Intern Med 151:775-783,2009. Original algorithm was validated without gestational diabetes as part of the model.

1. How old are you?
   Less than 40 years (0 points)
   40–49 years (1 point)
   50–59 years (2 points)
   60 years or older (3 points)

2. Are you a man or a woman?
   Man (1 point) Woman (0 points)

3. If you are a woman, have you ever been diagnosed with gestational diabetes?
   Yes (1 point) No (0 points)

4. Do you have a mother, father, sister, or brother with diabetes?
   Yes (1 point) No (0 points)

5. Have you ever been diagnosed with high blood pressure?
   Yes (1 point) No (0 points)

6. Are you physically active?
   Yes (0 points) No (1 point)

7. What is your weight status?
   (see chart at *left*)

Write your score in the box.

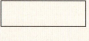

If you scored 5 or higher:
You are at increased risk for having type 2 diabetes. However, only your doctor can tell for sure if you do have type 2 diabetes or prediabetes (a condition that precedes type 2 diabetes in which blood glucose levels are higher than normal). Talk to your doctor to see if additional testing is needed.

Add up your score

Type 2 diabetes is more common in African Americans, Hispanics/Latinos, American Indians, and Asian Americans and Pacific Islanders.

Higher body weights increase diabetes risk for everyone. Asian Americans are at increased diabetes risk at lower body weights than the rest of the general public (about 15 pounds lower).

For more information, visit us at diabetes.org/resources or call 1-800-DIABETES (1-800-342-2383).

REVIEW QUESTIONS

(LO 10.1) 1. _____ occurs when the artery walls become constricted so that the force exerted as the blood flows through them is greater than it should be.
   a. Hypertension
   b. Diabetes mellitus
   c. Infiltration
   d. Myocardial infarction

(LO 10.1) 2. Which of the following statements is true of high-density lipoproteins?
   a. They cause the formation of plaque on arterial walls, leading to atherosclerosis and high blood pressure.
   b. They pick up excess cholesterol in the body and carry it back to the liver for removal from the body.
   c. They control the level of glucose in the blood.
   d. They reduce the levels of low-density lipoproteins in the blood by blocking the production of cholesterol in the liver.

(LO 10.2) 3. _____ is a cluster of disorders, including high blood pressure, high insulin levels, abdominal obesity, and abnormal cholesterol levels, that make a person more likely to develop diabetes, heart disease, or stroke.
   a. Down syndrome
   b. Metabolic syndrome
   c. Acute aortic syndrome
   d. Chronic fatigue syndrome

(LO 10.2) 4. Which of the following characteristics is a sign of metabolic syndrome?
   a. A higher-than-normal triglyceride level.
   b. A higher-than-normal high-density lipoprotein level.
   c. Lower-than-normal blood pressure.
   d. A lower-than-normal fasting blood sugar.

(LO 10.2) 5. Your BMI is 29 and you are found to have type 2 diabetes; what action should you take?
   a. Decrease your high glycemic index carbohydrate intake and lose weight.
   b. Eat only proteins.
   c. Increase water consumption.
   d. Have gastric bypass surgery.

(LO 10.2) 6. In _____, the body's immune system attacks the insulin-producing beta cells in the pancreas and destroys them.
   a. adult-onset diabetes
   b. type 2 diabetes
   c. gestational diabetes
   d. type 1 diabetes

(LO 10.3) 7. _____ occurs when blood pressure remains elevated over time and forces the heart to pump harder than is healthy.
   a. Atherosclerosis   c. Hypertension
   b. Arteriosclerosis   d. Myocardial infarction

(LO 10.3) 8. Which of the following statements about hypertension is true?
   a. Men and women are equally likely to develop hypertension.
   b. Low amounts of sodium in the diet lead to increased blood pressure in people with hypertension.
   c. Lack of blood supply to the myocardium is the primary cause of hypertension.
   d. Stage 1 hypertension is the most severe form.

(LO 10.3) 9. _____ are the blood fats released into the bloodstream after a meal.
   a. Monoglycerides   c. Phospholipids
   b. Diglycerides   d. Triglycerides

(LO 10.3) 10. Drugs called _____ work in the liver to block production of cholesterol.
   a. heparinoids   c. statins
   b. antibiotics   d. beta-blockers

(LO 10.4) 11. One-third of the cases of sudden cardiac death in young athletes is due to _____.
   a. stress
   b. high cholesterol
   c. the use of steroids
   d. excessive thickness of the heart muscle

(LO 10.3) 12. Which of the following is NOT a contributor to heart disease?
   a. Hostility
   b. Smoking
   c. Regular exercise
   d. Cocaine use

(LO 10.3) 13. _____ is a disease of the lining of the arteries in which plaque narrows the artery channels.
   a. Atherosclerosis
   b. Infiltration
   c. Epilepsy
   d. Metastasis

(LO 10.5) 14. _____ occurs when the blood supply to a portion of the brain is blocked.
   a. Melanoma
   b. Stroke
   c. Myocardial infarction
   d. Epilepsy

(LO 10.5) 15. _____ occurs when a diseased artery in the brain floods the surrounding tissue with blood.
a. Cerebral thrombosis
b. Ischemic stroke
c. Hemorrhagic stroke
d. Cerebral embolism

(LO 10.5) 16. Which of the following statements about risk factors of stroke is true?
a. Men are generally at higher risk.
b. Race is not a significant risk factor.
c. Low red blood cell count increases the risk.
d. Lowering LDL levels decreases the risk.

(LO 10.7) 17. _____ is a type of cancer that forms in the supporting, or connective, tissues of the body such as bones, muscles, and blood vessels.
a. Lymphoma
b. Carcinoma
c. Leukemia
d. Sarcoma

(LO 10.7) 18. Among gynecological cancers, the leading cause of death is _____.
a. HPV
b. cervical cancer
c. ovarian cancer
d. breast cancer

(LO 10.8) 19. A vector in an infectious process is _____.
a. the area in which the infection occurred
b. the biological or physical vehicle that carries the agent to the host
c. the organism that causes the infection
d. the person infected

(LO 10.8) 20. The time between the entry of a pathogen into your body and the first symptom is known as _____.
a. the incubation period
b. the prodromal period
c. the attack period
d. dormancy

(LO 10.8) 21. Which of the following statements about the immune system is true?
a. An antigen is a substance that is considered to be the same as a normal body cell, and they are therefore protected by the body's defense system.
b. The tonsils and lungs play a role in the body's immune system.
c. Inoculation with a vaccine confers active immunity.
d. Stress increases the effectiveness of the human immune system.

(LO 10.8) 22. As part of the body's immune response, macrophages _____.
a. act as specialist cells that respond to specific invaders
b. are part of the bone marrow
c. filter bacteria and many other agents of disease
d. are scavenger cells that consume foreign cells as well as diseased red blood cells

(LO 10.8) 23. Most vaccine-preventable deaths occur among _____.
a. infants
b. children
c. teenagers
d. adults

(LO 10.8) 24. The severity of common-cold symptoms can be lessened by _____.
a. vitamin C
b. vaccination
c. frequent handwashing
d. high doses of zinc

(LO 10.8) 25. Meningitis vaccination _____.
a. is recommended at 1–2 years of age.
b. protects against most common types of meningococcal bacteria
c. also protects against gonorrhea
d. may cause major side effects

(LO 10.8) 26. Early bacterial meningitis symptoms _____.
a. tend to be severe and develop within hours
b. resemble flu symptoms and take a couple of days to appear
c. take several days to appear
d. always include a red rash

(LO 10.8) 27. Hepatitis B _____.
a. is spread mainly through contaminated needles
b. infects mostly middle-aged people
c. does not have a preventive vaccine
d. can be spread in the sweat of athletes

(LO 10.8) 28. Which of the following is NOT true regarding hepatitis C (HCV)?
a. Many people with HCV do not know they have the disease.
b. HVC is spread by casual contact, such as hugging, kissing, or sharing food utensils.
c. Targeted antiviral drugs have proven highly effective in more than 95 percent of patients with chronic HCV.
d. There is controversy about whether HCV can be transmitted sexually.

(LO 10.8) 29. The primary danger posed by infection with the Zika virus is _____.
  a. fever
  b. birth defects
  c. severe fatigue
  d. breathing problems

(LO 10.8) 30. Lyme disease can be transmitted to humans by _____.
  a. a bite from an infected tick
  b. a bite from an infected mosquito
  c. contact with an infected bird
  d. a kiss from someone who is infected with the disease

(LO 10.8) 31. Avian influenza _____.
  a. often infects livestock
  b. cannot be passed to humans
  c. can spread only in tropical climates
  d. is usually passed to humans by other humans

Answers to these questions can be found on page 531.

tankist276/Shutterstock.com

LEARNING OBJECTIVES

After reading this chapter, you should be able to:

11.1 Assess the impact of health insurance legislation on access to health care.

11.2 Understand the benefits and terms of health insurance policies.

11.3 Explain the significance of personalized health care.

11.4 Describe what it means to be a savvy health-care consumer.

11.5 Outline your rights as a health-care consumer.

11.6 Discuss the pros and cons of elective treatments to enhance health or appearance.

11.7 Identify ways to recognize health hoaxes and medical quackery.

11.8 Weigh the benefits and potential risks of complementary and alternative medicine (CAM).

11.9 Review the components of the health-care system, including types of practitioners and health-care facilities.

WHAT DO YOU THINK?

- What do college students need to know about health insurance?

- Are you a savvy health-care consumer?

- What steps can you take to make sure you get quality health care?

- What do you need to know about complementary and alternative medicine?

11

Consumer Health

It sounded too good to be true: an herbal supplement that turned off appetite, burned up calories, melted away pounds. Of course it was safe, Mia's roommate reassured her. Lots of her friends had tried it. And anyone could get it online without a prescription.

Mia rarely took any medications, even over-the-counter ones, but a quick, easy way to lose weight seemed too good to resist. When her heart started beating rapidly, Mia blamed anxiety. Her head ached. She couldn't sleep. Her mouth felt dry. One day Mia got so dizzy that a classmate insisted on taking her to the campus health center. When the doctor inquired about drug use, she immediately said she didn't do drugs. But when asked about medications, she mentioned the diet pills—and where they came from.

It had never occurred to Mia that they might be the culprit or that she might have been taking counterfeit pills with unknown ingredients. "Never again!" Mia vows. She isn't going to take any more chances with her health—and she's going to make better health-care choices in the future.

Although you may not realize it, every day you, too, make crucial decisions that affect your health. You choose what you eat, whether you exercise, whether you smoke or drink, when to fasten your seat belt or put on a safety helmet. You determine when to see a doctor, what kind of doctor, and with what sense of urgency. You decide what to tell the physician and whether to follow his or her advice, take a prescribed medication as directed, or seek further help or a second opinion. The entire process of maintaining or restoring health depends on your decisions. It cannot start or continue without them.

This chapter helps you take greater responsibility for your personal well-being. Whether you are monitoring your blood pressure, taking medication, or deciding whether to try an alternative therapy, you need to gather information, ask questions, weigh advantages and disadvantages, and take charge of your health. The reason: No one cares more about your health than you do, and no one will do more to protect your well-being. <

✓check-in Do you take good care of yourself? If you say yes, how? If you say no, what do you think you should be doing?

Health Insurance

Health insurance, the subject of intense political debate, affects the well-being of Americans of every race, sex, age, and income level.

The Affordable Care Act

Initially referred to as Obamacare and signed into law in 2010, the Affordable Care Act (ACA) ushered in a new era in consumer health and provided insurance to more than 20 million people. It put a number of key reforms in place:

- Health insurance exchanges, or marketplaces, for individuals, families, and small businesses to purchase guaranteed health insurance plans with affordable premiums

- Subsidies for low-income purchasers to make buying health insurance more affordable

- A tax penalty for those who do not purchase coverage

- A prevention against insurance companies refusing coverage or charging higher premiums to people with a preexisting condition

- Elimination of annual and lifetime caps on how much an insurance company will pay a policyholder.

- No copayments, deductibles, or coinsurance for basic preventive care services (Table 11.1).

The ACA has helped millions of Americans receive and pay for medical care. Its positive impacts include the following:

- The number of uninsured working-age adults fell from a high of 22 percent in 2010 to 12 percent.[1]

- Prior to the ACA, one in three young adults lacked insurance. A significantly greater number, particularly African Americans and Hispanics, now have insurance coverage.[2]

- Access to primary care and medications has improved, as have positive health outcomes.

- Coverage of family planning has saved women a substantial amount—approximately 70 percent in government estimates—in out-of-pocket expenses for contraceptives.[3]

- Fewer adults report that concern about cost has kept them from going to a doctor when sick; filling a prescription; having a recommended test, treatment, or follow-up visit; or seeking needed care from a specialist.[4]

Since the passage of the ACA, legal and political controversy has continued. The Trump administration proposed various initiatives to invalidate the ACA or limit certain provisions. States, cities, advocates, and health plans sued to block these challenges. Issues related to the constitutionality of the ACA, either in whole or in part, continue to be argued in the courts.[5] Among the most intensely debated provisions are short-term plans that are renewable for up to three years but lack all ACA consumer protections, exemption for religious organizations for contraception coverage for their employees, and protection of transgender individuals from discrimination by insurers and health-care providers.[6]

✓check-in Do you have health insurance? If so, what type of coverage do you have?

How Health Care Insurance Works

Health insurance plans differ in actuarial value, the percentage of the cost of care that insurance will cover. If a plan has 60 percent actuarial value, then it covers 60 percent of your potential health-care spending, and you cover

TABLE 11.1 Free Preventive Services under the ACA

- Alcohol misuse screening and counseling
- Aspirin to prevent cardiovascular disease for men and women of certain ages
- Blood pressure screening for all adults
- Cholesterol screening for adults of certain ages or at higher risk
- Colorectal cancer screening for adults over age 50
- Depression screening for adults
- Diabetes (type 2) screening for adults with high blood pressure
- Diet counseling for adults at higher risk for chronic disease
- HIV screening for everyone ages 15 to 65
- Immunization vaccines for adults—doses, recommended ages, and recommended populations vary
- Obesity screening and counseling for all adults
- Sexually transmitted infection (STI) prevention counseling for adults at higher risk
- Syphilis screening for all adults at higher risk
- Tobacco use screening for all adults and cessation interventions for tobacco users

40 percent. Plans with higher actuarial value cost more. In the Affordable Care Act insurance exchanges, bronze plans had a 60 percent actuarial value; silver plans, 70 percent; and gold plans, 80 percent.

You pay for your health insurance up front with a premium that is usually charged monthly. Almost all plans come with deductibles. This is an amount of money that you are responsible for paying before insurance coverage kicks in. The reason plans have deductibles is that research shows that consumers are less likely to spend their own money than the insurance company's money. Plans with lower deductibles usually have higher premiums.

Even after you spend the deductible, most plans come with co-payments—set fees that you have to pay each time you use the health-care system; for instance, you pay $20 for a checkup with a doctor or $100 for an emergency room visit. Some plans offer co-insurance, in which you pay a percentage of your care instead of a set fee for each service.

The lower the actuarial value of your plan, the more you pay out of pocket in deductibles, co-pays, or co-insurance. Plans on the ACA exchanges are all subject to an out-of-pocket maximum, such as $6,850 for an individual. Even if you have insurance, you may be "underinsured," which means that you could be at significant financial risk because of such out-of-pocket payments.

At the time of publication of this text, it is not clear whether the ACA will remain law or be amended or repealed. However, it is expected that certain key provisions will be retained.

What You Need to Know

College students have several choices for health coverage:

- If you are enrolled in your school's student health plan, check to see if it qualifies as coverage under the health law.

- If you are under age 26, you can join or remain on a parents' plan even if you are married, attending school full or part time, not living at home, not financially dependent on your parents, or eligible to enroll in your employer's plan.

- Even if you have access to a student health plan, you can choose to buy a health plan at www.healthcare.gov. Based on your income, you may be able to obtain coverage at a lower cost.

✓**check-in** Do you know what your health insurance plan covers?

Carefully read and research advertisements and promotional material for insurance policies. Some cover only certain diseases or injuries and do not offer comprehensive insurance protection. Different policies offer different benefits; some limit which doctors, hospitals, or other providers you can use:

- **Prescriptions:** To find out which prescriptions are covered through a plan, visit an insurer's website to review a list of medications covered. Check the Summary of Benefits and Coverage that you received. You can also call your insurer. The number is on your insurance card and the insurer's website.

- **Doctor visits:** Most health plans give you the best deal on services when you see a doctor who has a contract with your health plan. While you may be able to see physicians who do not contract with your plan, visiting an "in-network" provider usually means you will have lower out-of-pocket costs. To find out if your current doctors and other health-care providers are covered through a new plan or to find a covered provider if you don't have one yet, visit your health plan's website and check the provider directory, which lists the doctors, hospitals, and other health-care providers that your plan contracts with to provide care.

- **Emergency care:** In an emergency, you should get care from the closest hospital that can help you. Your insurance company cannot require you to get prior approval before getting emergency services from a provider or hospital outside your plan's network or charge you more for such care.

- **Deductibles:** You may have to pay a deductible, which varies with different plans, each year before your insurance company begins to pay for care.

- **Copayments:** You may have to pay a share of the costs for specific services, such as a doctor visit or prescription. This may be a fixed amount of $10 or $20 or a percentage, such as 20 percent of the total cost.

If you are under age 30, you can buy a catastrophic health plan, which usually has lower monthly premiums but high deductibles. This means you pay for most of your care yourself, up to a certain amount. After that, the insurance company pays its share for covered services. Catastrophic plans are an affordable way to protect yourself from the high costs of worst-case scenarios, like an accident or a serious illness. They also cover three primary care visits per year before you meet your deductible, as well as certain preventive care benefits. For more information, log on to www.healthcare.gov.

Consumer-Driven Health Care

Increasingly Americans are approaching "purchases" of health care the same way as other major investments, like buying a car. More than ever, consumers need clear, concise, and accurate information, not just on specific health conditions but also on factors such as out-of-pocket expenses and the effectiveness of a particular treatment. By learning how to maintain your health, evaluate medical information, and spot early signs of a problem, you are more likely to get the best possible care.

The demand for this information coincides with the growth of personalized medicine, in which individuals' genetic profiles will help determine which drugs or cancer therapies to prescribe, as well as help predict the risk of future disease.

This means that you will have to be a savvier, more sophisticated health-care consumer. By learning how to maintain your health, evaluate medical information, and spot early signs of a problem, you're more likely to get the best possible care.

✓**check-in** How well informed a health-care consumer do you think you are?

Improving Your Health Literacy

According to federal estimates, about one-third of the population in the United States has limited ability to understand health information and to use that information to make good decisions about health and medical care. Because of poor **health literacy**, more than 90 million Americans may not understand how to take medication, monitor cholesterol levels or blood sugar, manage a chronic disease, find health providers and services, or fill out necessary forms. Individuals with limited health literacy are more likely to report poor health, to skip important preventive measures such as regular Pap smears, to have chronic conditions such as diabetes or asthma, to stop taking needed medications, and to have higher rates of preventable hospitalizations.

Regardless of their literacy skills, college students often do not seek out information on health concerns. In one study that tracked college students' communications for a 2-week period, they sought health-related advice and information in a little more than one-fourth of their communications about health. When they did seek help, they were most likely to turn to family members and friends. About half of students also turn to health educators for information, and most rank them and health center medical staff as trustworthy. Although students regularly get information from flyers, pamphlets, magazines, and television, they are less likely to consider these as authoritative, believable sources.

Evidence-Based Medicine

Large randomized, controlled trials and prospective studies provide the best evidence, or scientific proof, that a particular treatment is effective. **Evidence-based medicine**, now a fundamental part of medical education, is a way of improving and evaluating health care by combining the best research evidence with the patient's personal values.[7]

Reviewing all available medical studies pertaining to an individual patient or group of patients helps doctors diagnose illnesses more precisely, choose the best tests, and select the best treatments or methods of disease prevention. By using evidence-based medical techniques for large groups of patients with the same illness, doctors can develop **practice guidelines** for evaluating and treating particular illnesses.

Outcomes Research

Evidence-based medicine pays particular attention to **outcomes**—that is, the impact that a specific medication or treatment has on a patient's condition, overall health, and quality of life.

Outcomes research is designed to answer questions such as: Is treatment better or worse

---

health literacy Ability to understand health information and use it to make good decisions about health and medical care.

evidence-based medicine The choice of a medical treatment on the basis of large randomized, controlled research trials and large prospective studies.

practice guidelines Recommendations for diagnosis and treatment of various health problems, based on evidence from scientific research.

outcomes The ultimate impacts of particular treatments or absence of treatment.

YOUR STRATEGIES FOR PREVENTION

How to Boost Health Understanding

Always ask these questions of your doctor, nurse, or pharmacist:

- **What is my main problem?**

- **What do I need to do?**

- **Why is it important for me to do this?**

- **If you don't understand, say,** "This is new to me. Can you explain it one more time?"

- **If you don't know the meaning of a medical term, don't hesitate to ask what it means.** Health professionals sometimes forget they're using technical terms, such as "myocardial infarction" for heart attack.

- **Write down a list of your health concerns,** and bring it with you whenever you seek health care.

than no treatment? Is one treatment better than another? If a treatment is effective, is a little just as good as a lot? Does quality of life change because of treatment? Are the benefits of treatment worth the cost or the risks to the patient?

Studies of outcomes look at how patients fared with or without a specific treatment, the costs involved, and the impact of undergoing or not undergoing treatment in terms of the patients' quality of life. Outcomes research can help determine which of several therapies or approaches provides the best results at the most reasonable costs.

If you are diagnosed with a serious health problem, ask your doctor if the suggested treatment is based on the latest evidence and clinical guidelines. The National Guideline Clearinghouse provides a comprehensive database of evidence-based clinical practice guidelines for many common health problems, available at www.guideline.gov.

Personalizing Your Health Care

Thanks to advances in genomics (the study of the entire set of human genes), physicians are tailoring tests and treatments to individual patients. "Personalized" medicine can alert your doctor to potential threats that might be prevented, delayed, or detected at an earlier, more treatable stage and, if you do develop a disease, pinpoint the medications that will do the most good and cause the least harm.

"Personalizing" health care is also a personal responsibility. You can take charge of your own health by compiling a family health history and informing yourself about risks related to your gender, race, and ethnicity.

Your Family Health History

Someday a DNA scan from a single drop of blood may tell you the diseases you're most likely to develop. A family history can do the same—now.

Mapping your family **medical history** can help identify health risks you may face in the future. One way of charting your health history is to draw a medical family "tree" that includes your parents and siblings (who share your genes), as well as grandparents, uncles, aunts, and cousins. Depending on how much information you're able to obtain for each relative, your medical family tree can include health issues each family member has faced, including illnesses with a hereditary

❗ CONSUMER ALERT

Too Good to Be True?

Almost every week you're likely to see an ad for a new health product that promises better sleep, more energy, clearer skin, firmer muscles, lower weight, brighter moods, longer life—or all of these combined. But you can't believe every promise you read or hear. Keep these general guidelines in mind the next time you come across a health claim.

Facts to Know

- **Do your own research.** Check with your doctor or with the student health center. Go to the library or do some online research to gather as much information as you can.

- **Check credentials.** Anyone can claim to be a scientist or a health expert. Find out if advocates of any type of therapy have legitimate degrees from recognized institutions and are fully licensed in their fields.

Steps to Take

- **Look for objective evaluations.** If you're watching an infomercial for a treatment or technique, you can be sure that the enthusiastic endorsements have been skillfully scripted and rehearsed. Even ads that claim to be presenting the science behind a new breakthrough are really sales pitches in disguise.

- **Consider the sources.** Research findings from carefully controlled scientific studies are reviewed by leading experts in the field and published in scholarly journals. Just because someone has conducted a study doesn't mean it was a valid scientific investigation.

- **If it sounds too good to be true, it probably is.** If a magic pill could really trim off excess pounds or banish wrinkles, the world would be filled with thin people with unlined skin. Look around, and you'll realize that's not the case.

component, such as high blood pressure, diabetes, some cancers, and certain psychiatric disorders.

Although having a relative with a certain disease may mean you face increased risk for the condition, this likelihood also depends on your health habits, such as diet and exercise. Realizing that you have a relative with, say, colon cancer could mean that you should start screening tests 10 years before others because you're at risk of developing a tumor at an earlier age.

✓**check-in** Do you know your family's health history? For guidance on compiling a family health history, check this website from the office of the Surgeon General: https://familyhistory.hhs.gov/FHH/html/-index.html.

Sex Differences

The sexes differ significantly in the way they use health-care services in the United States. On average, women see doctors more often than men, take more prescription drugs, are hospitalized more often, and control the spending of three of every four health-care dollars.

medical history Health-related information that a health-care professional collects while interviewing a patient.

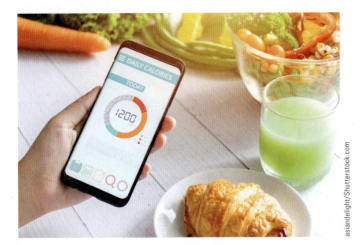

Apps providing basic nutritional information can help you make healthier food choices.

self-care Head-to-toe maintenance, including good oral care, appropriate screening tests, knowing your medical rights, and understanding the health-care system.

vital signs Measurements of physiological functioning—specifically temperature, blood pressure, pulse rate, and respiration rate.

Many experts believe that the need for birth control and reproductive health services gets women into the habit of making regular visits to health-care professionals, primarily gynecologists. There are no comparable specialists for men, who tend to visit urologists, specialists in male reproductive organs, only when they develop problems. In addition, men are conditioned to take a stoic, tough-it-out attitude to early symptoms of a disease. The length of time they wait to go for treatment may be one reason men die earlier than women.

In a survey of nearly 2 million patients who had recently been hospitalized, men tended to be more positive about their overall experiences. Women were less satisfied with staff responsiveness, discussions with nurses, communication about medications and discharge plans, and the general conditions of the hospital.

The genders also differ in the symptoms and syndromes they develop. For instance, men are more prone to back problems, muscle sprains and strains, allergies, insomnia, and digestive problems. Men develop heart disease about a decade earlier in life than women. More men develop ulcers and hernias; women are more likely to get migraines, gallbladder disease, and irritable bowel syndrome. Yet women and men spend similar proportions of their lifetimes—about 80 percent—free of disability.

Mobile Health (mHealth) Apps and Monitors

Do you want to check your vital signs? Track your workouts? Count your steps? Put yourself to sleep? There's a mobile health (mHealth) app for that! (Table 11.2). With almost 5 billion mobile phone users globally, the number of health-related apps is growing by about 40 percent every year.[8] Usually run on a smartphone or other handheld device, apps rely on an operating system and network connection to send and receive data.

Sensors or trackers consist of physical hardware with limited computing and communication capabilities that provide objective reporting of indicators such as blood glucose levels and heart rate. Some mHealth devices combine hardware and software to provide a comprehensive approach that physicians can use to diagnose problems such as an irregular heartbeat. The Food and Drug Administration (FDA) regulates only apps that turn smartphones into medical devices or accessories for measuring vital signs.

Can digital devices make you healthier? Medical scientists don't have definitive answers yet because research on their usefulness and impact on health outcomes remains limited.[9] Although they cannot replace a health professional, mobile apps and wearable monitors may offer significant benefits, including:

- Increased awareness of daily habits (healthful or not).
- Access to useful information when and where you need it.
- Reminders to take medications on time.
- A minute-by-minute record of your daily calories and activity.
- Better control of blood pressure and blood sugar in patients with hypertension or diabetes.
- More effective support for selecting healthful foods and losing weight.
- Greater success in smoking cessation.[10]
- Motivation to be more physically active.

TABLE 11.2 There's a mHealth app for that!

If you...	Recommended Apps
Want to start basic aerobic exercise	Fitbit, Couch to 5K Zombies, Run!, Map My Fitness, Map My Run, Strava Running and Cycling, Nike Running, RunKeeper, Runtastic
Want to build more lean muscle	Fitocracy Macros, Fitocracy
Have hypertension and want to reduce your cardiovascular risk	Fitbit, Map My Run
Want to lose weight and start exercising	Lose It!, Noom Weight Loss Coach, MyFitnessPal
Want to exercise and make a difference to the world	Charity Miles
Want to learn more about a medical condition	WebMD
Think you may have a sleep disorder	Sleep cycle alarm clock

Source: Higgins JP. Smartphone applications for patients' health and fitness. *Am J Med*. 2016;129(1):11–19.

- In breast cancer patients, decreased stress, positive behavioral changes (such as weight loss), improved early detection, help in managing care, and support for survivors.[11]

Skeptics argue that digital self-monitoring may create uncertainty and anxiety and cause healthy men and women needless worry. They are also expensive—often hundreds of dollars—and appeal to, as one analyst put it, "groups that might need them least."

Health apps that make deceptive claims—such as the capability to analyze skin moles to assess the risk of melanoma—could lead to false-negative diagnoses and a failure to get needed treatment. In one survey, more than half of people who bought a fitness tracker eventually stopped wearing it; of these, a third quit within 6 months.[12]

Other limitations include:

- Need to own a smartphone and have a sufficient WiFi data plan.

- Various conditions—sweat/water, extremes of weather, etc.—can interfere with the smartphone during an activity.

- Technical problems and app malfunctions.

- Smartphone sensors may not be as sensitive as stand-alone sensors.

- Apps require users to actively engage with them in order to benefit and may not work with users with certain disabilities.

- Most apps not yet peer reviewed by appropriately trained professionals.[13]

✓check-in Do you use a health-monitoring app or tracker? If so, what do you like/dislike about it? Has it had an impact on your behavior?

Self-Care

Self-care means head-to-toe maintenance, including good oral care, appropriate screening tests, knowing your medical rights, and understanding the health-care system.

Most people do treat themselves. You probably prescribe aspirin for a headache, chicken soup or orange juice for a cold, or a weekend trip to unwind from stress. At the very least, you should know what your **vital signs** are and how they compare against normal readings (Figure 11.1).

Hundreds of home tests are available to help consumers monitor everything from fertility to blood pressure to cholesterol levels (Table 11.3).

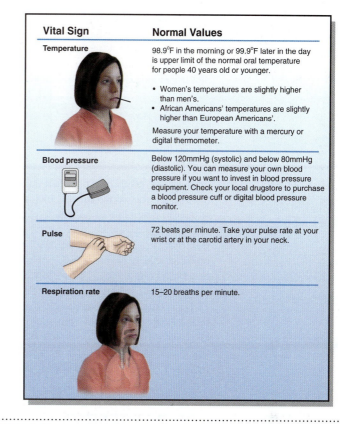

Vital Sign	Normal Values
Temperature	98.9°F in the morning or 99.9°F later in the day is upper limit of the normal oral temperature for people 40 years old or younger. • Women's temperatures are slightly higher than men's. • African Americans' temperatures are slightly higher than European Americans'. Measure your temperature with a mercury or digital thermometer.
Blood pressure	Below 120mmHg (systolic) and below 80mmHg (diastolic). You can measure your own blood pressure if you want to invest in blood pressure equipment. Check your local drugstore to purchase a blood pressure cuff or digital blood pressure monitor.
Pulse	72 beats per minute. Take your pulse rate at your wrist or at the carotid artery in your neck.
Respiration rate	15–20 breaths per minute.

FIGURE 11.1 Do you know your vital signs?

More convenient and less expensive than a visit to a clinic or doctor's office, the new tests are generally as accurate as those administered by a professional.

TABLE 11.3 Home Health Tests: A Consumer's Guide

Type of Test	What It Does
Pregnancy	Determines whether a woman is pregnant by detecting the presence of human chorionic gonadotropin in urine. Considered 99% accurate.
Fertility	Measures levels of luteinizing hormone (LH), which rise 24–36 hours before a woman ovulates. Can help women increase their odds of conceiving.
Blood pressure	Measures blood pressure by means of an automatically inflating armband or a cuff for the finger or wrist; helps people taking hypertension medication or suffering from high blood pressure to monitor their condition.
Cholesterol	Checks cholesterol in blood from a fingerprick; good for anyone concerned about cholesterol.
Colon cancer	Screening test to detect hidden blood in stool; recommended for anyone over age 40 or concerned about colorectal disease.
Urinary tract infection	Diagnoses infection by screening for certain white blood cells in urine; advised for women who get frequent UTIs and whose doctors will prescribe antibiotics without a visit.
HIV infection	Detects antibodies to HIV in a blood sample sent anonymously to a lab. Controversial because no face-to-face counseling is available for those who test positive.

Self-care can also mean getting involved in the self-help movement, which has grown into a major national trend. An estimated 20 million people participate in self-help support groups. Millions of others join virtual support communities online.

✓**check-in** How do you practice self-care?

Oral Health

Oral health involves more than healthy teeth; it refers to the entire mouth, including all the structures that allow us to talk, bite, chew, taste, swallow, smile, scream, and scowl. Oral health is a critical part of overall health. Research has revealed links between chronic oral infection and heart and lung diseases, stroke, low birth weight, premature births, and diabetes.

Poor oral health can lead to a variety of health problems. People with gum disease are at increased risk for developing heart disease, stroke, uncontrolled diabetes, preterm births, and respiratory disease. One recent study found an increased risk of pancreatic cancer in individuals who had experienced tooth loss.

Thanks to fluoridated water, toothpaste, and improved dental care, Americans' oral health is better today than in the past. However, without good self-care, you probably will lose some teeth to decay and gum disease. The best way to prevent such problems is through proper and regular brushing and flossing.

Gum disease, or periodontal disease, attacks the gums and bone that hold your teeth in place. The culprit is **plaque**, a sticky film of bacteria that forms on teeth. More than 300 species of bacteria live under the gum line, and about half a dozen have been linked to serious gum problems. The early stage of gum disease is called **gingivitis**. If untreated, it develops into a more serious form known as **periodontitis**, in which plaque moves down the tooth to the roots, which then become infected. In advanced periodontitis, the infection destroys the bone and fibers that hold teeth in place.

Taking care of your mouth isn't important only for dental health: It may affect how long you live. Gingivitis and periodontitis trigger an inflammatory response that causes the arteries to swell, which leads to a constriction of blood flow that can increase the incidence of cardiovascular disease. Periodontal disease also leads to a higher white blood cell count, an indicator that the immune system is under increased stress. The good news: You can prevent these problems by flossing daily and brushing your teeth and your tongue (to get rid of bacteria that can cause gum disease and bad breath).

✓**check-in** How would you rate your oral health care?

gum disease Infection of the gums and bones that hold teeth in place.

plaque A sticky film of bacteria that forms on teeth.

gingivitis Inflammation of the gums.

periodontitis Severe gum disease in which the tooth root becomes infected.

YOUR STRATEGIES FOR PREVENTION

How to Take Care of Your Mouth

- **Brush your teeth every morning and every night.** Oral bacteria reach their highest count during sleep because fluids in the mouth accumulate. Nighttime cleaning reduces the bacterial population; morning cleaning reduces the buildup.

- **Use a toothpaste that has the American Dental Association (ADA) seal of acceptance and a toothbrush with soft, rounded bristles.** Replace your toothbrush after an illness or every 3 months.

- **Hold the brush at a 45-degree angle from your gums.** Pay particular attention to the space between your teeth and gums, especially on the inside, toward your tongue. Brush for 2 to 5 minutes. Don't brush too vigorously. If you scrub as hard as you can, you may damage your teeth and gums. Abrasion—a problem for more than half of American adults—erodes tooth surfaces, weakens teeth, and increases sensitivity to hot and cold foods. There is some evidence that powered toothbrushes are better at removing plaque and reducing the risk of gum disease than are ordinary manual toothbrushes.

- **Because brushing can't reach plaque and food trapped between teeth, daily flossing is essential.** Using waxed or unwaxed floss, start behind the upper and lower molars at one side of your mouth and work toward the other side.

- **See your dentist twice a year for routine cleaning and examination.** Your dentist should take a complete medical history from you and update it every 6 months, examine your mouth for signs of cancer, and thoroughly outline all treatment options.

- **Make sure that everyone who works on the inside of your mouth wears a mask and rubber gloves.** Such measures reduce the risk of disease transmission (i.e., bacterial and viral infections, such as hepatitis, herpes, and HIV).

Becoming a Savvy Health-Care Consumer

Because physicians today have less time and less autonomy than they once had, patients today must do more. Your first step should be learning more about your body, any medical conditions or problems you develop, and your options for treatment. You can find a great deal of information online, via patient advocacy and support organizations, and from libraries.

Making the Most of a Medical Visit

Your visit to a health-care professional is an opportunity to learn, to share information, to get needed help, and to improve your health now and in the future. Here is how to ensure you get the greatest value from your health-care providers.

Scheduling the Appointment
When you schedule the appointment, you need to both get and give information:

- Always check to see if a health-care provider accepts your insurance plan.
- When you make your appointment, explain why you need to see the health-care provider.
- Are you scheduling a checkup?
- Have you developed a new problem?
- Is it urgent? Do you need to see a health-care provider right away?
- If you want to see a specialist, find out if you need a referral from your primary care provider.
- If you prefer a female provider for religious or cultural reasons, make this clear.

Before Your Appointment
To get the most out of your appointment, you need to do some homework ahead of time:

- Write down your questions, organize them in a logical fashion, and select the top 10 queries you want answered. Start with your main problem so you can bring it up right away. Then list other concerns that you want to discuss. Make a copy of all your questions to review and leave with your doctor.
- Make a list of all medications you take, including over-the-counter drugs, vitamins, and herbal supplements.
- Write down any symptoms or pain you are experiencing.
- If you are visiting a new health-care provider, download and bring any past medical records or test results you have. You will need the names and contact information of your past health-care providers.
- Sum up your medical and surgical history. You can give it to the health-care provider or use it to fill out a standardized form.
- Provide the names and contact information of other doctors you've seen recently.

- Be sure you can describe what your symptoms feel like, when they started, and what makes them better.
- Think about bringing a support person who can act as your advocate. Choose someone who knows you and who has your best interests in mind.
- If English is not your first language or if you are hearing impaired, you may need an interpreter. Ask the office staff whether they can find someone who is experienced in medical terms.
- Be sure to bring your health insurance card.

At Your Appointment
Provide a complete health history, including:

- Illnesses and injuries.
- Hospitalizations.
- Surgical procedures.
- Drugs (ones you take now or have taken in the past).
- Allergies, including bad reactions to drugs and foods.
- Immunizations.
- Also bring personal information, including:
- Exercise habits, diet, and alcohol use.
- Relevant factors such as experiencing stress at work, getting married, or moving.
- Harmful health behaviors such as smoking and drug use.
- Family history of disease (include aunts, uncles, cousins, and grandparents as well as parents, brothers and sisters, and children).
- When a staff member checks your height, weight, blood pressure, and pulse, ask for the readings. Remember that you have a right to ask questions of anyone who is involved in your health care.

The Physical Examination
Typically, your doctor will begin an exam by inspecting your body for any unusual marks or growths. Next, he or she may palpate your abdomen and other parts of your body to assess the consistency, location, size, tenderness, and texture of individual organs. Your doctor will use a stethoscope to listen to your heart and lungs as you take deep breaths. By using a technique known as *percussion*—tapping around the body as if it were a drum—your doctor checks for fluid in areas where it should not be and locates the borders, consistency, and size

of organs. Here are some other important points about a physical examination:

- Your health-care provider should make your physical examination as comfortable as possible. Speak up if something bothers or frightens you. Be clear about your modesty needs.

- A health-care professional (such as a nurse or nursing assistant) may remain throughout the exam. Let your doctor know if you want a friend or family member in the room.

- If you do not see your health-care providers wash their hands, you might ask, "Have you washed your hands?" Handwashing is the most important way your health-care provider can prevent the spread of infections.

Talking with Your Health-Care Provider

With the clues obtained during the *history* and *physical examination*, a health-care provider can formulate a differential diagnosis—that is, a list of potential causes of the symptoms. Specific diagnostic tests generally confirm the cause or reveal other, previously unsuspected causes. When you

Take charge of your health by educating yourself and asking your doctor questions about your health and treatments.

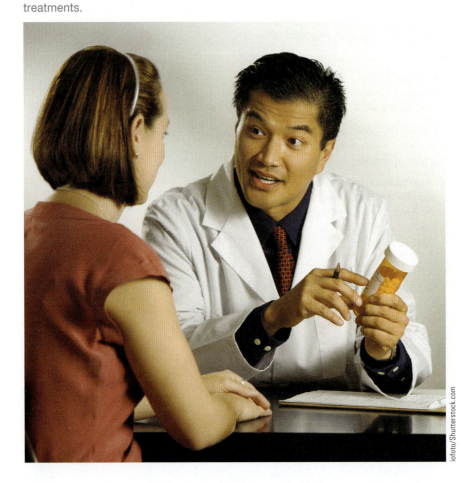

iofoto/Shutterstock.com

are talking with your health-care provider, keep these points in mind:

- **If you have questions, ask them.** If the health-care provider asks you questions, answer them as best you can. Be honest.

- **Make sure you understand everything your health-care provider says.** Ask for simple, clear explanations. Take careful notes. If you have a friend or relative with you, ask that person to take notes so that you can listen more closely to what the health-care provider says.

- **If you are given a diagnosis and need further care, ask about the different treatments that are available. You may want to ask the following questions:**
  - What might have caused this condition?
  - What are the treatment choices?
  - What are the benefits and risks of each treatment?
  - How might the treatment affect my life?
  - Why is it important that I follow a certain treatment plan?
  - What might happen if I do not get treated?

- **If you need a test, procedure, or surgery, the following are good questions to ask:**
  - Why do I need it?
  - What does it involve? What do I need to do to get ready?
  - What should I expect? What are the side effects?
  - How will I find out the results?
  - How long will it take to recover?

- **If a medication is prescribed, make sure you find out the following:**
  - The brand and generic (common) names.
  - Instructions for taking the drug.
  - When you should take it and whether you should take it with food or on an empty stomach.
  - Whether you should avoid alcohol.
  - How much you should take.
  - For how long you should take it.
  - Any side effects that may occur and what you should do about them (see Health on a Budget).

- **Ask about a "question hour."** Many health facilities set aside a specific time of day for patients with call-in questions. Find out if your college health center offers this service. Does a nurse or physician's assistant field all calls? Can you get specific advice?

$ HEALTH ON A BUDGET

Getting Your Money's Worth from the Health-Care System

The value of medical care depends not just on health-care professionals but also on you:

- **If you receive a diagnosis,** make sure you understand what may be wrong with you, as well as what medications you must take and why.

- **When your doctor writes a prescription for you,** know why and how you are to take the medication.

- **If your doctor recommends a screening test, ask**
  - **Am I at higher risk than the average person and, if so, why?**

- **How often does the test give false alarms?** How often does it provide falsely reassuring results?

- **Are any other tests just as good?**

- **If the test results reveal a problem, are treatments available? What impact will they have on my life?**

- **If you must undergo surgery** and you can choose a hospital, select one at which many patients have had the procedure or surgery you need.

- **Go online.** Many medical offices answer queries by e-mail. Ask your doctor or physician's assistant if you can e-mail follow-up questions or progress reports on how you're feeling.

- **Interrupt the interrupter.** If you're having difficulty explaining what's wrong, say so. If your doctor tries to put words in your mouth, say, "Please just listen so I can tell you the whole story without getting sidetracked."

- **Ask for access to your medical record.** With the advent of electronic records, more health-care institutions are using secure Internet portals to offer patients online access to test results, medication lists, and other parts of their records. Health-care providers report some reservations, but patients express considerable enthusiasm and few fears.

At the end of your appointment, repeat what you have learned to the health-care provider. This recap will give your health-care provider a chance to correct any misunderstandings. If you need more time to talk about something, tell your health-care provider or see if you can schedule another appointment to continue your talk.

After Your Visit

At college health centers, clinics, and some health-care organizations, consumers may be assigned to a primary physician or restricted to certain doctors. Even if your choices are limited, don't suspend your critical judgment. If your assigned physician does not listen to your concerns or is not providing adequate care, you can—and should—request another physician. Your rapport with your primary physician and the feelings of mutual trust and respect that develop between you can have as

much of an impact on your well-being as your doctor's technical expertise.

One key to making the health-care system work for you lies in choosing a good physician. After seeing your primary care physician, ask yourself the following questions to evaluate the quality of care you are getting.

- Did your physician take a comprehensive history? Was the physical examination thorough?

- Did your physician explain what he or she was doing during the exam?

- Did he or she spend enough time with you?

- Did you feel free to ask questions? Did your physician give you straight answers? Did he or she reassure you when you were worried?

- Does your physician seem willing to admit that he or she doesn't know the answers to some questions?

- Does your physician hesitate to refer you to a specialist even when you have a complex problem that warrants such care?

Look back at your answers. If they make you feel uneasy, have a talk with your physician. Or find a physician or a health plan that provides better service. If you question the diagnosis or recommended treatment, seek a second opinion about your problem and its treatment from another health-care provider.

✓**check-in** Do you have a good, ongoing relationship with a primary care physician?

Diagnostic Tests If you are a woman, your physician will provide counseling on birth control and, if indicated, preconception care. Your doctor should also screen for

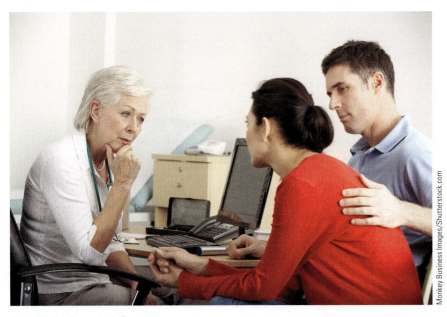

A patient advocate informs individuals of their rights and deals with specific concerns about their treatment.

intimate partner violence (discussed in Chapter 18) and, if you are at risk, for sexually transmitted infections.

Besides the diagnostic tests just listed, the physician may order some laboratory and other tests, including:

- **Chest X-ray:** A chest X-ray can reveal abnormalities of the heart and lungs; if you're a smoker, the physician may insist on one.

- **Urinalysis:** Your urine may be analyzed by a medical laboratory. If sugar (glucose) is found in your urine, your physician may order a separate blood test to check for diabetes. The presence of blood cells may indicate infection of the bladder or kidneys. Abnormal amounts of albumin (protein) in the urine may also suggest kidney disease.

- **Blood tests:** A baseline blood test, an important part of your health record, may include analyses of your lipids, or blood fats, including cholesterol and triglycerides; glucose; kidney and liver function; and minerals such as potassium and calcium. An excess of white blood cells most often indicates an infection; a deficiency of red blood cells may indicate anemia. High levels of glucose can indicate diabetes, and high levels of uric acid may point to gout or kidney stones.

Screening Tests In recent years, the medical profession has changed its recommendations for many tests used to screen for or detect disease at early stages.

Here are the current recommendations for some of the most common screening tests:

pap smears A test in which cells are removed from the cervix for microscopic examination for signs of cancer.

- **Low-back pain:** No imaging for low-back pain within the first 6 weeks, unless there may be serious underlying conditions. Imaging of the lower spine before 6 weeks does not improve outcomes but does increase costs.

- **Osteoporosis screening:** No dual-energy X-ray absorptiometry (DEXA) screening for osteoporosis in women younger than 65 or men younger than 70 if they have no risk factors. DEXA is not cost-effective in younger, low-risk patients but is cost-effective in older patients.

- **Cardiac screening:** No annual electrocardiograms (EKGs), echocardiograms, or any other cardiac screening for low-risk patients without symptoms. False-positive tests are likely to lead to harm through unnecessary invasive procedures, overtreatment, and misdiagnosis.

- **Mammography:** Breast cancer screening with mammography may be considered in women 40 to 49 years of age, based on patients' values and on potential benefits and harms. Mammography is recommended every two years in women 50 to 74 years of age.

- **Pap testing: Pap smears** are not recommended for women younger than age 21. In teenage girls, most abnormalities regress (clear up) spontaneously; therefore, Pap smears for this age group can lead to unnecessary anxiety, additional testing, and cost. See Chapter 13 for the most recent guidelines for cervical cancer screening.

- **Pelvic exams:** Although pelvic exams have traditionally been performed to screen for sexually transmitted infections (STIs) and gynecologic cancers and to evaluate women before prescribing hormonal contraceptives, there is no scientific justification for such testing on a routine basis. Some physicians continue to perform routine pelvic examinations for several reasons, including standard medical practice, patient reassurance, and identification of uterine and ovarian conditions. If you have questions about your need for a pelvic exam, raise them directly with your health care provider.

During a pelvic examination, a woman lies on her back, with her heels in stirrups at the end of the examining table and her legs spread out to the sides. The physician inspects the labia, clitoris, and vaginal opening. Using two gloved, lubricated fingers, the physician will check for abnormalities in the vagina, uterus, fallopian tubes, and ovaries. Many physicians will also perform a rectal or rectovaginal (one finger in the rectum and one in the vagina) examination.

A nurse or other health-care worker should be present throughout the exam.

The *speculum* is a medical instrument that spreads the walls of the vagina so that the inside can be seen.

✓**check-in** Which screening or diagnostic tests have you had?

Preventing Medical Errors

People die more often from medical errors than from motor vehicle accidents, breast cancer, or AIDS. Medical errors occur when a planned part of medical care doesn't work properly or when the wrong plan was used in the first place. These errors can happen anywhere in the health-care system, from doctors' offices to pharmacies to hospitals to patients' homes. They may involve medications, diagnoses, tests, lab equipment, surgery, or infection. They are most likely to occur when doctors and patients have problems communicating.

Your best defense against medical errors is information. Asking questions about your treatments can keep you safe and ensure that you get high-quality health care.

✓**check-in** Do you take any prescription medications on a regular basis? If so, are you taking precautions to avoid mistakes or complications?

Your Medical Rights

As a consumer, you have basic rights that help ensure that you know about any potential dangers, receive competent diagnosis and treatment, and retain control and dignity in your interactions with health-care professionals. Many hospitals publish a Patient's Bill of Rights, including your rights to know whether a procedure is experimental; to refuse to undergo a specific treatment; to designate someone else to make decisions about your care if and when you cannot; and to leave the hospital, even against your physician's advice.

Your Right to Be Treated with Respect and Dignity

Make clear how you would like health-care providers to address you—for example, as "Mr." or "Ms." or by your first name or whatever you wish. If you feel that health-care professionals are being condescending or inconsiderate, say so—in the same tone and manner that you would like others to use with you. If you're hospitalized, find out if there's a patient advocate or representative at your hospital. These individuals can help you communicate with physicians, make any special arrangements, and get answers to questions or complaints.

Your Right to Information

By law, a patient must give consent for hospitalization, surgery, and other major treatments. **Informed consent** is a right, not a privilege. Use this right to its fullest. Ask questions. Seek other opinions. Make sure that your expectations are realistic and that you understand the potential risks, as well as the possible benefits, of a prospective treatment.

Your Right to Privacy and Access to Medical Records

Your medical records are your property. You have the right to see them whenever you choose and to limit who else can see them. Federal standards protecting the privacy of patients' medical information guarantee patients access to their medical records, give them more control over how personal health information is disclosed, and limit the ways that health plans, pharmacies, and hospitals can use personal medical information.

Key provisions include:

- **Access to medical records:** As a patient, you should be able to see and obtain copies of your medical records and request corrections if there are errors. Health-care providers must provide these within 30 days; they may charge for the cost of copying and mailing records.

- **Notice of privacy practices:** Your providers must inform you of how they use personal medical information. Doctors, nurses, and other providers may not disclose information for purposes not related to your health care.

- **Prohibition on marketing:** Pharmacies, health plans, and others must obtain specific authorization before disclosing patient information for marketing.

- **Confidentiality:** Patients can request that doctors take reasonable steps to ensure confidential communications, such as calling a cell phone rather than a home or office number.

informed consent Permission (to undergo or receive a medical procedure or treatment) given voluntarily, with full knowledge and understanding of the procedure or treatment and its possible consequences.

A growing concern involves data breaches of protected health information. Since 2010, breaches involving more than 29 million health records have been reported, most accessed through laptops, portable devices, e-mail, and electronic health records. Health professionals worry that patients concerned about their information being stolen or leaked may withhold certain details from their providers, which could seriously undermine efforts to improve health.

✓**check-in** Think back on your health-care experiences. Were your rights as a patient respected? If not, what might you do differently in the future to ensure that they are?

Your Right to Quality Health Care

The essence of a *malpractice* suit is the claim that the physician failed to meet the standard of quality care required of a reasonably skilled and careful medical doctor. Although physicians don't have to guarantee good results to their patients and aren't held liable for unavoidable errors, they are required to use the same care as other physicians in the same specialty would use under similar circumstances. To protect themselves financially, physicians, particularly those in surgical specialties who are most likely to be sued, pay tens of thousands of dollars a year in malpractice insurance premiums. Some of this cost is passed on to patients.

Most lawsuits are based on negligence and assert that a physician failed to render diagnosis and treatment with appropriate professional knowledge and skill. Other cases are brought for failure to provide information, obtain consent, or respect a patient's confidentiality. However, analysis of malpractice cases has shown that, in 70 to 80 percent of cases, a doctor's attitude and inability to communicate effectively—by devaluing patients' views, delivering information poorly, failing to understand patients' perspectives, or displaying an air of superiority—also played a role.

Elective Treatments

As medical technology has developed new options, millions of Americans are trying elective procedures and products that are not medically necessary but that promise to enhance health or appearance. Some are new alternatives for correcting common problems, such as poor vision, while others offer the promise of looking younger or more attractive. In some cases, the procedures are scams or hoaxes.

Vision Surgery

Millions of people in the United States have undergone laser surgery to correct their vision. In lasik (laser-assisted in situ keratomileusis) surgery, the most common technique, a surgeon uses a razorlike instrument to lift a flap of the cornea—the clear, stiff outer layer over the colored iris—and then reshapes the exposed area using a laser. The surgery alters the way the eye focuses light, correcting nearsightedness, farsightedness, and some astigmatism. Lasik surgery cannot, however, make an aging eye's lens flexible again to improve close-up vision in middle-aged adults.

Other types of vision surgery include:

- PRK, photorefractive keratectomy, uses a laser to reshape the cornea but does not affect the tissue underneath.

- RLE (refractive lens exchange), similar to cataract surgery, replaces the natural lens with a plastic lens implant to correct extreme farsightedness or nearsightedness.

- PRELEX, short for presbyopic lens exchange, corrects presbyopia (loss of flexibility in the eye) by replacing the natural lens with a multifocal lens.

Although vision surgery is generally safe and effective, there are side effects and negative consequences, such as:

- Infection.

- Undercorrection or overcorrection, which may require a second operation.

- A haze over the cornea that may affect vision and require treatment.

- Regression or loss of improvement over time.

- Worse vision, which is rare but can happen.

Prices for lasik surgery have fallen, but ophthalmologists have warned consumers that some laser surgery centers have cut corners to reduce prices, such as hiring inexperienced surgeons or using optometrists or technicians rather than doctors for preoperative and postoperative checkups. A qualified eye surgeon should have a record of 100 or more lasik procedures and at least 25 enhancements—but no more than 20 percent of his or her patients should require enhancements.[14] Ideally, the surgeon should also be the one doing your preprocedure and postprocedure checks.

When Is Vision Surgery Not for You? You are probably *not* a good candidate for refractive surgery if:

- **You are not a risk-taker.** Certain complications are unavoidable in a percentage of patients, and there are no long-term data available for current procedures.

- **Cost is an issue.** Most medical insurance will not pay for refractive surgery. Although the cost is coming down, it is still significant.

- **You required a change in your contact lens or glasses prescription in the past year.** This is called refractive instability. Patients who are in their early 20s or younger, whose hormones are fluctuating due to disease such as diabetes, who are pregnant or breastfeeding, or who are taking medications that may cause fluctuations in vision are more likely to have refractive instability and should discuss the possible additional risks with their doctor.

- **You have a disease or are on medications that may affect wound healing.** Certain conditions, such as autoimmune diseases and diabetes, and some medications may prevent proper healing after a refractive procedure.

- **You actively participate in contact sports.** If you participate in boxing, wrestling, martial arts, or other activities in which blows to the face and eyes are a normal occurrence, lasik surgery is probably not right for you.

- **You are under 18.** Currently, no lasers are approved for vision surgery on persons under the age of 18.

- **It will jeopardize your career.** Some jobs, including certain military assignments, prohibit refractive procedures.

Cosmetic Surgery

The number of cosmetic, dermatologic, and surgical procedures continues to increase. More men, more adults under age 30, and more minorities, including black Americans and Asian Americans, are undergoing cosmetic treatments.[15] The most popular include laser/light treatments, Botox, and injectable fillers.[16]

Other common procedures include:

- Liposuction, the removal of fatty tissue by means of a vacuum device, can be performed on many areas of the body, from sagging jowls to midsection "love handles" or "muffin tops." The doctor first flushes the target area with a solution of lidocaine (a local anesthetic with a numbing effect), saline, and epinephrine (a drug that reduces bleeding by constricting blood vessels). Inserting a hollow, wandlike cannula under the skin, the doctor breaks up fatty deposits and suctions them, along with other body fluids, with a vacuum device. Risks and complications include infection, numbness, bleeding, discoloration, lumpiness, and, if too much tissue is removed without proper caution, potentially fatal complications. The American Society of Plastic Surgeons estimates that the mortality rate is 1 in 5,000 liposuction patients.

- Breast augmentation includes various approaches to increase the size or change the shape and texture of a woman's breasts. The Institute of Medicine, after reviewing all available evidence, has reported that there appears to be no link between breast implants and autoimmune disease, connective tissue disorders, or cancer. Patients still face possible complications, including rupture, scarring, infection, and leaking or hardening of their implants. Women with implants also may run the risk of being diagnosed with more advanced breast cancer and of dying of the disease because implants can make early diagnosis more difficult.

- Buttock augmentation with fat grafting, implants, and lifts is becoming increasingly popular. The number of men having plastic surgery continues to rise. The top male-focused procedures are pectoral (chest) implants and male breast reduction.

Body Art Perils

About one in five American adults has a tattoo; 14 percent say they regret having gotten tattoos. As discussed in Chapter 13, "body art" such as piercings and tattoos presents unique dangers, including adverse reactions to tattoo inks and bacterial and viral infections. Piercings of the lip or tongue have particularly high rates of complications, including injuries to teeth and recession of the gums.[17]

Dermatologists report about 100,000 tattoo removals a year; removal is a painful and painstaking process that typically requires 6 to 10 treatments, with a few weeks of healing required between each.

Temporary tattoos that use henna and other dyes, meant to last several days to several weeks, also present risks. According to the FDA's adverse-effects watch list, adverse effects include redness, blistering, raised red weeping lesions, loss of pigmentation, increased sun sensitivity, and permanent scarring. Dyes using so-called black henna present greater risks because many contain a coal-tar derivative.

✓**check-in** Do you have a tattoo or piercing? If so, what precautions were taken to prevent complications? Did you experience any adverse effects?

Health Hoaxes and Medical Quackery

Every year millions of Americans search for medical miracles that never happen. In all, they spend more than $10 billion on medical **quackery**, unproven health products and services. Those who lose only money are the lucky ones. Many also waste precious time, during which their conditions worsen. Some suffer needless pain, along with crushed expectations.

Promoters of fraudulent health products often make claims and use particular practices to trick consumers into buying their products. Be suspicious when you see the following:

- Claims that a product is a "scientific breakthrough," "miraculous cure," "secret ingredient," or "ancient remedy."

- Claims that the product is an effective cure for a wide range of ailments. No product can cure multiple conditions or diseases.

- Claims that use impressive-sounding medical terms. They're often covering up a lack of good science.

- Personalized genetic cancer tests, which have not proven useful in guiding cancer treatment.

- Undocumented case histories of people who've had amazing results. It's too easy to make them up. And even if true, they can't be generalized to the entire population. Anecdotes are not a substitute for valid science.

- Claims that the product is available from only one source and payment is required in advance.

- Claims of a "money-back" guarantee.

- Websites that fail to list the company's name, physical address, phone number, or other contact information.

To keep from risking your life on false hope, follow these guidelines:

- Arm yourself with up-to-date information about your condition or disease from appropriate organizations, such as the American Cancer Society or the Arthritis Foundation, which keep track of unproven and ineffective methods of treatment.

- Ask for a written explanation of what a treatment does and why it works, evidence supporting all claims (not just testimonials), and published reports of the studies, including specifics on numbers treated, doses, and side effects. Be skeptical of self-styled "holistic practitioners," treatments supported by crusading groups, and endorsements from self-proclaimed experts or authorities.

- Don't part with your money quickly. Insurance companies won't reimburse for unproven therapies.

- Don't discontinue your current treatment without your physician's approval. Many physicians encourage supportive therapies—such as relaxation exercises, meditation, or visualization—as a supplement to standard treatments.

✓**check-in** Have you ever been taken in by a health "con"? Do you know anyone who has?

Nontraditional Health Care

Complementary and alternative medicine (CAM) refers to various medical and health-care systems, practices, and products that are not considered part of conventional medicine because there is not yet sufficient proof of their safety and effectiveness. CAM's varied healing philosophies, approaches, and therapies include preventive techniques designed to delay or prevent serious health problems before they start and **holistic** methods that focus on the whole person and the physical, mental, emotional, and spiritual aspects of well-being. Some approaches are based on the same physiological principles as traditional Western methods; others, such as acupuncture, are based on different healing systems.

Many medical schools now include training in CAM in their curricula. **Integrative medicine**, which combines selected elements of both conventional and alternative medicine in a comprehensive approach to diagnosis and treatment, has gained greater acceptance within the medical community, including insurance coverage for more CAM therapies.[18]

✓**check-in** Have you ever used any CAM treatments? If so, which ones?

About half of Americans have tried CAM; more seek help from CAM practitioners than from primary care doctors.[19] (See Table 11.4 for the most popular CAM approaches.)

Women use CAM more often than men. Young adults ages 18 to 44 are more likely to use CAM than older Americans. White adults use CAM more often than Hispanic or African American men and

quackery Medical fakery; unproven practices claiming to cure diseases or solve health problems.

complementary and alternative medicine (CAM) A term applied to all health-care approaches, practices, and treatments not widely taught in medical schools, not generally used in hospitals, and not usually reimbursed by medical insurance companies.

holistic An approach to medicine that takes into account body, mind, emotions, and spirit.

integrative medicine An approach that combines traditional medicine with alternative/complementary therapies.

Complementary and Alternative Medicine on Campus

Used CAM within the last year	67 percent
Would use CAM for a current health condition	27 percent
Would consider CAM if they were more knowledgeable	51.9 percent

Source: Nguyen J et al. Use and interest in complementary and alternative medicine among college students seeking healthcare at a university campus student health center. *Complementary Therapies in Clinical Practice*. 2016;24:103–108. doi:http://dx.doi.org/10.1016/j.ctcp.2016.06.001.

women. Adults with a college degree or higher use CAM more often than those with less education. The majority of undergraduates report that they have tried CAM. (See Snapshot: On Campus Now.)

The reasons that consumers try CAM vary. Some want relief from common problems such as insomnia and anxiety. Others with serious diseases such as cancer may seek a cure or relief from symptoms. Among patients with breast cancer, college-educated women are more likely to use CAM, most often in addition to conventional treatments.[20]

Types of CAM

The National Center for Complementary and Alternative Medicine (NCCAM) has classified CAM therapies into the following five categories (see Figure 11.2):

- Alternative medical systems.
- Mind–body medicine.

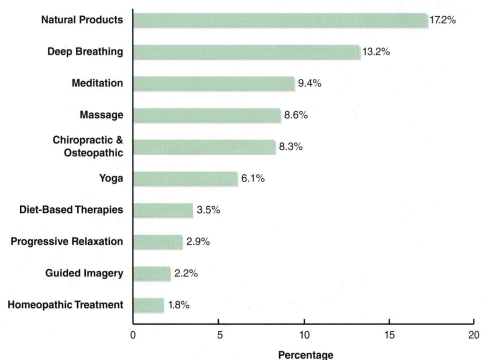

Andrey_Popov/Shutterstock.com

TABLE 11.4 The Most Popular CAM Approaches

Approach	Percentage
Natural Products	17.2%
Deep Breathing	13.2%
Meditation	9.4%
Massage	8.6%
Chiropractic & Osteopathic	8.3%
Yoga	6.1%
Diet-Based Therapies	3.5%
Progressive Relaxation	2.9%
Guided Imagery	2.2%
Homeopathic Treatment	1.8%

Percentage

Source: NIH MedlinePlus Magazine, www.nlm.nih.gov/medlineplus/magazine/.

The ancient Chinese practice of acupuncture produces healing through the insertion and manipulation of needles at specific points, or meridians, throughout the body.

acupuncture A Chinese medical practice of puncturing the body with needles inserted at specific points to relieve pain or cure disease.

Ayurveda A traditional Indian medical treatment involving meditation, exercise, herbal medications, and nutrition.

homeopathy A system of medical practice that treats a disease by administering dosages of substances that would in healthy persons produce symptoms similar to those of the disease.

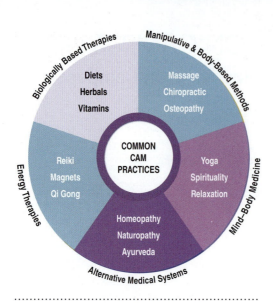

FIGURE 11.2 The Five Categories of CAM

Source: NCCAM, http://nccam.nih.gov.

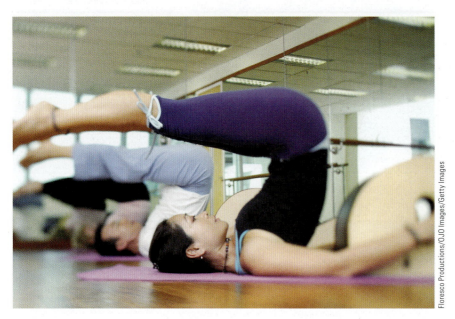

Floresco Productions/OJO Images/Getty Images

Yoga is one of the oldest and most popular mind–body approaches to health and wellness.

naturopathy An alternative system of treatment of disease that emphasizes the use of natural remedies such as sun, water, heat, and air. Therapies may include dietary changes, steam baths, and exercise.

- Biologically based therapies.
- Manipulative and body-based methods.
- Energy therapies.

Alternative Medical Systems

Systems of theory and practice other than traditional Western medicine are included in this group. They include acupuncture, Eastern medicine, t'ai chi, external and internal qi, Ayurvedic medicine, naturopathy, and unconventional Western systems such as homeopathy and orthomolecular medicine (see Health Now).

Acupuncture is an ancient Chinese form of medicine, based on the philosophy that a cycle of energy circulating through the body controls health. Pain and disease are the result of a disturbance in the energy flow, which can be corrected by inserting long, thin needles at specific points along longitudinal lines, or meridians, throughout the body. Each point controls a different corresponding part of the body. Once inserted, the needles are rotated gently back and forth or charged with a small electric current for a short time. Western scientists aren't sure exactly how acupuncture works but some believe that the needles alter the functioning of the nervous system.

Since the 1990s, studies have looked at acupuncture's effect on specific health conditions and how it affects the brain and nervous system, the neurological properties of meridians and acupuncture points, and methods for improving the quality of acupuncture research.

High-quality, randomized, controlled trials have shown that various forms of acupuncture, including so-called sham acupuncture during which no needles actually penetrate the skin, are equally effective for low-back pain—and more beneficial than standard care. However, even sham acupuncture can produce adverse effects, including infection and trauma.

Recent studies have found that acupuncture:

- Helps alleviate nausea in cancer patients undergoing chemotherapy.
- Relieves pain and improves function for some people with osteoarthritis of the knee.
- Helps in treating chronic lower-back pain.
- May or may not be of value for many other conditions, including irritable bowel syndrome and some neurologic disorders.

Considered alternative in this country, **Ayurveda** is a traditional form of medical treatment in India, where it has evolved over thousands of years. Its basic premise is that illness stems from incorrect mental attitudes, diet, and posture. Practitioners use a discipline of exercise, meditation, herbal medication, and proper nutrition to cope with such stress-induced conditions as hypertension, the desire to smoke, and obesity.

Homeopathy is based on three fundamental principles: like cures like; treatment must always be individualized; and less is more—the idea that increasing dilution (and lowering the dosage) can increase efficacy. By administering doses of animal, vegetable, or mineral substances to a large number of healthy people to see if they all develop the same symptoms, homeopaths determine which substances may be given, in small quantities, to alleviate the symptoms. Some of these substances are the same as those used in conventional medicine: nitroglycerin for certain heart conditions, for example, although the dose is minuscule.

Naturopathy emphasizes natural remedies, such as sun, water, heat, and air, as the best treatments for disease. Therapies might include dietary changes (such as more vegetables and no salt or stimulants), steam baths, and exercise. Some naturopathic physicians (who are not medical doctors) work closely with medical doctors in helping patients.

Mind–Body Medicine

Mind–body medicine uses techniques designed to enhance the mind's capacity to affect bodily function and symptoms. Some techniques that were considered alternative in the past have become mainstream (e.g., patient support groups and cognitive-behavioral therapy). Other mind–body approaches are still considered CAM, including meditation, prayer, yoga, t'ai chi, visual imagery, mental healing, and therapies that use creative outlets such as art, music, or dance. About 30 percent of Americans report using relaxation techniques and imagery, biofeedback, and hypnosis; 50 percent use prayer.

The physical and emotional risks of using mind–body interventions are minimal. However, some approaches, such as yoga can cause injury if not properly supervised and customized to individual patients. But there is also considerable evidence that mind–body interventions have positive effects on psychological functioning and quality of life and may be particularly helpful for patients coping with chronic illnesses.

Mind–body approaches definitely have won some acceptance in modern medical care. Techniques such as hypnosis have proved helpful in reducing discomfort and complications during and after various surgical procedures and in relieving hot flashes in breast cancer survivors. With biofeedback, people can learn to control usually involuntary functions, such as circulation to the hands and feet, tension in the jaws, and heartbeat rates. Biofeedback has been used to treat dozens of ailments, including asthma, epilepsy, pain, and Raynaud's disease (a condition in which the fingers become painful and white when exposed to cold) and has produced small reductions in blood pressure. Biofeedback has become accepted as a mainstream therapy, and many health insurers now cover biofeedback treatments.

Creative visualization helps patients heal, including some diagnosed as terminally ill with cancer. Other patients use visualization to create a clear idea of what they want to achieve, whether the goal is weight loss or relaxation.

Biologically Based Therapies

Biologically based CAM therapies use substances such as herbs, foods, and vitamins. They include **herbal medicine** (botanical medicine or phytotherapy), the use of individual herbs or combinations; special diet therapies, such as macrobiotics, Ornish, Atkins, and high fiber; orthomolecular medicine (use of nutritional and food supplements for preventive or therapeutic purposes); and use of other products (such as shark cartilage) and procedures applied in an unconventional manner.

In a recent review of herbal, complementary, and alternative approaches to prevent colds and flus, probiotics were found better than placebo in reducing the number and rate of episodes of acute upper respiratory tract infections. Other herbal remedies that require further study include maoto, licorice roots, Antiwei, North American ginseng, berries, Echinacea, plant-extracted carnosic acid, pomegranate, guava tea, and Bai Shao.[21]

Dietary supplements include vitamins, minerals, herbs, botanicals, amino acids, and enzymes and are sold as tablets, capsules, softgels, or gelcaps (see Table 11.5). The most popular is fish oil (discussed in Chapter 5). More people are using probiotics and melatonin, while fewer are taking Echinacea, glucosamine, chondroitin, garlic, ginseng, ginkgo biloba, and saw palmetto than in the past.

Unlike drugs, supplements are not intended to treat, diagnose, prevent, or cure diseases. Many contain active ingredients that have strong and potentially unsafe biological effects in the body.

TABLE 11.5 Evidence-Based Evaluations of Herbal Supplements

Herb	Evidence
Saw palmetto	Reduces an enlarged prostate, but the effect is small compared with that of prescription medication
Ginseng	Improves energy of cancer patients
Echinacea and vitamin C	Mixed results in warding off colds
Kava	May reduce anxiety but can cause liver damage
Ginkgo biloba	No improvement in memory or thinking in healthy older adults but has a small benefit for patients with dementia
Garlic	Not effective in lowering cholesterol
Black cohosh	No more effective than placebo for hot flashes; long-term effects unknown
Primrose oil	No benefit in treating eczema

HEALTH NOW!

Is a CAM Therapy Right for You?

You should never decide on any treatment—traditional or CAM—without fully evaluating it. Here are some key questions to ask:

- **Is it safe?** Be particularly wary of unregulated products.

- **Is it effective?** Check the website of the National Center for CAM: at http://nccam.nih.gov.

- **Will it interact with other medicines or conventional treatments?** Many widely used alternative remedies can interact with prescription medications in dangerous ways.

- **Is the practitioner qualified?** Find out if your state licenses practitioners who provide acupuncture, chiropractic services, naturopathy, herbal medicine, homeopathy, and other treatments.

- **What has been the experience of others?** Talk to people who have used CAM for a similar problem, both recently and in the past.

- **Can you talk openly and easily with the practitioner?** You should feel comfortable asking questions and confident in the answers you receive. And the practitioner's office should put you at ease.

- **What are the costs?** Many CAM services are not covered by health maintenance organizations (HMOs) or health insurers.

Answer these questions in your online journal.

herbal medicine An ancient form of medical treatment using substances derived from trees, flowers, ferns, seaweeds, and lichens to treat disease.

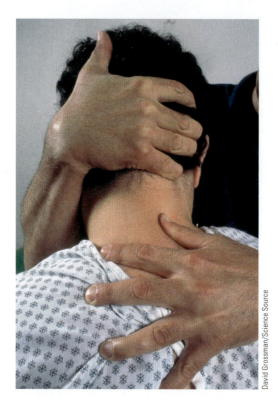

David Grossman/Science Source

Manipulative therapies are among the most widespread forms of complementary and alternative medicine.

demonstrated its efficacy for acute lower-back pain. The National Institutes of Health is funding research on other potential benefits, including headaches, asthma, middle-ear inflammation, menstrual cramps, and arthritis.

Chiropractors, who emphasize wellness and healing without drugs or surgery, may use X-rays and magnetic resonance imaging (MRI) as well as orthopedic, neurologic, and manual examinations in making diagnoses. However, chiropractic treatment consists solely of the manipulation of misaligned discs that may be putting pressure on nerve tissue and affecting other parts of the body. Many health maintenance organizations (HMOs) offer chiropractic services, which are the most widely used alternative treatment among managed-care patients.

Massage Therapy. This type of therapy includes osteopathic manipulation, Swedish massage, Alexander technique, reflexology, Pilates, acupressure, and rolfing. The limited research available suggests that massage therapy may relieve low-back and neck pain, relax and boost the spirits of cancer patients, help reduce depression, and temporarily reduce pain, fatigue, and other symptoms associated with fibromyalgia.[22]

Unconventional Physical Therapies. This category includes colonics, hydrotherapy, and light and color therapies.

Energy Therapies Various approaches focus on energy fields believed to exist in and around the body. Some use external energy sources, such as electromagnetic fields. Magnets are marketed to relieve pain, but there is little scientific evidence of their efficacy. Others, such as therapeutic touch, use a therapist's healing energy to repair imbalances in an individual's biofield.

This makes them particularly dangerous when used with medications (whether prescription or over-the-counter) or taken in high doses.

Liver injury related to herbal and dietary supplements has more than doubled in the past 10 years. Echinacea may cause liver damage if taken in combination with anabolic steroids. Several widely used herbs, including ginger, garlic, and ginkgo biloba, are dangerous if taken prior to surgery.

Canadian health authorities have pulled products containing a chemical called BMPEA off store shelves and warned that this amphetamine-like compound can increase blood pressure, heart rate, and body temperature; lead to serious cardiovascular complications (including stroke) at high doses; suppress sleep and appetite; and be addictive. Consumer groups and state attorneys have accused major retailers of selling contaminated herbal supplements and called on Congress to provide the FDA with more power to regulate supplements.

Manipulative and Body-Based Methods

CAM therapies based on manipulation and/or movement of the body are divided into three subcategories.

Chiropractic Medicine. This treatment method is based on the theory that many human diseases are caused by misalignment of the spine (subluxation). Chiropractors are licensed in all 50 states, but some consider **chiropractic** a mainstream therapy while others view it as a form of CAM. Significant research in the past 10 years has

The Health-Care System

As a college student, you may turn to the student health service if one is available on campus. There, a nurse, nurse practitioner, physician's assistant, or medical doctor may evaluate your symptoms and provide basic care. However, you may rely on a primary care physician in your hometown to perform regular checkups or manage a chronic condition such as asthma. If you're injured in an accident, you probably will be treated at the nearest emergency room. If you become seriously ill and require highly specialized care, you may have to go to a university-affiliated medical center to receive state-of-the-art treatment.

chiropractic A method of treating disease, primarily through manipulating the bones and joints to restore normal nerve function.

Under the ACA, students can usually continue their health-care coverage under their parents' policy until age 26. However, if your parent belongs to an HMO with a local network of providers, you may not be covered for anything outside the plan's service area except for emergency care. A more open plan, like a preferred provider organization, may allow students to see doctors near school, but the costs may be high. Most colleges offer some type of health insurance plan, with the student health center acting as the primary care provider. Many schools require participation if the student is not covered under any other plan. Check the plan carefully to see what is and is not covered.

✓**check-in** Does your school offer a health-care plan? If so, have you chosen to enroll in it?

Health-Care Practitioners

Fewer than 10 percent of health-care practitioners are physicians; other types of health professionals are assuming more important roles in delivering primary, or basic, health services. As a consumer, you should be aware of the range and special skills of the most common types of health-care providers.

Physicians A medical doctor (MD) trained in American medical schools usually takes at least 3 years of premedical college courses (with an emphasis on biology, chemistry, and physics) and then completes 4 years (but sometimes 3 or 5) of medical school. The first 2 years of medical school are devoted to the study of human anatomy, embryology, pharmacology, and similar basic subjects. During the last 2 years, students work directly with physicians in hospitals. Medical students who pass a series of national board examinations then enter a 1-year internship in a hospital, followed by another 2 to 5 years of residency (depending on their specialty), which leads to certification in a particular field, or specialty.

The Health-Care Team More than 60 types of health practitioners work together in providing medical services. Physician assistants (PAs), nationally certified and state-licensed medical professionals, provide a broad range of health-care services under the direction of medical doctors. They may conduct physical exams, diagnose and treat illnesses, order and interpret tests, prescribe medications, advise on preventive health care, and assist in surgery.[23]

Registered nurses (RNs), who may have a bachelor's or associate degree from an accredited school of nursing, may specialize in certain areas such as intensive care or nurse-midwifery. Nurse practitioners, RNs with advanced training and experience, may run community clinics or provide screening and preventive care at group medical practices.

PAs serve on a health-care team under the supervision of physicians and surgeons. Formally educated to examine patients, diagnose injuries and illnesses, and provide treatment, they typically need a master's degree from an accredited educational program and a state license.

Licensed practical nurses (LPNs), also called licensed vocational nurses, are graduates of state-approved schools of practical nursing, who work under the supervision of RNs or physicians. Certified nursing assistants (CNAs), nursing aides, and orderlies assist in providing services directly related to the comfort and well-being of hospitalized patients.

Allied health professionals may specialize in a variety of fields. Clinical psychologists have graduate degrees and provide a wide range of mental health services but don't prescribe medications—as do psychiatrists. Optometrists, trained in special schools of optometry, diagnose visual abnormalities and prescribe lenses or visual aids; however, they don't prescribe drugs, diagnose or treat eye diseases, or perform surgery—functions performed by ophthalmologists. Podiatrists are specially trained, licensed health-care professionals who specialize in problems of the feet.

Dentists Most dental students earn a bachelor's degree and then complete 2 more years of training in the basic sciences and 2 years of clinical work before graduating with a degree of Doctor of Dental Surgery (DDS) or Doctor of Medical Dentistry (DMD) and taking licensing exams. Dentists may work in general practice or choose a specialty, such as orthodontics (straightening teeth).

Chiropractors Chiropractors hold the degree of Doctor of Chiropractic (DC), which signifies that they have had 2 years of college-level training, plus 4 years in a health-care school specializing in chiropractic, described earlier in this chapter.

Health-Care Facilities

As a prospective patient, you can choose from various options: a physician's office, a clinic, an emergency room, or a hospital. Most **primary care**—also referred to as ambulatory or outpatient care—is provided by a physician in an office, an emergency room, or a clinic. Secondary care usually is provided by specialists or subspecialists in either an outpatient or inpatient (hospital) setting. Tertiary care, available at university-affiliated hospitals and regional referral centers, includes

primary care Ambulatory or outpatient care provided by a physician in an office, an emergency room, or a clinic.

special procedures such as kidney dialysis, open-heart surgery, and organ transplants.

College Health Centers The American College Health Association estimates that 1,500 institutions of higher learning provide direct health services. Student health centers, initially developed by departments of physical education and hygiene, range in size from small dispensaries staffed by nurses to large-scale, multispecialty clinics that provide both inpatient and outpatient care and are fully accredited by the Joint Commission. Some serve only students; others provide services for faculty, staff, and family members.

On some campuses, health educators work with student health centers to provide counseling on such topics as nutrition; tobacco, drug, and alcohol abuse; exercise and fitness; sexuality; and contraception. Some college health centers provide psychological counseling, as well as dental, pharmacy, and optometric services and sports-medicine services for student athletes. Services are paid for by various combinations of prepaid health fees, general university funds, fee-for-service charges, and health-insurance reimbursements.

Outpatient Treatment Centers Increasingly, procedures that once required hospitalization, such as simple surgery, are being performed at outpatient centers, which may be freestanding or affiliated with a medical center. Patients have any necessary tests performed beforehand, undergo surgery or receive treatment, and return home after a few hours to recuperate. Outpatient centers can handle many common surgical procedures, including cataract removal, tonsillectomy, breast biopsy, dilation and curettage (D and C), vasectomy, and cosmetic procedures such as liposuction.

Freestanding emergency or urgent-care centers (those that are not part of a hospital) claim that they deliver high-quality medical treatment with maximum convenience in minimal time. Rather than go to a crowded hospital emergency room when they slice a finger in the kitchen, patients can go to a freestanding emergency center and receive prompt attention.

Hospitals and Medical Centers Different types of hospitals offer different types of care:

- The most common type of hospital is the private, or community, hospital, which may be run on a profit or a nonprofit basis, generally contains 50 to 400 beds, and provides more personalized care than public hospitals do. The quality of care individual patients receive depends mostly on the physicians themselves.

- Public hospitals include city, county, public health service, military, and Veterans Administration hospitals. The quality of patient care depends on the overall quality of the institution.

- Of the more than 6,500 hospitals nationwide, about 300 are major academic medical centers or teaching hospitals. Affiliated with medical schools, they generally provide the most up-to-date and experienced care because staff physicians must stay current in order to teach their students. These centers, with the best equipment, researchers, and resources, offer high-technology care—at a price. At major teaching hospitals with large graduate training programs for physicians and other health providers, the costs are as much as 45 percent higher than those at nonteaching hospitals.

The Joint Commission reviews all hospitals every 3 years. Eighty percent of hospitals qualify for Joint Commission accreditation, an important indicator of quality assurance.

Emergency Services Hospital emergency rooms should be used only in a true emergency. Most are overwhelmed, understaffed, and underfinanced—particularly in big cities. Patients usually see a different physician each time, who deals with a patient's main complaints but doesn't have time for a full examination. Arranging extensive tests and procedures in an emergency room is difficult, and patients who don't have truly urgent problems may have to wait a long time. Emergency-room fees are higher than those for standard office visits and are not always covered by medical insurance.

Inpatient Care Inpatient hospital care remains the most expensive form of health care. Health-insurance companies and health-care plans (discussion to follow) often demand a second opinion or make their own evaluation before approving coverage of an elective, or nonemergency, hospital admission.

Because hospital stays are shorter today than in the past, patients often leave "quicker and sicker"—after a shorter stay and not as far along in their recovery. Nevertheless, the benefits of shorter hospital stays, including reduced risk of infection (discussed in Chapter 16) and more rapid resumption of normal life activities, may outweigh the slightly increased risks associated with early discharge.

Home Health Care With hospitals discharging patients sooner, **home health care**—the provision of equipment and services to patients in the home to restore or maintain comfort, function, and health—has become a major industry. Advances in technology have made it possible for treatments once administered only in hospitals—such as kidney dialysis, chemotherapy, and traction—to be performed at home at 10 to 40 percent of the cost of providing these treatments in a hospital.

home health care provision of equipment and services to patients in their homes.

- What do college students need to know about health insurance?

- Are you a savvy health-care consumer?

- What steps can you take to make sure you get quality health care?

- What do you need to know about complementary and alternative medicine?

Reflection

This chapter provides instruction on evaluating and obtaining quality health care. Identify at least two specific steps that you can take to become a savvy health-care consumer. When can you put them into action?

TAKING CHARGE OF YOUR HEALTH

Taking Charge of Your Health

You can do more to safeguard and enhance your well-being than any health-care provider. Here are some recommendations to keep in mind. Check the ones you have used or plan to use in the future.

____ **Trust your instincts.** You know your body better than anyone else. If something is bothering you, it deserves medical attention. Don't let your health-care provider—or your health plan administrator—dismiss it without a thorough evaluation.

____ **Do your homework.** Go to the library or online and find authoritative articles that describe what you're experiencing. The more you know about possible causes of your symptoms, the more likely you are to be taken seriously.

____ **Find a good primary care physician who listens carefully and responds to your concerns.** Look for a family doctor or general internist who takes a careful history, performs a thorough exam, and listens and responds to your concerns.

____ **See your doctor regularly.** If you're in your 20s or 30s, you may not need an annual exam, but it's important to get checkups at least every 2 or 3 years so you and your doctor can get to know each other and develop a trusting, mutually respectful relationship.

____ **Get a second opinion.** If you are uncertain of whether to undergo treatment or which therapy is best, see another physician and listen carefully for any doubts or hesitation about what you're considering.

____ **Seek support.** Patient support and advocacy groups can offer emotional support, information on many common problems, and referral to knowledgeable physicians.

____ **If your doctor cannot or will not respond to your concerns, get another one.** Regardless of your health coverage, you have the right to replace a physician who is not meeting your health-care needs.

____ **Speak up.** If you don't understand, ask. If you feel that you're not being taken seriously or being treated with respect, say so. Sometimes the only difference between being a patient or becoming a victim is making sure your needs and rights are not forgotten or overlooked.

____ **Bring your own advocate.** If you become intimidated or anxious talking to physicians, ask a friend to accompany you, to ask questions on your behalf, and to take notes.

SELF-SURVEY

Are You a Savvy Health-Care Consumer?

1. You want a second opinion, but your doctor dismisses your request for other physicians' names as unnecessary. What do you do?
   a. Assume that he or she is right and you would merely be wasting time.
   b. Suspect that your physician has something to hide and immediately switch doctors.
   c. Contact your health plan and request a second opinion.

2. As soon as you enter your doctor's office, you get tongue-tied. When you try to find the words to describe what's wrong, your physician keeps interrupting. When giving advice, your doctor uses such technical language that you can't understand what it means. What do you do?
   a. Prepare better for your next appointment.
   b. Pretend that you understand what your doctor is talking about.
   c. Decide you'd be better off with someone who specializes in complementary/alternative therapies and seems less intimidating.

3. You feel like you're running on empty, tired all the time, worn to the bone. A friend suggests some herbal supplements that promise to boost energy and restore vitality. What do you do?
   a. Immediately start taking them.
   b. Say that you think herbs are for cooking.
   c. Find out as much as you can about the herbal compounds and ask your doctor if they're safe and effective.

4. Your hometown physician's office won't give you a copy of your medical records to take with you to college. What do you do?
   a. Hope you won't need them and head off without your records.
   b. Threaten to sue.
   c. Politely ask the office administrator to tell you the particular law or statute that bars you from your records.

5. Your doctor has been treating you for an infection for 3 weeks, and you don't seem to be getting any better. What do you do?
   a. Talk to your doctor, by phone or in person, and say, "This doesn't seem to be working. Is there anything else we can try?"
   b. Stop taking the antibiotic.
   c. Try an herbal remedy that your roommate recommends.

6. Your doctor suggests a cutting-edge treatment for your condition, but your health plan or HMO refuses to pay for it. What do you do?
   a. Try to get a loan to cover the costs.
   b. Settle for whatever treatment options are covered.
   c. Challenge your health plan.

7. You call for an appointment with your doctor and are told nothing is available for 4 months. What do you do?
   a. Take whatever time you can get whenever you can get it.
   b. Explain your condition to the nurse or receptionist, detailing any symptoms and pain you're experiencing.

   c. Give up and decide you don't need to see a doctor at all.

8. Even though you've been doing situps faithfully, your waist still looks flabby. When you see an ad for waist-whittling liposuction, what do you do?
   a. Call for an appointment.
   b. Talk to a health-care professional about a total fitness program that may help you lose excess pounds.
   c. Carefully research the risks and costs of the procedure.

9. You have a condition that you do not want anyone to know about, including your health insurer and any potential employer. What do you do?
   a. Use a false name.
   b. Give your physician a written request for confidentiality about this condition.
   c. Seek help outside the health-care system.

10. Your doctor suggests a biopsy of a funny-looking mole that's sprouted on your nose. Rather than using a laboratory that specializes in skin analysis, your HMO requires that all samples be sent to a general lab, where results may not be as precise. What do you do?
    a. Ask your doctor to request that a specialty pathologist at the general lab perform the analysis.
    b. Hope that in your case, the general lab will do a good-enough job.
    c. Threaten to change HMOs.

Answers: 1. c; 2. a; 3. c; 4. c; 5. a; 6. c; 7. b; 8. b or c; 9. b; 10. a. Count up the answers you got right. **Scoring:** *3 or less: not yet health savvy; 4 to 6: savvy about some elements of health care; 7 to 10: congratulations you are a savvy health care consumer! To increase your consumer knowledge reread the section on page 362 on becoming a savvy health-care consumer.*

REVIEW QUESTIONS

(LO 11.1) 1. Which of the following is a change implemented under the Affordable Care Act?
   a. Fewer individuals will receive health care under Medicaid.
   b. Preventive services are no longer free.
   c. Insurance companies cannot deny coverage on the basis of preexisting medical conditions.
   d. Insurance companies can terminate coverage if a policyholder becomes ill.

(LO 11.1) 2. Which of the following statements is true of the Affordable Care Act?
   a. You cannot remain on your parent's health insurance plan if you are married.
   b. You can be covered under a parent's health insurance plan until you are 28.

   c. You can buy a catastrophic health plan if you are over 30.
   d. You may have to pay a deductible.

(LO 11.2) 3. In a health insurance plan, what is a *deductible*?
   a. The fee that you pay on each doctor visit.
   b. The amount of money you pay each month for plan membership.
   c. The amount of money you pay before your insurance begins paying.
   d. What you pay for benefits that your health insurance does not cover.

(LO 11.3) 4. Which of the following statements is true of periodontitis?
   a. It can result from excessive plaque on the teeth.

b. Periodontitis can increase the risk of cardiovascular disease.

c. If left untreated, it can turn into gingivitis.

d. It is an early stage of gum disease.

(LO 11.3) 5. The FDA monitors personal health apps that _____.

e. monitor vital signs

a. provide reminders about when to take medication

b. give instructions for the correct use of asthma inhalers

c. track food intake and give tips for making healthier food choices

(LO 11.4) 6. Before an appointment with a health-care professional, you should _____.

a. dress to look good

b. expect the clinic to locate a copy of your medical history

c. make a list of all medications you take, including vitamins and herbal supplements

d. keep track of everything you have eaten and drunk for the last week

(LO 11.5) 7. As a health-care consumer, you have the right to _____.

a. know about your doctor's record as a practitioner

b. obtain your medical records at no cost

c. information on how providers use your personal medical information

d. know if your physician is paying a malpractice insurance premium

(LO 11.5) 8. To avoid medical malpractice suits, doctors must _____.

a. not make any errors

b. prescribe treatments with good results

c. help their patients live as long as possible

d. use the same standard of care that other physicians would

(LO 11.6) 9. Which of the following statements is true of vision surgery?

a. It can be done by optometrists as well as surgeons.

b. It does not use cutting instruments other than lasers.

c. It may result in poor night vision.

d. It can make an aging eye lens flexible again.

(LO 11.6) 10. Getting breast implants can lead to _____.

a. connective tissue disorders

b. rupture and scarring

c. autoimmune diseases

d. cancer

(LO 11.7) 11. Which of the following is one of the signs that a health product may be fraudulent?

a. Claims that a product is a "scientific break-through," "miraculous cure," "secret ingredient," or "ancient remedy."

b. No guarantee is offered.

c. Lack of consumer testimonials.

d. A cited list of medical publications.

(LO 11.7) 12. How can you protect yourself against medical hoaxes?

a. Ask for a money-back guarantee.

b. Choose products that cure a wide range of ailments.

c. Choose products that are sold exclusively at one source.

d. Ask for published reports of the studies.

(LO 11.8) 13. Besides joint and back pain, acupuncture can also alleviate _____.

a. heart conditions

b. irritable bowel syndrome

c. neurological disorders

d. nausea for those undergoing chemotherapy

(LO 11.8) 14. Which of the following forms of complementary and alternative medicine (CAM) is a "mind–body medicine" approach?

a. Naturopathy

b. Homeopathy

c. Biofeedback

d. Energy therapy

(LO 11.8) 15. Biologically based therapies may include _____.

a. vitamins and herbs

b. massage therapy

c. hypnosis

d. acupuncture

(LO 11.9) 16. Which of the following statements is true of health-care practitioners?

a. One-third of health-care practitioners are medical doctors.

b. Nurse practitioners can run community clinics.

c. Registered nurses can prescribe medication.

d. Podiatrists specialize in problems of the stomach.

(LO 11.9) 17. In the current health-care system, which of the following is true?

a. Primary care is usually provided by specialists in a hospital.

b. Nurses can perform simple surgical procedures if they are board-certified.

c. Most hospitals in the United States are teaching hospitals affiliated with medical schools.

d. Hospital stays are generally shorter today than they were 10 years ago.

Answers to these questions can be found on page 531.

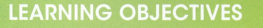
Katy Pack/Shutterstock.com

LEARNING OBJECTIVES

After reading this chapter, you should be able to:

12.1 Explain how substance abuse and other self-destructive behaviors can affect health.

12.2 Discuss the ill effects of problem gambling and gambling disorder.

12.3 Outline the key indicators and effects of substance abuse on college campuses.

12.4 Summarize the effects that drugs have on the brain, body, and behavior.

12.5 Discuss the origins and impact of the opioid epidemic.

12.6 Identify the benefits and the adverse effects of caffeine.

12.7 Describe the harmful effects of inappropriate use of over-the-counter drugs and prescription drugs.

12.8 Classify the characteristics and harmful effects of common drugs of abuse.

12.9 Explain how substance dependence and abuse can be treated.

WHAT DO YOU THINK?

- Is caffeine good or bad for you?
- What is the "opioid epidemic"?
- What are the dangers of prescription drug abuse?
- Does marijuana, even when legal, pose risks to well-being?

12

Addictive Behaviors and Drugs

Tyler had too many papers to write and too little time to finish them. One of his fraternity brothers suggested that he try a prescription stimulant a friend took for an attention-deficit disorder. The jolt felt like just what Tyler needed. During midterms he bought another prescription stimulant from a classmate. As finals approached, Tyler started hoarding stimulants from several people. He popped the final ones to rev up for the big end-of-school-year parties. Without realizing the consequences of what he was doing, Tyler put himself at risk for drug-related problems—physical, psychological, and legal.

Although prescription drug abuse remains widespread on campuses, the drug scene across the United States may be changing. The use of many illicit drugs—including MDMA (Ecstasy), inhalants, synthetic marijuana, the hallucinogen salvia, and the amphetamine-like stimulants known as bath salts—has declined among adolescents and young adults.[1] This is also true for college students—except for marijuana use, which has risen.[2] Nonetheless, according to the American College Health Association (ACHA) National College Health Assessment, 6 in 10 undergraduates have never tried marijuana.[3] (see Snapshot: On Campus Now in this chapter).

No one ever sets out to become an addict. Drug users believe they are smart enough, strong enough, and lucky enough not to get caught or hooked. However, addictions produce changes in an individual's body, brain, and behavior. In time, the grip of addiction can outweigh everything else a person values and holds dear.

This chapter provides information about and insights into how addictions start, why students use and abuse drugs, the nature and effect of drugs, and the most commonly used, misused, and abused drugs. It also offers practical strategies for preventing, recognizing the signs of, and seeking help for addictions. <

Student Marijuana Use

Percent (%)	Actual Use			Perceived Use		
	Male	Female	Total	Male	Female	Total
Never used	58.6	58.8	58.5	9.9	6.7	7.8
Used, but not in the past 30 days	19.6	21.1	20.6	6.9	4.4	5.1
Used 1–9 days	12.5	13.4	13.2	45.2	39.9	41.4
Used 10–29 days	5.5	4.1	4.5	26.5	32.4	30.6
Used all 30 days	3.8	2.7	3.1	11.5	16.6	15.1
Any use within the last 30 days	21.8	20.2	20.9	83.2	88.9	87.1

Did you know that about 6 in 10 undergraduates have never used marijuana? What has been your experience? If you are among the majority, what are the factors that have enabled you to say no to pot? If you have used drugs, what were your reasons? What role do drugs now play in your life? What has been their impact? Write in your online journal your feelings about how drugs might affect your health and your life.

Source: American College Health Association. American College Health Association-National College Health Assessment II: Reference Group Executive Summary Spring 2018. Silver Spring, MD: American College Health Association, 2018.

Understanding Addiction

Once people thought of **addiction**—a compulsive need for and reliance on a habit-forming substance or behavior—as a moral issue. We now understand that addiction is a chronic illness that affects brain, body, and spirit. According to the American Society of Addiction Medicine, its characteristics are[4]:

- Inability to abstain from use of a substance.

- Craving or "hunger" for a substance or rewarding experience.

- Diminished recognition of significant problems with one's behavior and interpersonal relationships.

- Dysfunctional or unhealthy emotional response.

Without treatment, addiction becomes progressively more severe and can lead to disability, illness, or premature death. Like other chronic diseases, addiction often involves cycles of relapse frequently triggered by environmental cues and emotional stressors. These triggers also heighten activity and, as a recent landmark report from the Office of the Surgeon General documented, can and should be treated with evidence-based, compassionate care.[5]

addiction A behavioral pattern characterized by compulsion, loss of control, and continued repetition of a behavior or an activity in spite of adverse consequences.

Addiction and the Dimensions of Health

Young adults have the highest rates of illicit drug use. Many do not realize that substance abuse and other self-destructive behaviors, such as gambling or compulsive eating, can affect every dimension of health. Some of the harmful effects are as follows:

- **Physical health.** Abuse of alcohol, tobacco, and drugs takes a toll on every organ system in the body, increasing the likelihood of disease, disability, and premature death. People who start using hard drugs, such as cocaine and amphetamines, as young adults and continue to use them in middle age have a fivefold increased risk of early death.

- **Psychological health.** Sometimes people begin abusing substances or engaging in addictive behavior as a way of "self-medicating" symptoms of anxiety or depression. However, alcohol and drugs provide only temporary relief. As abuse continues, shame and guilt increase, and coping with daily stressors becomes more difficult. Depression and anxiety are as likely to be consequences as causes of substance abuse.

- **Spiritual health.** Addictive behavior blocks the pursuit of meaning and inner fulfillment. As they rely more on a chemical or behavioral escape, individuals lose their sense of self and of connection with other people and with a spiritual higher power.

- **Social health.** Addictive behavior strains and, in time, severs ties to family, friends, colleagues, and classmates. The primary relationship in the life of alcoholics or addicts is with a behavior or a drug. As addicts withdraw from others, they become increasingly isolated.

- **Intellectual health.** The brain is one of the targets of alcohol and drugs. Under their influence, logic and reasoning break down. Impulses become more difficult to control. Judgment falters. Certain substances, such as Ecstasy, can lead to permanent changes in brain chemistry.

- **Environmental health.** The use of some substances, such as tobacco, directly harms the environment. Abusers of alcohol and drugs also pose indirect threats to others because their behavior can lead to injury and damage.

✓**check-in** Have alcohol or drugs affected any dimension of your health?

Preventing Addictions

Most college students do not engage in addictive behaviors. One fundamental reason is that they have better things to do. "Substance-free reinforcement"—in simpler terms, a positive addiction to anything from rock-climbing to snowboarding to Zumba—can produce very real "highs," often for very little money. Without passions to pursue, young adults are more likely to use and abuse multiple substances, including marijuana, alcohol, and emerging tobacco products (discussed in Chapter 13).[6]

Such "polysubstance abuse" greatly increases their risk of physical, social, legal, and academic problems and pushes them deeper into drug involvement.[7]

The more that students use mind-altering substances, the less they engage in drug-free activities. This may be because substance abuse diminishes the brain's chemical response to other forms of pleasure. As a result, the deliciousness of chocolate or the excitement of bungee-jumping fails to trigger the normal surge in dopamine, the brain's "feel-good" chemical. Instead, chronic substance abusers develop anhedonia, an inability to experience pleasure.

Fortunately, this condition is reversible. When college students increase physical or creative activities, they often simultaneously reduce their drug and alcohol use, even if not directed to do so.[8] So the next time you're feeling bored, restless, anxious, frustrated, or overwhelmed, don't think a drug might offer a quick fix. Go for the longer-lasting, more fulfilling high of a positive addiction (see Health on a Budget).

Gambling and Behavioral Addictions

Addictions are not limited to brain-altering substances. Researchers have described a similar process of dependence, tolerance, and withdrawal with a variety of behaviors, including

$ HEALTH ON A BUDGET
Develop a Positive Addiction

There is a crucial difference between a positive addiction and drug dependency: One is real, the other is chemical. With one, you're in control; with the other, drugs are. Here are some examples:

- **If you feel a need for physical relaxation,** or if you want more energy or distraction from physical discomforts, you can turn to athletics, exercise (including walking and hiking), dance, or outdoor hobbies.

- **If you want to stimulate your senses,** enhance sexual stimulation, or magnify the sensations of sight, sound, and touch, train yourself to be more sensitive to nature and beauty. Take time to appreciate the sensations you experience when you're walking in the woods or embracing a person

you love. Through activities like sailing or sky-diving, you can literally fill up your senses without relying on chemicals.

- **If you want to escape mental boredom,** gain new understanding of the world around you, study better, experiment with your levels of awareness, or indulge your intellectual curiosity, you can challenge your mind through reading, classes, creative games, discussion groups, memory training, or travel.

- **If you're looking for kicks,** adventure, danger, and excitement, sign up for a wilderness survival course. Take up an adventurous sport, like hang-gliding or rock-climbing. Set a challenging professional or personal goal and direct your energies to meeting it.

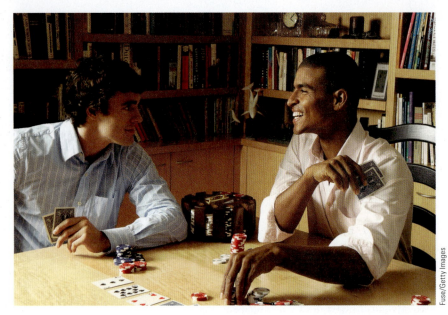

College students who gamble say they do so for fun or excitement, to socialize, to win money, or "just to have something to do."

video gaming,[9] indoor tanning,[10] night eating,[11] texting and smartphone use,[12] and Internet addiction.[13] **Gambling disorder** is the only "behavioral" addiction officially recognized as a psychiatric diagnosis.[14] However, Internet use, video game playing, shopping, eating, and other behaviors also bear a resemblance to alcohol and drug dependence. Researchers are investigating their causes, characteristics, and impact on psychological and physical well-being.[15]

Gambling is an act of risking a sum of money on the outcome of a game or an event that is determined by chance. Although most people who gamble limit the time and money they spend, some cross the line and lose control of their gambling "habit."

Problem Gambling

The term *problem gambling* refers to all gambling-related problems, including mild or occasional ones. Here are some relevant key points:

- Problem gambling has become more common than alcohol dependence among American adults. Two factors associated with higher risk are male gender and lack of family engagement.

- Levels of gambling, frequent gambling, and problem gambling increase during the teen years (even though underage gambling is illegal in most states), then peak in the 20s and 30s, and decline after age 70.[16]

- Men are more than twice as likely as women to be frequent gamblers and reach their highest gambling rates in their late teens.

gambling disorder Persistent and recurrent problematic gambling that leads to significant impairment or distress.

- Whites are much more likely to report gambling in the past year than blacks or Asians, but both African Americans and Native Americans report higher levels of frequent gambling.

Gamblers typically progress through various stages:

- **Winning.** In the winning phase, they feel empowered by their winnings and success.

- **Losing.** Next comes the losing phase, during which gamblers try to win back their losses.

- **Desperation.** During the desperation phase, a gambler may resort to illegal activity, including stealing, to continue gambling.

- **Giving up.** In the giving-up phase, gamblers may desperately try to stay afloat in a game even though they realize they can't win.

Gambling Disorder

The American Psychiatric Association's *Diagnostic and Statistical Manual of Mental Disorders, Fifth Edition (DSM-5)*, classifies persistent and recurrent problematic gambling that leads to significant impairment or distress as a gambling disorder, similar to other addictive disorders in its effects on brain and behavior. A diagnosis is made if individuals exhibit four or more of the following symptoms in a 12-month period:

- Need to gamble with increasing amounts of money to achieve excitement.

- Becoming restless or irritable if they cut down or stop gambling.

- Repeated unsuccessful attempts to control, reduce, or stop gambling.

- Preoccupation with gambling.

- Gambling when feeling guilty, anxious, or distressed.

- After losing money, trying to recoup by "chasing" losses.

- Lying to conceal the extent of gambling.

- Putting a significant relationship, job, or opportunity in jeopardy because of gambling.

- Reliance on others for money to relieve desperate financial situations caused by gambling.[17]

A gambling disorder can begin during adolescence or young adulthood but generally develops over the course of years. Many college students "grow out" of the disorder over time, although it remains a lifelong problem for some. Gambling disorders are more common among young men than among young women. Younger individuals prefer forms of gambling such as sports betting and Internet poker, whereas older adults are more likely to play slot machines or games of chance like bingo.

Psychological interventions can improve outcomes and reduce symptom severity for individuals with a gambling disorder. These include behavioral and cognitive treatment with a professional therapist as well as self-directed workbooks and computer-facilitated programs. No specific approach has consistently proven more effective than other alternatives, but cognitive-behavioral therapy has the most empirical support for the treatment of gambling disorder.[18]

✓**check-in** Do you buy lottery or scratch tickets? Bet on sporting events? Play poker online? Do you consider any or all of these forms of gambling?

Gambling on Campus

Gambling has become a more serious and widespread problem on college campuses. About half of students who gamble at least once a month experience significant problems related to their gambling, including poor academic performance, heavy alcohol consumption, illicit drug use, unprotected sex, and other risky behaviors. An estimated 3 to 6 percent of college students engage in "pathological gambling," which is characterized by "persistent and recurrent maladaptive gambling behavior."

Researchers have identified key indicators associated with "pathological" gambling:

- Gambling more than once a month.
- Gambling more than 2 hours at a time.
- Wagering more than 10 percent of monthly income.
- A combination of parental gambling problems, gambling frequency, and psychological distress.

College students who gamble say they do so for fun or excitement, to socialize, to win money, or to "just have something to do"—reasons similar to those of other adults who gamble. Simply having access to casino machines, ongoing card games, or Internet gambling sites increases the likelihood that students will gamble.

Researchers view problem or pathological gambling as an addiction that runs in families. Individuals predisposed to gambling because of their family history are more likely to develop a problem if they are regularly exposed to gambling. Alcoholism and drug abuse often occur along with gambling, leading to chaotic lives and greater health risks.[19]

Risk Factors for Problem Gambling

Among young people (ages 16 to 25), the following behaviors indicate increased risk of problem gambling:

- Being male.
- Gambling at an early age (as young as age 8).
- Having a big win early in one's gambling career.
- Consistently chasing losses (betting more to recover money already lost).
- Gambling alone.
- Feeling depressed before gambling.
- Feeling excited and aroused during gambling.
- Behaving irrationally during gambling.
- Having poor grades at school.
- Engaging in other addictive behaviors (smoking, drinking alcohol, and using illegal drugs).
- Lower socioeconomic class.
- Parent with a gambling or other addiction problem.
- A history of delinquency or stealing money to fund gambling.
- Skipping class to go gambling.

Drug Use on Campus

Marijuana remains the most widely used illicit drug on campuses, but the nonmedical use of prescription drugs now outranks other forms of substance abuse. About 11 percent of college students report that they misused prescription drugs in the last year.[20] Here are more statistics on campus drug use from the Monitoring the Future study[21]:

- More than a third of college students— 38 percent—report marijuana use in the previous year.
- Fifty-five percent of students report use of an illicit drug during their lifetimes. Far fewer— 26 percent—report use of drugs other than marijuana.
- Nonmedical use of prescription opioid, or narcotic, drugs, such as Oxycontin, Vicodin, Percocet, and fentanyl, in the previous year has fallen from nearly 9 percent a decade ago to around 3 percent.

- Use of heroin, another opioid, is low—about 1 percent.

- Thirteen percent of college students report that they have used amphetamines, 7 percent hallucinogens, 6.5 percent cocaine, and 5 percent LSD or Ecstasy.

- Use of synthetic marijuana products, such as salvia, "K-2," and "Spice," has fallen significantly.

- There has been little change in nonprescribed use of tranquilizers and sedatives in recent years.

Substance abuse remains a serious health risk for the minority of undergraduates who do use drugs. Drugs can threaten students' physical and psychological health as well as their academic futures. Pot smoking in particular is strongly linked with "discontinuous enrollment"—in lay terms, dropping out of school.

✓**check-in** How widespread is drug use on your campus?

Why Students Don't Use Drugs

The majority of undergraduates do not use illegal drugs or abuse prescription drugs. In general, students are more influenced by fear of negative consequences than by barriers such as not having money for drugs.[22] Here are other factors that keep them drug-free:

- **Lack of interest.** At one liberal arts college in the Northeast, 8 in 10 of the undergraduates who reported never taking prescription drugs for nonmedical reasons said they simply had no interest in doing so.[23]

- **Timing of enrollment.** Students who delay enrollment or enter college at an older age are less likely to use drugs than those who enroll in college directly from high school.[24]

- **Spirituality and religion.** The greater a student's religiousness or religiosity—terms that encompass prayer, attendance at religious services, and reading spiritual materials—the less likely the student is to use alcohol, illegal drugs, or tobacco.

- **Academic engagement.** Illicit drug use is much less common among students who actively participate in classes and feel connected with the subject matter.

- **Socioeconomic status.** Students from lower socioeconomic status are less likely to use illicit drugs or misuse prescription drugs than those from more affluent families.[25]

- **Athletics.** Although male and female college athletes drink at higher rates than nonathletes,

they are less likely to use illegal drugs. One exception is the use of anabolic steroids (discussed in Chapter 6), which college athletes use more than other students.

✓**check-in** What do you think is the best reason not to use drugs?

Why Students Use Drugs

Various factors influence which students use drugs, including the following:

- **Genetics and family history.** Some college students inherit a genetic or biological predisposition to substance abuse. Researchers have identified specific genes tied to all types of addictions. Some genes associated with alcohol dependence are closely linked with addictions to marijuana, nicotine, cocaine, heroin, and other substances. Also, the risk for problem drinking and alcohol abuse is higher among children of substance abusers.

- **Parental attitudes and behavior.** Parents' concerns or expectations influence whether and how much most students drink, smoke, or use drugs. Those who perceive that their parents approve of their drinking, for instance, are more likely to report a drinking-related problem, such as memory loss or missing class.

✓**check-in** How would you describe your parents' attitudes toward alcohol and drugs?

- **Substance use in high school.** Many students start abusing drugs or alcohol well before getting to college. Misusing alcohol or drugs before age 15 increases by four times the risk of a substance abuse disorder later in life.[26]

- **Social norms.** College students tend to overestimate drug use on campus. In the ACHA survey, students reported believing that 10.4 percent of undergraduates had never used marijuana. In fact, 66.5 percent never had.[27]

- **Positive expectations.** Many students expect a drug to make them feel less stressed or anxious, more relaxed or confident, less shy or inhibited. Among students who use illicit drugs, many say that they do so to relieve stress.

- **Self-medication.** Some students take drugs to relieve depression or anxiety. Some abuse prescription medications, such as Adderall and Ritalin, because they mistakenly think these drugs will energize them to study longer or perform better.

- **Risk perception.** Individuals who view marijuana as not harmful, for instance, are more than nine times as likely to report having used the drug in the past.[28]

- **Mental health problems.** Students with feelings of hopelessness, sadness, depression, and anxiety as well as those with clinical mental disorders have higher rates of prescription drug abuse and illegal drug use. Students diagnosed with depression in the past school year have higher rates of marijuana, cocaine, alcohol, and tobacco use. Those with a history of ADHD (discussed in Chapter 2) are more likely to report having used marijuana and other illicit drugs, to begin use at a younger age, and to suffer higher levels of impairment.

- **Social influences.** More than 9 in 10 students who use illegal drugs were introduced to the habit through friends; most use drugs with friends. Sorority and fraternity members, who tend to socialize more often than their peers, are more likely to abuse prescription stimulants, but students who live off campus have higher rates of marijuana and cocaine use.

- **Alcohol use.** Often individuals engage in more than one risky behavior. Researchers have found that students who report binge drinking are much more likely than other students to report current or past use of marijuana, cocaine, or other illegal drugs.

- **Race/ethnicity.** In general, white students have higher levels of alcohol and drug use than do African American students. African American students at historically black colleges tend to have lower rates of alcohol and drug use than did either white or African American students at predominantly white schools. The reason may be that these colleges provide a greater sense of self-esteem, which helps prevent alcohol and drug use.

- **Sexual identity.** Gay, lesbian, and bisexual teens may rely on alcohol and marijuana to lessen social anxiety and boost self-confidence when they first come out. However, once they become more involved in the gay community, many are less likely to do so. Nonetheless, lesbians are significantly more likely than heterosexual women to use marijuana, Ecstasy, and other drugs. Gay and bisexual men are significantly less likely than heterosexual men to drink heavily but more likely to use drugs.[29]

- **Media influences.** In a recent survey, watching reality television and identifying with drug-using characters were associated with greater illegal drug use by college students.[30]

Understanding Drugs and Their Effects

A **drug** is a chemical substance that affects the way you feel and function. In some circumstances, taking a drug can help the body heal or relieve physical and mental distress. In others, taking a drug can distort reality, undermine well-being, and threaten survival.

No drug is completely safe; all drugs have multiple effects that vary greatly in different people at different times. Knowing how drugs affect the brain, body, and behavior is crucial to understanding their impact and making responsible decisions about their use:

- **Drug abuse** is a pattern of substance use resulting in negative consequences or impairment.

- **Drug dependence** is a pattern of continuing substance use despite cognitive, behavioral, and physical symptoms.

- **Drug misuse** is the taking of a drug for a purpose other than that for which it was intended or by a person other than for whom it was intended or not taking the recommended doses.

- **Drug diversion** is the transfer of a medication from the individual to whom it was prescribed to another person.

All forms of drug use involve risk. Even medications that help cure illnesses or soothe symptoms have side effects and can be misused. Some substances that millions of people use every day, such as caffeine, pose some health risks. Others—like the most commonly used drugs in our society, alcohol and tobacco—can lead to potentially life-threatening problems. With some illicit drugs, any form of use can be dangerous. Death rates related to drug overdose have tripled since 1990, with most of the increase tied to the growing abuse of prescription pain medications.

Many factors determine the effects a drug has on an individual. These include how the drug enters the body, the dosage, the drug action, and

drug Any substance, other than food, that affects bodily functions and structures when taken into the body.

drug abuse The excessive use of a drug in a manner inconsistent with accepted medical practice.

drug dependence Continued substance use even when its use causes cognitive, behavioral, and physical symptoms.

drug misuse The use of a drug for a purpose (or person) other than that for which it was medically intended.

drug diversion The transfer of a drug from the person for whom it was prescribed to another individual.

the presence of other drugs in the body—as well as the physical and psychological makeup of the person taking the drug and the setting in which the drug is used.

Routes of Administration

Drugs can enter the body in a number of ways (see Figure 12.1):

- **By swallowing:** The most common way of taking a drug is by swallowing a tablet, capsule, or liquid. However, drugs taken orally don't reach the bloodstream as quickly as drugs introduced into the body by other means and may not have any effect for 30 minutes or more.

- **By inhaling:** Drugs can enter the body through the lungs either by inhaling smoke (e.g., from marijuana) or by inhaling gases, aerosol sprays, or fumes from solvents or other compounds that evaporate quickly. Young users of such inhalants, discussed later in this chapter, often soak a rag with fluid and press it over their nose. Or they may place inhalants in a plastic bag, put the bag over their nose and mouth, and take deep breaths—a practice called *huffing* that can produce serious, even fatal, consequences.

- **By injecting:** Drugs can be injected with a syringe subcutaneously (beneath the skin), intramuscularly (into muscle tissue, which is richly supplied with blood vessels),

or intravenously (directly into a vein). **Intravenous** (IV) injection gets the drug into the bloodstream immediately (within seconds, in most cases); **intramuscular** injection involves moderately fast results (within a few minutes); and **subcutaneous** injection, more slowly (within 10 minutes).

Injecting drugs is extremely dangerous because many diseases, including hepatitis and infection with human immunodeficiency virus (HIV), can be transmitted by sharing contaminated needles. Injection-drug users who are HIV-positive are a major source of transmission of HIV among heterosexuals.

Dosage and Toxicity

The effects of any drug depend on the amount that an individual takes. Increasing the dose usually intensifies the effects produced by smaller doses. Also, the kind of effect may change at different dose levels. For example, low doses of barbiturates may relieve anxiety, while higher doses can induce sleep, loss of sensation, and even coma and death.

The dosage level at which a drug becomes poisonous to the body, causing either temporary or permanent damage, is called its **toxicity**. In most cases, drugs are eventually broken down in the liver by special body chemicals called *detoxification enzymes*.

Individual Differences

Each person responds differently to different drugs, depending on circumstances or setting. The enzymes in the body reduce drug levels in the bloodstream; because there can be 80 variants of each enzyme, every person's body may react differently.

Drugs often intensify a person's emotional state. If you're feeling depressed, a drug may make you feel more depressed. A generalized physical problem, such as having the flu, may make your body more vulnerable to the effects of a drug. Genetic differences among individuals also may account for varying reactions.

Personality and psychological attitude play a role in drug effects. Each user's *mind-set*—his or her expectations or preconceptions about using the drug—affects the experience. Someone who takes a club drug (discussed further later in this chapter) to feel more "connected" may feel more sociable simply because that's what he or she expects.

Sex and Drugs

Beginning at a very early age, males and females show different patterns in drug use:

intravenous Into a vein.

intramuscular Into or within a muscle.

subcutaneous Under the skin.

toxicity Poisonousness; the dosage level at which a drug becomes poisonous to the body, causing either temporary or permanent damage.

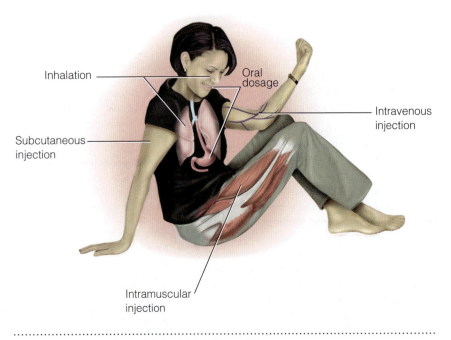

Inhalation

Oral dosage

Intravenous injection

Subcutaneous injection

Intramuscular injection

FIGURE 12.1 Routes of Administration of Drugs

- Men generally encounter more opportunities to use drugs than women do and are more likely to use drugs to fit into a group.

- Women abusing certain drugs tend to "escalate" or increase use more rapidly than men and to suffer more negative effects.[31]

- Women often encounter more barriers to treatment for substance use disorders, but both men and women have similar outcomes after treatment.[32]

- Given an opportunity to use drugs for the first time, both sexes are equally likely to do so and to progress from initial use to dependence.

- Men and women are equally likely to become addicted to or dependent on cocaine, heroin, hallucinogens, tobacco, and inhalants.

- Women are more likely than men to become addicted to or dependent on sedatives and drugs designed to treat anxiety or sleeplessness.

- Men are more likely than women to abuse alcohol and marijuana.

- Male and female long-term cocaine users showed similar impairment in tests of concentration, memory, and academic achievement.

- Female cocaine users are more vulnerable to poor nutrition and below-average weight, depression, physical abuse, and, if pregnant, preterm labor or early delivery. Smoking marijuana, taking prescription painkillers, or using illegal drugs during pregnancy is associated with double or even triple the risk of stillbirth.[33]

Setting

The setting for drug use also influences its effects. Passing around a marijuana joint at a friend's house is not a healthy or safe behavior, but the experience of going to a crack house is very different—and entails greater dangers.

Types of Action

A drug can act *locally*, as novocaine does to deaden pain in a tooth; *generally*, throughout a body system, as barbiturates do on the central nervous system; or *selectively*, as a drug does when it has a greater effect on one specific organ or system than on others, such as a spinal anesthetic. A drug that accumulates in the body because it's taken in faster than it can be metabolized and excreted is called *cumulative*; alcohol is such a drug.

Interaction with Other Drugs or Alcohol

A drug can interact with other drugs in four different ways:

- An **additive** interaction is one in which the resulting effect is equal to the sum of the effects of the different drugs used.

- A **synergistic** interaction is one in which the total effect of the two drugs taken together is greater than the sum of the effects the two drugs would have had if taken by themselves on separate occasions. Mixing barbiturates and alcohol, for example, has up to four times the depressant effect that either drug has alone.

- A drug can be **potentiating**—that is, one drug can increase the effect of another. Alcohol, for instance, can increase the drowsiness caused by antihistamines (antiallergy medications).

- Drugs can interact in an **antagonistic** fashion—that is, one drug can neutralize or block another drug with opposite effects. Tranquilizers, for example, may counter some of the nervousness and anxiety produced by cocaine.

The danger of mixing alcohol with other drugs cannot be emphasized too strongly. Alcohol and marijuana intensify each other's effects, making driving and many other activities extremely dangerous. Some people who have mixed sedatives or tranquilizers with alcohol never regained consciousness.

Caffeine and Its Effects

Caffeine, which has been drunk, chewed, and swallowed since the Stone Age, is the most widely used **psychoactive** (mind-affecting) drug in the world. Genetics may determine how much caffeine one craves. Scientists have identified the genes that drive people to consume more—or less—of this stimulant.

More than 85 percent of Americans consume caffeine. Coffee is our principal caffeine source, with Americans drinking an average of 3.5 cups a day. Coffee contains 100 to 150 milligrams of caffeine per cup; tea, 40 to 100 milligrams; cola, about 45 milligrams. Most medications that contain caffeine are one-third to one-half the strength

additive Characterized by a combined effect that is equal to the sum of the individual effects.

synergistic Characterized by a combined effect that is greater than the sum of the individual effects.

potentiating Making more effective or powerful.

antagonistic Opposing or counteracting.

psychoactive Mind-affecting.

of a cup of coffee. However, some, such as Excedrin, are very high in caffeine. (See Table 12.1 for caffeine counts of various products.)

As a stimulant, caffeine relieves drowsiness, helps in the performance of repetitive tasks, and improves the capacity for work. Caffeine improves performance and endurance during prolonged, exhaustive exercise and, to a lesser degree, enhances short-term, high-intensity athletic performance. Additional benefits include improved concentration, reduced fatigue, and sharpened alertness.

You'll stay more alert, particularly if you are fighting sleep deprivation, if you spread your coffee consumption over the course of the day. For instance, rather than drinking two 8-ounce cups in the morning, try consuming smaller servings of an ounce or two during the course of the day.

In recent decades, some 19,000 studies have examined caffeine's impact on the body and the brain. Their conclusion: For most people, caffeine poses few serious health risks. Drinking up to six cups a day of caffeinated or decaffeinated coffee won't shorten your lifespan and may convey some health benefits. Researchers have found no significant relationship between coffee and tea consumption and the risk of breast cancer or of miscarriage.[34] Contrary to common belief, regular caffeine consumption also does not cause dangerous racing of the heart.[35]

✓**check-in** Where do you get your coffee?
A typical cup of coffee at home contains only 5 ounces of caffeine, but the smallest size available at most coffee shops contains 8 to 12 ounces, and larger ones even more.

As documented in numerous studies, caffeine can:

- Relieve drowsiness.
- Boost performance at repetitive tasks.
- Improve memory for up to 14 hours after consumption.[36]
- Improve performance and endurance during prolonged, exhaustive exercise.
- Enhance, to a lesser degree, short-term, high-intensity athletic performance.
- Sharpen concentration.
- Reduce fatigue.
- Increase alertness.
- Lower the risk of type 2 diabetes and cardiovascular disease.
- Possibly protect against Parkinson's disease, colon cancer, liver cirrhosis, gallstones, and stroke.
- Possibly relieve migraines, boost mood, and prevent cavities.
- Protect against depression.[37]
- Possibly reduce the risk of endometrial cancer in women who drink four or more cups a day.
- Possibly lower the likelihood of multiple sclerosis in people drinking about six cups a day.[38]
- Possibly delay or protect against late-life cognitive impairment or decline, especially in women, although researchers describe the evidence to date as "inconclusive."[39]

Despite these positive findings, doctors advise pregnant women, heart patients, and those at risk for osteoporosis to limit or avoid coffee. Too much caffeine, particularly in high-powered energy drinks, can be dangerous for everyone and particularly harmful for children.[40] A single dose of 5 grams can be fatal.

✓**check-in** If you normally drink a couple of 8-ounce cups of coffee in the morning, try smaller servings of an ounce or two during the course of the day. You'll feel more alert and less jittery.

TABLE 12.1 Caffeine Content in Selected Soft Drinks and Energy Drinks

Drink	Company	Milligrams of Caffeine in 12 oz.
Soft Drinks		
JOLT	Wet Planet	72
Mountain Dew Code Red	PepsiCo	55
Mountain Dew	PepsiCo	55
Mello Yello	Coca-Cola	51
Diet Coke	Coca-Cola	45
Dr Pepper	Keurig Dr Pepper	41
Pepsi-Cola	PepsiCo	38
Energy Drinks		
Redline Power Rush	Vital Pharmaceuticals	1,680
JOLT Endurance Shot	Wet Planet	900
Cocaine Energy Drink	Redux Beverages	400
Blow (Energy Drink Mix)	Kingpin Concepts	360
Monster	Monster Beverage	120
Red Bull	Red Bull	116

Jeffrey Blackler/Alamy

Caffeine Intoxication

Doctors recommend that all adults limit their caffeine intake to 500 milligrams a day, with lesser amounts for those who have heart problems, high blood pressure, or trouble sleeping or who are taking medications. The recommended maximum for adolescents is 100 milligrams of caffeine a day. Ingesting more than 250 milligrams of caffeine may produce caffeine intoxication, which is diagnosed on the basis of five or more of the following signs and symptoms:

- Restlessness.
- Nervousness.
- Excitement.
- Insomnia.
- Flushed face.
- Increased urination.
- Digestive disturbances.
- Muscle twitching.
- Rambling thoughts or speech.
- Rapid or irregular heart rate.
- Periods of inexhaustibility.
- Agitation.

College students tend to be aware of the potential side effects of too much caffeine, but they generally continue to drink coffee and other caffeinated beverages.[41] Higher doses may also produce ringing in the ears or flashes of light. Among the potentially life-threatening conditions that can result from caffeine intoxication are acute kidney injury, hepatitis, seizures, strokes, coronary artery spasms, and heart attack.

Caffeine withdrawal for those dependent on this substance can cause headaches and other neurological symptoms. Those who must cut back should taper off gradually. One approach is to mix regular and decaffeinated coffee, gradually decreasing the quantity of the former.

Caffeine-Containing Energy Drinks

Caffeine-containing energy drinks (CCEDs, in the medical literature) have become extremely popular, especially in Western and Asian countries. These fortified beverages differ from soft drinks or sports drinks in that they contain higher levels of caffeine—typically 500 milligrams or more—as well as sugars and dietary supplements.[42] As consumption has increased, especially among adolescents and young adults, medical

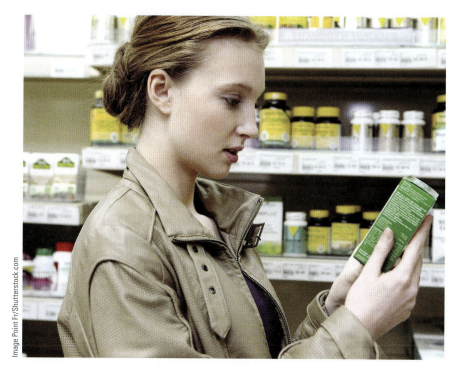

Always read the consumer-information label before using an over-the-counter drug.

professionals have raised concerns about health impacts, including the following:

- Disrupted sleep.
- Increased heart rate and blood pressure.
- Overweight and obesity.
- Heightened anxiety and tension.
- Hallucinations (with the equivalent of seven or more cups of coffee a day).
- Dehydration.
- Dental erosion.
- Possible contribution to seizures or stroke.

Many of these drinks contain herbs that enhance the effects of caffeine and can interact with medication, causing harmful effects. Emergency department visits related to energy drinks have more than doubled in recent years.

Alcohol mixed with energy drinks (AmED, in the medical literature) presents even greater dangers. About a third of college students report having consumed AmED in the past year.

Students mixing alcohol and caffeine engage in more high-risk drinking behaviors and are twice as likely to report being hurt or injured as those who don't.[43] (See Chapter 13 for a discussion on alcohol mixed with energy drinks.)

✓**check-in** Do you drink high-energy beverages? If so, do you know how much caffeine is in a single bottle or can?

Image Point Fr/Shutterstock.com

Medications

As many as half of all patients take the wrong medications, in the wrong doses, at the wrong times, or in the wrong ways. Every year these inadvertent errors lead to an estimated 125,000 deaths and more than $8.5 billion in hospital costs. Mistakes occur among people of all ages, both sexes, and every race, occupation, level of education, and personality type. Their number-one cause: not understanding directions.

Doctors occasionally make errors when it comes to prescription drugs. The most frequent are:

- Over dosing or underdosing.
- Omitting information from prescriptions.
- Ordering the wrong dosage form (a pill instead of a liquid, for example).
- Not recognizing a patient's allergy to a drug.

Over-the-Counter Drugs

More than half a million health products—remedies for everything from bad breath to bunions—are readily available without a doctor's prescription. This doesn't mean that they're necessarily safe or effective. Like other drugs, **over-the-counter (OTC)** medications can be used improperly, often simply because of a lack of education about proper use. Among those most often misused are the following:

- **Painkillers.** Federal regulators have issued warnings for many popular painkillers, including OTC pills such as Advil (ibuprofen) and Aleve (naproxen). Their labels cite risks to the heart, stomach, and skin. Tylenol (acetaminophen) and aspirin are generally considered safe for people with temporary pain such as headaches and muscle aches. However, aspirin can cause stomach irritation and bleeding, and Tylenol, which is found in more than 600 OTC and prescription medications, poses multiple dangers (see Table 12.2).

- **Nasal sprays.** Nasal sprays relieve congestion by shrinking blood vessels in the nose. If they are used too often or for too many days in a row, the blood vessels widen instead of contract, and the surrounding tissues become swollen, causing more congestion. To make the vessels shrink again, many people use more spray more often. The result can be permanent damage to nasal membranes, bleeding, infection, and partial or complete loss of smell.

- **Laxatives.** Believing that they must have one bowel movement a day (a common misconception), many people rely on laxatives. Brands that contain phenolphthalein irritate the lining of the intestines and cause muscles to contract or tighten, often making constipation worse rather than better. Bulk laxatives are less dangerous, but regular use is not advised. A high-fiber diet and more exercise are safer and more effective remedies for constipation.

- **Eye drops.** Eye drops make the blood vessels of the eye contract. However, as in the case of nasal sprays, with overuse (several times a day for several weeks), the blood vessels expand, making the eye look redder than before.

- **Sleep aids.** Although OTC sleeping pills are widely used, there has been little research on their use and possible risks. A national consensus panel on insomnia concluded that they are not effective and cause side effects such as morning-after grogginess. Medications such as Tylenol PM and Excedrin PM combine a pain reliever with a sleep-inducing antihistamine, the same ingredient that people take for hay fever or cold symptoms. Although they make people drowsy, they can leave a groggy feeling the next day, and they dry out the nose and mouth.

- **Cough syrup.** Many of the "active" ingredients in OTC cough preparations may be ineffective. Young people may chug cough syrup (called *roboing*, after the OTC medication Robitussin) because they think of dextromethorphan (DXM), a common ingredient in cough medicine, as a "poor man's version" of the popular drug Ecstasy.

✓**check-in** Which OTC painkillers have you used? Have you experienced any adverse effects?

Prescription Drugs

Like OTC drugs, many prescribed medications aren't taken the way they should be; millions simply aren't taken at all. As many as 70 percent of adults have trouble understanding dosage information, and 30 percent can't read standard labels, according to the FDA, which has called for larger, clearer drug labeling.

The dangers of nonadherence (not properly taking prescription drugs) include:

- Recurrent infections.
- Serious medical complications.
- Emergency hospital treatment.

over-the-counter (OTC)
Medications that can be obtained legally without a prescription from a medical professional.

The drugs most likely to be taken incorrectly are those that treat problems with no obvious symptoms (such as high blood pressure), require complex dosage schedules, treat psychiatric disorders, or have unpleasant side effects.

The most common reason that college students fail to take medicines as directed is forgetting. Others are concerned about cost, or they stop when they feel better.

Physical Side Effects Most medications, taken correctly, cause only minor complications. No drug is entirely without side effects for all individuals taking it. Serious complications that may occur include heart failure, heart attack, seizures, kidney and liver failure, severe blood disorders, birth defects, blindness, memory problems, and allergic reactions. Overdoses of opioid painkillers now cause more deaths than heroin and cocaine combined—one fatality every 19 minutes, according to the Centers for Disease Control and Prevention (CDC).

Allergic reactions to drugs are common. The drugs that most often provoke allergic responses are penicillin and other antibiotics (drugs used to treat infection). Aspirin, nonsteroidal anti-inflammatory drugs (NSAIDs), sulfa drugs, barbiturates, anticonvulsants, insulin, and local anesthetics can also provoke allergic responses.

✓**check-in** Do you have any drug allergies? If so, what symptoms do they provoke?

Psychological Side Effects Dozens of drugs—both OTC and prescription—can cause changes in the way people think, feel, and behave. Unfortunately, neither patients nor their physicians usually connect such symptoms with medications. Doctors may not even mention potential mental and emotional problems because they don't want to scare patients away from what otherwise may be a very effective treatment. What you don't know about a drug's effects on your mind *can* hurt you.

Among the medications most likely to cause psychiatric side effects are drugs for high blood pressure, heart disease, asthma, epilepsy, arthritis, Parkinson's disease, anxiety, insomnia, and depression. Some drugs—such as the powerful hormones called *corticosteroids*, used for asthma, autoimmune diseases, and cancer—can cause different psychiatric symptoms, depending on dosage and other factors. The older you are, the sicker you are, and the more medications you're taking, the greater your risk of developing some psychiatric side effects.

TABLE 12.2 Acetaminophen Alert!

The FDA has issued the following guidelines for safe use of acetaminophen:

- Do not exceed 4,000 milligrams or 4 grams (the equivalent of eight 500-mg Tylenol Extra Strength pills) a day.
- Carefully read all labels for prescription and OTC medications and ask if any prescription medicine contains acetaminophen.
- Don't take more than one acetaminophen-containing product (including OTC medications) at the same time.
- Avoid drinking alcohol while taking acetaminophen.
- Stop taking acetaminophen and seek medical help immediately if you experience allergic reactions such as rash, itching, swelling of the face, and/or difficulty breathing.
- Seek medical help right away if you think you have taken more than the directed dosage of acetaminophen. Tylenol and other products containing acetaminophen account for 40 to 50 percent of all acute cases of liver failure, many resulting from unintentional overdose.
- Men younger than age 50 who take acetaminophen more than two times a week have roughly double the risk of hearing loss compared to men who do not. Men of similar ages who take ibuprofen (the main ingredient in Motrin or Advil) at least twice a week have a nearly two-thirds higher risk of hearing loss. Men who take aspirin twice a week have a one-third higher risk. However, the absolute risk of hearing loss remains small in young and middle-aged men.

Source: www.fda.gov.

Drug Interactions OTC and prescription drugs can interact in a variety of ways. For example, mixing some cold medications with tranquilizers can cause drowsiness and coordination problems, thus making driving dangerous. Moreover, what you eat or drink can impair or completely wipe out the effectiveness of drugs or lead to unexpected effects on the body. For instance, aspirin takes 5 to 10 times as long to be absorbed when taken with food or shortly after a meal than when taken on an empty stomach. If tetracyclines encounter calcium in the stomach, they bind together and cancel each other out.

To avoid potentially dangerous interactions, do the following:

- Check the label(s) for any instructions on how or when to take a medication, such as "with a meal."
- If the directions say that you should take a drug on an empty stomach, take it at least 1 hour before eating or 2 to 3 hours after eating.
- Don't drink a hot beverage with a medication; the temperature may interfere with the effectiveness of the drug.

Drugs and Alcohol About 4 in 10 current drinkers in the United States take prescription drugs that interact with alcohol. Depending on the medication, the combination could cause side effects that range from drowsiness to depressed breathing and lower heart rate.[44]

Alcohol can change the rate of metabolism and the effects of many different drugs. Because it dilates the blood vessels, alcohol can add to the dizziness sometimes caused by drugs for high blood pressure, angina, or depression. Also, its irritating effects on the stomach can worsen stomach upset from aspirin, ibuprofen, and other anti-inflammatory drugs.

Generic Drugs

The **generic** name is the chemical name for a drug. A specific drug may appear on the pharmacist's shelf under a variety of brand names, which tend to cost far more than the generic equivalent. About 75 percent of all prescriptions specify a brand name, but pharmacists may—and in some states must—switch to a generic drug unless the doctor specifically tells them not to. Prescriptions filled with generic drugs cost 20 to 85 percent less than their brand-name counterparts.

Generic drugs have the same active ingredients as brand-name prescriptions, but their fillers and binders, which can affect the absorption of a drug, may be different. For some serious illnesses, the generics may not be as effective; some experts recommend sticking with brand names for heart medications, psychiatric drugs, and anticonvulsant drugs (for epilepsy and other seizure disorders).

> ✓**check-in** Should you buy the generic version of a drug? Ask your physician if switching to a generic or from one generic to another might affect your condition in any way.

Buying Drugs Online

Millions of people in the United States purchase prescription medications online. Although some websites fill only faxed prescriptions from medical doctors, others ignore or sidestep traditional regulations and safeguards.

Cyberspace distributors often ship pills across state lines without requiring a physical examination by a medical doctor. Instead, a "cyberdoc," who may or may not be qualified or up to date in a given specialty, reviews information submitted by a "patient." International pharmacies sometimes sell drugs that are not available or approved in the United States. And patients themselves use bulletin boards and other online resources to sell unused or unwanted medications to each other.

Many individuals turn to the Internet for "lifestyle" drugs such as pills for erectile dysfunction, weight control, and smoking cessation. Customers like the convenience and anonymity of buying drugs online. Although many people assume that drugs cost less on the Internet, shipping costs tend to drive prices up to the same amount as or more than the price at a pharmacy.

> ✓**check-in** Have you ever bought a medication online?

Consumers have to be wary. Ordering a drug like Accutane, an acne treatment, online may seem harmless. However, without close monitoring by a physician, you could develop complications, such as a bad reaction that aggravates hepatitis or inflames the pancreas.

Quality control is another concern. Counterfeit drugs, increasingly sold online, may do little, if any, good and could be harmful. Cyberspace pharmacies provide no information on how the drug was stored or whether its expiration date has passed. In addition, since importing medications without a prescription is against the law, you could find yourself in legal trouble.

Substance Use Disorders

An estimated 20.8 million Americans have a substance use disorder,[45] defined by the American Psychiatric Association as "a cluster of cognitive, behavioral, and physiological symptoms indicating that the individual continues using the substance despite significant substance-related problems"[46] (see Health Now!). Only 1 in 10 receives treatment. A key characteristic is an underlying change in brain circuits that may persist beyond detoxification, particularly in individuals with severe disorders. These brain changes may result in repeated relapses and intense craving for the drug.

The characteristics of a substance use disorder include:

- Taking a substance in larger amounts or over a longer period than was originally intended.
- A persistent desire to cut down or stop substance use.
- Unsuccessful efforts to decrease or discontinue use.
- A great deal of time given to obtaining the substance, using the substance, or recovering from its effects.

generic A consumer product with no brand name or registered trademark.

- Cravings, which may be so strong that a user cannot think of anything else.
- Failure to fulfill major obligations at work, school, or home because of substance use.
- Recurrent substance use in physically hazardous situations.[47]

Dependence

Substance users may develop **psychological dependence** and feel a strong craving for a drug because it produces pleasurable feelings or relieves stress and anxiety. **Physical dependence** occurs when a person develops *tolerance* to the effects of a drug and needs larger and larger doses to achieve intoxication or another desired effect. Individuals who are physically dependent and have a high tolerance to a drug may take amounts many times those that would produce intoxication or an overdose in someone who was not a regular user.

Men and women with a substance dependence disorder may use a drug to avoid or relieve withdrawal symptoms, or they may consume larger amounts of a drug or use it over a longer period than they'd originally intended.

Specific symptoms of dependence vary with particular drugs. Some drugs, such as marijuana, hallucinogens, and phencyclidine, do not cause withdrawal symptoms. The degree of dependence also varies. In mild cases, a person may function normally most of the time. In severe cases, the person's entire life may revolve around obtaining, using, and recuperating from the effects of a drug.

Individuals with drug dependence become intoxicated or high on a regular basis—whether every day, every weekend, or several binges a year. They may try repeatedly to stop using a drug and yet fail, even though they realize that their drug use is interfering with their health, family life, relationships, and work.

Misuse

Some drug users do not develop the symptoms of tolerance and withdrawal that characterize dependence, yet they use drugs in ways that clearly have a harmful effect on them. These individuals are diagnosed as having a *psychoactive substance abuse disorder*. They continue to use drugs despite their awareness of persistent or repeated social, occupational, psychological, or physical problems related to drug use, or they use drugs in dangerous ways or situations (before driving, for instance).

Intoxication and Withdrawal

Intoxication refers to maladaptive behavioral, psychological, and physiologic changes that occur as a result of substance use. **Withdrawal** is the development of symptoms that cause significant psychological and physical distress when an individual reduces or stops drug use. (Intoxication and withdrawal from specific drugs are discussed later in this chapter.)

Polyabuse

Most users prefer a certain type of drug but also use several others; this behavior is called **polyabuse**. The average user who enters treatment is on five different drugs. The more drugs anyone uses, the greater the chance of side effects, complications, and possibly life-threatening interactions.[48]

Coexisting Conditions

Mental disorders and substance use disorders have a great deal of overlap. Many individuals with substance use disorders also have another psychiatric disorder, such as depression. Individuals with such *dual diagnoses* require careful evaluation and appropriate treatment for the complete range of complex and chronic difficulties they face.

Causes of Substance Use Disorders

No one fully understands why some people develop drug dependence or substance use disorders, whereas others, who may experiment briefly with drugs, do not. Inherited body chemistry, genetic factors, and sensitivity to drugs may make some individuals more susceptible than others. These disorders may stem from many complex causes.

The Neurobiology of Dependence

Drug dependence is a brain disease triggered by frequent use of drugs that change the biochemistry and anatomy of neurons and alter the way they work. A major breakthrough in understanding dependence has been the discovery that certain mood-altering substances and experiences—a puff of marijuana, a slug of whiskey, a snort of cocaine, a big win at blackjack—trigger a rise in a brain chemical called **dopamine**, which is associated with feelings of satisfaction and euphoria. This brain chemical or neurotransmitter is one of the crucial messengers that link nerve cells in the brain, and its level rises during

HEALTH NOW!

Recognizing Substance Abuse

How can you tell if a friend or loved one has a substance use disorder? Look for the following warning signs:

- An abrupt change in attitude
- Mood swings
- A decline in performance
- Increased sensitivity
- Secrecy
- Physical changes
- Money problems
- Changes in appearance
- Defiance of restrictions
- Changes in relationships

Does someone you care about show signs of substance abuse? If so, write down your observations in your online journal. Describe your feelings, and list some options for what to do next. If not, create a hypothetical situation in which you discover that a friend or family member is abusing drugs.

psychological dependence Strong craving for a drug because it produces pleasurable feelings or relieves stress and anxiety.

physical dependence Physiological attachment to, and need for, a drug.

intoxication Maladaptive behavioral, psychological, and physiologic changes that occur as a result of substance abuse.

withdrawal Development of symptoms that cause significant psychological and physical distress when an individual reduces or stops drug use.

polyabuse The misuse or abuse of more than one drug.

dopamine A brain chemical associated with feelings of satisfaction and euphoria.

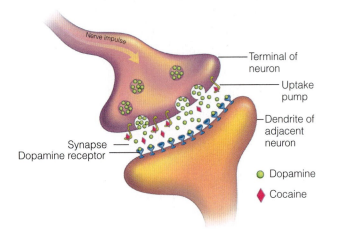

FIGURE 12.2 Dopamine Levels for Cocaine

Within the synapses between adjacent neurons, cocaine binds to the dopamine uptake pumps and thus allows the neurotransmitter dopamine to build up in the synapse and bind to more dopamine receptors.

any pleasurable experience, whether it be a loving hug or a taste of chocolate.

The mechanism governing the rise in dopamine levels is not the same for all drugs. Figure 12.2 shows the one for cocaine. Normally, after dopamine is released from the axon terminal of a neuron and activates dopamine receptors on the adjacent neuron, the dopamine is then transported back to its original neuron by "uptake pumps." Cocaine binds to the uptake pumps and prevents them from transporting dopamine back into the neuron terminal. So more dopamine builds up in the synapse and is free to activate more dopamine receptors.

The Psychology of Vulnerability

Although scientists do not believe there is an addictive personality, certain individuals are at increased risk of drug dependence because of psychological factors, including:

- Difficulty controlling impulses.
- A lack of values that might constrain drug use (whether based in religion, family, or society).
- Low self-esteem.
- Feelings of powerlessness.
- Depression.

The one psychological trait most often linked with drug use is denial. Young people in particular are absolutely convinced that they will never lose control or suffer in any way as a result of drug use.

People with mental illness such as depression, anxiety, schizophrenia, or bipolar disorder have an increased risk for substance use. Individuals may self-administer drugs to treat psychiatric symptoms; for example, they may take sedating drugs to suppress a panic attack. An estimated 8.4 million adults in the United States have both a mental and substance use disorder.[49]

Users of illicit drugs are much more likely than the general population to think about suicide, according to the U.S. Substance Abuse and Mental Health Services Administration's (SAMHSA's) most recent National Survey on Drug Use and Health.

The Opioid Epidemic

The United States is experiencing a deadly epidemic caused by addiction to opioids. These drugs, also discussed on page 397, are chemically similar to the neurotransmitters and other brain chemicals naturally produced by our bodies. They reduce the intensity of pain perception by interacting with opioid receptors in the spinal cord and brain.

Opioids are classified into categories according to how they are manufactured:

- Natural opiates, made from the opium poppy, such as morphine and codeine.
- Semisynthetic opioids, such as hydrocodone from codeine.
- Fully synthetic opioids, such as fentanyl and methadone.

The most prescribed opioids in the United States are hydrocodone and extended- and immediate-release oxycodone. According to federal estimates, 4.7 million individuals use prescription opioids nonmedically every month. Another 1.9 million are addicted to prescription opioids.[50]

How the Epidemic Started

Medications derived from the opium poppy have been used for centuries to treat pain, cough, and diarrhea. Before the 1990s, doctors often prescribed opioids to treat cancer and postsurgery pain. In 1996, Purdue Pharma began promoting Oxycontin (extended-release oxycodone) to relieve chronic noncancer pain, despite a lack of quality studies demonstrating the drug's safety and efficacy.

Initially, Oxycontin—whose active ingredient is twice as potent as morphine—was marketed as a safe drug that would not lead to addiction "if taken as prescribed." Health-care providers without adequate training in pain management became the largest prescribers of Oxycontin, and manufacturers sold billions of dollars of this and similar medications every year.

Health policy analysts blame the spread of the opioid epidemic on a combination of factors, including:

- A successful marketing campaign to promote the use of prescription opioids for pain.

- Misleading messages that opioids carry a low risk of addiction and overdose.

- Exaggerated claims of efficacy.

- Weak regulation in some states to control nonmedical use of opioids.

- Social and political factors, including rising unemployment, declining local economies, and poor access to behavioral health treatment.

During its early stages, the opioid epidemic took its highest toll in rural areas and small towns. Over time, larger cities also have been affected, with a sharp increase in opioid-related emergency department visits, hospitalizations, and overdose deaths. Demographic characteristics of heroin users have also changed, from younger nonwhite individuals in more urban areas to older white men and women in nonurban areas, many of whom first used prescription opioids prior to using heroin.

In 2017, the Department of Health and Human Services declared the opioid epidemic "a public health emergency" and outlined the five following strategies to address it:

- Improve access to prevention, treatment, and recovery support services.

- Target the availability and distribution of overdose-reversing drugs.

- Strengthen public health data reporting and collection.

- Support cutting-edge research on addiction and pain.

- Advance the practice of pain management.

The Impact of the Epidemic

The following statistics summarize the toll of the epidemic in the United States:

- On average, 130 Americans die every day from an opioid overdose. The rate of

overdose deaths involving opioids has risen by 200 percent over the last 10 years.

- In the past decade, more than 700,000 people have died from a drug overdose. More than two-thirds of fatal drug overdoses involve an opioid.

- The number of overdose deaths involving opioids (including prescription opioids and illegal opioids like heroin and illicitly manufactured fentanyl) is six times higher than it was in 1999.

- Non-Hispanic whites, American Indians/Alaskan Natives, and people from lower socioeconomic backgrounds have experienced a higher prevalence of opioid misuse, addiction, and overdoses (see Figure 12.3).

The impact of the opioid epidemic extends beyond addiction and fatal overdoses. Sharing

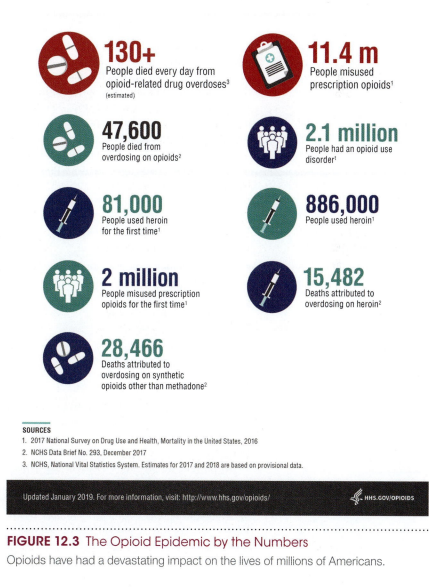

130+ People died every day from opioid-related drug overdoses[3] (estimated)

11.4 m People misused prescription opioids[1]

47,600 People died from overdosing on opioids[2]

2.1 million People had an opioid use disorder[1]

81,000 People used heroin for the first time[1]

886,000 People used heroin[1]

2 million People misused prescription opioids for the first time[1]

15,482 Deaths attributed to overdosing on heroin[2]

28,466 Deaths attributed to overdosing on synthetic opioids other than methadone[2]

SOURCES

1. 2017 National Survey on Drug Use and Health, Mortality in the United States, 2016
2. NCHS Data Brief No. 293, December 2017
3. NCHS, National Vital Statistics System. Estimates for 2017 and 2018 are based on provisional data.

Updated January 2019. For more information, visit: http://www.hhs.gov/opioids/   HHS.GOV/OPIOIDS

FIGURE 12.3 The Opioid Epidemic by the Numbers

Opioids have had a devastating impact on the lives of millions of Americans.

drug-injection equipment has tripled the prevalence of hepatitis C infections. Babies of pregnant women addicted to opioids are born with opioid withdrawal syndrome, which makes them more likely to suffer low birth weight and respiratory and central nervous system complications.[51]

The total economic burden of the opioid epidemic is estimated to be around $78.5 billion, comprised of increased health care and substance abuse treatment, crime-related costs, and lost productivity.

Who Is at Risk?

An estimated 35.5 percent of Americans suffer from chronic pain of some kind; 11 percent, with severe chronic pain. They are most likely to take prescription opioids. An estimated one in four patients receiving long-term opioid therapy struggles with opioid addiction.

Anyone who takes prescription opioids, including those using them for nonmedical reasons, can become addicted to them. Once addicted, it can be hard to stop. As tolerance develops, users may take more medication for the same pain relief and may suffer withdrawal symptoms if they cut back or stop. Taking too many prescription opioids can stop a person's breathing and cause death.

As discussed later in this chapter, abuse of these medications can cause serious, potentially fatal side effects, including:

- Drowsiness.
- Increased sensitivity to pain.
- Constipation.
- Nausea, vomiting, and dry mouth.
- Sleepiness and dizziness.
- Confusion.
- Depression.
- Confusion.
- Slowed breathing.
- Death.

Other health effects include miscarriage, low birth weight, risk of drug interactions, and spreading of HIV, hepatitis, and other infectious diseases from shared needles.

To prevent misuse, the CDC has issued recommendations for clinicians prescribing opioids. They include starting treatment with nondrug or nonopioid options, using opioids only in the lowest effective doses, and limiting opioid use to three days or fewer.

Recovery

Health professionals describe opioid addiction as "a chronic relapsing brain disease." Because of the high rate of relapse, maintenance therapy is usually needed to prevent consumption of illegal opioids, such as heroin, and potentially fatal overdoses. The most effective maintenance therapies include methadone, buprenorphine, and extended-release naltrexone, combined with psychosocial therapy. Researchers are continuing to develop new approaches, including cannabinoids, to aid in recovery.[52]

Prescription Drug Abuse

Nonmedical use of any prescription medication is highest among young adults between the ages of 18 and 25, compared with other age groups.

Prescription Drugs on Campus

About 12 percent of college students report using drugs that were not prescribed for them, including stimulants, painkillers, sedatives, and antidepressants.[53] Among painkillers, oxycodone—the active ingredient in OxyContin—and hydrocodone are the most widely used. College women use more antidepressants; college men, more painkillers and stimulants (see Table 12.3).

✓**check-in** Have you ever taken a medication that was not prescribed for you?

Abuse of prescription medications on college campuses has increased in the last 15 years. Here is what we know about it:

- Only marijuana use is more widespread on campus than prescription drug abuse.
- College men have higher rates of prescription drug abuse than women.
- White and Hispanic undergraduates are significantly more likely to abuse medications than are African American and Asian students.

- Undergraduates who misuse or abuse prescription medications are much more likely to report heavy binge drinking and use of illicit drugs.
- College women who abuse prescription drugs are at increased risk for sexual victimization and assault.

Prescription Stimulants

Stimulants are among the most widely abused prescription drugs on campus, with about 6 percent of students reporting their misuse.[54] The most widespread are Adrenal, Benzedrine, Concerta, and Ritalin. Their street names include Bennies, Black Beauties, Crosses, Hearts, Users, Truck Drivers, Skippy, and Vitamin R (for Ritalin). Misuse of the prescription drug Adderall, which increases brain chemicals linked with better cognitive functioning and has a false reputation for making people smarter, has surged among young adults ages 18 to 25.[55] (See page 407 for more on stimulants.)

Users generally obtain these drugs from peers with prescriptions for the treatment of attention-deficit/hyperactivity disorder (ADHD), which affects an estimated 2 to 8 percent of undergraduates. They are more likely than other students to be Caucasian, male upperclassmen rather than freshmen or sophomores, from higher-income families, and members of fraternities and sororities.

Students generally take stimulants to focus better while studying, stay awake to study longer, and improve their grades. However, a meta-analysis of existing research found no scientific basis for these alleged benefits.[56] The lower a student's GPA, the greater the odds of stimulant misuse, which is also associated with skipping class and studying less. Other reasons for stimulant misuse include wanting to get high, to prolong the effects of alcohol and other drugs, and to lose weight.

Students who misuse stimulants typically perceive them as relatively safe, but they produce a range of effects.[57]

Short-Term Effects

- Increased alertness, attention, and energy.
- Increased blood pressure and heart rate.
- Narrowed blood vessels.
- Increased blood sugar.
- With high doses: dangerously high body temperature and irregular heartbeat, heart failure, and seizures.

TABLE 12.3 Nonmedical Prescription Drug Use by College Students

Percentage of college students who reported using medications that were not prescribed to them within the past 12 months:

	Percent (%)		
	Male	Female	Total
Antidepressants	2.0	3.1	2.9
Erectile dysfunction drugs	0.9	0.6	0.7
Pain killers	4.0	4.2	4.2
Sedatives	3.0	2.9	3.0
Stimulants	6.6	5.4	5.8
Used one or more of the above	11.0	10.8	11.0

Source: American College Health Association. American College Health Association-National College Health Assessment II: Reference Group Executive Summary Spring 2018. Silver Spring, MD: American College Health Association, 2018.

Long-Term Effects

- Heart problems.
- Psychosis.
- Anger.
- Paranoia.
- Use of alcohol and other drugs.
- Risky behaviors, including unsafe sex and reckless driving.

Overdoses can cause delirium, confusion, aggressiveness, hallucinations, and psychotic symptoms. Combining stimulants with alcohol increases the likelihood of blackouts, accidents, and unprotected or unplanned sex. In individuals with certain cardiac conditions, stimulant medications can cause serious, even fatal, complications.[58]

Some universities are setting strict regulations for ADHD medications, including confirmation of

YOUR STRATEGIES FOR PREVENTION

How to Say No to Drugs

If people offer you a drug, here are some ways to say no.

- **Let them know you're not interested.** If the pressure seems threatening, leave.
- **Have something else to do: "No, I'm going for a walk now."**
- **Be prepared for different types of pressure.** If your friends tease you, tease them back.
- **Keep it simple.** "No, thanks," "No," or "No way," all get the point across.
- **Hang out with people who won't offer you drugs.**

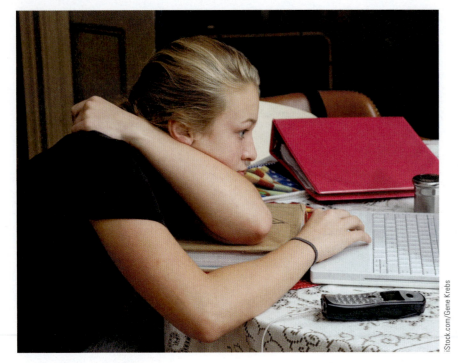

Some college students try stimulants to stay alert while cramming for exams, but these medications do not improve academic performance and can cause harmful effects.

iStock.com/Gene Krebs

the diagnosis through a medical evaluation and a formal written promise to submit to drug testing and not to share the pills.

Prescription Painkillers

An estimated 2 million Americans abuse or are dependent on prescription painkillers. Each day an estimated 1,000 people are treated for misusing prescription opioids in emergency departments across the United States.[59]

The most commonly abused prescription painkillers are codeine (sold under various brand names), Vicodin, Dilaudid, Demerol, OxyContin, Percodan, and Percocet. About 5 percent of undergraduates report use of Vicodin or OxyContin.[60] Students who are members of fraternities and sororities, who are enrolled at more competitive schools, who earn lower grade-point averages, and who engage in substance use and other risky behaviors are more likely to abuse these drugs.

Like other addictions, a prescription painkiller "habit" is a treatable brain disease but not an easy habit to break. Recovery usually requires carefully supervised detoxification, appropriate medications (similar to those used for opioid dependence), behavioral therapy, and ongoing support.

✓**check-in** How widespread do you think prescription drug abuse is on your campus?

marijuana The drug derived from the cannabis plant, containing the psychoactive ingredient THC, which causes a mild sense of euphoria when inhaled or eaten.

hashish A concentrated form of a drug derived from the cannabis plant that contains the psychoactive ingredient THC, which causes a sense of euphoria when inhaled or eaten.

cannabinoids A group of closely related compounds that include cannabinol and the active constituents of cannabis (marijuana).

Commonly Abused Drugs

The common drugs of abuse fall within these categories: cannabinoids, herbal drugs, club drugs, stimulants, dissociative drugs, hallucinogens, opioids, and other compounds.

Cannabinoids

Marijuana (pot) is derived from several species of the cannabis plant. **Hashish** is more potent than cannabis sativa, the most widespread cannabis plant. The major psychoactive ingredient in the **cannabinoids** is THC (delta-9-tetrahydrocannabinol).

More than 100 million Americans have tried marijuana, the third most popular recreational drug in the United States (after alcohol and tobacco). According to government surveys, some 12 million Americans use cannabis; more than 1 million cannot control this use. An estimated 12.5 percent of adults report using marijuana in the previous year.[61] On college campuses, marijuana remains the most widely used illicit drug. (See Student Snapshot in this chapter.)

✓**check-in** How widespread do you think marijuana use is on your campus?

Because of careful cultivation, the strength of today's marijuana is much greater than that used in the 1960s and 1970s. Today, a marijuana joint contains 150 milligrams of THC, compared to 10 milligrams in the 1960s.

CBD

Cannabidiol, or CBD, the second most-abundant cannabinoid in cannabis, comes in various strains, including some that are not psychoactive and do not produce the euphoric highs associated with THC. Although research is limited, CBD is being widely marketed as a treatment for pain, inflammation, anxiety, and other chronic conditions.

CBD can be consumed like other cannabinoids—by smoking or vaporizing a CBD-rich flower, eating a CBD-infused edible, swallowing a CBD oil capsule, applying a CBD lotion, or using a CBD tincture under the tongue. The strongest scientific evidence has been in treating a rare form of childhood epilepsy.

Street Names Marijuana: Blunt, Bud, Dope, Ganja, Grass, Green, Herb, Joint, Mary Jane, Pot, Reefer, Trees, Smoke, Sinsemilla, Skunk, and Weed; Hashish: Boom, Gangster, Hash, and Hemp.

How Administered Swallowed or smoked in a joint (hand-rolled cigarette) or pipe. It may also be drunk in tea or eaten as an ingredient in other foods (as when baked in brownies), though with a less predictable effect.

How Users Feel The circumstances in which marijuana is smoked, the communal aspects of its use, and the user's experience, all can affect the way a marijuana-induced high feels.

In low to moderate doses, marijuana typically creates[62]:

- A mild sense of euphoria.
- Slowed thinking and reaction time.
- A dreamy sort of self-absorption.
- Confusion.
- Some impairment in thinking and communicating.
- Heightened sensations of color, sound, and other stimuli.
- Impaired balance and coordination.
- Increased pulse rate, bloodshot eyes, and dry mouth and throat.
- Slowed reaction times.
- Impaired motor skills.
- Increased appetite.
- Diminished short-term memory and problems learning.

Some users—particularly those smoking marijuana for the first time or taking a high dose in an unpleasant or unfamiliar setting—experience acute anxiety, which may be accompanied by a panicky fear of losing control. They may believe that their companions are ridiculing or threatening them and experience a panic attack, a state of intense terror.

All the reactions experienced with low doses are intensified with higher doses, leading to sensory distortion and, in the case of hashish, vivid hallucinations and LSD-like, psychedelic reactions.

The sense of being stoned peaks within half an hour and usually lasts about 3 hours. Even when alterations in perception seem slight, it is not safe to drive a car for as long as 4 to 6 hours after smoking a single joint. The drug remains in the body's fat cells 50 hours or more after use, so people may experience psychoactive effects for several days afterward. Drug tests may produce positive results for days or weeks after last use.

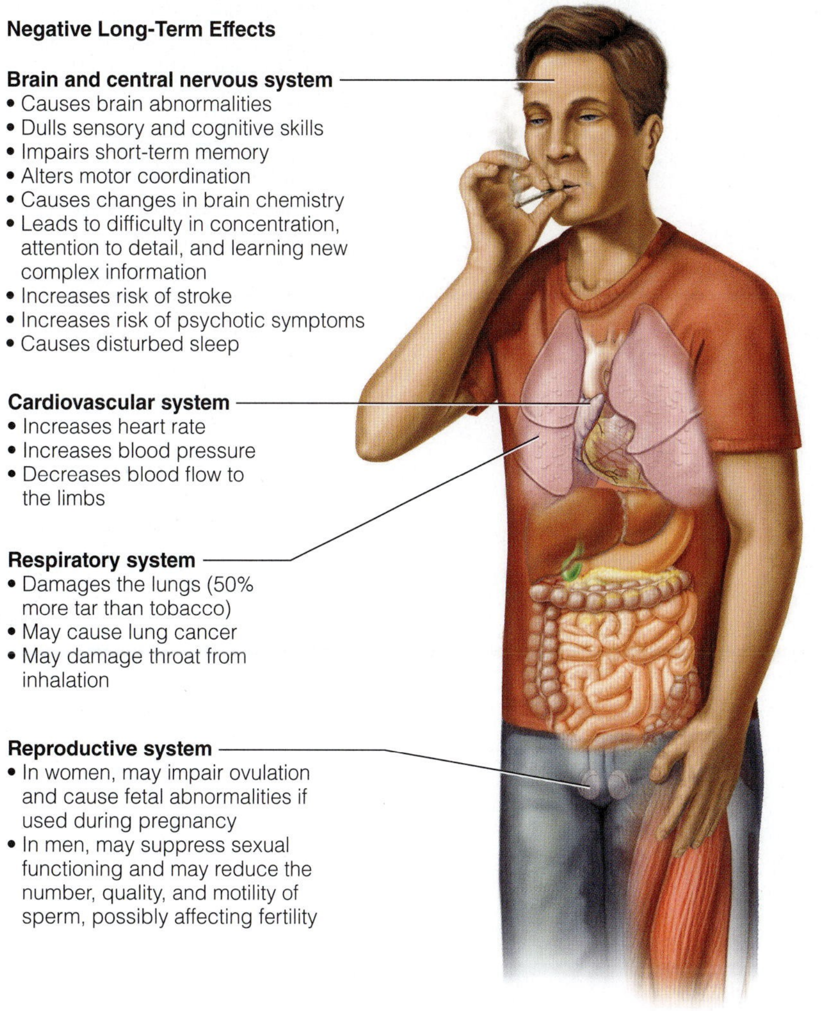

Negative Long-Term Effects

Brain and central nervous system
- Causes brain abnormalities
- Dulls sensory and cognitive skills
- Impairs short-term memory
- Alters motor coordination
- Causes changes in brain chemistry
- Leads to difficulty in concentration, attention to detail, and learning new complex information
- Increases risk of stroke
- Increases risk of psychotic symptoms
- Causes disturbed sleep

Cardiovascular system
- Increases heart rate
- Increases blood pressure
- Decreases blood flow to the limbs

Respiratory system
- Damages the lungs (50% more tar than tobacco)
- May cause lung cancer
- May damage throat from inhalation

Reproductive system
- In women, may impair ovulation and cause fetal abnormalities if used during pregnancy
- In men, may suppress sexual functioning and may reduce the number, quality, and motility of sperm, possibly affecting fertility

FIGURE 12.4 Impact of Marijuana

Marijuana has negative long-term effects on many systems of the body.

Risks and Potential Health Consequences Marijuana produces a range of effects in different organs (see Figure 12.4):

Brain

- Problems with memory and learning.
- Distorted perceptions.
- Difficulty thinking and solving problems.
- Loss of coordination.
- Increased anxiety.
- Panic attacks.
- Impaired verbal fluency, memory, and coordination.
- Disrupted sleep.
- Impaired brain development and possible lower IQ in adolescents and young adults.[63]

- Psychotic symptoms (particularly in young users)[64] and worsening of symptoms in those diagnosed with psychosis.[65]
- Five times greater risk of alcohol abuse and addiction.[66]
- Double the risk of stroke in young adults, even in those with no other risk factors.
- Significant brain abnormalities, including shrinkage of key structures involved in memory, learning, and emotion, that can lead to memory loss, difficulty learning new information, and psychotic symptoms. Younger users seem most susceptible.[67]
- Cognitive impairment. Marijuana lowers performance in tests measuring memory, attention, reaction time, tracking, and motor function. The effects depend on the dose and are highest in the first hour after smoking marijuana or within 1 to 2 hours after oral intake. Frequent or heavy users show greater impairment than those who smoked marijuana an average of once a month.
- Psychological symptoms. Some users experience feelings of anxiety and/or paranoia, with hallucinations and other psychotic symptoms that may last for minutes, hours, or, in some cases, days. Studies have also linked marijuana use with an earlier age of onset and increased incidence of schizophrenia and other psychiatric disorders (discussed in Chapter 2).

Lungs

- Effects similar to those of smoking tobacco, although long-term effects on pulmonary function may vary.
- Frequent respiratory infections.
- Chronic bronchitis.
- Emphysema.

Heart

- Heart attacks and sudden death, even in healthy persons, shortly after smoking marijuana.
- Risk of elevated blood pressure and decreased oxygen supply to the heart muscle.
- If combined with cocaine, potentially deadly increases in heart rate and blood pressure.

Brain and Central Nervous System

- Causes brain abnormalities.
- Dulls sensory and cognitive skills.
- Impairs short-term memory.
- Alters motor coordination.
- Causes changes in brain chemistry.
- Leads to difficulty in concentration, attention to detail, and learning new complex information.
- Increases risk of stroke.
- Increases risk of psychotic symptoms.
- Causes disturbed sleep.

Cardiovascular System

- Increases heart rate.
- Increases blood pressure.
- Decreases blood flow to the limbs.

Respiratory System

- Damages the lungs (50 percent more tar than tobacco).
- May cause lung cancer.
- May damage throat from inhalation.

Reproductive System

- In women, may impair ovulation and cause fetal abnormalities if used during pregnancy.
- In men, may suppress sexual functioning and may reduce the number, quality, and motility of sperm, possibly affecting fertility.

Pregnancy

- Lower birth weight.
- More health problems after birth.
- Impaired motor development in nursing infants whose mothers smoke pot.

Cancer. Marijuana smoke contains known cancer-causing chemicals. Some studies have suggested a link with cancers of the head and neck, lungs, and testicles, but most of the subjects also smoked tobacco, so the findings are inconclusive.

Motor Vehicle Accidents. Fatal crashes have increased among drivers who tested positive for marijuana after the drug was legalized in their states.

Medical Marijuana A growing number of states have passed voter referenda or legislative actions making marijuana available for a variety of medical conditions upon a doctor's recommendation. There is limited scientific evidence supporting the use of cannabis or cannabinoid drugs as a medical therapy. A recent comprehensive meta-analysis of clinical trials of medical marijuana found some benefits for relieving nausea and vomiting related to chemotherapy, specific pain syndromes, and spasticity from multiple sclerosis.[68]

Research has shown little or weak evidence for the use of marijuana in treating conditions such as hepatitis C, Crohn's disease, Parkinson's disease, and Tourette's syndrome. Common adverse effects among patients treated with marijuana included dizziness, dry mouth, nausea, fatigue, sleepiness, euphoria, vomiting, disorientation, drowsiness, confusion, loss of balance, and hallucinations. There is also a risk of dependence.

Legalized Marijuana
Residents of more than 33 states and the District of Columbia are considering or have voted to remove criminal and civil penalties for the adult possession of up to 1 ounce of cannabis. However, the possession and sale of marijuana remain illegal under federal law.

Medical scientists and policy experts are monitoring the effects of marijuana decriminalization on health, safety, crime, and other dimensions of daily life, but the impact is not yet clear. Some see legalized marijuana as no more (or less) perilous than alcohol; others fear that legalization will increase use by young people under age 21, marijuana-related accidents, and serious health consequences. Colorado, for instance, has reported a steep increase in pot-related emergencies.[69]

The American Academy of Pediatrics has officially opposed legalizing marijuana because greater access may lead to greater use by teens and increased risks, including:

- Impaired memory and concentration.
- Interference with learning.
- Lower odds of completing high school or obtaining a college degree.
- Impaired motor control, coordination, and judgment, which may contribute to unintentional deaths and injuries.
- Psychological problems, poorer lung health, and a higher likelihood of drug dependence in adulthood.[70]

✓check-in Do you think marijuana should be legalized in more states?

Dependence
Although marijuana is less addictive than heroin or tobacco, it can cause dependence. One in six of those who start smoking pot at younger ages may become addicted. Young users also show significant impairment in brain development and functioning. Marijuana also increases the risk of respiratory problems, stroke, and cancer in users of all ages.

Withdrawal
Marijuana users can develop a compulsive, often uncontrollable craving for the drug. Stopping after long-term marijuana use can produce *marijuana withdrawal syndrome*, which is characterized by insomnia, restlessness, loss of appetite, and irritability. People who smoke marijuana daily for many years may become aggressive after they stop using it and may relapse to prevent aggression and other symptoms.

Herbal Drugs

Salvia
An herb, **salvia** (*Salvia divinorum*) is grown in southern Mexico and Central and South America. Its main active ingredient, salvinorin A, activates kappa opioid receptors that differ from those activated by the more commonly known opioids, such as heroin and morphine.

Street Names: Diviner's Sage, Magic Mint, Maria Pastora, Sally-D, and Shepherdess's Herb.

How Administered: Although it is traditionally ingested by chewing fresh leaves or drinking their extracted juices, *S. divinorum* can also be dried and smoked as a joint or in a water pipe or vaporized and inhaled.

How Users Feel:

- Hallucinations or "psychotomimetic" episodes (a transient experience that mimics a psychosis) that occur in less than a minute and last less than 30 minutes.
- Emotional swings.
- Laughter and euphoria.
- Feelings of detachment.

Risks and Potential Health Consequences:

- Psychedelic-like changes in visual perception.
- Mood changes.
- Dizziness.
- Slurred speech, emotional swings, and a greatly altered perception of external reality and the self.

Khat
For centuries people in East Africa and the Arabian Peninsula consumed the fresh young leaves of the *Catha edulis* shrub in ways similar to our drinking coffee. Its active ingredients are two controlled substances, cathinone and cathine.

Street Names: Abyssinian Tea, Catha, Chat, and Kat.

How Administered: Chewed.

How Users Feel:

- Less fatigue.
- More energy.
- Reduced appetite.

Risks and Potential Health Consequences:

- Increased risk of death and stroke in those with heart disease.
- With compulsive use, manic behavior, grandiose illusions, paranoia, and hallucinations.

Synthetic Designer Drugs

Unregulated psychoactive substances, often referred to as **designer drugs**, include marijuana-like smoking blends frequently branded as "K2" or "Spice," designer stimulant preparations of powders generally termed "bath salts," and various tablets or capsules frequently described as "party pills" or "research chemicals." Their use on college campuses has fallen in recent years.

✓**check-in** Do you think that synthetic drugs are widely used on your campus?

These compounds, many available legally via the Internet, may be sold as bath salts, plant food, insecticides, chicken feed, and research chemicals, often labeled "not for human consumption." Some are highly toxic industrial chemicals with potentially life-threatening adverse effects.

Specific agents include methoxetamine, sold on the Internet as "legal ketamine"; piperazine derivatives, amphetamine-like compounds known as BZP, TMFPP, or "legal Ecstasy"; and Kratom, a legal plant product derived from a Southeast Asian tree with opium-like effects, as well as the drugs described in the following sections.[71]

Synthetic Marijuana Synthetic versions of the active ingredient in marijuana, developed for medical use, act on the brain like the THC in smoked marijuana but eliminate the need to inhale harmful chemicals. Various herbal mixtures, marketed as safe and legal alternatives to pot yet labeled "not for human consumption," contain dried, shredded plant material and chemical additives. The majority of users are young men in their teens.[72] U.S. poison control centers have experienced an exponential increase in emergency calls regarding synthetic marijuana.

Street Names: Fake Weed, K2, Moon Rocks, Skunk, Spice, and Yucatan Fire.

How Administered: Some products are sold as incense, but they are mainly smoked or drunk in an herbal infusion.

How Users Feel:

- Elevated mood.
- Relaxation.

- Altered perception.
- Effects similar to those of marijuana but in some cases much more intense.

Risks and Potential Health Consequences:

- Confusion.
- Anxiety and paranoia.
- Hallucinations.
- Agitation.
- Extreme nervousness.
- Nausea and vomiting.
- Fast heartbeat.
- Elevated blood pressure.
- Tremors.
- Seizures.
- Heart attack.
- Acute, potentially fatal kidney failure.

Users of synthetic marijuana have required emergency treatment for reactions such as paranoia, anxiety, agitation, high blood pressure, profuse sweating, palpitations, elevated heart rate, dizziness, slowed speech, confusion, muscle rigidity, and catatonia (an inability to respond to verbal or physical stimulation).

✓**check-in** Do you know anyone who has had an adverse reaction to synthetic marijuana?

Synthetic Cathinone "Bath salts" are a new family of drugs that contain one or more synthetic chemicals related to **cathinone**, an amphetamine-like stimulant found naturally in the khat plant. They should not be confused with products like Epsom salts, which have no druglike properties. The majority of users are young men, most often between ages 20 and 29. Bath salts are usually a white or brown crystalline powder in small plastic or foil packages labeled "not for human consumption," may be labeled as "plant food"—or, more recently, as "jewelry cleaner" or "phone screen cleaner"— and sold online and in drug product stores under a variety of brand names.

Street and Brand Names: Bath salts, Bloom, Cloud Nine, Cosmic Blast, Flakka, Ivory Wave, Lunar Wave, Scarface, Vanilla Sky, and White Lightning.

How Administered: Typically swallowed, inhaled, or injected; the worst dangers are

designer drugs Illegally manufactured psychoactive drugs that have dangerous physical and psychological effects.

cathinone An amphetamine-like stimulant derived from the khat plant.

associated with snorting and needle injection. Bath salts contain various amphetamine-like chemicals, such as methylenedioxypyrovalerone (MDPV), mephedrone, and pyrovalerone.

How Users Feel:

- Intense stimulation.
- Alertness.
- Euphoria.
- Increased sociability.
- Heightened sex drive.

Risks and Possible Health Consequences:
The most common synthetic cathinone found in the blood and urine of patients admitted to emergency departments after taking bath salts raises brain dopamine in the same way as cocaine but is at least 10 times stronger. Its effects include.

- Paranoia.
- Agitation.
- Hallucinations.
- Depression.
- Panic attacks.
- Cloudy thinking.
- Break with reality.
- Reduced motor control.
- Increased heart rate and blood pressure.
- Nausea and vomiting.
- Nosebleeds.
- Sweating.
- Insomnia.
- Irritability.
- Dizziness.
- Suicidal thoughts.
- Violent behavior.
- Heart problems (such as racing heart, high blood pressure, and chest pains).
- Kidney failure.
- "Excited delirium," characterized by dehydration, breakdown of skeletal muscle tissue, and kidney failure.
- Suicide; those who survive suicide attempts may suffer long-term psychiatric symptoms.

Club Drugs

A variety of drugs—MDMA, GHB, GBL, ketamine, fentanyl, Rohypnol, and nitrites—called **club drugs**—first became popular among teens and young adults at nightclubs, bars, and raves (i.e., night-long dances often held in warehouses or

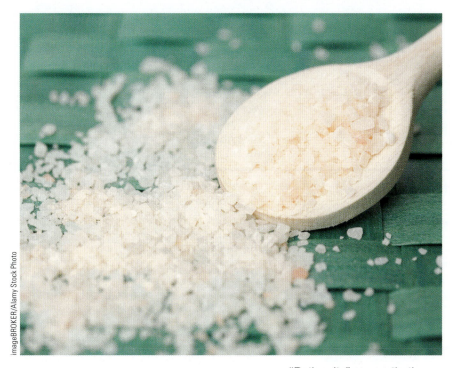

imageBROKER/Alamy Stock Photo

"Bath salts" are synthetic stimulants, often sold legally, that can cause dangerous physical and psychological effects.

other unusual settings). Their use by teenagers has been dropping in recent years.

Young people may take club drugs to relax, energize, and enhance their social interactions, but a large number also experience negative consequences. As many as three in four report side effects such as:

- Profuse sweating.
- Hot and cold flashes.
- Tingling or numbness.
- Blurred vision.
- Trouble sleeping.
- Hallucinations.
- Depression.
- Confusion.
- Anxiety.
- Irritability.
- Paranoia.
- Loss of libido (sex drive).
- Difficulty with their usual daily activities.
- Financial and work troubles.

Ecstasy Methylenedioxymethamphetamine (**MDMA**) is more commonly called **Ecstacy** on the streets. It is a synthetic compound with both stimulant and mildly hallucinogenic properties that belongs to a family of drugs called *enactogens*, which literally means "touching within." MDMA increases the activity of three brain chemicals:

club drugs A variety of drugs including MDMA, GHB, GBL, ketamine, fentanyl, Rohypnol, and nitrites that first became popular at nightclubs, bars, and raves.

MDMA/Ecstacy A synthetic compound, also known as methylenedioxymethamphetamine, that is similar in structure to methamphetamine and has both stimulant and hallucinogenic effects.

dopamine, norepinephrine, and serotonin. Medical emergencies related to the drug have increased 75 percent in recent years. Most Ecstasy users requiring emergency care were between ages 18 and 29.

Street Names: Adam, Clarity, E, Lover's Speed, Peace, Uppers, X, and XTC.

How Administered: Although it can be smoked, inhaled (snorted), or injected, Ecstasy is almost always taken as a pill or tablet. Its effects begin in 45 minutes and last for 3 to 6 hours. Ecstasy pills often contain a variety of other chemicals that increase the danger to users.

How Users Feel:

- Relaxation and euphoria.
- Lower inhibitions.
- Sense of connectedness with others; in some settings, they reveal intimate details of their lives (which they may later regret), and in other settings, they join in collective rejoicing.
- Enhanced sensory experience.
- In rare cases, visual distortions, sudden mood changes, or psychotic reactions.
- In regular users, depression and anxiety the week after taking MDMA.

The psychological effects of Ecstasy become less intriguing with repeated use, and the physical side effects become more uncomfortable.

Risks and Potential Health Consequences: Ecstasy is more likely than other stimulants, such as methamphetamine, to kill young, healthy people between the ages of 16 and 24 who are not known to be regular drug users. Researchers theorize that young people's brains, which are still developing in late adolescence and early adulthood, may be more vulnerable to the effects of the drug.

Ecstasy poses risks similar to those of cocaine and amphetamines, including[73]:

- Long-lasting confusion.
- Depression.
- Problems with attention, memory, and sleep.
- Drug craving.
- Severe anxiety.
- Paranoia.
- Muscle tension.
- Involuntary teeth clenching.
- Nausea and vomiting.
- Dizziness.
- Blurred vision.
- Rapid eye movement.

- Faintness.
- Chills.
- Sweating.
- Less interest in sex.
- Increases in heart rate and blood pressure, which pose a special risk for people with circulatory or heart disease.
- When combined with extended physical exertion, like dancing, hyperthermia (severe overheating), severe dehydration, serious increases in blood pressure, stroke, and heart attack.
- Without sufficient water, dehydration and heat stroke, which can be fatal; individuals with high blood pressure, heart trouble, or liver or kidney disease are in the greatest danger.
- Fatal damage and death when users drink large amounts of water to counteract drug-induced hyperthermia.
- Acute hepatitis, which can lead to liver failure; even after liver transplantation, the mortality rate for individuals with this condition is 50 percent.
- If combined with the antidepressants known as SSRIs (see Chapter 2), which modulate the mood-altering brain chemical serotonin, jaw-clenching, nausea, tremors, and, in extreme cases, potentially fatal elevations in body temperature.
- Although not a sexual stimulant (if anything, MDMA has the opposite effect), strong feelings of intimacy that may lead to risky sexual behavior.
- Risks to a developing fetus, including a greater likelihood of heart and skeletal abnormalities and long-term learning and memory impairments in children born to women who used MDMA during pregnancy.

✓**check-in** Do you think that Ecstasy is widely used on your campus?

Herbal Ecstasy   Herbal Ecstasy, also known as Cloud Nine, Herbal Bliss, and Herbal X, is a mixture of stimulants such as ephedrine, pseudoephedrine, and caffeine. Sold in tablet or capsule form as a "natural" and safe alternative to Ecstasy, its ingredients vary greatly. Herbal Ecstasy can have dangerous and unpleasant side effects, including stroke, heart irregularities, and a disfiguring skin condition.

GHB and GBL   Once sold in health-food stores for its muscle-building and alleged fat-burning properties, **gamma hydroxybutyrate (GHB)**—also known as G, Georgia Home Boy, Grievous Bodily Harm, Liquid Ecstasy, Liquid X, Soap, and Scoop—was banned because of its effects on the brain and nervous system. The main ingredient is **gamma butyrolactone (GBL)**, an industrial solvent often used to strip floors, which converts into GHB once ingested. GHB acts as a sedative while producing feelings of euphoria and heightened sexuality as well as confusion and impaired memory. Because of its amnesic properties, GHB has been used as a "date-rape" drug, similar to Rohypnol. Alcohol intensifies its effects, which typically last up to 4 hours.

Large doses can cause someone to pass out in 15 minutes and fall into a coma within half an hour. Death can occur. Other side effects include aggressive behavior, nausea, amnesia, hallucinations, decreased heart rate, convulsions, and sometimes blackouts. Long-term use at high doses can lead to a withdrawal reaction: rapid heartbeat, tremor, insomnia, anxiety, and psychotic thoughts and hallucinations that last a few days to a week.[75]

GHB is addictive. Users who attempt to quit may experience significant withdrawal symptoms, including anxiety, tremors, and insomnia. Most symptoms decrease within 1 to 2 weeks of cessation, but severe psychological effects can last for weeks to months.

Nitrites Nitrites (amyl, butyl, and isobutyl nitrite) are clear, amber liquids that have had a history of abuse for more than three decades, especially in gay and bisexual men. Popular in dance clubs, they are used recreationally for a high feeling, a slowed sense of time, a carefree sense of well-being, and intensified sexual experiences.

Sold in small glass ampoules containing individual doses, nitrites are usually inhaled and rapidly absorbed into the bloodstream. Users feel their physiological and psychological impact in seconds. Acute adverse effects include headache, dizziness, a drop in blood pressure, changes in heart rate, increased pressure within the eye, and skin flushing. Some individuals develop respiratory irritation and cough, sneezing, or difficulty breathing. Chronic use can lead to crusty skin lesions and chemical burns around the nose, mouth, and lips.

Stimulants

Central nervous system **stimulants** are drugs that increase activity in some portion of the brain or spinal cord. Some stimulants increase motor activity and enhance mental alertness, and some combat mental fatigue. Amphetamine, methamphetamine, caffeine, cocaine, and khat are stimulants. As discussed on page 400, some college students use stimulant medications prescribed for others to boost their concentration and alertness.

Amphetamines Drugs that trigger the release of epinephrine (adrenaline) and therefore stimulate the central nervous system include **amphetamines** such as benzedrine, dextroamphetamin, methamphetamine, Desoxyn, and related *uppers* such as the prescription drugs methylphenidate (Ritalin), pemoline (Cylert), and phenmetrazine (Preludin). They were once widely prescribed for weight control because they suppress appetite, but they have emerged as a global danger.

Street Names: Bennies, Copilots, Crank, Dex, Meth, and Speed.

How Administered: Taken orally or injected.

How Users Feel:

- Agitated and restless.
- Talkative, moody, and irritable.
- Confused and anxious.
- Confident in one's ability to perform exceptionally well—although amphetamines do not boost performance or thinking.
- Violent.

If taken intravenously, a rush of elation and confidence as well as adverse effects, occur, including:

- Tremors.
- Rambling or incoherent speech.
- Headache.
- Palpitations.
- Paranoia.
- Excessive sweating.
- Unusual perceptions, such as ringing in the ears, a sensation of insects crawling on the skin, or hearing one's name called.
- High blood pressure.
- Convulsions.
- Cardiac arrest.

Risks and Possible Health Consequences:

- Dependence with episodic or daily use.
- Bingeing—taking high doses over a period of several days—can lead to an extremely intense and unpleasant *crash*, characterized by a craving for the drug, shakiness, irritability, anxiety, and depression.

gamma hydroxybutyrate (GHB) A brain messenger chemical that stimulates the release of human growth hormone; commonly abused for its high and its alleged ability to trim fat and build muscles. Also known as "blue nitro" or the "date rape drug."

gamma butyrolactone (GBL) The main ingredient in gamma hydroxybutyrate (GHB); once ingested, GBL converts to GHB and can cause the ingestor to lose consciousness.

stimulants Agents, such as drugs, that temporarily relieve drowsiness, help in the performance of repetitive tasks, and improve capacity for work.

amphetamines Any of a class of stimulants that trigger the release of epinephrine, which stimulates the central nervous system; users experience a state of hyperalertness and energy, followed by a crash as the drug wears off.

Amphetamine intoxication can lead to:

- Feelings of grandiosity, anxiety, tension, hypervigilance, anger, social hypersensitivity, fighting, jitteriness or agitation, paranoia, and impaired judgment in social or occupational functioning.
- Increased heart rate, dilated pupils, elevated blood pressure, perspiration or chills, and nausea or vomiting.
- Less frequent effects, such as speeding up or slowing down of physical movement; muscular weakness; impaired breathing, chest pain, heart arrhythmia; confusion, seizures, impaired movements or muscle tone; or even coma.
- In high doses, a rapid or irregular heartbeat, tremors, loss of coordination, and collapse.

The long-term effects of amphetamine abuse include:

- Malnutrition.
- Skin disorders.
- Ulcers.
- Insomnia.
- Depression.
- Vitamin deficiencies.
- Brain damage that results in speech and thought disturbances.
- Sexual dysfunction.
- Withdrawal, characterized by fatigue, disturbing dreams, much more or less sleep than usual, increased appetite, and speeding up or slowing down of physical movements; depression and irritability may persist for months.
- Significantly increased risk of suicide.[74]

··

✓**check-in** Do you think many students at your school have tried stimulants?

··

Methamphetamine Methamphetamine, an addictive stimulant that is less expensive and possibly more addictive than cocaine or heroin, has become America's leading problem drug. More than 12 million Americans have tried methamphetamine, and 1.5 million are regular users, according to federal estimates. The estimated annual economic cost of methamphetamine is $23.4 billion.

Made in illegal laboratories, methamphetamine is chemically related to amphetamine, but its effects on the central nervous system are greater. The release of large amounts of dopamine creates a sensation of euphoria, increased self-esteem, and alertness. Users also report a marked increase in sexual appetite, which often leads to risky sexual behaviors while under the drug's influence.

Street Names: Chalk, Crank, Crystal, Fire, Meth, and Speed; methamphetamine hydrochloride, clear chunky crystals resembling ice that can be inhaled by smoking, is called Crystal, Glass, Ice, and Tina.

How Administered: Snorted, smoked, injected, or ingested orally.

How Users Feel:

- Smoking or injection causes an intense pleasurable sensation, called a rush or flash, that lasts only a few minutes.
- Oral or intranasal use produces a high but not a rush.
- Increased wakefulness and physical activity.
- Decreased appetite.
- Increased breathing, heart rate, blood pressure, and temperature.
- Irregular heartbeat.

Risks and Possible Health Consequences: Users may become addicted quickly, using more methamphetamine more and more frequently. Despair and suicidal thinking can develop when the stimulant effect wears off.

Even small amounts of methamphetamine can increase wakefulness and physical activity, depress appetite, and raise body temperature. Other effects on the central nervous system include[75]:

- Irritability.
- Insomnia.
- Confusion.
- Aggressive behavior.
- Tremors.
- Convulsions.
- Anxiety.
- Paranoia.
- Intellectual impairment.
- Intense itching leading to skin sores from scratching.
- Depression.
- Increased heart rate and blood pressure.
- Irreversible damage to blood vessels in the brain, producing strokes.
- Damage to the frontal cortex of developing teen brains.[76]

- Respiratory problems.
- Irregular heartbeat.
- Extreme loss of appetite and weight.
- Elevated body (and probably brain) temperature, sometimes resulting in convulsions and high fevers that can be fatal.
- Inability to cope with everyday problems.
- High risk of psychotic symptoms, such as hallucinations and delusions that may persist for months or years after use stops.
- "Meth mouth," with teeth turning a grayish-brown, twisting, falling out, and taking on a peculiar texture; about 40 percent of meth users have serious dental problems.
- Risky sex; meth has been linked to an increase in unsafe practices, including needle-sharing with partners, which has led to a spike in HIV and hepatitis C infections in gay communities.
- Abnormalities in brain regions associated with selective attention and in those associated with memory; the brain may recover somewhat after months of abstinence, but problems often remain.
- With long-term use, changes in brain chemistry that may lead to compulsive drug-seeking and that make addiction especially hard to overcome.
- Significantly increased risk of Parkinson's disease.
- Even after stopping use, chronic apathy and anhedonia (inability to experience pleasure).

The Toll on Society: Law enforcement officials consider methamphetamine their biggest drug problem. Meth addicts are pouring into prisons and recovery centers at an ever-increasing rate. "Meth babies" are crowding the foster-care system. Meth-making operations, which have been uncovered in all 50 states, involve the release of poisonous gases and toxic waste that is often dumped down household drains, in backyards, or by the side of the road. The cost of cleaning up the environmental impacts of meth is a growing problem for many communities.

OTC cold medicines (ephedrine and pseudo-ephedrine) are commonly used in meth production, which is one reason for federal and state restrictions on their sale.

✓**check-in** Do you believe that methamphetamine can be a threat to a community?

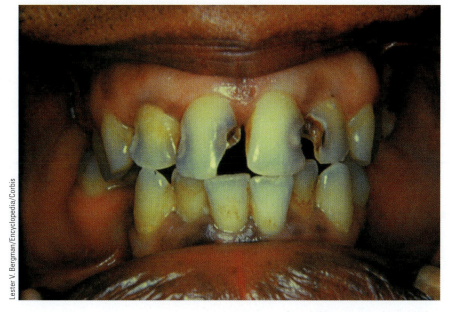

Lester V. Bergman/Encyclopedia/Corbis

In addition to causing respiratory problems, brain damage, and mental impairment, methamphetamine damages teeth. This is how "meth mouth" looks.

Withdrawal: Methamphetamine addiction is difficult to treat. As with cocaine, coming off methamphetamine causes intense distress, so users often seek out the drug to relieve their pain. Treatment usually requires the intervention of the patient's family as well as a substance abuse specialist team experienced in treating individuals with methamphetamine addiction.

Standard substance abuse treatment methods such as education, behavior therapy, individual and family counseling, and support groups may be effective for some. Methamphetamine abusers often use other illicit drugs as well, a problem that can be addressed as part of a comprehensive program.

Cocaine
A white crystalline powder, **cocaine** is extracted from the leaves of the South American coca plant.

Street Names: Blow, Bump, C, Coke, Crack, Flake, Lady, Rock, Snow, and Toot.

How Administered: Usually mixed with various sugars and local anesthetics like lidocaine and procaine, cocaine powder is generally inhaled. When sniffed or snorted, cocaine anesthetizes the nerve endings in the nose and relaxes the lung's bronchial muscles.

Cocaine can be dissolved in water and injected intravenously. The drug is rapidly metabolized by the liver, so the high is relatively brief, typically lasting only about 20 minutes. This means that users commonly inject the drug repeatedly, increasing the risk of infection and damage to their veins.

cocaine A white crystalline powder extracted from the leaves of the coca plant that stimulates the central nervous system and produces a brief period of euphoria followed by a depression.

Cocaine alkaloid, or *freebase*, is obtained by removing the hydrochloride salt from cocaine powder. *Freebasing* is smoking the fumes of the alkaloid form of cocaine. *Crack*, pharmacologically identical to freebase, is a cheap, easy-to-use, widely available, smokable, and potent form of cocaine named for the popping sound it makes when burned. Because it is absorbed rapidly into the bloodstream and large doses reach the brain very quickly, it is particularly dangerous. However, its low price and easy availability have made it a common drug of abuse in poor urban areas.

How Users Feel: A powerful stimulant to the central nervous system, cocaine targets several chemical sites in the brain, producing:

- Feelings of soaring well-being.
- Boundless energy.
- Restlessness and anxiety, although users feel that they have enormous physical and mental ability.

After a brief period of euphoria, users slump into a depression. They often go on cocaine binges, lasting from a few hours to several days, and consume large quantities of cocaine.

Crack cocaine is produced by mixing cocaine with baking soda and water and then heated to produce small chunks or rocks, which can be smoked. It was dubbed "crack" because smoking rocks produces a crackling sound. Crack cocaine can be injected as well as smoked. Dependence develops quickly. As soon as crack users come down from one high, they want more crack. Whereas heroin addicts may shoot up several times a day, crack addicts need another hit within minutes. Thus, a crack habit can quickly become more expensive than heroin addiction.

··

✓**check-in** What do you think are the dangers of crack cocaine?

··

Risks and Potential Health Consequences: Cocaine dependence is an easy habit to acquire. With repeated use, the brain becomes tolerant of the drug's stimulant effects, and users must take more of it to get high. Those who smoke or inject cocaine can develop dependence within weeks. Those who sniff cocaine may not become dependent on the drug for months or years. It is thought that 5 to 20 percent of all coke users—a group as large as the estimated total number of heroin addicts—are dependent on the drug.

The physical effects of cocaine use include:

- Narrowed blood vessels.
- Dilated pupils.
- Elevated or lowered blood pressure.
- Perspiration or chills.
- Increased body temperature.
- Nausea and vomiting.
- Speeding up or slowing down of physical activity.
- Muscular weakness.
- Impaired breathing.
- Chest pain.
- Impaired movements or muscle tone.
- With prolonged snorting, ulceration of the mucous membrane of the nose and damage to the nasal septum (the membrane between the nostrils) severe enough to cause it to collapse.
- Sexual side effects. At low doses, delayed orgasm and heightened sensory awareness. With regular use, problems maintaining erections and ejaculating, low sperm counts, less active sperm, more abnormal sperm than in nonusers. Both male and female chronic cocaine users tend to lose interest in sex and have difficulty reaching orgasm.
- Increased risk of stroke, bleeding in the brain, coma, and potentially fatal brain seizures.
- Psychiatric or neurological complications with repeated or high doses, including impaired judgment, hyperactivity, panic attacks, nonstop babbling, feelings of suspicion and paranoia, and violent behavior (see Figure 12.5). The brain never learns to tolerate cocaine's negative effects; users may become incoherent and paranoid and may experience unusual sensations.
- Damage to the liver and lungs in freebasers. Smoking crack causes bronchitis and may promote the transmission of HIV through burned and bleeding lips. Some smokers have died of respiratory complications, such as pulmonary edema (buildup of fluid in the lungs).
- Rapid rise in heart rate and blood pressure, which can trigger the symptoms of a heart attack in young people
- Other cardiac complications, including arrhythmia (disruption of heart rhythm), angina (chest pain), and acute myocardial infarction (heart attack).
- Dangers to pregnant women and their babies, including miscarriages, developmental disorders, and life-threatening complications during birth; reduced fetal oxygen supply may

interfere with the development of the fetal nervous system.

- Greatly increased risk of suicide.

The combination of alcohol and cocaine is particularly lethal. The liver combines the two agents and manufactures cocaethylene, which intensifies cocaine's euphoric effects, while possibly increasing the risk of sudden death. Cocaine users who inject the drug and share needles put themselves at risk for another potentially lethal problem: HIV infection.

Withdrawal: When addicted individuals stop using cocaine, they often become depressed. This may lead to further cocaine use to alleviate depression. Other symptoms of cocaine withdrawal include:

- Fatigue.
- Vivid and disturbing dreams.
- Excessive or inadequate sleep.
- Irritability.
- Increased appetite.
- Physical slowing down or speeding up.

The initial crash may last 1 to 3 days after cutting down or stopping heavy use of cocaine. Some individuals become violent, paranoid, and suicidal.

Withdrawal symptoms usually reach a peak 2 to 4 days after cutting down or stopping heavy use of cocaine, although depression, anxiety, irritability, lack of pleasure in usual activities, and low-level cravings may continue for weeks. As memories of the crash fade, the desire for cocaine intensifies. For many weeks after stopping, individuals may feel an intense craving for the drug.

Treatment: Overcoming an addiction to cocaine or another stimulant drug can be challenging. The FDA has not approved any medications for addictions to cocaine and other stimulants, but several drugs have shown promise. These include Antabuse, widely used for alcohol dependence; the muscle relaxant baclofen (Lioresal); the anticonvulsant topiramate (Topamax); and the stimulant modafinil (Provigil), used to treat narcolepsy. Among the behavioral approaches that have shown the greatest success are contingency management, which uses tangible rewards, such as vouchers for movies, to encourage abstinence, and the Matrix Model, which combines a 12-Step program, behavioral therapy, family education, and individual counseling. Exercise may help reduce craving and impulsivity.[77]

Depressants

Depressants depress the central nervous system, reduce activity, and induce relaxation, drowsiness,

Central nervous system
- Repeated use or high dosages may cause severe psychological problems
- Suppresses desire for food, sex, and sleep
- Can cause strokes, seizures, and neurological damage

Nose
- Damages mucous membrane

Cardiovascular system
- Increases blood pressure by constricting blood vessels
- Causes irregular heartbeat
- Damages heart tissue

Respiratory system
- Freebasing causes lung damage
- Overdose can lead to respiratory arrest

Reproductive system
- In men, affects ability to maintain erections and to ejaculate; also causes sperm abnormalities
- In women, may affect ability to carry pregnancy to term

FIGURE 12.5 Some Effects of Cocaine on the Body

or sleep. They include the benzodiazepines and barbiturates, the opioids, and alcohol.

Benzodiazepines and Barbiturates

These depressants are the sedative-hypnotics, also known as anxiolytic or antianxiety drugs. They include chlordiazepoxide (Librium), diazepam (Valium), oxazepam (Serax), lorazepam (Ativan), flurazepam (Dalmane), and alprazolam (Xanax). Benzodiazepines and barbiturates are most often prescribed for tension, muscular strain, sleep problems, anxiety, panic attacks, and anesthesia. They are also used to treat alcohol withdrawal. As prescriptions for these agents have increased, so have deaths from overdoses of Xanax, Valium, Ativan, and other sedatives, which can slow breathing, particularly if taken with alcohol or narcotics such as Oxycontin.[78]

Benzodiazepine sleeping pills have largely replaced the **barbiturates**, which were used medically in the past for inducing relaxation and sleep, relieving tension, and treating epileptic seizures. These drugs are usually taken by mouth in tablet, capsule, or liquid form. When used as a general anesthetic, benzodiazepines are administered intravenously. They differ widely in their mechanism of action, absorption rate, and metabolism, but all produce similar intoxication and withdrawal symptoms.

benzodiazepine An anti-anxiety drug that depresses the central nervous system, reduces activity, and induces relaxation, drowsiness, or sleep; often prescribed to relieve tension, muscular strain, sleep problems, anxiety, and panic attacks; also used as an anesthetic and in the treatment of alcohol withdrawal.

barbiturates Anti-anxiety drugs that depress the central nervous system, reduce activity, and induce relaxation, drowsiness, or sleep; often prescribed to relieve tension and treat epileptic seizures or as a general anesthetic.

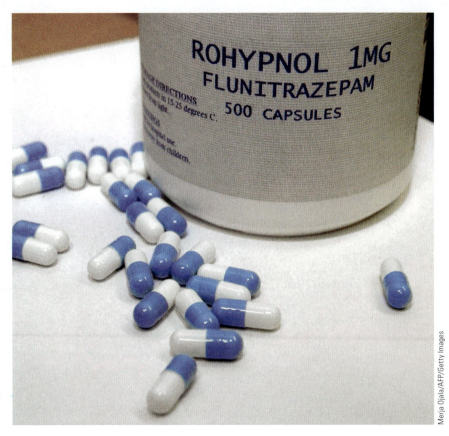

Merja Ojala/AFP/Getty Images

Because Rohypnol is colorless, tasteless, and odorless, it can be added to beverages without your knowledge.

Rohypnol, a trade name for flunitrazepam (called Circles, Forget-Me Pill, Lunch Money, Mexican Valium, Mind Eraser, Pings, R2, Reynolds, Rib, Roach, Rocha, Roofies, Rope, Rophie, Ruffles, Trip-And-Fall, and Wolfs) is one of the benzodiazepines that has been of particular concern for the past few years because of its abuse in date rape. When mixed with alcohol, Rohypnol, which is flavorless and odorless, can incapacitate victims and prevent them from resisting sexual assault. It produces "anterograde amnesia," which means individuals may not remember events they experienced while under the effects of the drug.

How Users Feel:

- Reduced or relieved tension with low doses.
- Loosening of sexual or aggressive inhibitions with increasing doses.
- Rapid mood changes.
- Impaired judgment.
- Impaired social or occupational functioning.

Risks and Potential Health Consequences: All sedative-hypnotic drugs can produce physical and psychological dependence within 2 to 4 weeks. A complication specific to sedatives is *cross-tolerance* (cross-addiction), which occurs

when users develop tolerance for one sedative or become dependent on it and develop tolerance for other sedatives as well. Adverse effects include[79]:

- Decreased blood pressure.
- Drowsiness and sedation.
- Visual disturbances.
- Headache.
- Slowed breathing and heart rate.
- Dizziness.
- Blacking out.
- Confusion.
- Urinary retention.
- Digestive problems.
- Changes in mood or behavior, such as inappropriate sexual or aggressive acts.
- Mood swings.
- Impaired judgment.
- Slurred speech.
- Poor coordination.
- Unsteady gait.
- Involuntary eye movements.
- Impaired attention or memory.
- Stupor or coma.

Sedative-hypnotic drugs and alcohol together have a synergistic effect that can be dangerous or even lethal. For example, an individual's driving ability, already impaired by alcohol, will be made even worse, increasing the risk of an accident. Alcohol in combination with sedative-hypnotics leads to respiratory depression and may result in respiratory arrest and death.

Withdrawal: Regular users of any of these drugs who become physically dependent should not try to cut down or quit on their own. If they try to quit suddenly, they run the risk of seizures, coma, and death.

Withdrawal from sedative-hypnotic drugs may range from relatively mild discomfort to a severe syndrome with grand mal seizures, depending on the degree of dependence. Symptoms include:

- Malaise or weakness.
- Sweating.
- Rapid pulse.
- Coarse tremors (of the hands, tongue, or eyelids).
- Insomnia.
- Nausea or vomiting.

- Temporary hallucinations or illusions.
- Physical restlessness.
- Anxiety or irritability.
- Grand mal seizures.

Withdrawal may begin within 2 to 3 days after stopping drug use, and symptoms may persist for many weeks.

Opioids The **opioids** include opium and its derivatives (morphine, codeine, and heroin) and synthetic drugs that have similar sleep-inducing and pain-relieving properties. The opioids come from a resin taken from the seedpod of the Asian poppy. Synthetic opioids, such as meperidine (Demerol), methadone, and propoxyphene (Darvon), are synthesized in a chemical laboratory. Whether natural or synthetic, these drugs are powerful *narcotics*, or painkillers.

Heroin use has soared in the last decade, with an estimated 914,000 reported users in the United States and a spike in overdose deaths.[80] Male addicts outnumber female addicts by three to one. Among people ages 18 to 25, the percentage of heroin users who inject the drug has doubled in the past decade. Nearly 80 percent of people who recently started using heroin had previously used prescription pain relievers illegally.[81] Among the risk factors for transitioning to heroine are starting pill use at an early age, using pills to get high rather than to treat a health problem, and injecting or snorting a prescription opiate.[82]

Street Names: Brown Sugar, China White, Dope, H, Horse, Junk, Skag, Smack, and White Horse.

How Administered: Heroin users typically inject the drug into their veins. However, individuals who experiment with recreational drugs often prefer *skin-popping* (subcutaneous injection) rather than *mainlining* (intravenous injection); they also may snort heroin as a powder or dissolve it and inhale the vapors. To try to avoid addiction, some users begin by *chipping*, taking small or intermittent doses. Regardless of the method of administration, tolerance can develop rapidly.

Morphine, used as a painkiller and anesthetic, acts primarily on the central nervous system, eyes, and digestive tract. By producing mental clouding, drowsiness, and euphoria, it does not decrease the physical sensation of pain as much as it alters a person's awareness of the pain; in effect, the morphine user no longer cares about the pain.

How Users Feel: All opioids relax the user. When injected, they can produce an immediate

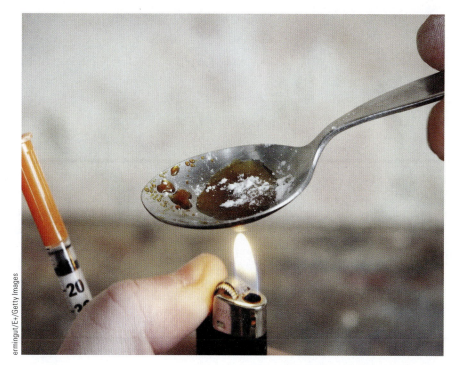

ermingut/E+/Getty Images

Opioid drugs, made from the Asian poppy, come in both legal and illegal forms. All are highly addictive.

rush (high) that lasts 10 to 30 minutes. For 2 to 6 hours thereafter, users may feel indifferent, lethargic, and drowsy; they may slur their words and have problems paying attention, remembering, and going about their normal routine. The primary attractions of heroin are the euphoria and pain relief it produces. However, some people experience very unpleasant feelings, such as anxiety and fear. Other effects include:

- Sensation of warmth or heaviness.
- Clouded thinking.
- Itching.
- Alternate wakeful and drowsy states.
- Dry mouth.
- Facial flushing.
- Nausea and vomiting (particularly in first-time users).

Risks and Potential Health Consequences: Addiction is common. Almost all regular users of opioids rapidly develop drug dependence, which can lead to lethargy, weight loss, loss of sex drive, and the continual effort to avoid withdrawal symptoms through repeated drug administration. Users continue taking opioids as much to avoid the discomfort of withdrawal, a classic sign of opioid addiction, as to experience pleasure. In addition, they may experience adverse effects, including[83]:

- Anxiety.
- Insomnia.

opioids Drugs that have sleep-inducing and pain-relieving properties, including opium and its derivatives and nonopioid, synthetic drugs.

- Restlessness.
- Craving for the drug.
- Constricted pupils (although pupils may dilate from a severe overdose).
- Drowsiness.
- Slurred speech.
- Impaired attention or memory.
- Collapsed veins.
- Infection of the lining and valves in the heart.
- Pneumonia.
- Liver or kidney disease.
- In pregnant women, increased risk of miscarriage, stillbirth, or low birth weight; babies born to addicted mothers experience withdrawal symptoms after birth.

Morphine affects blood pressure, heart rate, and blood circulation in the brain. Both morphine and heroin slow the respiratory system; overdoses can cause fatal respiratory arrest.

Over time, users who inject opioids may develop infections of the heart lining and valves, skin abscesses, and lung congestion. Infections from unsterile solutions, syringes, and shared needles can lead to hepatitis, tetanus, liver disease, and HIV. Depression is common and may be both an antecedent and a risk factor for needle sharing.

Heroin overdose deaths have skyrocketed in recent years, quadrupling since 2000. More than 70,200 Americans died from drug overdoses in 2017, a twofold increase in a single decade.[84]

Withdrawal: If a regular user stops taking an opioid, withdrawal begins within 6 to 12 hours. The intensity of the symptoms depends on the degree of the addiction; they may grow stronger for 24 to 72 hours and gradually subside over a period of 7 to 14 days, though some symptoms, such as insomnia, may persist for several months. Individuals may develop craving for an opioid, irritability, nausea or vomiting, muscle aches, runny nose or eyes, dilated pupils, sweating, diarrhea, yawning, fever, and insomnia. Opioid withdrawal is usually not life threatening.

....
✓**check-in** Do you view heroin addicts as different from other drug users?
....

Fentanyl A synthetic narcotic, fentanyl (the generic name for Sublimaze) was developed as an anesthetic. It may be 50 to 100 times more potent than morphine. Injected when used in surgery,

hallucinogens Drugs that cause hallucinations.

LSD (lysergic acid diethylamide) A synthetic psychoactive substance originally developed to explore mental illness.

fentanyl (called Apache, Cash, China Girl, China White, Dance Fever, Friend, Goodfella, Jackpot, Murder 8, Tango, and TNT) is usually snorted or smoked by abusers. It depresses the respiratory system, decreases blood pressure and heart rate, and slows the digestive tract, causing constipation.

Side effects include nausea, dizziness, delirium, decreased blood pressure, vomiting, blurred vision, and respiratory and cardiac arrest, which can be fatal. Fentanyl is often combined with other drugs, especially heroin, which increases the potential for adverse reactions. The potential for addiction is extremely high.

Hallucinogens

The drugs known as **hallucinogens** produce vivid and unusual changes in thought, feeling, and perception. Hallucinogens do not produce dependence in the same way as cocaine or heroin. Individuals who have an unpleasant experience after trying a hallucinogen may stop using the drug completely without suffering withdrawal symptoms. Others continue regular or occasional use because they enjoy the effects.

LSD (lysergic acid diethylamide), commonly known as acid, was initially developed as a tool to explore mental illness. It became popular in the 1960s and resurfaced among teenagers in the 1990s. Its street names include Acid, Blotter, Blue Heaven, Cubes, Microdot, and Yellow Sunshine. LSD is taken orally, usually blotted onto pieces of paper that are held in the mouth or chewed along with another substance, such as a sugar cube. Peyote (whose active ingredient is mescaline) is another hallucinogen, but it is much less commonly used in this country.

Its health effects include:

- Rapid mood swings.
- Distorted perceptions.
- Impaired rational thinking and ability to communicate.
- Dry mouth.
- Sweating.
- Numbness, weakness, tremors, and enlarged pupils.
- Frightening flashbacks.
- Ongoing visual disturbances.
- Paranoia.

Dissociative Drugs

Drugs such as PCP (phencyclidine) and ketamine, initially developed as general anesthetics for surgery, distort perceptions of sight and sound and produce feelings of dissociation or detachment from the environment and self. They alter distribution of the neurotransmitter glutamate—which is involved in perception of pain, responses to the environment, and memory—in the brain.

Because these mind-altering effects are not hallucinations, scientists refer to PCP and ketamine as "dissociative anesthetics." High doses of dextromethorphan, a widely available cough suppressant, and the herb salvia can produce effects similar to those of PCP and ketamine.

Ketamine Ketamine—called K, Special-K, and Vitamin K—is an anesthetic used by veterinarians. When cooked, dried, and ground into powder for snorting, ketamine blocks chemical messengers in the brain that carry sensory input. As a result, the brain fills the void with hallucinations. Users may report an "out-of-body" experience, with distorted perceptions of time and space. The effects typically begin within 30 minutes and last for approximately 2 hours.

Ketamine has become common in clubs and has been used as a date-rape drug. Low doses can cause:

- Impaired attention and memory.
- Anxiety.
- Agitation.
- Paranoia.
- Vomiting.

Higher doses can cause:

- Delirium.
- Amnesia.
- Impaired motor function.
- High blood pressure.
- Depression.
- Potentially deadly breathing problems.

Repeated ketamine use can be addictive, and even a single use can occasionally produce audiovisual "flashbacks," similar to those described by PCP users, and long-term memory loss.

PCP The illicit drug **phencyclidine (PCP)** has a brand name Sernyl; and street names Angel Dust, Hog, Love Boat, and Peace Pill. It is manufactured as a tablet, capsule, liquid, flake, spray, or crystal-like white powder that can be swallowed, smoked, sniffed, or injected. Sometimes it is sprinkled on crack, marijuana, tobacco, or parsley and smoked. A fine-powdered form of PCP can be snorted or injected.

PCP use peaked in the 1970s, but it remains a popular drug of abuse in both inner-city ghettos and suburban high schools. Users often think that the PCP they take together with another illegal psychoactive substance, such as amphetamines, cocaine, or hallucinogens, is responsible for the highs they feel, so they seek it out specifically.

The effects of PCP are utterly unpredictable. It may trigger violent behavior or irreversible psychosis the first time it is used, or the 20th time, or never. In low doses, PCP produces changes similar to those produced by other psychoactive drugs, including:

- Hallucinations.
- Delusions.
- Feelings of emptiness or numbness.
- Impaired thinking.
- Anxiety.
- Increased breathing rate, blood pressure, and heart rate.
- Shallow breathing.
- Facial redness.
- Sweating.
- Numbness in hands and feet.
- Problems with coordination and movement.

Higher doses may produce:

- A stupor that lasts several days.
- Lower heart rate and blood pressure.
- Paranoia.
- Dizziness.
- Nausea and vomiting.
- Blurred vision.
- Eye flickering.
- Drooling.
- Loss of balance.
- Violence.
- Self-injury.
- Suicidal thoughts.
- Seizures, coma.
- Death.

Some people experience repetitive motor movements (such as facial grimacing), hallucinations, and paranoia. Suicide is a definite risk. Intoxication typically lasts 4 to 6 hours, but some effects can linger for several days. Delirium may occur within 24 hours of taking PCP or after recovery from an overdose and can last as long as a week.

phencyclidine (PCP)
A synthetic psychoactive substance that produces effects similar to those of other psychoactive drugs when swallowed, smoked, sniffed, or injected and also may trigger unpredictable behavioral changes.

Inhalants

Inhalants or *deliriants* (called Poppers, Snappers, or Whippets) are chemicals that produce vapors with psychoactive effects. The most commonly abused inhalants are solvents, aerosols, model-airplane glue, fabric protectors, cleaning fluids, and petroleum products such as kerosene and butane. Some anesthetics and nitrous oxide (laughing gas) are also abused.

✓**check-in** Do you know anyone who experimented with inhalants when they were younger?

Only alcohol is a more widely used intoxicant among preteens and teens. Young people who have been treated for mental health problems, have a history of foster care, or already abuse other drugs have an increased risk of abusing or becoming dependent on inhalants. In addition, adolescents who first begin using inhalants at an early age are more likely to become dependent on them. Approximately 11 percent of adolescents nationwide report having used inhalants in their lifetime. Many report coexisting multiple drug abuse and dependence, mental health treatment, and delinquent behaviors.

Inhalants very rapidly reach the lungs, bloodstream, and other parts of the body. At low doses, users may feel slightly stimulated; at higher doses, they may feel less inhibited. Intoxication often occurs within 5 minutes and can last more than an hour. Inhalant users do not report the intense rush associated with other drugs, nor do they experience the perceptual changes associated with LSD. However, inhalants interfere with thinking and impulse control, so users may act in dangerous or destructive ways.

Often there are visible external signs of use, such as:

- Rash around the nose and mouth.
- Breath odor.
- Residue on the face, hands, and clothing.
- Redness, swelling, and tearing of the eyes, and
- Irritation of the throat, lungs, and nose that leads to coughing and gagging.
- Nausea and headache.

Regular use of inhalants leads to tolerance, so the sniffer needs more and more to attain the desired effects. Younger children who use inhalants several times a week may develop dependence. Older users who become dependent may use the drugs many times a day.

Although some young people believe inhalants are safe, this is far from true. Inhalation of butane from cigarette lighters displaces oxygen in the lungs, causing suffocation. Users can also suffocate while covering their heads with a plastic bag to inhale a substance or from inhaling vomit into their lungs while high. The effects of inhalants are unpredictable, and even a single episode can trigger asphyxiation or cardiac arrhythmia, leading to disability or death. Other adverse effects include:

- Difficulties with memory and abstract reasoning.
- Lack of coordination.
- Uncontrollable movements of the extremities.
- Confusion.
- Hallucinations.
- Convulsions or seizures.
- Liver and kidney damage.
- Damage to bone marrow.
- Sudden "sniffing" deaths due to heart failure, asphyxiation, suffocation, and choking.

Treatment of Substance Dependence and Misuse

Most Americans with a substance use disorder never get professional help. The first step for a drug user is to admit that he or she *is* in fact an addict. If drug users are not forced to deal with their problem through some unexpected trauma, such as being fired or going bankrupt, those who care—family, friends, coworkers, and doctors—may have to confront them and insist that they do something about their addiction. Often such an *intervention* can be the turning point for an addict and his or her family.

Treatment has proved equally successful for young people and for older adults. It also yields economic benefits. According to the Surgeon General, every dollar invested in treatment saves $4 in health-care costs and $7 in criminal justice system costs. Undergraduates who enter substance abuse treatment programs are more likely to complete them successfully than nonstudents, often in a shorter period. The reason may be that academics provides a source of external goals and optimism

inhalants Substances that produce vapors having psychoactive effects when sniffed.

that improves motivation to change and enhances a sense of urgency to complete treatment.

✓**check-in** Do you know anyone who has been treated for substance abuse?

Treatment may take place in an outpatient setting, a residential facility, or a hospital. Increasingly, treatment thereafter is tailored to address coexisting or dual diagnoses. A personal treatment plan may consist of individual psychotherapy, marital and family therapy, medication, and behavior therapy. Once an individual has made the decision to seek help for substance abuse, the first step is usually detoxification, which involves clearing the drug from the body.

The aim of chemical dependence treatment is to help individuals establish and maintain their recovery from alcohol and drugs of abuse. Recovery is a dynamic process of personal growth and healing in which the drug user makes the transition from a lifestyle of active substance use to a drug-free lifestyle. Anti-addiction medications that target neurotransmitters in the brain are becoming safer and more effective. With treatment, substance abusers are less prone to relapse. If they do return to drug use, their relapses tend to be shorter and less frequent.

Principles of Drug Addiction Treatment

Decades of scientific research have shown that treatment can help drug-addicted individuals stop drug use, avoid relapse, and successfully recover their lives. Based on this research, the National Institute on Drug Abuse (NIDA) has developed fundamental principles that characterize effective drug abuse treatment. They include the following:

- Addiction is a complex but treatable disease that affects brain function and behavior.

- No single treatment is appropriate for everyone.

- Treatment needs to be readily available.

- Effective treatment attends to multiple needs of an individual, not just his or her drug abuse.

- Remaining in treatment for an adequate period of time is critical.

- Counseling—individual and/or group—and other behavioral therapies are the most commonly used forms of drug abuse treatment.

- Medications are an important element of treatment for many patients, especially when combined with counseling and other behavioral therapies.

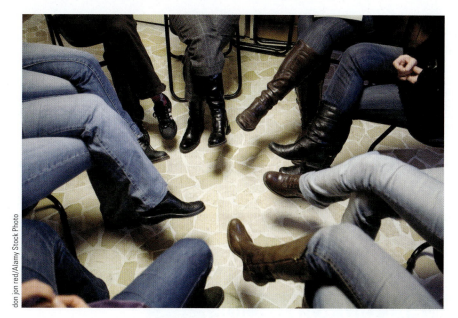

don jon red/Alamy Stock Photo

- Many drug-addicted individuals also have other mental disorders.

- Medically assisted detoxification is only the first stage of addiction treatment and by itself does little to change long-term drug abuse.

- Treatment does not need to be voluntary to be effective.

- Drug use during treatment must be monitored continuously, as lapses during treatment do occur.

12-Step Programs

Since its founding in 1935, Alcoholics Anonymous (AA)—the oldest, largest, and most successful self-help program in the world—has spawned a worldwide movement. Participation in **12-Step programs** for drug abusers, such as Substance Anonymous, Narcotics Anonymous, and Cocaine Anonymous, is of fundamental importance in promoting and maintaining long-term abstinence.

The basic precept of 12-Step programs is that members have been powerless when it comes to controlling their addictive behavior on their own. Meetings are held daily in almost every city in the country. Some chapters, whose members often include disabled individuals or those in remote areas, meet via Internet chat rooms or electronic bulletin boards. There are no dues or fees for membership.

Many individuals belong to several programs because they have several problems, such as alcoholism, substance abuse, and pathological gambling. All these programs have only one requirement for membership: a desire to stop an addictive behavior.

Based on the Alcoholics Anonymous model, "12 Step" programs have helped many people overcome addiction. The one requirement for membership is a desire to end a pattern of addictive behavior.

12-Step programs Self-help group program based on the principles of Alcoholics Anonymous.

Relapse Prevention

The most common clinical course for substance abuse disorders involves a pattern of relapses over the course of a lifespan. It is important for individuals with these problems and their families to recognize this fact. When relapses occur, they should be viewed as neither a mark of defeat nor evidence of moral weakness. While painful, relapses do not erase the progress that has been achieved and ultimately may strengthen self-understanding. They can serve as reminders of potential pitfalls to avoid in the future.

One key to preventing relapse is learning to avoid obvious cues and associations that can set off intense cravings. This means staying away from the people and places linked with past drug use.

As therapists emphasize, every lapse does not have to lead to a full-blown relapse. Users can turn to the skills acquired in treatment—calling people for support and going to meetings—to avoid a major relapse. Ultimately, users must learn much more than how to avoid temptation; they must examine their entire view of the world and learn new ways to live in it without turning to drugs. This is the underlying goal of the recovery process.

WHAT DID YOU DECIDE?

- Is caffeine good or bad for you?
- What is the "opioid epidemic"?
- What are the dangers of prescription drug abuse?
- Does marijuana, even when legal, pose risks to your well-being?

Reflection

People with substance abuse disorders and addictive behaviors lose control of their choices and their lives. Their compulsion to gamble or to use a drug seems irresistible. You, in contrast, have a choice. Reflect on the impact an addiction could have on your options now and in the future.

TAKING CHARGE OF YOUR HEALTH
Choosing an Addiction-Free Lifestyle

You can create a life and a lifestyle with no need and no room for reliance on a substance or a self-destructive behavior. Check those that you have already implemented. Are there others you plan to incorporate into your life? In your online journal, discuss the ways in which you are creating an addiction-free lifestyle.

____ Set goals for yourself. Think about who you want to become, what you'd like to do, and the future you wish for yourself. Focus on what it will take—years of education, perhaps, or specialized training—to achieve these goals. Understand that drugs can only get in the way and diminish your potential.

____ Participate in drug-free activities. If you're bored or unfocused, drugs may appeal to you simply as something to do. Take charge of your time. Play a sport. Work out at the gym. Join a club. Volunteer. Start a blog.

____ Educate yourself. Much of the information that young people hear from friends, particularly drug-using friends, is incorrect. Drugs that are used as medicines are not safe for recreational use. The fact that many people at a party or club are having fun doesn't mean that some aren't endangering their brains and their lives by taking club drugs.

____ Choose friends who have a future. The world of drug users shrinks. Nothing matters more than the next hit, the next high, the next fix. Losing all sense of tomorrow, they focus on getting through the day, with the help of drugs. Are these the people you want to spend time with? Choose friends who can broaden your world with new ideas, ambitious plans, and great dreams for tomorrow.

SELF-SURVEY

Do You Have a Substance Use Disorder?

Check the statements that apply to you.

____ Use more of an illegal drug or a prescription medication or use a drug for a longer period of time than you desire or intend.

____ Try, repeatedly and unsuccessfully, to cut down or control drug use.

____ Spend a great deal of time doing whatever is necessary in order to get drugs, taking them, or recovering from their use.

____ Are so high or feel so bad after drug use that you often cannot work or fulfill other responsibilities.

____ Give up or cut back on important social, work, or recreational activities because of drug use.

____ Continue to use drugs even though you realize that they are causing or worsening physical or mental problems.

____ Use a lot more of a drug in order to achieve a "high" or desired effect or feel fewer such effects than in the past.

____ Use drugs in dangerous ways or situations.

____ Have repeated drug-related legal problems, such as arrests for possession.

____ Continue to use drugs, even though the drug causes or worsens social or personal problems, such as arguments with a spouse.

____ Develop hand tremors or other withdrawal symptoms if you cut down or stop drug use.

____ Take drugs to relieve or avoid withdrawal symptoms.

Scoring

The more blanks that you (or someone close to you) checks, the more reason you have to be concerned about drug use. The most difficult step for anyone with a substance use disorder is to admit that he or she has a problem. Sometimes a drug-related crisis, such as being arrested or fired, forces individuals to acknowledge the impact of drugs. If not, those who care—family, friends, boss, physician—may have to confront them and insist that they do something about it. This confrontation, planned beforehand, is called an intervention and can be the turning point for drug users and their families.

REVIEW QUESTIONS

(LO 12.1) 1. Which of the following statements about risky addictive behaviors among adults is true?
   a. Women are more likely to indulge in risky behaviors than men.
   b. Non-Hispanic white males are least likely to indulge in substance abuse.
   c. The vast majority of college students do not engage in addictive behaviors.
   d. There are no promising treatments for addictions.

(LO 12.1) 2. As neuroscientists have shown, the brain's "reward center" responds to both pleasurable and exciting experiences, such as eating chocolate or bungee jumping, by producing _____, a "feel-good" chemical in the brain.
   a. acetaminophen
   b. dopamine
   c. serotonin
   d. amphetamine

(LO 12.2) 3. Which of the following statements is true about problem gambling?
   a. It is primarily a brain disorder.
   b. It is an addiction that runs in families.

   c. Individuals who have high academic grades are most likely to exhibit problem gambling.
   d. Having access to casino machines, ongoing card games, or Internet gambling sites does not increase the likelihood that students will gamble.

(LO 12.2) 4. Which of the following behaviors indicates an increased risk of problem gambling?
   a. Being very spiritual.
   b. Feeling depressed during gambling.
   c. Belonging to a high socioeconomic class.
   d. Gambling at an early age.

(LO 12.3) 5. _____ is/are the most widely used illicit drug(s) on campuses.
   a. Marijuana
   b. Opioids
   c. Tranquilizers
   d. Ecstasy

(LO 12.3) 6. Which of the following factors can influence students to use drugs?
   a. Reading spiritual material.
   b. Participating actively in class activities.

c. Understanding the risks associated with drug usage.
d. Consuming alcohol.

(LO 12.4) 7. Drug _____ is a pattern of continuing substance use despite cognitive, behavioral, and physical symptoms.
a. misuse
b. diversion
c. dependence
d. abuse

(LO 12.4) 8. Which of the following is one of the sex-based differences in patterns of drug use?
a. Men are more likely to become addicted to cocaine or heroin.
b. Men are more likely to begin using drugs if given the opportunity.
c. Women are more likely to abuse alcohol and marijuana.
d. Women who abuse drugs are more likely to experience negative effects.

(LO 12.5) 9. Which of the following statements is true regarding the opioid epidemic?
a. Opioids first became available in 1996.
b. OxyContin is not as strong as morphine.
c. One in four patients who receive long-term opioid therapy become addicted to opioids.
d. The Centers for Disease Control and Prevention has not yet developed recommendations on the amount of opioids physicians should be prescribing.

(LO 12.6) 10. Which of the following statements is true about caffeine?
a. It increases fatigue even when taken in very small amounts.
b. It provides relief from anxiety and digestive disturbances.
c. It lowers the risk of cardiovascular disease.
d. It increases the risk of type 2 diabetes.

(LO 12.6) 11. Which of the following statements about caffeine intoxication is true?
a. Doctors recommend that all adults limit their caffeine intake to 250 milligrams per day.
b. The recommended maximum dosage for adolescents is 500 milligrams of caffeine a day.
c. Ingesting 50 milligrams of caffeine may produce caffeine intoxication.
d. It is diagnosed on the basis of five or more specific symptoms.

(LO 12.7) 12. Psychological side effects of over-the-counter and prescription drugs _____.
a. do not include mental or emotional problems
b. decrease as people get older
c. can include changes in the way people think, feel, and behave
d. remain the same regardless of the dosage

(LO 12.7) 13. _____ occurs when a person develops tolerance to the effects of a drug and needs larger and larger doses to achieve intoxication or another desired effect.
a. Drug diversion
b. Drug interaction
c. Physical dependence
d. Psychological dependence

(LO 12.7) 14. Which of the following is a characteristic of substance use disorder?
a. A persistent desire to cut down or stop substance use.
b. Developing intolerance toward the substance.
c. Adhering to prescribed medications.
d. Absence of cravings and withdrawal symptoms.

(LO 12.8) 15. Which of the following is an herbal drug?
a. K2
b. Tylenol
c. Acetaminophen
d. Khat

(LO 12.8) 16. Which of the following is an example of a stimulant?
a. Tylenol
b. Phenolphthalein
c. Aspirin
d. Amphetamine

(LO 12.9) 17. What is the first step in substance abuse treatment?
a. Removing access to drugs.
b. The user admitting that he or she is an addict.
c. Providing a source of external motivation.
d. Beginning a 12-Step program.

(LO 12.9) 18. Which of the following statements is true about preventing relapses in substance abuse?
a. Relapses tend to result from moral weakness.
b. Lapses usually lead to full-blown relapses.
c. The ultimate goal of treatment is learning how to avoid temptation.
d. Relapses do not erase the progress that has been achieved.

Answers to these questions can be found on page 531.

Cagkan Sayin/Shutterstock.com

LEARNING OBJECTIVES

After reading this chapter, you should be able to:

13.1 Outline the patterns of alcohol consumption among different populations in America.

13.2 Discuss the patterns, reasons, and perils of drinking on campus.

13.3 Describe the characteristics of alcohol and its effects on human health.

13.4 Explain how alcohol is associated with serious health risks and disorders.

13.5 Review racial, ethnic, and sex differences in alcohol-related risks.

13.6 Examine the health consequences of alcohol-related disorders.

13.7 Compare the patterns of tobacco consumption among the populations in America.

13.8 Outline the patterns of tobacco consumption among different groups of students.

13.9 Discuss sex, racial, and ethnic differences in tobacco consumption.

13.10 Identify the immediate effects of tobacco consumption on body and brain functions.

13.11 Evaluate the serious health risks and dangers associated with cigarette smoking.

13.12 Review the health risks posed by different forms of tobacco.

13.13 Compare the different ways of quitting to show advantages and disadvantages of each.

13.14 Analyze the harmful effects of environmental tobacco smoke on health.

WHAT DO YOU THINK?

• Why do people smoke even when they're aware of the risks?

• What are the short- and long-term effects of tobacco on health?

• Why are secondhand and thirdhand smoke dangerous to nonsmokers' health?

• Do you agree with experts who see alcohol as the greatest single threat to college students' health?

• What are the most dangerous forms of campus drinking?

• Are "emerging tobacco products" like electronic cigarettes safe to use?

13

Alcohol and Tobacco

At first glance, the Friday night get-together looks like any other college party. Music booms. Clusters of undergraduates, plastic cups in hand, chat and laugh. A few couples dance. But there is one crucial difference: no alcohol. At hundreds of campuses across the United States—including some infamous "party schools"—students are finding ways to get together and have a good time without getting drunk, high, or wasted.

Seth, a third-year student at a large state university, couldn't imagine partying without alcohol. "In my freshman year, I carried a flask so I could take a few swigs and loosen up before going out," he recalls. Most evenings ended the same way—with him throwing up on the way back to his dorm.

"It all got old—the drinking games, the crazy fights, the hangovers," Seth says. With the help of a campus counseling program and local support groups, he stopped drinking. "For a while, I'd just hole up in my room and stream videos on weekends. Everyone else was out drinking." Not everyone, he discovered. As he met other students in various stages of recovery, Seth joined in a wide range of alcohol-free adventures: hikes, bike rides, tailgating, volleyball games, dances, film screenings, and evenings at trendy "dry" bars.

Many other students, as well as school officials, are rethinking their attitudes toward alcohol. Alcohol-linked sexual assaults and violence have triggered renewed focus on the negative,

sometimes tragic, consequences of excessive campus drinking. Universities are banning liquor at many campus events. Local police in many communities are cracking down on underage drinkers. And more students like Seth are choosing not to let alcohol take control of their lives.

Long before the creation of alcohol-free zones, many schools banned tobacco—for good reason. Any exposure to tobacco smoke can cause both immediate and long-term damage to the body. Tobacco continues to kill more people than AIDS, alcohol, drug abuse, motor vehicle accidents, murders, suicides, and fires combined. According to the Centers for Disease Control and Prevention (CDC), more than 480,000 Americans die each year from smoking or exposure to secondhand smoke, while 16 million suffer from smoking-related illnesses.

Fewer college students smoke cigarettes than in the past, but more are trying other forms of tobacco, including e-cigarettes and hookahs (water pipes). Yet these too pose a real and significant danger to health. <

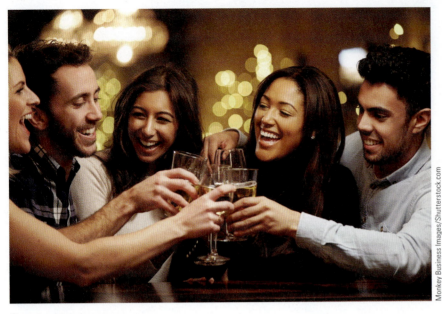

People drink for many reasons, including celebrating and socializing.

Monkey Business Images/Shutterstock.com

• White men and women are more likely to drink than other adults: 70 percent of white men say they drink, compared to 57 percent of black men, 55 percent of Asian men, and 58 percent of American Indian or Alaska Native men.

• Among women, 59 percent of white women drink, compared with 40 percent of blacks, 32 percent of Asians, and 45 percent of American Indian or Alaska Natives.

• The median age of first alcohol use is 15. Drinking typically increases in the late teens, peaks in the early 20s, and decreases as people age. The median age of onset for alcohol use disorders is 19 to 20.[3]

✓**check-in** Have you ever had an alcoholic drink? If so, how old were you when you had your first drink?

Alcohol and tobacco, the most widely used mind-altering substances in the world, are each dangerous on their own, but drinking and smoking tend to go together. And the more that individuals drink or smoke, the less likely they are to follow a healthy lifestyle.

Even if you never abuse alcohol or smoke, you live with the consequences of others' drinking and smoking. That's why it's important for everyone to know about the health risks of alcohol and tobacco. This chapter provides information that can help you understand, avoid, and change behaviors that could undermine your health, happiness, and life.

Drinking in America

More than 170 million Americans—about two-thirds of the population—report drinking alcohol in the previous year.[1] Most do not misuse alcohol. According to the National Institute on Alcohol Abuse and Alcoholism.

• 56 percent of adults over age 18 are current regular drinkers.

• 13 percent are in frequent drinkers.

• 6 percent are former regular drinkers.

• 9 percent are former infrequent drinkers.

• About 14 percent have never drunk alcohol.[2]

Why People Don't Drink

More Americans are choosing not to drink, and alcohol consumption is at its lowest level in decades. About a quarter of adults—31 percent of women and 18 percent of men—report drinking no alcohol in the past year.

With fewer people drinking alcohol, nonalcoholic beverages have grown in popularity. They appeal to drivers, boaters, individuals with health problems that could worsen with alcohol, older individuals who can't tolerate alcohol, anyone taking medicines that interact with alcohol (including antibiotics, antidepressants, and muscle relaxers), and everyone interested in limiting alcohol intake. Under federal law, these drinks can contain some alcohol but a much smaller amount than regular beer or wine. Nonalcoholic beers and wines on the market also are lower in calories than alcoholic varieties.

Certain people should not drink at all. These include:

• Anyone younger than age 21. Underage drinking (discussed later in this chapter) poses many medical, behavioral, and legal dangers.

• Anyone who plans to drive, operate motorized equipment, or engage in other activities that require alertness and skill (including sports and recreational activities).

• Women who are pregnant or trying to become pregnant.

• Individuals taking certain over-the-counter (OTC) or prescription medications.

- People with medical conditions that can be made worse by drinking.
- Recovering alcoholics.

Why People Drink

The most common reason people drink alcohol is to relax and relieve stress. Because it depresses the central nervous system, alcohol can make people feel less tense. Here are some other reasons men and women drink:

- **Social ease.** When people use alcohol, they may seem bolder, wittier, or sexier. At the same time, they become more relaxed and seem to enjoy each other's company more. Because alcohol lowers inhibitions, some people see it as a prelude to seduction.
- **Happiness.** In a study that used smartphones to check on drinkers' moods, individuals reported feeling happier at the moment of drinking, but this sense of euphoria didn't persist for long.[4]
- **Role models.** Athletes, musicians, and other famous people who write, sing, or talk about drinking can make alcohol abuse seem normal or acceptable.
- **Advertising.** Brewers and beer distributors spend millions of dollars every year promoting the message: If you want to have fun, have a drink. Young people may be especially responsive to such sales pitches.
- **Relationship issues.** Single, separated, or divorced men and women drink more and more often than married ones.
- **Early exposure to alcohol.** A first drink—even a first sip—of alcohol in the middle-school years has been linked to later alcohol misuse.[5]
- **Childhood traumas.** Female alcoholics often report that they were physically or sexually abused as children or suffered great distress because of poverty or a parent's death. Individuals being treated for alcoholism are likely to have experienced sexual, physical, or emotional abuse as well as physical or emotional neglect.
- **Unemployment.** Individuals who lose their jobs are at increased risk of alcohol use and misuse, including more daily consumption and more binge drinking.

√**check-in** If you drink alcohol, when and why do you drink?

Drinking on Campus

Young adults are the most frequent users of alcohol in the United States. The highest proportion of heavy drinkers and individuals with diagnosable alcohol use disorders are 18 to 25 years old. According to the 2017 National Survey on Drug Use and Health, 53.6 percent of college students between the ages of 18 and 22 drank alcohol during the past month, compared with 48.2 percent of their non–college-attending peers. About 35 percent of students reported binge drinking, defined as consuming five or more drinks on the same occasion[6] (see Snapshot: On Campus Now).

Many health experts consider the use and abuse of alcohol the primary health concern for college students. Here are some reasons:

- Although the percentage of students who drink hasn't changed much over the years, drinking patterns have. At many schools, students' social lives revolve around parties, games, and bar crawls. More students drink simply to get drunk and drink a lot during each drinking episode.
- About one-third of students increase alcohol use and encounter more related problems throughout the college years, one-third do not change previous patterns, and one-third decrease drinking.
- More college women drink now than in the past, and they drink more than in the past.
- In the American College Health Association survey, 30 percent of female students reported drinking more than four drinks the last time they socialized or partied.[7] College women who drink are at greatly increased risk of unwanted sexual activity.
- Alcohol can affect every aspect of a student's life. Nearly 160,000 freshmen drop out of college after their first year for alcohol- or drug-related reasons, according to the Core Institute, which surveys drinking practices on campuses.
- College drinking is responsible for an estimated 1,700 annual alcohol-related deaths, 599,000 injuries, more than 696,000 physical attacks, and more than 97,000 sexual assaults.[8]
- Binge drinking (discussed later in this chapter) has been linked with lower grades,

SNAPSHOT: ON CAMPUS NOW

Student Drinking

Alcohol Consumption	Percent (%)					
	Actual Use			Perceived Use		
	Male	Female	Total	Male	Female	Total
Never used	23.6	20.0	21.2	5.7	3.7	4.4
Used, but not in the past 30 days	15.9	17.4	17.1	3.0	2.2	2.5
Used 1–9 days	45.2	51.3	49.3	43.0	39.0	40.2
Used 10–29 days	13.9	10.7	11.6	37.1	41.3	39.9
Used all 30 days	1.5	0.5	0.8	11.4	13.8	13.0
Any use within the past 30 days	60.6	62.5	61.7	91.4	94.1	93.2

As the figures above show, most undergraduates overestimate the number of students who drink—and drink frequently—and underestimate the number who don't drink often or at all. How do your perceptions and actual behavior compare?

Source: American College Health Association. American College Health Association-National College Health Assessment II: Reference Group Executive Summary Spring 2018. Silver Spring, MD: American College Health Association, 2018.

---

poorer performance on memory tests, and higher levels of both depression and anxiety.

- College men drink more, and more often, and more intensely than college women. They report consuming an average of almost six drinks the last time they partied or socialized; 29 percent drank six or more.[9]
- Caucasians drink more than African Americans or Asian Americans.
- Fraternity and sorority members, athletes, and vigorous exercisers use more alcohol more often than other students.
- The students who drink the least are those attending two-year institutions, religious schools, commuter schools, and historically black colleges and universities. (See Health on a Budget for ways to drink less.)

✓**check-in** How widespread is drinking on your campus?

Why Students Don't Drink

According to the ACHA, 21 percent of students have never used alcohol.[10] African American students are more likely than white undergraduates to abstain and to report never having had an alcoholic drink or not having a drink in the past 30 days. They also drink less frequently and consume fewer drinks per occasion than whites.

Students who don't drink give various reasons for their choice, including:

- Under age 21.
- Not having access to alcohol.
- Parental or peer pressure.
- Cost.
- Not liking the taste.
- Spiritual and religious values. Students who place high importance on religion consume less alcohol, even when in an environment where drinking is the norm.

✓**check-in** Do you choose not to drink? If so, why?

Why Students Drink

Alcohol has been part of campus life for a very long time. Away from home, often for the first time, many students are excited by and apprehensive about their newfound independence. Social motives are the most common reason for drinking—and for problem drinking—on campus. When students feel overwhelmed, awkward, or insecure or when they just want to let loose and have a good time, they reach for a drink. Being less engaged in their studies and more willing to risk negative academic consequences for the sake of partying increase the likelihood of excessive drinking.[11]

$ HEALTH ON A BUDGET

Drink Less, Save More

Yet another good reason to control how much you drink is economic. The less spending money that college students have, the less they drink—and the less likely they are to get drunk and to suffer alcohol-related negative consequences. Here are some simple ways to spend less on alcohol:

- **Pace yourself.** Start with a soft drink and have a non-alcoholic drink every second or third drink.

- **Stay busy.** You will drink less if you play pool or dance rather than just sit and drink.

- **Try low-alcohol alternatives,** such as light beers and low- or no-alcohol wines.

- **Have alcohol-free days.** Don't drink at all at least two days a week.

- **Drink slowly.** Take sips and not gulps. Put your glass down between sips.

- **Avoid salty snacks.** Salty foods like chips or nuts make you thirsty, and then you drink more.

- **Have one drink at a time.** Don't let people top up your drinks. It makes it harder to keep track of how much alcohol you're consuming.

The following list summarizes key influences on student drinking:

- **Social norms.** Compared with other factors, such as race, sex, year in school, and fraternity/sorority membership, social norms (discussed in Chapter 1) have the strongest association with how much college students drink. In a recent study, more than eight in ten students overestimated how many and how much their peers drink. Overestimation of heavy drinking by peers is associated with more frequent heavy drinking.[12]

- **Coping.** Students turn to alcohol to cope with everyday problems and personal issues. Those with symptoms of depression who lack skills to cope with daily problems, particularly males, are more likely to drink than others, as are those who feel anxious, angry, hostile, nervous, guilty, or ashamed.

- **Social anxiety.** Both traditional-age and older undergraduates who report social anxiety are more likely to drink, including heavy episodic drinking, as a way of coping.[13]

- **Party schools.** Colleges and universities in the Northeast, those with a strong Greek system, and those where athletics predominate have higher drinking rates than others. Students who never join or who drop out of a fraternity or sorority report less risky drinking behavior than those who go Greek.

- **Living arrangements.** Drinking rates are highest among students living in fraternity and sorority houses, followed by those in on-campus housing (dormitories, residence halls) and off-campus apartments or houses. Study-abroad students are at risk for increased and problematic drinking behavior.

Undergraduates living at home with their families drink the least.[14]

- **Weekends and special occasions.** Students drink more heavily on weekends and holidays than on typical weekdays.[15] The highest drinking days include Halloween, New Year's Eve, and St. Patrick's Day. Alcohol consumption typically soars on big-game days for various sports, when a significant number of students engage in "extreme ritualistic alcohol consumption," defined as consuming 10 or more drinks on the same day for a male and 8 or more for a female.[16] Many students celebrate their 21st birthday by drinking—and those who party with fraternity or sorority members drink more than those who toast the big day with romantic partners.[17]

- **Spring break.** Annual excursions devoted to nonstop partying with thousands of other young people have become notorious for extreme drinking.[18] Frequent consequences include intoxication, alcohol poisoning, accidents, and risky sexual behavior. Students who overestimate their peers' alcohol consumption during spring break drink more than those who don't assume that everyone else is drinking heavily.

- **Participation in sports.** Students who place a higher moral priority on loyalty to a group, such as a team, fraternity, or sorority, tend to have more favorable attitudes toward drinking.[19] College athletes, who generally drink more alcohol more often than nonathletes, may be at greater risk because many are younger than 21, belong to Greek organizations, have lower GPAs, or spend more time socializing than other students.[20] Those who play team sports tend to drink heavily. Male hockey and female soccer players drink the most; male basketball players and cross-country or track athletes of both sexes, the least.

- **Parental attitudes.** Students who believe that their parents approve of drinking are more likely to drink and to report having a drinking-related problem. Those whose parents communicate clear zero-tolerance messages about alcohol are least likely to drink. Parents also influence stopping or limiting drinking.

- **First-year transition.** Some students who drank less in high school than classmates who weren't headed for college start drinking, and drinking heavily, in college—often during their first 6 weeks on campus and during school breaks. But heavy drinkers often continue to maintain or increase their risky drinking behaviors, and some nondrinkers or light drinkers also increase their alcohol consumption throughout college.[21]

- **Sexual victimization.** Women who've experienced sexual assault are at greater risk of binge drinking.[22] Risky drinking, including bingeing, in itself increases the risk of sexual victimization.

✓**check-in** About one in five college students tends to overestimate how much alcohol he or she has consumed; about one in ten underestimates his or her alcohol consumption.[23] How accurately do you think you can estimate how much you've had to drink?

High-Risk Drinking on Campus

The most common types of undergraduate high-risk drinking are binge drinking, bingeing combined with disordered eating, predrinking, underage drinking, and consumption of caffeinated alcoholic beverages. Obviously, many factors influence students' drinking behaviors.

Binge Drinking According to the National Institute of Alcohol Abuse and Alcoholism, a **binge** is a pattern of drinking alcohol that brings blood-alcohol concentration (BAC) (discussed later in this chapter) to 0.08 gram-percent or above. For a typical adult man, this pattern corresponds to consuming five or more drinks in about 2 hours; for a woman, four or more drinks in the same amount of time.

According to the Surgeon General's report on addiction in America, 66.7 million people in the United States engaged in binge drinking in the previous month. On average, binge drinkers

binge For a man, having five or more alcoholic drinks at a single sitting; for a woman, having four or more drinks at a single sitting.

consume eight drinks during a drinking episode, with men consuming more drinks than women and those between ages 18 and 34 drinking more than older binge drinkers. According to various reports, binge-drinking rates range from 1 percent to more than 70 percent at different campuses. The average is 40 percent.

✓**check-in** Is binge drinking common on your campus?

Who Binge-Drinks in College? An estimated four in ten college students drink at binge levels or greater. They consume 91 percent of all alcohol that undergraduates report drinking.[24] Hundreds of studies have created a portrait of who binge drinkers are and how they differ from others:

- Binge drinkers are more likely to be male than female, although one in three women—up from one in four—reports binge drinking.[25]

- Binge drinkers are more likely to be white than any other ethnic or racial group. (African American women are least likely to binge.)

- Most are under age 24.

- More binge drinkers are enrolled in four-year colleges than in two-year ones.

- Binge drinkers tend to be residents of states with fewer alcohol control policies.

- Binge drinkers tend to be involved in athletics and socialize frequently.

- They often belong to a fraternity or sorority.

- They are more likely to be dissatisfied with their bodies, not prone to exercise, eat poorly, and go on unhealthy diets.

- Binge drinkers tend to be behind in schoolwork or miss class.

- They are often users of other substances, including nicotine, marijuana, cocaine, and LSD.

- Binge drinkers are likely to black out, be injured or hurt, to engage in unplanned or unprotected sexual activity, or to get in trouble with campus police.[26]

Why Students Binge-Drink Young people who came from, socialized within, or were exposed to "wet" environments—settings in which alcohol is cheap and accessible and drinking is prevalent—are most likely to engage in binge drinking. Students who report drinking at least once a month during their final year of high school are more likely to binge-drink in college than those who drank less frequently in high school.

The factors that most influence students to binge-drink are:

- **Low price for alcohol.** Beer, which is cheap and easy to obtain, is the beverage of choice among binge drinkers.

- **Easy access to alcohol.** In one study, the density of alcohol outlets (such as bars) near campus affected the drinking of students.

- **Proximity to other binge drinkers.** Students who attend a school or live in a residence with many binge drinkers tend to become binge drinkers themselves.

- **Peer pressure.** Those who believe that close friends are likely to binge end up bingeing themselves.

- **Family attitudes.** Students whose parents drank or did not disapprove of their children drinking are more likely to binge.

- **Early access to alcohol.** Places with lower drinking ages are associated with more frequent binge episodes.

- **Campus environment.** Students tend to binge-drink at the beginning of the school year and then cut back as the semester progresses and academic demands increase. Binge drinking also peaks following exam times, during home football weekends, and during spring break.

- **Drinking games.** Two-thirds of college students engage in drinking games—such as beer pong or "Beirut"—that involve binge drinking. Although these games vary in many ways, all share a common theme: becoming intoxicated in a short period of time. Men are more likely to participate than women and to consume larger amounts of alcohol, often six drinks or more.[27] Drinking game players who don't monitor or regulate how much they're drinking are at risk of extreme intoxication. Drinking games have been implicated in alcohol-related injuries and deaths from alcohol poisoning.

✓**check-in** Have you ever played drinking games?

Binge Drinking and Disordered Eating

The combination of two risky behaviors—disordered eating and heavy drinking—poses special dangers to students. As discussed in Chapter 5, disordered eating can range from excessive concern about weight to binge eating to extreme weight-control methods, such as purging. In some studies, as many as 60 percent of college women reported binge eating and

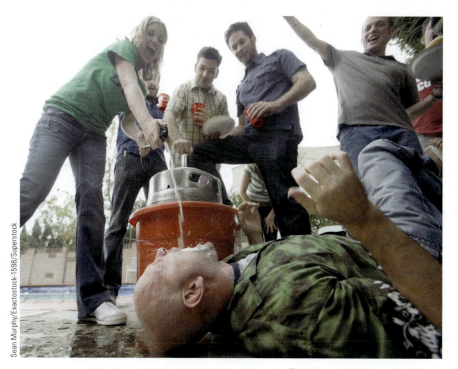

Sean Murphy/Exactostock-1598/Superstock

Drinking games can lead to extreme intoxication, alcohol-related injuries, and alcohol poisoning.

purging, while 9 percent of college men reported some form of disordered eating. In women, the combination of these behaviors increases the risk of many negative consequences, including blackouts, unintended sexual activity, and forced sexual intercourse.

Some students restrict calories from food prior to planned drinking—some to avoid weight gain and others to enhance the effects of alcohol. The popular media have created the term "drunkorexia" to describe this risky behavior, but it is not an official psychiatric term.

Predrinking/Pregaming

Drinking before going out has become increasingly common on college campuses, where **predrinking** (also called pregaming, preloading, or front-loading) is announced and celebrated in text messages, e-mails, blogs, YouTube videos, and Facebook posts.

In various studies, a greater proportion of white than Hispanic/Latino, African American, and Pacific Islander American students reported prepartying in the previous month. Within all ethnic groups, prepartyers consumed more drinks per week and experienced a higher number of alcohol-related consequences than non-prepartyers.

Predrinkers consistently report much higher alcohol consumption during the evening and more negative consequences, such as getting into fights, being arrested, or being referred to a university's mandatory alcohol intervention program.

predrinking Consuming alcoholic beverages, usually with friends, before going out to bars or parties; also called pregaming, preloading, or front-loading.

Why Is Predrinking Popular?
College students predrink for a variety of reasons, including:

- **Economy.** Many say they want to avoid paying for expensive drinks at a bar, although most end up drinking at least as much when they're out as they do when they don't predrink.

- **Intoxication.** A growing number of students seem to want to get drunk as quickly as possible.

- **Socializing.** Predrinking gives students a chance to chat with their friends, which often isn't possible in noisy, crowded clubs or bars.

- **Anxiety reduction.** By drinking alone before meeting strangers, students say they feel less shy or self-conscious—but their risk of alcohol-related problems increases.[28]

- **Group bonding.** For some young men, drinking together may serve as a way of bonding and building confidence prior to interacting with the opposite sex.

The Perils of Predrinking
When students get together to drink before a game or a night out, they usually consume large quantities of alcohol quite rapidly. In part that's because they're drinking in places without restraints on how much they can drink. Various studies have shown that students drink more and have higher blood-alcohol concentrations on days when they predrink. They also are at greater risk of blackouts, passing out, hangovers, and alcohol poisoning.

In addition to drinking more alcohol, predrinkers are more likely to use other drugs, such as marijuana and cocaine. The combined effects of these substances further increase the risks of injury, violence, or victimization.

✓**check-in** Have you ever engaged in predrinking?

Underage Drinking on Campus
Each year, approximately 5,000 young people under age 21 die as a result of underage drinking. This figure includes about 1,900 deaths from motor vehicle crashes, 1,600 homicides, and 300 suicides, as well as hundreds due to other injuries, such as falls, burns, and drownings.

Students under age 21 drink less often than older students but tend to drink more heavily and to experience more negative alcohol-related consequences. More underage students report drinking "to get drunk" and drinking at binge levels when they consumed alcohol.

Underage college students are most likely to drink if they can easily obtain cheap alcohol, especially beer. They tend to drink in private settings, such as dorms and fraternity parties, and to experience negative drinking-related consequences, such as doing something they regretted, forgetting where they were or what they did, causing property damage, getting into trouble with police, and being hurt or injured. The drinking behavior of underage students also depends on their living arrangements. Those in controlled settings, such as their parents' home or a substance-free dorm, are less likely to binge-drink. Students living in fraternities or sororities are most likely to binge-drink, regardless of age.

A number of university chancellors and presidents have signed a public statement calling for informed, dispassionate discussion of the *Amethyst Initiative*, a proposal that supports a series of educational and policy-level efforts to enable 18- to 20-year-old adults to purchase, possess, and consume alcoholic beverages at their own discretion. Opponents note that the minimum legal drinking age of 21 has reduced alcohol-related deaths, injuries, and traffic crashes. Various factors may inhibit the ability of underage students to drink responsibly, including less self-efficacy.

✓**check-in** What do you think the minimum legal drinking age should be?

Alcohol Mixed with Energy Drinks
AmED (alcohol mixed with energy drinks) refers to any combination of alcohol with caffeine and other stimulants. Energy drinks themselves can increase cardiovascular and metabolic risks for young adults.[29] Alcohol adds to the dangers.

Premixed beverages, often malt-based or distilled spirits–based, usually have a higher alcohol content (5 to 12 percent) than beer (4 to 5 percent). Some states classify them as liquor, thereby limiting the locations where they can be sold.

Like the energy drinks discussed in Chapter 4, AmEDs have surged in popularity among teens and young adults. The Food and Drug Administration (FDA) has banned some premixed AmEDs, but young people continue to combine energy drinks like Red Bull with vodka or other forms of alcohol.

AmED users are most likely to be younger men who score higher on measures of risk-taking propensity.[30] In a recent study of college students, most had neutral or negative views of AmED.[31]

AmED (alcohol mixed with energy drinks) Any combination of alcohol with caffeine and other stimulants.

The most frequent users had positive expectations, such as being able to party longer.[32]

The caffeine in these drinks may mask the depressant effects of alcohol, but it has no effect on the liver's metabolism of alcohol and thus does not reduce blood-alcohol concentrations or reduce alcohol-related risks.

Various studies have linked AmED use to risky behaviors on campus, including:

- Unprotected sex and sex under the influence of drugs or alcohol.

- More high-risk drinking behaviors, such as consuming large amounts of alcohol.

- Increased danger of becoming alcohol dependent.

- Twice the likelihood of being hurt or injured as those who don't consume AmEDs.

✓**check-in** Have you ever had an alcoholic energy drink?

Why Students Stop Drinking

Only 1 percent of students ages 18 to 24 receive treatment for alcohol or drug abuse. Nonetheless, as many as 22 percent of alcohol-abusing college students "spontaneously" reduce their drinking as they progress through college. Unlike older adults, who often hit bottom before they change their drinking behaviors, many college students go through a gradual process of reduced drinking. Researchers refer to this behavioral change as early cessation, natural reduction, natural recovery, or spontaneous recovery.

As with other behavioral changes, individuals must be ready to change their drinking patterns. In one study, students who binged frequently, who experienced more alcohol-related interpersonal and academic problems, who did not also use marijuana, and who lived in a residence hall where binge drinking was the norm showed a greater readiness to change.

Why do students stop heavy drinking? Here are some common responses:

- "It was just getting old."
- Vomiting.
- Urinating in hallways.
- Being physically fondled.
- Sexual assault.
- Violence.
- Accidents.
- Injuries.

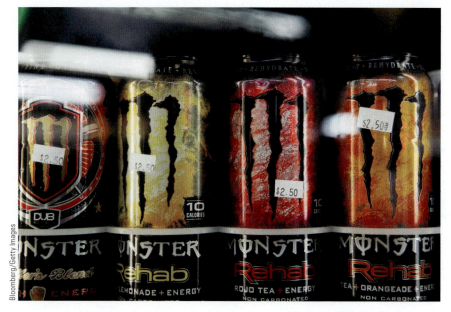

Bloomberg/Getty Images

- Unprotected intercourse.
- Emergency room visits.
- Vicarious experiences, such as a roommate's arrest for driving under the influence or a sorority sister's date rape.

Psychologists have found that students "mature out" of heavy drinking as they become less impulsive and develop healthier coping behaviors. Several interventions have proven effective in reducing alcohol consumption and alcohol-related problems on college campuses.[33] They include getting personalized feedback about drinking habits, learning moderation strategies, challenging expectations, identifying risky situations, and setting goals for responsible drinking.

✓**check-in** Has your attitude toward drinking changed since you entered college?

Alcohol-Related Problems on Campus

In a recent study, about 9 in 10 undergraduates reported "secondhand exposure" to alcohol abuse in the previous month, including interpersonal harm as well as greater anxiety, stress, and depression. Women were at greater risk of mental health consequences.[34] Men were more likely than women to injure themselves, have unprotected sex, get involved in a fight, or physically injure another person. Women were more likely to have someone use force or threat of force to have sex with them (see Table 13.1). Students who drink heavily also are much more likely to abuse prescription drugs (see Chapter 12).

Mixing caffeinated beverages with alcohol can increase the risk of harmful consequences.

TABLE 13.1 Consequences of Drinking

College students who drank alcohol reported experiencing the following in the past 12 months when drinking alcohol:

	Percent (%)		
	Male	Female	Total
Did something you later regretted	31.8	32.0	31.9
Forgot where you were or what you did	28.3	26.8	27.1
Got in trouble with the police	2.7	1.4	1.8
Someone had sex with you without your consent	1.3	2.9	2.5
Had sex with someone without their consent	0.4	0.2	0.3
Had unprotected sex	22.0	21.4	21.5
Physically injured yourself	12.4	11.6	11.9
Physically injured another person	1.8	0.8	1.1
Seriously considered suicide	4.2	3.7	4.0
Reported one or more of the above	50.6	48.8	49.3

Source: American College Health Association. American College Health Association-National College Health Assessment II: Reference Group Executive Summary Spring 2018. Silver Spring, MD: American College Health Association, 2018.

Consequences of Drinking Among the other problems linked to drinking are:

- **Atypical behavior.** Under the influence of alcohol, students behave in ways they normally wouldn't. Some sext or post comments and photos they later regret on social media.[35] Male heavy drinkers are more prone to behave in ways that are considered "antisocial," or contrary to the standards of our society, such as forcing or trying to force unwanted sexual contact, driving drunk, exposing themselves, or having sex with a stranger. Although some college students "mature out" of heavy drinking once they leave college, others do not and are at risk for poor adaptation to adulthood, including continued problem drinking and associated health outcomes.[36]

- **Academic problems.** The more that students drink, the more likely they are to fall behind in schoolwork, miss classes, have lower GPAs, and face suspensions. In general, students with an A average have three to four drinks per week, whereas students with D or F averages drink almost ten drinks a week (see Figure 13.1).

- **Risky sexual behavior.** About one in five college students reports engaging in unplanned sexual activity, including having sex with someone he or she just met and having unprotected sex. Drinking, including social drinking, increases the likelihood of risky sex and unwanted sexual experiences.[37]

- **Sexual assault.** In a recent survey, almost 20 percent of undergraduate women reported some type of completed sexual assault since entering college. Most occurred after women voluntarily consumed alcohol; a few occurred after they were unknowingly given a drug in their drinks.[38]

- **Intimate partner violence.** Each year an estimated 80 percent of college men perpetrate psychological aggression; 20 to 30 percent, physical aggression; and 15 to 20 percent, sexual aggression against a dating partner. Heavy drinking increases the likelihood of all three forms, especially physical violence. Alcohol increases the likelihood that women will be either perpetrators or victims of partner aggression.

- **Unintentional injury.** More than 30 percent of college drinkers have been injured as a result of drinking. Increased alcohol use increases their likelihood of causing injury to others, having a car accident, and suffering burns or a fall serious enough to require medical attention.[39] The costs of emergency treatment for alcohol-related injuries can be more than half a million dollars a year at schools with 40,000 or more students.

- **Consequences beyond college.** Alcohol-related convictions, including carrying a false I.D. or driving under the influence of alcohol, remain on an individual's criminal record and could affect a student's graduate school and professional opportunities. In a recent study, students who had planned to attend graduate school were less likely to enroll if they abused or became dependent on alcohol.[40]

- **Illness and death.** Many students suffer short-term health consequences of drinking, such as headaches and hangovers. Heavy alcohol use in college students is associated with immunological problems and digestive and upper respiratory disorders. Even moderate drinking can contribute to infertility in women. Longer-term consequences of heavy drinking include liver disease, stroke, heart disease, and certain types of cancer. About 300,000 of today's college students will eventually die from alcohol-related causes, including drunk-driving accidents, cirrhosis of the liver, various cancers, and heart disease.

✓**check-in** Have you experienced any alcohol-related problems on campus?

Drinking and Driving

Drunk driving, the most frequently committed crime in the United States, claims almost 10,000 lives a year.[41] In the ACHA survey, 19.8 percent of students reported driving after having had any alcohol; 1.4 percent reported driving after five or more drinks.[42] Traditional-age undergraduates typically are more likely to drink and drive as they get older, with the biggest jump between ages 21 and 23. Colleges have reported some success in using text messages and emails to reduce the risk of driving under the influence.[43]

Alcohol impairs driving-related skills regardless of the age of the driver or the time of day it is consumed. However, younger students who drink and drive are at greatest risk:

• Underage drinkers are more likely to drive after drinking, to ride with intoxicated drivers, and to be injured after drinking—at least in part because they believe that people can drive safely and legally after drinking.

• More young women than ever before are driving drunk and getting into fatal car accidents. More young women than men involved in deadly crashes had high blood-alcohol levels, according to a recent analysis of data from the National Highway Traffic Safety Administration (NHTSA).

• According to national surveys, men have higher rates of alcohol-impaired driving than women. The highest rates are among those ages 18 to 29 and 35 to 44 and those with higher education and income.[44]

• Of the 5,000 alcohol-related deaths among 18- to 24-year-olds, 80 percent were caused by alcohol-related traffic accidents. A young person dies in an alcohol-related traffic crash an average of once every 3 hours.

Since states began setting the legal drinking age at 21, the NHTSA estimates that more than 26,000 lives have been saved. Safety groups, such as Mothers Against Drunk Driving (MADD) and Students Against Destructive Decisions (SADD), attribute the decline in alcohol-related deaths to enforcement tools such as sobriety checkpoints and to the states' adoption of a uniform drunken driving standard of a BAC of 0.08 percent. Since courts have held establishments that serve alcohol liable for the consequences of allowing drunk customers to drive, many bars and restaurants have joined the campaign against drunk driving.

✓**check-in** What steps do you take to prevent drunk driving disasters? Do you always designate a driver who won't drink at all? Do you never get behind the wheel if you've had more than two drinks within 2 hours, especially if you haven't eaten? Do you never allow intoxicated friends to drive home?

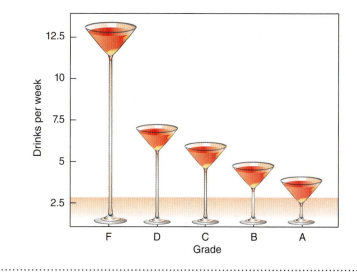

FIGURE 13.1 Alcohol and Academic Success

Source: SIU's Core Institute and SDSU's eCHECKUP TO GO, http://core.siuc.edu and www.echeckuptogo.com.

"Secondhand" Drinking Problems

Heavy alcohol use can endanger both drinkers and others. Secondhand problems caused by others' alcohol use include:

• Loss of sleep.
• Interruption of studies.
• Assaults.
• Vandalism.
• Unwanted sexual advances.

Students living on campuses with high rates of binge drinking are two or more times as likely to experience these secondhand effects as those living on campuses with low rates. In one study, nearly three-quarters of campus rapes happened when the victims were so intoxicated that they were unable to consent or refuse.

Understanding Alcohol

Pure alcohol is a colorless liquid obtained through the fermentation of a liquid containing sugar. **Ethyl alcohol**, or *ethanol*, is the type of alcohol in alcoholic beverages.

Hospitals have reported cases of alcohol poisoning, some fatal, after consumption of hand sanitizers, such as Purell, which contain 60 percent ethyl alcohol. Some people drink it straight as a "Purell shot," and others use salt to separate the ethyl alcohol from the glycerin in the gel.

ethyl alcohol The intoxicating agent in alcoholic beverages; also called ethanol.

Another type—methyl, or wood, alcohol—is a poison that should never be consumed.

Any liquid containing 0.5 to 80 percent ethyl alcohol by volume is an alcoholic beverage; however, different drinks contain different amounts of alcohol. The types of alcohol consumed vary around the world. Beer accounts for most of the alcohol consumed in the United States. People in southern European countries such as France, Spain, Italy, and Portugal prefer wine.

Do you know what a "drink" is? Most students—particularly freshmen, sophomores, and women—don't. In one experiment undergraduates defined a "drink" as one serving, regardless of how big it was or how much alcohol it contained. In fact, one standard drink can be any of the following:

- **One bottle or can** (12 ounces) of beer, which is 5 percent alcohol.
- **One glass** (4 or 5 ounces) of table wine, such as burgundy, which is 12 percent alcohol.
- **One small glass** (2.5 ounces) of fortified wine, which is 20 percent alcohol.
- **One shot** (1 ounce) of distilled spirits (such as whiskey, vodka, or rum), which is 50 percent alcohol.

All of these drinks contain close to the same amount of alcohol—that is, if the number of ounces in each drink is multiplied by the percentage of alcohol, each drink contains the equivalent of approximately 0.5 ounce of 100 percent ethyl alcohol.

Drinks at college parties vary greatly in their alcoholic content. It may be impossible for students to monitor their alcohol intake simply by counting the number of drinks they consume. In one study, when asked to pour a liquid into cups of various sizes to reflect what they perceived to be one beer, one shot, or the amount of liquor in one mixed drink, undergraduates overpoured beer by 25 percent, shots by 26 percent, and mixed drinks by 80 percent.

The words *bottle* and *glass* also can be deceiving:

- Drinking a 16-ounce bottle of malt liquor, which is 6.4 percent alcohol, is not the same as drinking a 12-ounce glass of light beer (3.2 percent alcohol): The malt liquor contains 1 ounce of alcohol and is the equivalent of two drinks.
- Two bottles of high-alcohol wines (such as Cisco), packaged to resemble much less powerful wine coolers, can lead to alcohol poisoning, especially in those who weigh less than 150 pounds.

With distilled spirits (such as bourbon, scotch, vodka, gin, and rum), alcohol content is expressed in terms of **proof**, a number that is twice the percentage of alcohol—for example, 100-proof bourbon is 50 percent alcohol, and 80-proof gin is 40 percent alcohol. Many mixed drinks are equivalent to one and a half or two standard drinks; for instance, see the margarita in Figure 13.2.

Palcohol, the first powdered alcohol product to be marketed and sold in the United States, is sold in individual-serving size packets that, when added to 6 ounces of liquid, are equivalent to a standard drink. This study assessed awareness of powdered alcohol and likelihood to use and/or misuse powdered alcohol among college students. In a recent study of college students, 16.4 percent had heard of powdered alcohol, but after reading a brief description, 23 percent indicated that they would use the product if available. Of these, 62 percent also indicated likelihood of misusing the product—for example, by snorting it or mixing it with alcohol. Hazardous drinkers were six times more likely to say they might misuse the product.[45]

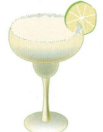

Margarita:

1½ oz tequila (80 proof) = 1.5 oz × 40 percent alcohol = 0.6 oz alcohol

¾ oz triple sec (60 proof) = 0.75 oz × 30 percent alcohol = 0.23 oz alcohol

Splash of sour mix

Dash of lime juice

Salt for the rim

0.83 oz alcohol = 1½ drinks

Malt liquor:

16 oz × 6.4 percent alcohol = 1 oz alcohol = 2 drinks

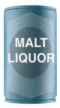

proof The alcoholic strength of a distilled spirit, expressed as twice the percentage of alcohol present.

FIGURE 13.2 How many standard drinks are you drinking?

Blood-Alcohol Concentration

The amount of alcohol in your blood at any given time is your **blood-alcohol concentration (BAC)**. It is expressed in terms of the percentage of alcohol in the blood and is often measured from breath or urine samples.

Law enforcement officers use BAC to determine whether a driver is legally drunk. All the states have followed the recommendation of the federal Department of Transportation to set 0.08 percent—the BAC that a 150-pound man would have after consuming about three mixed drinks within an hour—as the threshold at which a person can be cited for drunk driving (see Figure 13.3).

Using a formula for blood-alcohol concentration developed by highway transportation officials, researchers calculate that when college students drink, their typical BAC is 0.079, dangerously close to the legal limit.

A BAC of 0.05 percent indicates approximately 5 parts alcohol to 10,000 parts other blood components. Most people reach this level after consuming one or two drinks and experience all the positive sensations of drinking—relaxation, euphoria, and well-being—without feeling intoxicated. If they continue to drink past the 0.05 percent BAC level, they start feeling worse rather than better, gradually losing control of speech, balance, and emotions. At a BAC of 0.2 percent, they may pass out. At a BAC of 0.3 percent, they could lapse into a coma; at 0.4 percent, they could die.

Many factors affect your BAC and response to alcohol, including the following:

- **How much and how quickly you drink.** The more alcohol you put into your body, the higher your BAC. If you chug drink after drink, your liver, which metabolizes about 0.5 ounce of alcohol an hour, won't be able to keep up—and your BAC will soar.

- **What you're drinking.** The stronger the drink, the faster and harder the alcohol hits. Straight shots of liquor and cocktails such as martinis get alcohol into your bloodstream faster than beer or table wine. Beer and wine not only contain lower concentrations of alcohol but also contain nonalcoholic substances that slow the rate of **absorption** (passage of the alcohol into body tissues).

- **Mixers.** Carbon dioxide—whether in champagne, ginger ale, or a cola—whisks alcohol into your bloodstream. Also, the alcohol in warm drinks—such as a hot rum toddy or warmed sake—moves into your bloodstream more quickly than the alcohol in chilled wine or scotch on the rocks. Mixing alcohol with a diet soft drink causes higher alcohol concentrations, as measured by breath analysis, in both women and men, compared to mixing alcohol with a nondiet beverage.

- **Your size.** If you're a large person (whether due to fat or to muscle), you'll get drunk more slowly than someone smaller who's drinking the same amount of alcohol at the same rate. Heavier individuals have a larger water volume, which dilutes the alcohol they drink.

- **Your sex.** Women have lower quantities of a stomach enzyme that neutralizes alcohol, so one drink for a woman has the impact that two drinks have for a man. Hormone levels also affect the impact of alcohol. Women are more sensitive to alcohol just before menstruation, and birth control pills and other forms of estrogen can intensify alcohol's impact (see Figure 13.3).

- **Your age.** The same amount of alcohol produces higher BACs in older drinkers, who have lower volumes of body water to dilute the alcohol than younger drinkers do. People over 50 may become impaired after only one or two drinks.

- **Your race.** Many members of certain ethnic groups, including Asians and Native Americans, are unable to break down alcohol as quickly as Caucasians. This can result in higher BACs, as well as uncomfortable reactions, such as flushing and nausea, when they drink.

- **Other drugs.** Some common medications—including aspirin, acetaminophen (Tylenol), and ulcer medications—can cause blood-alcohol levels to increase more rapidly. Individuals taking these drugs can be over the legal limit for blood-alcohol concentration after as little as a single drink.

- **Family history of alcoholism.** Some children of alcoholics don't develop any of the usual behavioral symptoms that indicate someone is drinking too much. It's not known whether this behavior is genetically caused or is a result of growing up with an alcoholic.

- **Eating.** Food slows the absorption of alcohol by diluting it, by covering some of the membranes through which alcohol would be absorbed, and by prolonging the time the stomach takes to empty. Eating while consuming alcohol can significantly reduce alcohol concentrations.

- **Expectations.** In various experiments, volunteers who believed they were given alcoholic beverages but were actually given

blood-alcohol concentration (BAC) The amount of alcohol in the blood, expressed as a percentage.

absorption The passage of substances into or across membranes or tissues.

FIGURE 13.3 Alcohol Impairment
Chart

Source: Adapted from data supplied by the Pennsylvania Liquor Control Board.

Men	Approximate blood alcohol percentage								
	Body weight in pounds								
Drinks	100	120	140	160	180	200	220	240	
0	.00	.00	.00	.00	.00	.00	.00	.00	Only safe driving limit
1	.04	.03	.03	.02	.02	.02	.02	.02	Impairment begins
2	.08	.06	.05	.05	.04	.04	.03	.03	Driving skills significantly affected
3	.11	.09	.08	.07	.06	.06	.05	.05	
4	.15	.12	.11	.09	.08	.08	.07	.06	Possible criminal penalties
5	.19	.16	.13	.12	.11	.09	.09	.08	
6	.23	.19	.16	.14	.13	.11	.10	.09	
7	.26	.22	.19	.16	.15	.13	.12	.11	Legally intoxicated
8	.30	.25	.21	.19	.17	.15	.14	.13	
9	.34	.28	.24	.21	.19	.17	.15	.14	Criminal penalties
10	.38	.31	.27	.23	.21	.19	.17	.16	

Subtract 0.01 percent for each 40 minutes of drinking.
One drink is 1.25 oz of 80 proof liquor, 12 oz of beer, or 5 oz of table wine.

Women	Approximate blood alcohol percentage									
	Body weight in pounds									
Drinks	90	100	120	140	160	180	200	220	240	
0	.00	.00	.00	.00	.00	.00	.00	.00	.00	Only safe driving limit
1	.05	.05	.04	.03	.03	.03	.02	.02	.02	Impairment begins
2	.10	.09	.08	.07	.06	.05	.05	.04	.04	Driving skills significantly affected
3	.15	.14	.11	.10	.09	.08	.07	.06	.06	
4	.20	.18	.15	.13	.11	.10	.09	.08	.08	Possible criminal penalties
5	.25	.23	.19	.16	.14	.13	.11	.10	.09	
6	.30	.27	.23	.19	.17	.15	.14	.12	.11	
7	.35	.32	.27	.23	.20	.18	.16	.14	.13	Legally intoxicated
8	.40	.36	.30	.26	.23	.20	.18	.17	.15	
9	.45	.41	.34	.29	.26	.23	.20	.19	.17	Criminal penalties
10	.51	.45	.38	.32	.28	.25	.23	.21	.19	

Subtract 0.01 percent for each 40 minutes of drinking.
One drink is 1.25 oz of 80 proof liquor, 12 oz of beer, or 5 oz of table wine.

.01–.06 BAC	.06–.10 BAC	.11–.20 BAC	.21–.29 BAC	.30–.39 BAC	.40+ BAC
Relaxation, sense of well-being, loss of inhibition, lowered alertness

Some impact on thought, judgment, coordination, concentration | Blunted feelings, disinhibition, extroversion, reduced sexual pleasure

Impaired reflexes, reasoning, depth perception, distance acuity, peripheral vision, glare recovery | Emotional swings, anger, sadness, boisterous

Impaired reaction time, gross motor control, staggering, slurred speech | Stupor, impaired sensations

Severe motor impairment, memory blackouts | Not responsive, slowed heart rate, breathing, risk of death | Not responsive, death |

nonalcoholic drinks acted as if they were guzzling the real thing and became more talkative, relaxed, and sexually stimulated.

- **Physical tolerance.** If you drink regularly, your brain becomes accustomed to a certain level of alcohol. You may be able to look and behave in a seemingly normal fashion, even though you drink as much as would normally intoxicate someone your size. However, your driving ability and judgment will still be impaired.

- **Your drinking companions.** According to new research, the people around you can influence your sense of inebriation. If surrounded by others who are also drunk, you are more likely to underestimate how drunk you are. If your companions are sober, you are more aware of alcohol's impact on you.[46]

- **Tolerance.** Once you develop tolerance, you may drink more to get the desired effects from alcohol. In some people, this can lead to abuse and alcoholism. On the other hand, after years of drinking, some people become exquisitely sensitive to alcohol. Such reverse tolerance means that they can become intoxicated after drinking only a small amount of alcohol.

✓**check-in** Which of these above-mentioned factors may influence your BAC when you drink?

Moderate Alcohol Use

Many people describe themselves as "light" or "moderate" drinkers. However, these are not scientific terms. It is more precise to think in terms of the amount of alcohol that seems safe for most people. The federal government's Dietary Guidelines for Americans recommend no more than one drink a day for women and no more than two drinks a day for men. The American Heart Association (AHA) advises that alcohol account for no more than 15 percent of the total calories consumed by an individual every day, up to an absolute maximum of 1.75 ounces of alcohol a day—the equivalent of three beers, two mixed drinks, or three and a half glasses of wine.

Moderate alcohol use has been linked with some positive health benefits, including lower risks of heart disease. In addition, middle-aged women who report light to moderate drinking are less likely to put on excessive weight over time. However, even occasional binges of four to five drinks a day can undo alcohol's positive effects.

The benefits of alcohol also are related to age. Below age 40 drinking at all levels is associated with an increased risk of death. Among people older than 50 or 60, moderate drinkers have the lowest risk of death.

Using a mathematical model, researchers have determined that alcohol-related problems occur at every drinking level, including just two drinks, but increase fivefold at three drinks and more gradually thereafter. Individuals who drink heavily have a higher mortality rate than those who have two or fewer drinks a day. However, the boundary between moderate and heavy drinking isn't the same for everyone. For some people, the upper limit of safety is zero: Once they start, they can't stop.

✓**check-in** If you drink, do you consider yourself a moderate drinker?

Alcohol Intoxication

If you drink too much, the immediate consequence is that you get drunk—or, more precisely, intoxicated. Alcohol intoxication, which can range from mild inebriation to loss of consciousness, is characterized by at least one of the following signs: slurred speech, poor coordination, unsteady gait, abnormal eye movements, impaired attention or memory, stupor, or coma.

Medical risks of intoxication include falls, hypothermia in cold climates, and increased risk of infections because of suppressed immune function. Time and a protective environment are the recommended treatments for alcohol intoxication.

✓**check-in** Do you know how best to help someone who's intoxicated?

To help an intoxicated person, follow these guidelines:

- Continually monitor the individual.

- If the person is "out," check breathing and wake the person often to be sure he or she is not unconscious.

- Do not force the person to walk or move around.

- Do not allow the person to drive a car or ride a bicycle.

- Do not give the person food, liquid (including coffee), medicines, or drugs to "sober up."

- Do not give the person a cold shower; the shock of the cold could cause unconsciousness.

Alcohol Poisoning

In large enough doses, alcohol can and does kill. Alcohol depresses nerves that control involuntary actions, such as breathing and the gag reflex (which prevents choking). A fatal dose of alcohol will eventually suppress these functions. Because alcohol irritates the stomach, people who drink an excessive amount often vomit. If intoxication has led to a loss of consciousness, a drinker is in danger of choking on vomit, which can cause death by asphyxiation. Blood-alcohol concentration can rise even after a drinker has passed out because alcohol in the stomach and intestine continues to enter the bloodstream and circulate throughout the body.

The signs of alcohol poisoning include:

- Mental confusion, stupor, coma, or the inability to be roused.
- Vomiting.
- Seizures.
- Slow breathing (fewer than eight breaths per minute).
- Irregular breathing (10 seconds or more between breaths).
- Hypothermia (low body temperature), bluish skin color, paleness.

Alcohol poisoning is a medical emergency requiring immediate treatment. Black coffee, a cold shower, and letting a person "sleep it off" do not help. Without medical treatment, breathing slows, becomes irregular, or stops. The heart beats irregularly. Body temperature falls, which can cause cardiac arrest. Blood sugar plummets, which can lead to seizures. Vomiting creates severe dehydration, which can cause seizures, permanent brain damage, or death. Even if the victim lives, an alcohol overdose can result in irreversible brain damage.

✓check-in Do you know what to do if you suspect alcohol poisoning? Call 911 immediately for help.

The Impact of Alcohol on the Body

Unlike food or drugs in tablet form, alcohol is directly and quickly absorbed into the bloodstream through the stomach walls and upper intestine. The alcohol in a typical drink reaches the bloodstream in 15 minutes and rises to its peak concentration in about an hour. The bloodstream carries the alcohol to the liver, heart, and brain (see Figure 13.4).

Most of the alcohol you drink can leave your body only after metabolism by the liver, which converts about 95 percent of the alcohol to carbon dioxide and water. The other 5 percent is excreted unchanged, mainly through urination, respiration, and perspiration.

Alcohol is a diuretic, a drug that speeds up the elimination of fluid from the body, so it's a good idea to drink water when you drink alcohol to maintain your fluid balance. Also, alcohol lowers body temperature, so you should never drink in an attempt to get or stay warm.

Digestive System

Alcohol first reaches the stomach, where it is partially broken down. The remaining alcohol is absorbed easily through the stomach tissue into the bloodstream. In the stomach, alcohol triggers the secretion of acids, which irritate the stomach lining. Excessive drinking at one sitting may result in nausea; chronic drinking may result in peptic ulcers (breaks in the stomach lining) and bleeding from the stomach lining.

The alcohol in the bloodstream eventually reaches the liver. The liver, which bears the major responsibility of fat metabolism in the body, converts this excess alcohol to fat. After a few weeks of four or five drinks a day, liver cells start to accumulate fat. Alcohol also stimulates liver cells to attract white blood cells, which normally travel throughout the bloodstream, engulfing harmful substances and wastes. If white blood cells begin to invade body tissue, such as the liver, they can cause irreversible damage. More than 2 million Americans have alcohol-related liver diseases, such as alcoholic hepatitis and cirrhosis of the liver.

Weight and Waists

At 7 calories per gram, alcohol has nearly as many calories as fat (9 calories per gram) and significantly more than carbohydrates or protein (which have 4 calories per gram). Since a standard drink contains 12 to 15 grams of alcohol, the alcohol in a single drink adds about 100 calories to your daily intake. A glass of wine contains as many calories as some candy bars; you would have to walk a mile to burn them off. In addition to being a calorie-dense food, alcohol stimulates the appetite, so you're likely to eat more. Obesity plus daily drinking boosts the risks of liver disease in men and women.

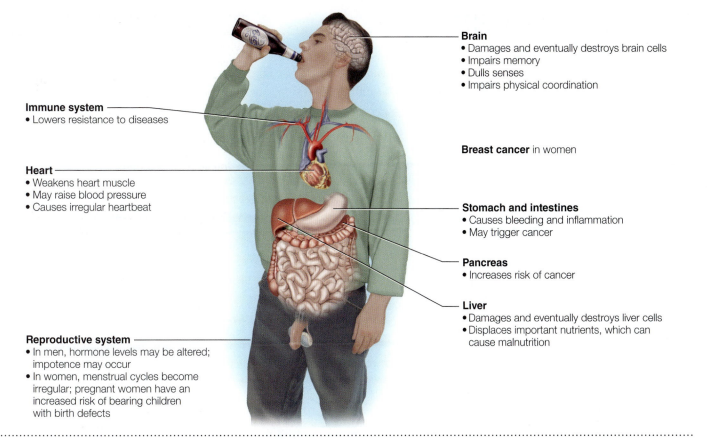

Immune system
• Lowers resistance to diseases

Heart
• Weakens heart muscle
• May raise blood pressure
• Causes irregular heartbeat

Reproductive system
• In men, hormone levels may be altered; impotence may occur
• In women, menstrual cycles become irregular; pregnant women have an increased risk of bearing children with birth defects

Brain
• Damages and eventually destroys brain cells
• Impairs memory
• Dulls senses
• Impairs physical coordination

Breast cancer in women

Stomach and intestines
• Causes bleeding and inflammation
• May trigger cancer

Pancreas
• Increases risk of cancer

Liver
• Damages and eventually destroys liver cells
• Displaces important nutrients, which can cause malnutrition

FIGURE 13.4 The Effects of Alcohol Abuse on the Body

Alcohol has a major effect on the brain, damaging brain cells, impairing judgment and perceptions, and often leading to accidents and altercations. Alcohol also damages the digestive system, especially the liver.

Source: National Institute on Alcohol Abuse and Alcoholism.

Cardiorespiratory System

Alcohol gets mixed reviews regarding its effects on the cardiorespiratory system. Several studies have shown that people who drink moderate amounts of alcohol have lower mortality rates after a heart attack as well as a lower risk of heart attack compared to abstainers and heavy drinkers. However, new research suggests that alcohol may not be as healthy for everyone's heart as previously believed. Light or moderate drinking does not improve cardiovascular health in men and may have only a slight beneficial effect, if any, on women.[47] Heavy drinkers remain at greater risk even after reducing their alcohol intake[48] (see Chapter 10).

However, some cardiologists contend that the benefits of moderate drinking may be overstated, especially because of alcohol's contribution to the epidemic of obesity around the world. Heavier drinking triggers the release of harmful oxygen molecules called free radicals, which can increase the risks of heart disease, stroke, and cirrhosis of the liver. Alcohol use can weaken the heart muscle directly, causing a disorder called cardiomyopathy. The combined use of alcohol and other drugs, including tobacco and cocaine, greatly increases the likelihood of damage to the heart.

Cancer

Overall past and current drinking may contribute to about 10 percent of all cancer cases in men and 3 percent in women. Alcohol consumption has been specifically implicated as a cause of cancers of the oral cavity, pharynx, larynx, esophagus, liver, colon-rectum, pancreas, and female breast.

According to a recent analysis, alcohol use accounts for approximately 3.5 percent of cancer deaths, or about 1 in 30, each year in the United States. Each alcohol-attributable cancer death results in about 18 years of potential life lost. Although cancer deaths are more common among persons who consume an average of three drinks or more per day, approximately 30 percent of deaths occur among people who drink less than

Alcohol and Drug Interactions

Drug	Possible Effects of Interaction
Allergy, cold, flu medicines (Allegra, Benadryl, Claritin, Dimetapp, Sudafed, Tylenol Cold & Flu)	Drowsiness, dizziness, increased risk for overdose
Analgesics (painkillers) Narcotic (Codeine, Demerol, Percodan, Vicodin)	Increase in central nervous system depression, possibly leading to respiratory failure and death
Non-narcotic (aspirin, acetaminophen, ibuprofen)	Irritation of stomach resulting in bleeding and increased susceptibility to liver damage
Antabuse (disulfiram: an aid to quit drinking)	Nausea, vomiting, headache, high blood pressure, and erratic heartbeat
Antianxiety drugs (Valium, Librium, Ativan, Xanax)	Increase in central nervous system depression; decreased alertness and impaired judgment
Antidepressants (Prozac, Zoloft, Celexa, Lexapro, Paxil, Wellbutrin, Luvox, and others)	Increase in central nervous system depression; certain antidepressants in combination with red wine could cause a sudden increase in blood pressure
Antihistamines (Actifed, Dimetapp, and other cold medications)	Increase in drowsiness; decrease in ability to drive
Antibiotics	Nausea, vomiting, headache; some medications rendered less effective
Central nervous system stimulants (caffeine, Dexedrine, Ritalin)	Stimulant effects of these drugs may reverse depressant effect of alcohol but do not decrease its intoxicating effects
Cocaine	Intensification of cocaine's effects; increased risk of sudden death
Sedatives (Dalmane, Nembutal, Quaalude)	Increase in central nervous system depression, possibly leading to coma, respiratory failure, and death

three drinks per day. About 15 percent of breast cancer deaths among women in the United States may be attributable to alcohol consumption.

Alcohol may make women more vulnerable to cancer by increasing estrogen levels. Health officials recommend that women should not exceed one drink a day, and those at an elevated risk for breast cancer, perhaps because of family history, should avoid alcohol or consume alcohol only occasionally.

Brain and Behavior

At first when you drink, you feel up. In low dosages, alcohol affects the regions of the brain that inhibit or control behavior, so you feel looser and act in ways you might not otherwise act. However, you also experience losses of concentration, memory, judgment, and fine motor control, and you have mood swings and emotional outbursts.

Moderate amounts of alcohol can have disturbing effects on perception and judgment, including the following:

- **Impaired perceptions.** You're less able to adjust your eyes to bright lights or to distinguish between sounds or judge their direction well.
- **Dulled smell and taste.** Alcohol may cause some vitamin deficiencies, and the poor eating habits of heavy drinkers result in further nutrition problems.
- **Diminished sensation.** On a freezing winter night, you may walk outside without a coat and not feel the cold.
- **Altered sense of space.** You may not realize, for instance, that you have been in one place for several hours.
- **Impaired motor skills.** Writing, typing, driving, and other abilities involving your muscles are impaired. This is why law enforcement officers sometimes ask suspected drunk drivers to touch their nose with a finger or to walk a straight line.
- **Sleep problems.** Even a single drink can increase snoring in normal sleepers and worsen sleep apnea in those with this disorder. Among young adults, binge drinking increases the frequency and severity of sleep problems.
- **Impaired sexual performance.** While drinking may increase your interest in sex, it may also impair sexual response, especially a man's ability to achieve or maintain an erection. As Shakespeare wrote, "It provokes the desire, but it takes away the performance."

✓**check-in** Have you ever experienced any of these alcohol-induced effects?

Moderate and heavy drinkers show signs of impaired intelligence, slowed reflexes, and difficulty remembering. Because alcohol is a central nervous system depressant, it slows down the activity of the neurons in the brain, gradually dulling the responses of the brain and nervous system. One or two drinks act as a tranquilizer or relaxant. Additional drinks result in a progressive reduction in central nervous system activity, leading to sleep, general anesthesia, coma, and even death.

Heavy alcohol use may pose special dangers to the brains of drinkers at both ends of the age spectrum. Adolescents who drink regularly show impairments in their neurological and cognitive functioning. Elderly people who drink heavily appear to have more brain shrinkage, or atrophy, than those who drink lightly or not at all. In general, moderate drinkers have healthier brains and a lower risk of dementia than those who don't drink and those who drink to excess.

Interaction with Other Drugs

Alcohol can interact with other drugs—prescription and nonprescription, legal and illegal. Of the 100 most frequently prescribed drugs, more than half contain at least one ingredient that interacts adversely with alcohol. Because alcohol and other psychoactive drugs may work on the same areas of the brain, their combination can produce an effect much greater than that expected of either drug by itself. For example, the liver combines alcohol and cocaine to produce cocaethylene, which intensifies the drug's effects and may increase the risk of sudden death. Alcohol is particularly dangerous when combined with other depressants and antianxiety medications (see Consumer Alert).

Immune System

Chronic alcohol use can inhibit the production of both white blood cells, which fight off infections, and red blood cells, which carry oxygen to all the organs and tissues of the body. Alcohol may increase the risk of infection with human immunodeficiency virus (HIV) by altering the judgment of users so that they more readily engage in activities such as unsafe sex that put them in danger. If you drink when you have a cold or the flu, alcohol interferes with the body's ability to recover. It also increases the chance of bacterial pneumonia in flu sufferers.

Health Problems Later in Life

Young adults who drink heavily put themselves at risk of health problems later in life. On average, men with alcohol dependence in young adulthood have an average of three medical conditions in their 60s, compared with two for nondrinkers. Men who experienced alcoholism for at least 5 years in early adulthood scored lower on standard measures of both physical and mental health once they reached their 60s. This increased risk persisted whether or not the person quit drinking by age 30 or continued to drink.[49]

Increased Risk of Dying

Alcohol kills. Drinking, which claims 100,000 lives each year, is the third leading cause of death after tobacco and improper diet and lack of exercise, and involves the following:

- The leading alcohol-related cause of death is injury. Alcohol plays a role in almost half of all traffic fatalities, half of all homicides, and a quarter of all suicides.

- The second leading cause of alcohol-related deaths is cirrhosis of the liver, a chronic disease that causes extensive scarring and irreversible damage.

- As many as half of patients admitted to hospitals and 15 percent of those making office visits seek or need medical care because of direct or indirect effects of alcohol.

- Young drinkers—teens and those in their early 20s—are at highest risk of dying from injuries, mostly car accidents.

- Drinkers over age 50 face the greatest danger of premature death from cirrhosis of the liver, hepatitis, and other alcohol-linked illnesses.

Most studies of the relationship between alcohol consumption and death from all causes show that moderate drinkers—those who consume approximately seven drinks per week—have a lower risk of death than abstainers, while heavy drinkers have a higher risk than either group. In one 10-year study, never-drinkers showed no elevated risk of dying, while consistent heavier drinkers were at higher risk than other men of dying of any cause.

Alcohol, Gender, and Race

Experts in alcohol treatment are increasingly recognizing racial and ethnic differences in risk factors for drinking problems, patterns of drinking, and most effective types of treatment.

Gender

Historically, men have been far more likely to drink alcohol and to drink in ways that affect their health, but this gender gap is closing. Women across the globe are now nearly as likely to drink and to engage in excessive, harmful drinking. Researchers have not identified any single reason why more women are drinking although

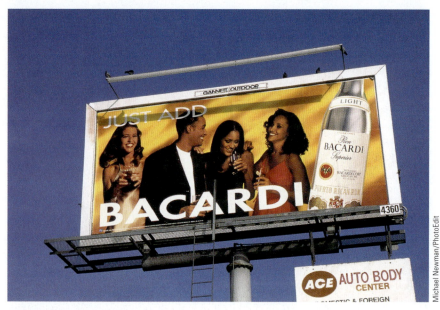

Advertisers often target particular types of alcohol to different ethnic communities.

fetal alcohol effects (FAE)
Milder forms of FAS, including low birth weight, irritability as newborns, and permanent mental impairment as a result of the mother's alcohol consumption during pregnancy.

fetal alcohol syndrome disorders (FASD) A cluster of serious physical and mental defects linked with alcohol consumption during pregnancy.

they speculate that drinking has become more socially acceptable as women have gained more education, greater job opportunities, and financial independence.[50]

The bodies of men and women respond to alcohol in different ways:

- Because they have a far smaller quantity of a protective enzyme in the stomach to break down alcohol before it's absorbed into the bloodstream, women absorb about 30 percent more alcohol into their bloodstream than men (see Table 13.2). The alcohol travels through the blood to the brain, so women become intoxicated much more quickly.

- Blood-alcohol concentration rises faster and stays elevated longer in women than in men. This increases negative health consequences, including increased risk of alcohol-related heart disease, immune disorders (which include autoimmune diseases) and infectious diseases, breast cancer, and liver damage.[51]

- Nearly 14 million American women—one in eight—binge drink about three times a month, averaging about six drinks per binge. The risks to girls and women include injuries, sexual assault, chronic diseases, unintended pregnancy, learning and memory problems, and alcohol dependence. A poor body image and expectations that alcohol will enhance social confidence are risk factors for women's excessive drinking.[52]

- An estimated 15 percent of women drink alcohol while pregnant, most having one drink or less per day. Even light consumption of alcohol can lead to **fetal alcohol effects (FAE)**: low birth weight, irritability as newborns, and permanent mental impairment. Drinking in the latter part of the first trimester may be most likely to cause the physical characteristics typical of FAE.[53]

- A few drinking binges of four or more drinks a day during pregnancy may significantly increase the risk of childhood mental health and learning problems. One of every 750 newborns has a cluster of physical and mental defects called **fetal alcohol syndrome disorders (FASD)**: small head, abnormal facial features, jitters, poor muscle tone, sleep disorders, sluggish motor development, failure to thrive, short stature, delayed speech, mental retardation, and hyperactivity.[54]

- Alcohol interferes with male sexual function and fertility through direct effects on testosterone and the testicles. Damage to the nerves in the penis by heavy drinking can lead to impotence. In women who drink heavily, a drop in female hormone production may cause menstrual irregularity and infertility.

Race

African American Community   Overall, African Americans consume less alcohol per person than whites, yet twice as many blacks die of cirrhosis of the liver each year. In some cities, the rate of cirrhosis is 10 times higher among African American men than among white men. Alcohol also contributes to high rates of hypertension, esophageal cancer, and homicide among African American men.

TABLE 13.2 How Alcohol Discriminates

	Women	Men
Ability to dilute alcohol	Average total body water: 52%	Average total body water: 61%
Ability to metabolize alcohol	Women have a smaller quantity of dehydrogenase, an enzyme that breaks down alcohol.	Men have a larger quantity of dehydrogenase, which allows them to more quickly break down the alcohol they take in.
Monthly fluctuations	Premenstrual hormonal changes cause intoxication to set in faster during the days right before a woman gets her period.	Their susceptibility to getting drunk does not fluctuate dramatically at certain times of the month.
Estrogen levels	Alcohol increases estrogen levels. Birth control pills and other medicines containing estrogen increase intoxication.	Alcohol also increases estrogen levels in men. Chronic alcoholism has been associated with loss of body hair and muscle mass, development of swollen breasts and shrunken testicles, and impotence.

Latino Community The various Hispanic cultures tend to discourage any drinking by women but encourage heavy drinking by men as part of *machismo*, or feelings of manhood. Hispanic men have higher rates of alcohol use and abuse than the general population and suffer a high rate of cirrhosis. Moreover, American-born Hispanic men drink more than those born in other countries.

Few Hispanics with severe alcohol problems enter treatment, partly because of a lack of information, language barriers, and poor community-based services. Hispanic families generally try to resolve problems themselves, and their cultural values discourage the sharing of intimate personal stories, which characterizes Alcoholics Anonymous and other support groups. Churches often provide the most effective forms of help.

Native American Community European settlers introduced alcohol to Native Americans. Because of the societal and physical problems resulting from excessive drinking, at the request of tribal leaders, the U.S. Congress in 1832 prohibited the use of alcohol by Native Americans. Many reservations still ban alcohol use, so Native Americans who want to drink may have to travel long distances to obtain alcohol, which may contribute to the high death rates from hypothermia and pedestrian and motor vehicle accidents among Native Americans. (Injuries are the leading cause of death among this group.)

Certainly, not all Native Americans drink, and not all who drink do so to excess. However, they have three times the general population's rate of alcohol-related injury and illness. Cirrhosis of the liver is the fourth leading cause of death among this cultural group. While many Native American women don't drink, those who do have high rates of alcohol-related problems, which affect both them and their children. Their rate of cirrhosis of the liver is 36 times that of white women. In some tribes, 10.5 of every 1,000 new borns have fetal alcohol syndrome, compared with an average 2 of 1,000 in the general population.

Asian American Community Asian Americans tend to drink very little or not at all, in part because of an inborn physiological reaction to alcohol that causes facial flushing, rapid heart rate, lowered blood pressure, nausea, vomiting, and other symptoms. A very high percentage of women of all Asian American nationalities abstain completely. Some sociologists have expressed concern, however, that as Asian Americans become more assimilated into American culture, they'll drink more—and possibly suffer very adverse effects from alcohol.

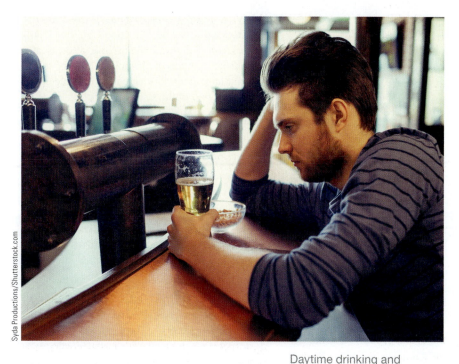

Syda Productions/Shutterstock.com

✓**check-in** Are you at higher risk of alcohol-related consequences because of your sex or race?

Daytime drinking and drinking alone can be signs of a serious problem, even though the drinker may otherwise appear to be in control.

Alcohol-Related Disorders

As many as one in six adults in the United States may have a problem with drinking, which means, by the simplest definition, that they use alcohol in any way that creates difficulties, potential difficulties, or health risks. Like alcoholics, problem drinkers are individuals whose lives are in some way impaired by their drinking. The only difference is degree. Alcohol becomes a problem, and a person becomes an alcoholic, when the drinker can't "take it or leave it." He or she spends more and more time anticipating the next drink, planning when and where to get it, buying and hiding alcohol, and covering up secret drinking.

Alcohol Use Disorder

An estimated 8.5 percent of adults in the United States—12.4 percent of men and 4.9 percent of women—have an **alcohol use disorder**. The prevalence of this problem is greatest among individuals ages 18 to 29 (16.2 percent) but declines over the lifetime to 1.5 percent of those age 65 or older.[55]

alcohol use disorder Problematic pattern of alcohol use leading to significant impairment or distress.

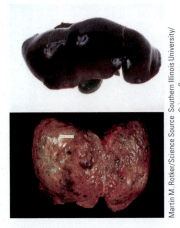

A normal liver (top) compared to one with cirrhosis.

In its most recent *Diagnostic and Statistical Manual (DSM-5)*, the American Psychiatric Association defines an alcohol use disorder as a problematic pattern of alcohol use leading to significant impairment or distress and characterized by at least two of the following:

- Drinking larger amounts of alcohol or drinking for a longer time than intended.

- A strong urge or craving to use alcohol.

- Persistent desire or unsuccessful efforts to cut down or control alcohol use.

- Spending a great deal of time obtaining or using alcohol or recovering from its effects.

- Use of alcohol in physically hazardous situations.

- Continued alcohol use despite social, interpersonal, or occupational problems caused by drinking.

- **Tolerance**, as defined by a need for markedly increased amounts of alcohol to achieve the desired effect or a markedly diminished effect with continued use of the same amount of alcohol.

- **Withdrawal**, including symptoms such as sweating, rapid pulse, increased hand tremors, insomnia, nausea or vomiting, temporary hallucinations or illusions, physical agitation or restlessness, anxiety, or seizures.

- **Alcoholism**, as defined by the National Council on Alcoholism and Drug Dependence and the American Society of Addiction Medicine, is a primary, chronic disease whose development and manifestations are influenced by genetic, psychosocial, and environmental factors. The disease is often progressive and fatal. Its characteristics include an inability to control drinking; a preoccupation with alcohol; continued use of alcohol despite adverse consequences; and distorted thinking, most notably denial. Like other diseases, alcoholism is not a matter of insufficient willpower but a complex problem that can have serious consequences yet can improve with treatment.

Causes

Although the exact cause of alcohol use disorders is not known, certain factors—including biochemical imbalances in the brain, heredity, cultural acceptability, and stress—all seem to play a role. They include the following:

- **Genetics.** Scientists have not yet identified conclusively a specific gene that puts people at risk for alcoholism. However, epidemiological studies have shown evidence of heredity's role. Studies of twins suggest that heredity accounts for two-thirds of the risk of becoming alcoholic in both men and women.

- **Parental alcoholism.** According to researchers, alcoholism is four to five times more common among the children of alcoholics, who may be influenced by the behavior they see in their parents.

✓**check-in** Do you have a family history of alcohol use disorders?

- **Drug abuse.** Alcoholism is associated with the abuse of other psychoactive drugs, including marijuana, cocaine, heroin, amphetamines, and various antianxiety medications.

- **Stress and traumatic experiences.** Many people start drinking heavily as a way of coping with psychological problems.

Medical Complications

As previously discussed, excessive alcohol use adversely affects virtually every organ system in the body, including the brain, the digestive tract, the heart, muscles, blood, and hormones (see Figure 13.4). In addition, because alcohol interacts with many drugs, it can increase the risk of potentially lethal overdoses and harmful interactions. A summary of the major risks and complications follows:

- **Liver disease.** Chronic heavy drinking can lead to alcoholic hepatitis (inflammation and destruction of liver cells) and, in the 15 percent of people who continue drinking beyond this stage, cirrhosis (irreversible scarring and destruction of liver cells). The liver eventually may fail completely, resulting in coma and death.

- **Cardiorespiratory disease.** Heavy drinking can weaken the heart muscle (causing cardiac myopathy), elevate blood pressure, and increase the risk of stroke.

- **Cancer.** Heavy alcohol use may contribute to cancer of the liver, stomach, and colon, as well as malignant melanoma, a deadly form of skin cancer.

- **Brain damage.** Long-term heavy drinkers may suffer memory loss and be unable to think abstractly, recall names of common objects, and follow simple instructions. Chronic brain damage resulting from alcohol consumption is second only to Alzheimer's disease as a cause of cognitive deterioration in adults.

- **Vitamin deficiencies.** Alcoholism is associated with vitamin deficiencies, especially of thiamin (B_1). Lack of thiamin may result in

tolerance A need for markedly increased amounts of alcohol or a drug to achieve the desired effect or a markedly diminished effect with continued use of a substance.

withdrawal Development of symptoms, such as sweating, rapid pulse, tremor, nausea, vomiting, temporary hallucinations, physical agitation, anxiety, or seizures, when substance use is stopped.

alcoholism A chronic, progressive, potentially fatal disease characterized by impaired control of drinking; a preoccupation with alcohol; continued use of alcohol despite adverse consequences; and distorted thinking, most notably denial.

Wernicke-Korsakoff syndrome, which is characterized by disorientation, memory failure, hallucinations, and jerky eye movements, and it can be disabling enough to require lifelong custodial care.

- **Digestive problems.** Alcohol triggers the secretion of acids in the stomach that irritate the mucous lining and cause gastritis. Chronic drinking may result in peptic ulcers (breaks in the stomach lining), bleeding from the stomach lining, and chronic pancreatitis.[56]

Alcoholism Treatments

Individuals whose drinking could be hazardous to their health may choose from a variety of approaches, including medication, behavioral therapy, or both. There is no one path to sobriety. A wide variety of treatments may offer help and hope to those with alcohol-related problems. Men and women who have remained sober for more than a decade credit a variety of approaches, including Alcoholics Anonymous (AA), individual psychotherapy, and other groups, such as Women for Sobriety.

Medications The most widely prescribed medications for alcoholism recovery include the following[57]:

- Disulfiram (Antabuse), in use for more than 50 years, causes unpleasant effects when even small amounts of alcohol are consumed. These include flushing of the face, headache, nausea, vomiting, chest pain, weakness, blurred vision, mental confusion, sweating, choking, breathing difficulty, and anxiety. These effects begin about 10 minutes after alcohol enters the body and last for an hour or more.

- Acamprosate (Campra), combined with counseling and social support, helps the brains of people who have consumed large amounts of alcohol to work normally again. Acamprosate does not prevent withdrawal symptoms and has not been shown to work in people who have not stopped drinking alcohol or who also abuse substances such as street drugs or prescription medications.

- Naltrexone (Revia, Decade, Vivitrol) reduces cravings, perhaps by blocking the normal pleasurable reaction of the part of the brain that reacts to alcohol or opioids.

12-Step Self-Help Programs The best-known and most commonly used self-help program for alcohol problems is AA, which offers support from others struggling with the same

YOUR STRATEGIES FOR PREVENTION
How to Recognize the Warning Signs of Alcoholism

- Experiencing the following symptoms after drinking: frequent headaches, nausea, stomach pain, heartburn, gas, fatigue, weakness, muscle cramps, irregular or rapid heartbeats

- Needing a drink in the morning to start the day

- Denying any problem with alcohol

- Doing things while drinking that are regretted afterward

- Experiencing dramatic mood swings, from anger to laughter to anxiety

- Having sleep problems

- Experiencing depression and paranoia

- Forgetting what happened during a drinking episode

- Changing brands or going on the wagon to control drinking

- Having five or more drinks a day

illness, from a sponsor available at any time of the day or night, and from fellowship meetings that are held every day of the year. Because anonymity is a key part of AA, it has been difficult for researchers to study its success, but it is generally believed to be a highly effective means of overcoming alcoholism and maintaining abstinence. Its 12 steps, which emphasize honesty, sobriety, and acknowledgment of a "higher power," have become the model for self-help groups for other addictive behaviors, including drug abuse (discussed in Chapter 12) and compulsive eating.

Recovery

Recovery from alcoholism is a lifelong process of personal growth and healing. The first two years are the most difficult, and relapses are extremely common. By some estimates, more than 90 percent of those recovering from substance use will use alcohol or drugs in any one 12-month period after treatment. However, approximately 70 percent of those who get formal treatment stop drinking for prolonged periods. Even without treatment, 30 percent of alcoholics are able to stop drinking for long periods. Those most likely to remain sober after treatment have the most to lose by continuing to drink: They tend to be employed, married, and upper-middle class. Recovering alcoholics who help other alcoholics stay sober are better able to maintain their own sobriety.

Increasingly, treatment programs focus on **relapse prevention**, which includes the development of coping strategies and learning

relapse prevention An alcohol recovery treatment method that focuses on social skills training to develop ways of preventing a relapse.

techniques that make it easier to live with alcohol cravings and rehearsal of various ways of saying "no" to offers of a drink. According to outcomes research, social skills training—a combination of stress management therapy, assertiveness and communication skills training, behavioral self-control training, and behavioral marital therapy—has proved effective in decreasing the duration and severity of relapses after one year in a group of alcoholics. A new approach to relapse behavior, Mindfulness-Based Relapse Prevention, teaches clients meditation techniques as a way of coping with cravings and high-risk relapse situations.

Tobacco

In the past, teenagers were most likely to take their first puff of tobacco from a cigarette. Now electronic cigarettes, or e-cigarettes, have become a common entry into tobacco use.[58] Among college students, 9 percent smoked cigarettes within the last 30 days, while about 4 percent used e-cigarettes.[59] About 3 percent of U.S. adults are current e-cigarette users.[60]

There is no risk-free method of using tobacco. Any exposure to tobacco smoke can cause both immediate and long-term damage to the body. Tobacco continues to kill more people than AIDS, alcohol, drug abuse, car crashes, murders, suicides, and fires combined. According to the Centers for Disease Control (CDC), more than 480,000 Americans die each year from smoking or exposure to secondhand smoke, while 16 million suffer from smoking-related illnesses.[61]

✓check-in Did you know that if you smoke and are under age 35, you can add 10 years to your lifespan by quitting?

Tobacco Use in America

Despite widespread awareness of the dangers of tobacco, about 14 percent of Americans smoke cigarettes.[62] The more and the longer that individuals smoke, the greater their risks of heart disease, respiratory problems, several types of cancer, and a shortened lifespan. Consider these facts:

- According to the CDC, 8.6 million Americans suffer from serious smoking-related illnesses.[63]

- Smoking rates are highest among the poor, the mentally ill, drug and alcohol abusers, Native Americans, and lesbian, gay, bisexual, and transgender persons.

- The groups with the lowest smoking rates include women with undergraduate or graduate degrees, men with graduate degrees, Hispanic and Asian women, people over age 65, and residents of Utah. Individuals with undergraduate and graduate degrees are least likely to smoke.

- Asians and Hispanics have the lowest smoking rates.

- Smoking rates vary in different states. Utah has the fewest smokers (about 12 percent); Kentucky has the most (29 percent).

$ HEALTH ON A BUDGET

The Toll of Tobacco

Whether or not you smoke, you indirectly pay the price of tobacco use around the world:

Global economic cost	$500 billion
U.S. economic cost	$193 billion
Annual global number of tobacco-caused deaths	6 million
Annual number of premature deaths due to tobacco in the U.S.	443,000
Property damage in fires caused by smoking, globally	$27 billion
Injuries in fires caused by smoking, globally	60,000
Deaths in fires caused by smoking, globally	17,300
Deaths caused by secondhand smoke in the U.S.	3,000

Source: www.tobaccoatlas.org.

- In the United States, 57 percent of adults have never been smokers; 22 percent are former smokers. Approximately 20 percent of current smokers do not smoke daily.
- Among adults over age 18, about 13 percent—14 percent of men and 12 percent of women—smoke to the extent that they are dependent on nicotine. Tobacco dependence is more prevalent among young adults between the ages of 18 and 29 (17 percent) than among those ages 65 and older (4 percent).[64]

✓check-in Have you ever smoked? If so, how old were you when you tried your first cigarette?

Why People Smoke

Most people are aware that an enormous health risk is associated with smoking, but many don't know exactly what that risk is or how it might affect them.

One of the key factors linked with the onset of a smoking habit is being young. Children who start smoking early in life are at greater risk of both nicotine and alcohol dependence later in life, as well as school failure, crime, injury, and premature death.[65]

According to a recent poll, nearly 90 percent of adults who smoke report that, if they could do it over again, they would not have started. In order to help adolescents avoid that regret as well as smoking's many dangers, some legislators have proposed raising the minimum legal age for purchasing tobacco products to 21.

✓check-in Do you think the minimal legal age for buying tobacco products should be raised to 21?

There are a number of other reasons why people smoke, which are discussed next.

Limited Education
People who have graduated from college are much less likely than high school graduates who have not also graduated from college to smoke; those with fewer than 12 years of education are more likely to smoke. An individual with 8 years or less of education is 11 times more likely to smoke than someone with postgraduate training.

Underestimation of Risks
Young people who think the health risks of smoking are fairly low are more likely than their peers to start smoking. In a 2-year study, teenagers who thought they had little chance of developing either short-term

problems—such as a higher risk of colds or a chronic cough—or long-term problems—such as heart disease, cancer, and respiratory diseases—were three to four times more likely to start smoking.

Adolescent Experimentation and Rebellion
For teenagers, smoking may be a coping mechanism for dealing with boredom and frustration; a marker of the transition into high school or college; a bid for adult status; a way of gaining admission to a peer group; or a way to have fun, reduce stress, or boost energy. The teenagers most likely to begin smoking are those least likely to seek help when their emotional needs are not met. They might smoke as a means of gaining social acceptance or to self-medicate when they feel helpless, lonely, or depressed.

Stress
In studies that have analyzed the impact of life stressors, depression, emotional support, marital status, and income, researchers have concluded that an individual with a high stress level is approximately 15 times more likely than a person with low stress to be a smoker.

Parent Role Models
Children who start smoking are 50 percent more likely than youngsters who don't smoke to have at least one smoker in their family. A mother who smokes seems to be a particularly strong influence in making smoking seem acceptable. The majority of youngsters who smoke say that their parents also smoke and are aware of their own tobacco use.

✓check-in Do your parents smoke? Did they smoke when you were growing up?

Addiction
Nicotine addiction is as strong as or stronger than addiction to drugs such as cocaine and heroin. The first symptoms of nicotine addiction can begin within a few days of starting to smoke and after just a few cigarettes, particularly in teenagers (see Self-Survey: Are You Addicted to Nicotine?).

Genetics
Researchers speculate that genes may account for about 50 percent of smoking behavior, with environment playing an equally important role. Studies have shown that identical twins, who have the same genes, are more likely than fraternal twins to have matching smoking profiles. If one identical twin is a heavy smoker, the other is also likely to be; if one smokes only occasionally, so does the other.

According to NIDA research, genetic factors play a more significant role for initiation of

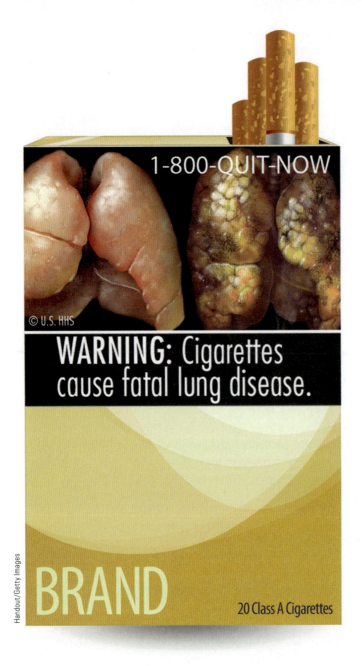

anxiety, and bipolar disorder. People with mental health conditions who smoke are at greater risk of dying prematurely of smoking-related disease and may find quitting more difficult without intensive support.[66]

Substance Abuse   Young adults who drink alcohol or abuse drugs are more likely to use a range of tobacco products, including cigarettes, cigars, e-cigarettes, and other forms of tobacco.[67]

Tobacco Use Disorder

In its *DSM-5*, the American Psychiatric Association defines a **tobacco use disorder** as "a problematic pattern of tobacco use leading to clinically significant impairment or distress," characterized by at least two of the following signs and symptoms within a 12-month period:

- Use of tobacco in larger amounts or over a longer period than was intended.
- Persistent desire or unsuccessful efforts to cut down or control tobacco use.
- A great deal of time spent in activities necessary to obtain or use tobacco.
- Craving, or a strong desire or urge to use tobacco.
- Interference with obligations at work, school, or home because of continued tobacco use.
- Persistent or recurrent social or interpersonal problems, such as arguments about smoking, caused or exacerbated by tobacco.
- Giving up or cutting back on important social, occupational, or recreational activities.
- Recurrent tobacco use in physically hazardous situations, such as smoking in bed.
- Continued tobacco use despite a persistent or recurrent physical or psychological problem caused or exacerbated by tobacco.
- Tolerance, as indicated by a need for markedly increased amounts of tobacco to achieve the desired effect or a markedly diminished effect with continued use of the same amount of tobacco.
- Withdrawal, as indicated by symptoms such as irritability, frustration, anger, anxiety, difficulty concentrating, increased appetite, restlessness, depressed mood, and insomnia, or use of tobacco or closely related substances to avoid such symptoms.

Some cigarette labels warn of the dangers of smoking; others emphasize the benefits of quitting.

smoking in women than in men, but they play a less significant role in smoking persistence for women.

Weight Control   Concern about weight is a significant risk factor for smoking among young women. Daily smokers are two to four times more likely to fast, use diet pills, and purge to control their weight than nonsmokers. Although black women smoke at substantially lower rates than white women, the common factor in predicting daily smoking among all women, regardless of race, is concern with weight.

Mental Disorders   About half of smokers report a mental illness, including depression,

tobacco use disorder A problematic pattern of tobacco use leading to clinically significant impairment or distress.

Student Smoking

Cigarettes	Actual Use			Perceived Use		
Percent (%)	Male	Female	Total	Male	Female	Total
Never used	73.8	81.6	79.1	16.2	11.4	12.9
Used, but not in the last 30 days	16.1	12.2	13.5	16.6	13.0	14.1
Used 1–9 days	6.6	4.0	4.8	45.7	45.0	45.1
Used 10–29 days	1.4	0.8	1.0	12.6	16.2	15.1
Used all 30 days	2.1	1.4	1.6	8.9	14.4	12.8
Any use within the last 30 days	10.1	6.2	7.5	67.3	75.6	73.0

Source: American College Health Association. American College Health Association-National College Health Assessment II: Reference Group Executive Summary Spring 2018. Silver Spring, MD: American College Health Association, 2018.

Tobacco Use on Campus

About one in every four to five students currently smokes, but a majority—77 percent—have never smoked[68] (see Snapshot on Campus Now: Student Smoking). Here is what we know about student smokers:

- Eight in 10 college smokers started smoking before age 18. They report smoking on twice as many days and smoke nearly four times as many cigarettes as those who began smoking at an older age.

- White students have the highest smoking rates, followed by Hispanic, Asian, and African American students. Although black students are least likely to smoke, more are doing so than in the past. Smoking rates remain consistently lower at predominantly black colleges and universities, however.

- About equal percentages of college men and women smoke, although women are somewhat more likely than men to report smoking daily.

- Many college students say they smoke as a way of managing depression or stress. Studies consistently link depression with the use of tobacco products, including electronic cigarettes.[69] Smokers are significantly more likely to have higher levels of perceived stress than nonsmokers. The more depressed students are (particularly women), the more likely they are to use nicotine as a form of self-medication.

- Male students who smoke are more likely to say that smoking makes them feel more masculine and less anxious.

- More than half of female smokers feel that smoking helps them control their weight, although only 3 percent say it is their primary reason for smoking. Overweight female students are more likely to smoke to lose weight and to see weight gain as a barrier to quitting.

- Students can and do change their smoking behavior. As psychologists have noted, often those who quit smoking between ages 18 and 26 become less impulsive and negative over time, so they may "mature out" of this unhealthy behavior.

✓**check-in** How widespread is smoking on your campus?

Social Smoking

Some college students who smoke say they are "social smokers" who average less than one cigarette a day and smoke mainly in the company of others. On the positive side, social smokers smoke less often and less intensely than other smokers and are less dependent on tobacco. However, they are still jeopardizing their health. The more they smoke, the greater the health risks they face. Even smokers who don't inhale or nonsmokers who breathe in secondhand smoke are at increased risk for negative health effects. Here are some examples:

- Smoking less than a pack of cigarettes a week has been shown to damage the lining of blood vessels and to increase the risk of heart disease as well as of cancer.

- In women taking birth control pills, even a few cigarettes a week can increase the likelihood of heart disease, blood clots, stroke, liver cancer, and gallbladder disease.

- Pregnant women who smoke only occasionally still run an increased risk of giving birth to unhealthy babies.

- Social smokers are less motivated than smokers with tobacco use disorder to quit and make fewer attempts to do so. Many end up smoking more cigarettes for many more years than they intended.

✓check-in If you smoke, do you consider yourself a social smoker?

College Tobacco-Control Policies

The American College Health Association (ACHA) has recommended that all forms of tobacco be banned on college campuses, both indoors and outdoors. Many schools have 100 percent smoke- or tobacco-free policies; others prohibit smoking everywhere but in designated areas. Universities that have banned smoking from designated residence halls report decreased damage to the buildings, increased retention of students, and improved enforcement of marijuana policies. Although a majority of students and faculty support restrictions on tobacco use, current and former smokers as well as users of non-cigarette combustible products, such as e-cigarettes, are most likely to oppose such bans.[70]

Enforcement of campus tobacco bans varies, and student smokers often ignore or disregard their schools' policies. Schools are experimenting with various ways to increase compliance, including passing out informational cards and training undergraduates as "ambassadors" to be advocates for no-tobacco policies.

✓check-in Does your school ban tobacco entirely or in certain areas? Would you like to see more or fewer restrictions? Would you ask students smoking in a restricted area to put out their cigarettes?

Smoking, Sex, and Race

Almost 1 billion men in the world smoke—about 35 percent of men in developed countries and 50 percent of men in developing countries. Male smoking rates are slowly declining, but tobacco still kills about 5 million men every year. Men also face specific risks because smoking:

- Increases the risk of aggressive prostate cancer.

- May affect male hormones, including testosterone.

- Can reduce blood flow to the penis, impairing a man's sexual performance and increasing the likelihood of erectile dysfunction.

- Is a risk factor for developing rheumatoid arthritis for men, but not for women.

About 250 million women in the world are daily smokers. Cigarette smoking among women is declining in the United States, but in several southern, central, and eastern European countries, cigarette smoking rates among women are either stable or increasing. On average, girls who begin smoking during adolescence continue smoking for 20 years, which is 4 years longer than boys.

Compared with men who smoke the same amount, women are at greater risk for developing smoking-related illnesses. Here are some examples:

- Lung cancer now claims more women's lives than breast cancer. As discussed later in this chapter, both active and passive smoking increase a woman's risk of breast cancer.

- Teenage girls who smoke may be at increased risk of osteoporosis because girls who smoke build up less bone during this critical growth period in their lives.

- Women who smoke are less fertile and experience menopause 1 or 2 years earlier than women who don't smoke. Smoking also greatly increases the possible risks associated with taking oral contraceptives.

- Women who smoke during pregnancy increase their risk of miscarriage and pregnancy complications, including bleeding, premature delivery, and birth defects such as cleft lip or palate. Smoking narrows the blood vessels and reduces blood flow to the fetus, resulting in lower birth weight, shorter length, smaller head circumference, and possibly lower IQ. Smoking may double or even triple the risk of stillbirth.

✓check-in How might you react if you saw a pregnant woman smoking?

- Youngsters whose mothers smoked during pregnancy tend to have problems with hyperactivity, inattention, and impulsivity. Some of these behavior problems persist through the teenage years and even into adulthood. At ages 16 to 18, children exposed to prenatal smoking have higher rates of conduct disorder, substance use, and depression than others.

- According to the U.S. Surgeon General, women account for 39 percent of smoking-related deaths each year, a proportion that has doubled since 1965. Each year, American women lose an estimated 2.1 million years of life due to premature deaths attributable to smoking. If she smokes, a woman's annual risk of dying more than doubles after age 45 compared with a woman who has never smoked.

- Compared with men, women seem to have a higher behavioral dependence on cigarettes. For them, wearing a nicotine patch or chewing nicotine gum does not substitute for the "hand-to-mouth" behaviors associated with smoking, such as lighting a cigarette, inhaling, and handling the cigarette. Women are more likely to quit successfully when they use a combination of nicotine replacement and a device like a nicotine inhaler to substitute for smoking behaviors.

- LGBTQIA young adults have higher smoking rates, with the heaviest smoking among transgender individuals.[71]

Cigarette smoking is a major cause of disease and death in racial and ethnic minority groups. Among adults, Native Americans and Alaska Natives have the highest rates of tobacco use. African American and Southeast Asian men also have a high smoking rate. Asian American and Hispanic women have the lowest rates of smoking. Tobacco use is significantly higher among white college students than among Hispanic, African American, and Asian American students.

Tobacco is the substance most abused by Hispanic youth, whose smoking rates have soared in the past 10 years. In general, smoking rates among Hispanic adults increase as they adopt the values, beliefs, and norms of American culture. Recent declines in the prevalence of smoking have been greater among Hispanic men with at least a high school education than among those with less education.

Tobacco's Immediate Effects

Tobacco, an herb that can be smoked or chewed, directly affects the brain. While its primary active ingredient is nicotine, tobacco smoke contains almost 400 other compounds and chemicals, including gases, liquids, particles, tar, carbon monoxide, cadmium, pyridine, nitrogen dioxide, ammonia, benzene, phenol, acrolein, hydrogen cyanide, formaldehyde, and hydrogen sulfide.

How Nicotine Works

A colorless, oily compound, **nicotine** is poisonous in concentrated amounts. If you inhale while smoking, 90 percent of the nicotine in the smoke is absorbed into your body. Even if you draw smoke only into your mouth and not into your lungs, you still absorb 25 to 30 percent of the nicotine. The FDA has concluded that nicotine is a dangerous, addictive drug that should be regulated. Yet in recent years tobacco companies have increased the levels of addictive nicotine by an average of 1.6 percent per year.

Faster than an injection, smoking speeds nicotine to the brain in seconds (see Figure 13.5). Nicotine affects the brain in much the same way as cocaine, opiates, and amphetamines, triggering the release of dopamine, a neurotransmitter associated with pleasure and addiction, as well as other messenger chemicals. Because nicotine acts on some of the same brain regions stimulated by interactions with loved ones, smokers subconsciously come to regard cigarettes as a friend that they turn to when they're stressed, sad, or mad.

Nicotine may enhance smokers' performance on some tasks but leaves other mental skills unchanged. Nicotine also acts as a sedative. How often you smoke and how you smoke determine nicotine's effect on you. If you're a regular smoker, nicotine will generally stimulate you at first and then tranquilize you. Shallow puffs tend to increase alertness because low doses of nicotine facilitate the release of the neurotransmitter *acetylcholine*, which makes the smoker feel alert. Deep drags, on the other hand, relax the smoker because high doses of nicotine block the flow of acetylcholine.

nicotine The addictive substance in tobacco; one of the most toxic of all poisons.

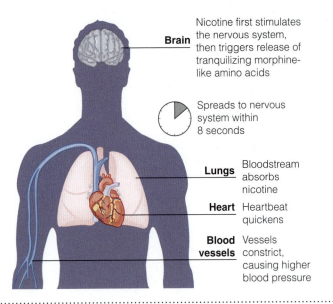

Brain Nicotine first stimulates the nervous system, then triggers release of tranquilizing morphine-like amino acids

Spreads to nervous system within 8 seconds

Lungs Bloodstream absorbs nicotine

Heart Heartbeat quickens

Blood vessels Vessels constrict, causing higher blood pressure

FIGURE 13.5 The Immediate Effects of Nicotine on the Body

The primary active ingredient in tobacco is nicotine, a fast-acting and potent drug.

Sources: American Cancer Society, National Cancer Institute.

Nicotine stimulates the adrenal glands to produce adrenaline, a hormone that increases blood pressure, speeds up the heart rate by 15 to 20 beats a minute, and constricts blood vessels (especially in the skin). Nicotine also inhibits the formation of urine, dampens hunger, irritates the membranes in the mouth and throat, and dulls the taste buds so foods don't taste as good as they would otherwise.

Nicotine withdrawal usually begins within hours. Symptoms include craving, irritability, anxiety, restlessness, and increased appetite.

Tar and Carbon Monoxide

As it burns, tobacco produces **tar**, a thick, sticky dark fluid made up of several hundred different chemicals—many of them poisonous, some of them *carcinogenic* (enhancing the growth of cancerous cells). As you inhale tobacco smoke, tar and other particles settle in the forks of the branchlike bronchial tubes in your lungs, where precancerous changes are apt to occur. In addition, tar and smoke damage the mucus and the cilia in the bronchial tubes, which normally remove irritating foreign materials from the lungs.

Smoke from cigarettes, cigars, and pipes also contains **carbon monoxide**, the deadly gas that comes out of the exhaust pipes of cars, in levels 400 times those considered safe in industry. Carbon monoxide interferes with the ability of the hemoglobin in the blood to carry oxygen, impairs normal functioning of the nervous

tar A thick, sticky dark fluid produced by the burning of tobacco, made up of several hundred different chemicals, many of them poisonous, some of them carcinogenic.

carbon monoxide A colorless, odorless gas produced by the burning of gasoline or tobacco; it displaces oxygen in the hemoglobin molecules of red blood cells.

system, and is at least partly responsible for the increased risk of heart attacks and strokes in smokers.

Health Effects of Cigarette Smoking

As many as 98 percent of tobacco-related deaths, including many due to secondhand smoke, are attributable to "combustible," or smokable, products. Figure 13.6 shows a summary of the physiological effects of tobacco and the other chemicals in tobacco smoke. If you're a smoker who inhales deeply and started smoking before age 15, you're trading a minute of future life for every minute you now spend smoking.

Health Effects on Students

An estimated 6.4 million young people will eventually suffer premature death or diminished quality of life, or both, as a result of smoking-related diseases:

- Although little research has focused specifically on college students, young people who smoke are less physically fit and suffer diminished lung function and growth.
- Young smokers frequently report symptoms such as wheezing, shortness of breath, coughing, and increased phlegm. They also are more susceptible to respiratory diseases.
- Young adults who smoke are three times more likely to have consulted a doctor or mental health professional because of an emotional or psychological problem and almost twice as likely to develop symptoms of depression.
- Frequent smoking has been linked to panic attacks and panic disorder in young people.
- Long-term health consequences of smoking in young adulthood include dental problems, lung disorders (including asthma, chronic bronchitis, and emphysema), heart disease, and cancer.
- Young women who smoke may develop menstrual problems, including irregular periods and painful cramps. If they use oral contraceptives, they are at increased risk of heart disease or stroke.
- Male smokers suffer a more rapid decline in brain function as they age so that early

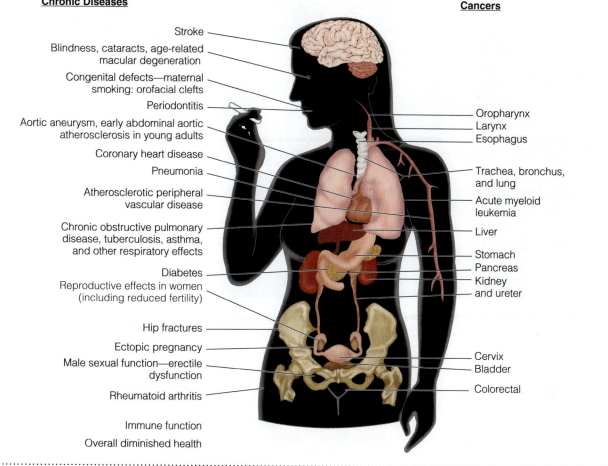

Chronic Diseases

Stroke

Blindness, cataracts, age-related macular degeneration

Congenital defects—maternal smoking: orofacial clefts

Periodontitis

Aortic aneurysm, early abdominal aortic atherosclerosis in young adults

Coronary heart disease

Pneumonia

Atherosclerotic peripheral vascular disease

Chronic obstructive pulmonary disease, tuberculosis, asthma, and other respiratory effects

Diabetes

Reproductive effects in women (including reduced fertility)

Hip fractures

Ectopic pregnancy

Male sexual function—erectile dysfunction

Rheumatoid arthritis

Immune function

Overall diminished health

Cancers

Oropharynx

Larynx

Esophagus

Trachea, bronchus, and lung

Acute myeloid leukemia

Liver

Stomach

Pancreas

Kidney and ureter

Cervix

Bladder

Colorectal

FIGURE 13.6 The Health Consequences of Smoking

Source: The Health Consequences of Smoking—50 Years of Progress: A Report of the Surgeon General. Atlanta, GA: U.S. Department of Health and Human Services, Centers for Disease Control and Prevention, National Center for Chronic Disease Prevention and Health Promotion, Office on Smoking and Health, 2014.

dementia-like symptoms may appear as early as age 45.

✓**check-in** If you smoke, have you experienced any effects on your health?

Premature Death

Smoking kills, robbing smokers of a decade of life. Smokers are half as likely to live to age 80 as nonsmokers. But smoking doesn't kill only the elderly. According to a CDC study, individuals who smoked between ages 12 and 39 have an 86 percent greater risk of dying before age 55 as compared with nonsmokers.

Heart Disease and Stroke

Although a great deal of publicity has been given to the link between cigarettes and lung cancer, heart attack is actually the leading cause of death

for smokers. The federal Office of the Surgeon General blames cigarettes for 1 in every 10 deaths attributable to heart disease.

Smoking is more dangerous than the two most notorious risk factors for heart disease: high blood pressure and high cholesterol. If smoking is combined with one of these, the chances of heart attack are four times greater. Women who smoke and use oral contraceptives have a 10 times greater risk of suffering heart attacks than women who do neither. In addition to contributing to heart attacks, cigarette smoking increases the risk of stroke two to three times in men and women, even after other risk factors are taken into account.

Even people who have smoked for decades can reduce their risk of heart attack if they quit smoking. However, studies indicate some irreversible damage to blood vessels. Progression of atherosclerosis (hardening of the arteries) among former smokers continues at a faster pace than among those who never smoked.

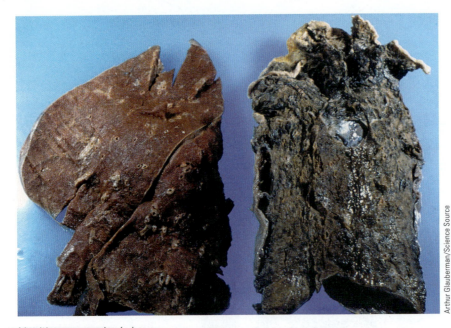

Arthur Glauberman/Science Source

Healthy nonsmoker's lung (left) and smoker's lung (right). Healthy lungs are pink, with a smooth but porous texture. A smoker's lungs show obvious signs of impairment. Bronchial tubes are inflamed, air passages are constricted, and tar coats the bronchial tubes.

Cancer

Smoking is linked to at least 10 different cancers and accounts for 30 percent of all deaths from cancer:

- Smoking is the cause of more than 80 percent of all cases of lung cancer. The more people smoke, the longer they smoke, and the earlier they start smoking, the more likely they are to develop lung cancer. At highest risk are those who have accumulated 30 "pack-years" of smoking—for example, by smoking 20 cigarettes a day for 30 years.

- Smoking causes about 130,000 lung cancer deaths each year. Smokers of two or more packs a day have lung cancer mortality rates 15 to 25 times greater than nonsmokers. If smokers stop smoking before cancer has started, their lung tissue tends to repair itself, even if there were already precancerous changes. However, their risk is never as low as that of individuals who never smoked.

- Cigarette smoking is associated with stomach and duodenal ulcers and with mouth, throat, and other types of cancer, including deadly bladder cancers.

- The risk of breast cancer increases among women who smoke, especially among those who start smoking early. In a recent study, the risks were highest among women who started smoking before their first menstrual cycle and those who started smoking after their first periods but before having their first child.

Respiratory Diseases

Smoking quickly impairs the respiratory system, including the cough reflex, a vital protective response. Cigarette smokers are up to 18 times more likely than nonsmokers to die of noncancerous diseases of the lungs. Even some teenage smokers show signs of respiratory difficulty—breathlessness, chronic cough, excess phlegm production—compared with nonsmokers of the same age.

✓**check-in** Do you know anyone who has developed smoking-related illnesses?

Other Smoking-Related Problems

Smoking, which affects almost every organ system in the body:

- Contributes to gum disease and the loss of teeth and teeth-supporting bone, even in individuals with good oral hygiene.

- Worsens the symptoms or complications of allergies, diabetes, hypertension, cirrhosis of the liver, peptic ulcers, and disorders of the lungs or blood vessels.

- Is an independent risk factor for high-frequency hearing loss and adds to the danger of hearing loss for those exposed to noise.

- May increase the likelihood of anxiety, panic attacks, and social phobias.

- May cause fires that claim thousands of lives.

E-Cigarettes and Vaping

E-cigarettes are battery-powered devices that deliver aerosolized nicotine and additives flavored with chocolate, mint, candy, and other sweetness. Designed to mimic the look and feel of smoking, they are marketed as a relatively benign alternative to cigarettes, without tar, carbon monoxide, and other harmful ingredients.

"Vaping," the term for using e-cigarettes, comes from the cloud of vapor released by electronic cigarettes. More than 100 brands are available, and sales have soared into the billions of dollars. Vaping has gained popularity not just among smokers but also among adolescents and young adults, including many who have never smoked cigarettes but are attracted to the sweet-flavored e-cigarettes.[72]

About 1 in every 5 high school students and 1 in every 20 middle school students report using e-cigarettes in the previous 30 days.[73] Health officials warn that vaping increases the likelihood of subsequent use of traditional cigarettes, marijuana, opioids, and other illicit drugs, as well as both short- and long-term health risks.[74] Some fear that young nonsmokers who start using e-cigarettes are setting themselves up for a lifetime of nicotine dependence.[75]

According to the ACHA, more than 8 in 10 students have never tried electronic cigarettes[76] (see Table 13.3). Nonetheless, vaping on campus has been linked with illicit drug use, mental health problems, and impulsivity in university students.[77] Students who use Juul, a popular e-cigarette brand, are more likely to be male, non-Hispanic white, freshmen or sophomores, and current cigarette smokers.[78] Their reasons for using include curiosity, a friend's recommendation, ease of use, and lack of a bad smell.[79]

Cigarette smokers report being attracted to e-cigarettes for several reasons, including lower cost, perceived lesser danger, freedom to use them in some places where cigarettes are banned, and enjoyment of the "smoking experience." However, puffing on e-cigarettes produces airway constriction and inflammation, might lead to serious lung diseases, including emphysema.[80] The smoke in brands such as Juul may expose users to ultrafine particles that can be inhaled deep into the lungs, cancer-causing chemicals, and heavy metals such as nickel, tin, and lead.[81] Other potential risks include headache, cough, dizziness, sore throat, nose bleeds, chest pain or other cardiovascular problems, and allergic reactions such as itchiness and swelling of the lips.[82] Regular use may lead to nicotine addiction[83] (see Consumer Alert). Health experts continue to debate the risks and benefits of e-cigarettes, as well as the need for greater regulation. Because the long-term effects of e-cigarettes on the cardiovascular system are not known, physicians do not consider them safe for use at any age.[84] E-cigarettes pose the greatest risk to teenagers and young adults, whose brains are still developing, and to pregnant women.[85]

Other Forms of Tobacco

Although cigarettes remain the most widely used form of tobacco, more college students are trying new or "alternative" tobacco products.[86] Especially popular among young adults ages

ⓘ CONSUMER ALERT

E-cigarettes

Electronic cigarettes first emerged as a form of nicotine substitute to help cigarette smokers break their habit. The first generation of "cigalikes," designed to look like conventional cigarettes, restricted the number of puffs and offered limited flavors. More sophisticated devices, perceived as more stylish and equipped with lithium batteries, deliver nicotine more efficiently. Vaping has gained popularity not just among smokers but also among adolescents and young adults, including many who have never smoked cigarettes but are attracted to sweet-flavored e-cigarettes. Serious respiratory problems, hospitalizations, and deaths have led to bans or restrictions on vaping products, particularly flavored e-cigarettes marketed to young people.

Facts to Know

● The sale, use, and advertising of e-cigarettes are permitted in the United States, but some individual states have imposed restrictions.

● There is not yet enough research to show whether e-cigarettes are any more or less toxic than traditional ones.

● E-cigarette smokers report mouth and throat irritation and dry cough with continuing use, and physiological tests reveal changes in respiratory function similar to those caused by cigarette smoking.

● Other potential risks include headache, cough, dizziness, sore throat, nosebleeds, chest pain or other cardiovascular problems, and allergic reaction such as itchiness and swelling of the lips.

● E-cigarette refill cartridges may contain toxic amounts of nicotine, which can remain on surfaces for weeks to months. This "environmental electronic smoke" may create the same dangers associated with secondhand and thirdhand smoke (see page 462).

Steps to Take

● If you are not a smoker, don't try electronic cigarettes as a "healthier" alternative. There is no safe form of tobacco use.

● If you are trying to quit smoking, e-cigarettes may lessen symptoms such as irritability, but it is not yet known whether they help with long-term abstinence.

● Advertisements for e-cigarettes or depictions of vaping serve as visual cues that can trigger nicotine cravings in smokers and former smokers.

● If you try e-cigarettes, use caution. There have been reports of the devices overheating, igniting, or exploding.

TABLE 13.3 E-Cigarettes on Campus

Percent (%)	Actual Use			Perceived Use		
	Male	Female	Average	Male	Female	Average
Never used	75.2	84.1	81.4	14.4	11.6	12.5
Used, but not in the last 30 days	12.0	8.6	9.6	10.9	8.6	9.4
Used 1–9 days	7.0	4.6	5.3	40.9	39.6	39.9
Used 10–29 days	2.5	1.2	1.6	20.8	21.8	21.4
Used all 30 days	3.3	1.4	2.0	13.0	18.4	16.8
Any use within the last 30 days	12.8	7.3	9.0	74.7	79.8	78.1

Source: American College Health Association. American College Health Association-National College Health Assessment II: Reference Group Executive Summary Spring 2018. Silver Spring, MD: American College Health Association, 2018.

18 to 24 are flavored non-cigarette tobacco products, including hookahs, cigars, and smokeless tobacco. Some use multiple products, including cigarettes, bidis, clove cigarettes, smokeless tobacco, and snus.[87] "Polytobacco use" is more likely than any single form of tobacco to lead to nicotine addiction as well as additional health risks.

Two percent of Americans smoke cigars; 2 percent use smokeless tobacco. Ingesting tobacco may be less deadly than smoking cigarettes, but it is dangerous. Smoking cigars, clove cigarettes, and pipes, and chewing or sucking on smokeless tobacco, all put the user at risk of cancer of the lip, tongue, mouth, and throat, as well as other diseases and ailments. Despite claims of lower risk, "safer" cigarettes still jeopardize smokers' health.

Water Pipes (Hookahs)

A water pipe (known by different terms, such as hookah, narghile, arghile, and hubble-bubble, in different parts of the world) allows smoke to pass through water prior to inhalation. Although also used to smoke other substances, including marijuana and hashish, water pipes are most often used with flavored tobacco, made by mixing shredded tobacco with honey or molasses and dried fruit. This mix is most commonly called *shisha* in the United States.

According to the ACHA, 23.2 percent of college students have smoked tobacco from a water pipe (see Table 13.4).[88] Individuals with Middle Eastern backgrounds and their friends are most likely to use hookahs.[89] As with conventional cigarettes, students overestimate their peers' use of hookahs.

Characteristics of users include the following:

- Male.
- 18 to 24 years old.
- White and, in some studies, Hispanic/Latino.
- Some college education.
- Belonging to a sexual minority.
- Also using cigarettes, cigars, and other tobacco products.

Hookah Use on Campus   Many students assume that water-pipe smoking is safer than cigarette smoking,[90] but the existing research indicates that the risks are similar, if not greater:[91]

- A typical 1-hour hookah smoking session involves inhaling 100 to 200 times the volume of smoke inhaled from a single cigarette.
- Waterpipe smoking can lead to nicotine dependence.[92]
- In a recent meta-analysis, water-pipe smoking was significantly associated with lung cancer, respiratory illnesses, low birth weight, and periodontal disease.
- Smoke from a water pipe contains the same harmful or potentially harmful substances as cigarette smoke, often at higher levels.[93]

Water-pipe smoking usually occurs in a group setting. Commercial water-pipe venues, offering ready-to-smoke water pipes, have proliferated in many college towns. Students who use water pipes tend to be younger, male, and white. They also are more likely than other undergraduates to perceive water-pipe tobacco smoking as less harmful and less addictive than cigarette smoking.

✓**check-in** Have you ever smoked a water pipe (hookah)?

The health effects of hookah use include the following[94]:

Short term
- Increased heart rate.
- Increased blood pressure.
- Impaired lung function.
- Carbon monoxide intoxication.

Long term
- Chronic bronchitis.
- Emphysema.
- Coronary artery disease.
- Periodontal (gum) disease.

TABLE 13.4 Tobacco from a Water Pipe (Hookah)

Percent (%)	Actual Use			Perceived Use		
	Male	Female	Average	Male	Female	Average
Never used	79.6	84.0	82.6	24.2	17.0	19.3
Used, but not in the last 30 days	17.1	13.6	14.7	21.1	17.4	18.6
Used 1–9 days	2.7	2.1	2.3	43.5	48.2	46.6
Used 10–29 days	0.4	0.2	0.3	7.7	12.1	10.7
Used all 30 days	0.2	0.1	0.2	3.5	5.3	4.8
Any use within the last 30 days	3.3	2.4	2.7	54.7	65.6	62.1

Source: American College Health Association. American College Health Association-National College Health Assessment II: Reference Group Executive Summary Spring 2018. Silver Spring, MD: American College Health Association, 2018.

Maksim Shmeljov/Shutterstock.com

- Osteoporosis.
- Increased risk of lung, stomach, and esophageal cancer.

Here are some of the facts you need to know about hookah use:

- The charcoal used to heat tobacco in the hookah produces smoke that contains high levels of carbon monoxide, metals, and cancer-causing chemicals.

- A hookah smoking session may expose the smoker to more smoke over a longer period of time than occurs when smoking a cigarette. The volume of smoke inhaled during a typical hookah session is about 90,000 milliliters, compared with 500 to 600 milliliters inhaled when smoking a cigarette. In a recent meta-analysis, water-pipe smoking was significantly associated with lung cancer, respiratory illnesses, low birth weight, and periodontal disease.

- Hookah smokers may absorb higher concentrations of the same toxins found in cigarettes.

- In a 6-month follow-up among college students, hookah users reported smoking more cigarettes more often over time.[95]

- When those who smoke both hookah and cigarettes try to quit, they have lower success rates than cigarette smokers.[96] The interventions that have proven most effective include providing information on the consequences of hookah smoking, assessing readiness to quit, and making individuals aware of withdrawal symptoms.[97]

- Hookah use increases secondhand and thirdhand smoke (discussed later in this chapter) in the room where smoking occurs as well as in adjacent rooms to levels higher than those associated with cigarette smoking.[98]

Cigars and Pipes

Cigar use has declined in the past few years; however, after cigarettes, cigars are the tobacco product most widely used by college students:

- About 2.3 percent of adults age 18 or older in the United States smoke cigars.[99]

- White and African American students are more likely to smoke cigars than Hispanic or Asian American students.

- About 4 in 10 cigar smokers—particularly those who are female, younger, and less wealthy—report using flavored cigars.

✓check-in Do you think that pipes or cigars are "healthier" alternatives to cigarettes?

Many cigarette smokers switch to pipes to reduce their risk of health problems. But former cigarette smokers may continue to inhale, even though pipe smoke is more irritating to the respiratory system than cigarette smoke. People who have smoked only pipes and who do not inhale are less likely to develop lung and heart disease than cigarette smokers. However, they are likely to suffer respiratory problems and to develop—and die of—cancer of the mouth, larynx, throat, and esophagus.

Bidis

Skinny, sweet-flavored cigarettes called **bidis** (pronounced "beedees") have become a smoking fad among teens and young adults. For centuries, bidis were popular in India, where they are known as the poor man's cigarette and sell for less than five cents a pack. They look strikingly like clove cigarettes or marijuana joints and are available in flavors like grape, strawberry, and mandarin orange. Bidis are legal for adults and even minors in some states and are sold on the Internet as well as in stores.

Although bidis contain less tobacco than regular cigarettes, their unprocessed tobacco is more potent. Smoke from bidis has about three times as much nicotine and carbon monoxide and five times as much tar as smoke from regular filtered cigarettes. Because bidis are wrapped in nonporous brownish leaves, they don't burn as easily as cigarettes, and smokers have to inhale harder and more often to keep them lit. In one study, smoking a single bidi required 28 puffs, compared to 9 puffs for a cigarette.

Clove Cigarettes (Kreteks)

Sweeteners have long been mixed with tobacco, and clove, a spice, is an ingredient commonly added to the recipe for cigarettes. Clove cigarettes typically contain two-thirds tobacco and one-third clove. Consumers of these cigarettes are primarily teenagers and young adults.

Many users believe that clove cigarettes are safer because they contain less tobacco, but this isn't necessarily the case. The CDC reports that people who smoke clove cigarettes may be at risk of serious lung injury. Regular kretek smokers have 13 to 20 times the risk for abnormal lung function as nonsmokers.

Clove cigarettes deliver twice as much nicotine, tar, and carbon monoxide as moderate-tar American brands. Eugenol, the active ingredient in cloves (which dentists have used as an anesthetic for years), deadens sensation in the throat, allowing smokers to inhale more deeply and hold smoke in their lungs for a longer time. Chemical relatives of eugenol can produce the kind of damage to cells that may lead to cancer.

bidis Skinny, sweet-flavored cigarettes.

HEALTH NOW!

Kicking the Habit

Here's a six-point program to help you or someone you love quit smoking. (Caution: Don't undertake the quit-smoking program until you have a 2- to 4-week period of relatively unstressful work or study as well as reduced social commitments.)

- **Identify your smoking habits.** Keep a daily diary (a piece of paper wrapped around your cigarette pack with a rubber band will do) and record the times you smoke, the activities associated with smoking (eating a meal, driving), and your urge for a cigarette (desperate, pleasant, or automatic).

- **Get support.** Find some ex-smokers who can give you support.

- **Begin by tapering off.** For a period of 1 to 4 weeks, aim at cutting down to, say, 12 or 15 cigarettes a day. As indicated by your diary, begin by cutting out the cigarettes you smoke automatically. In addition, restrict the times you allow yourself to smoke. Throughout this period, stay in touch, once a day or every few days, with your ex-smoker friend(s) to discuss your problems.

- **Set a quit date.** At some point during the tapering-off period, announce to everyone when you're going to quit.

- **Do it with flair.** Announce it to coincide with a significant date, such as your birthday or an anniversary.

- **Stop.** In the week before Q-day, smoke only five cigarettes a day.

- **Focus on the future.** Now that you've quit, you're becoming healthier, more mature, and better looking. Enjoy the new you.

snus A smokeless tobacco product similar to snuff and chewing tobacco.

✓**check-in** Have you ever tried bidis or clove cigarettes?

Smokeless Tobacco

An estimated 3 percent of adults in the United States use smokeless tobacco products (sometimes called "spit"). Use of chewing tobacco by teenage boys, particularly in rural areas, has surged 30 percent in the past decade. About 9 percent of college men (and 0.4 percent of women) use smokeless tobacco. These substances include snuff, finely ground tobacco that can be sniffed or placed inside the cheek and sucked; and chewing tobacco, tobacco leaves mixed with flavoring agents such as molasses. With both, nicotine is absorbed through the mucous membranes of the nose or mouth.

Smokeless tobacco causes a user's heart rate, blood pressure, and epinephrine (adrenaline) levels to jump. In addition, it can cause cancer and noncancerous oral conditions and lead to nicotine addiction and dependence. People who use smokeless tobacco, or "snuff," become just as hooked on nicotine as cigarette smokers—if not more. Those who both smoke and use snuff may be especially nicotine dependent.

Powerful carcinogens in smokeless tobacco include nitrosamines, polycyclic aromatic hydrocarbons, and radiation-emitting polonium. Its use can lead to the development of white patches on the mucous membranes of the mouth, particularly on the site where the tobacco is placed. Most lesions of the mouth lining that result from the use of smokeless tobacco dissipate 6 weeks after the use of the tobacco product is stopped. However, when first found, about 5 percent of these lesions are cancerous or exhibit changes that progress to cancer within 10 years if not properly treated. Cancers of the lips, pharynx, larynx, and esophagus have all been linked to smokeless tobacco. Nicotine replacement with gum or patches decreases cravings for smokeless tobacco and helps with short-term abstinence; however, it does not improve long-term abstinence. Behavioral approaches are more effective for long-term quitting.

Tobacco control programs, such as higher taxes on smokeless tobacco products, media campaigns, health warnings, and cessation programs, affect smokeless tobacco use but some individuals continue to use other forms of tobacco.[100]

Snus

Snus (rhymes with "loose") is a smokeless tobacco product similar to snuff and chewing tobacco. It was originally developed in Sweden

---

and banned elsewhere in Europe, but tobacco companies have introduced snus in the United States in recent years.[101]

Users, generally white males between the ages of 18 and 24, pack snus under their upper lip and then swallow the byproduct rather than spit it out.[102] Snus may pose less of a cancer risk than other forms of tobacco, but it can lead to or exacerbate other conditions, such as gastroesophageal reflux.[103]

✓**check-in** Have you ever used smokeless tobacco?

Quitting Tobacco Use

The U.S. Public Health Service's most recent guidelines for treating tobacco use and dependence recognize tobacco dependence as "a chronic disease that often requires repeated intervention and multiple attempts to quit." Once a former smoker takes a single puff, the odds of a relapse are 80 to 85 percent. Smokers are most likely to quit on the third, fourth, or fifth attempt. Some interventions aim at reducing exposure to tobacco, for example, by using less toxic products such as pharmaceutical nicotine and potentially reduced-exposure tobacco products as an alternative to cigarettes.[104] Smoking cessation, however, remains the only guaranteed way to reduce the harm caused by tobacco smoking.[105]

Numbers show the difficulty of quitting, but there are effective treatments:

- Two-thirds of smokers want to quit, but many make as many as 30 attempts before finally breaking their nicotine habit.[106]

- About half of whites who have smoked were able to kick the habit, compared with 45 percent of Asian Americans, 43 percent of Hispanics, and 37 percent of African Americans. About 8 in 10 African Americans choose menthol cigarettes, compared with just one-quarter of adults of other races, which may make quitting harder.

- Smokers who work with a counselor specially trained to help them quit and who also use medications or nicotine patches or gum are three times more likely to kick the habit than smokers who try to quit without any help, according to large recent study.

Physical Benefits of Quitting

Young adults who quit smoking see improvements in coughing and other respiratory symptoms within a few weeks, according to a recent study of college students ages 18 to 24. Quitting eliminates the excess risk of dying from heart disease fairly quickly. After 15 smoke-free years, the risk of smoking-related cancers drops to that of someone who never smoked. Table 13.5 provides a more complete list of reasons to quit smoking.

Psychological Benefits of Quitting

Quitting may be as good for your mental health as it is for your physical health, according to analysis of 3 years of data on 4,800 daily smokers in the United States. Significantly fewer of those who quit were less likely to report alcohol or drug problems or anxiety or depression than those who continued to smoke.

Quitting on Your Own

More than 90 percent of former smokers quit on their own—by throwing away all their cigarettes, by gradually cutting down, or by first switching to a less potent brand. One characteristic of successful quitters is that they see themselves as active participants in health maintenance and take personal responsibility for their own health.

Physically active smokers have greater success quitting, possibly because participating in one healthy behavior, such as exercise, leads to adoption of other positive behaviors. Often they experiment with a variety of strategies, such as learning relaxation techniques. In women, exercise has proved especially effective for quitting and avoiding weight gain. Making a home a smoke-free zone also increases a smoker's likelihood of successfully quitting.

Virtual Support

Electronic communications via cell phones, emails, text messages, blogs, and social networking sites may be particularly effective in helping young smokers quit. In the few research studies that have been done, these approaches generally resulted in higher quitting rates—but only if continued over time. Short text messages can help individuals track their smoking urges and provide encouragement in resisting them. Other options include apps for smartphones and online support groups. In one study, smokers who strictly adhered to a stop-smoking phone app were over four times more likely to quit successfully.[107]

TABLE 13.5 Why Quit?

Quitting is the smartest choice a smoker can make—and keeps paying off far into the future. Consider these facts:
• **20 minutes after quitting:** Your heart rate and blood pressure drop.
• **12 hours after quitting:** The carbon monoxide level in your blood drops to normal.
• **2 weeks to 3 months after quitting:** Your circulation improves and your lung function increases.
• **1 to 9 months after quitting:** Coughing and shortness of breath decrease; cilia (tiny hairlike structures that move mucus out of the lungs) regain normal function, increasing the ability to handle mucus, clean the lungs, and reduce the risk of infection.
• **1 year after quitting:** Your excess risk of coronary heart disease is half that of a smoker's.
• **5 years after quitting:** Your stroke risk is reduced to that of a nonsmoker.
• **10 years after quitting:** The lung cancer death rate is about half that of a continuing smoker's. Your risks of cancers of the mouth, throat, esophagus, bladder, cervix, and pancreas also decrease.
• **15 to 20 years after quitting:** Your risk of coronary heart disease is that of a nonsmoker's.

Source: American Cancer Society.

Darkkong/Shutterstock.com

Stop-Smoking Groups

Joining a support group doubles your chances of quitting for good. Options include the American Cancer Society's Freshstart program, the American Lung Association's Freedom from Smoking program, stop-smoking classes (available through student health services on many college campuses as well as through community public health departments), and commercial smoking-cessation programs.

Some smoking-cessation programs rely primarily on **aversion therapy**, which provides a negative experience every time a smoker has a cigarette. This may involve taking drugs that make tobacco smoke taste unpleasant, undergoing electric shocks, having smoke blown at you, or rapid smoking (inhaling smoke every 6 seconds until you're dizzy or nauseated).

Nicotine Anonymous, a nonprofit organization based on the 12-Step programs to recovery developed by Alcoholics Anonymous, acknowledges the power of nicotine and provides support to help smokers, chewers, and dippers live free of nicotine.

Nicotine Replacement Therapy (NRT)

NRT uses a variety of products that supply low doses of nicotine in a way that allows smokers to taper off gradually over a period of months. Nicotine replacement therapies include

aversion therapy A treatment that attempts to help a person overcome a dependence or bad habit by making the person feel disgusted or repulsed by that habit.

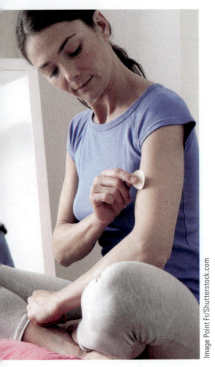

Image Point Fr/Shutterstock.com

A nicotine patch releases nicotine through the skin in measured amounts, which are gradually decreased over time.

nonprescription products (nicotine gum, lozenges, nicotine-free cigarettes, and nicotine patches) and prescription products (nicotine nasal spray, nicotine inhalers, and e-cigarettes).

The nasal spray, dispensed from a pump bottle, delivers nicotine to the nasal membranes and reaches the bloodstream faster than any other nicotine replacement therapy product. The inhaler delivers nicotine into the mouth and enters the bloodstream much more slowly than the nicotine in cigarettes. Electronic cigarettes, or e-cigarettes, mimic the experience of smoking, right down to the glowing tip and smokelike vapor.

The FDA has approved the use of nicotine replacement gums, lozenges, and skin patches for a longer period of time. None of these smoking cessation therapies appear to raise the risk of serious cardiovascular disease events. Although not without some risks, these products are substantially less dangerous than cigarettes and other combustible forms of tobacco.

Although NRT is touted as an aid to permanent cessation of smoking, recent studies have found equivalent rates of relapse among smokers, regardless of whether they used nicotine replacement therapy, with or without professional counseling.[108] Pregnant women and individuals with heart disease shouldn't use nicotine replacements.

The most effective approaches combine medication—nicotine patches or Chantix, for instance—with psychological intervention. Each doubles a person's chance of quitting successfully. Nicotine replacement therapy has proved more beneficial for men than for women—particularly with higher doses of nicotine.

Nicotine Gum

Nicotine gum (available in less expensive generic forms as well) contains a nicotine resin that's gradually released as the gum is chewed. Absorbed through the mucous membrane of the mouth, the nicotine doesn't produce the same rush as a deeply inhaled drag on a cigarette. However, the gum maintains enough nicotine in the blood to diminish withdrawal symptoms.

Although this gum is lightly spiced to mask nicotine's bitterness, many users say that it takes several days to become accustomed to its unusual taste. Its side effects include mild indigestion, sore jaws, nausea, heartburn, and stomachache. Also, because nicotine gum is heavier than regular chewing gum, it may loosen fillings or cause problems with dentures. Drinking coffee or other beverages may block absorption of the nicotine in the gum; individuals trying to quit smoking shouldn't ingest any substance immediately before or while chewing nicotine gum.

Most people use nicotine gum as a temporary crutch and gradually taper off (rather painlessly) until they can stop chewing it; however, 5 to 10 percent of users transfer their dependence from cigarettes to the gum. When they stop using nicotine gum, they experience withdrawal symptoms, although the symptoms tend to be milder than those prompted by quitting cigarettes. Intensive counseling to teach smokers coping methods can greatly increase success rates.

Nicotine Patches

Nicotine transdermal delivery system products, or patches, provide nicotine, their only active ingredient, via a patch attached to the skin by an adhesive. Like nicotine gum, the nicotine patch minimizes withdrawal symptoms, such as the intense craving for cigarettes. Nicotine patches help nearly 20 percent of smokers quit entirely after 6 weeks, compared with 7 percent on a placebo patch. Some insurance programs pay for patch therapy. Nicotine patches, which cost between $3.25 and $4 each, are replaced daily during therapy programs that run between 6 and 16 weeks. Extended use for 24 weeks provides added benefit.

Some patches deliver nicotine around the clock and others for just 16 hours (during waking hours). Those most likely to benefit from nicotine patch therapy are people who smoke more than a pack a day, are highly motivated to quit, and participate in counseling programs. While using the patch, 37 to 77 percent of people are able to abstain from smoking. When combined with counseling, the patch can be about twice as effective as a placebo, enabling 26 percent of smokers to abstain for 6 months. Occasional side effects include redness, itching, or swelling at the site of the patch application; insomnia; dry mouth; and nervousness.

Nicotine Inhaler

Available only by prescription, a nicotine inhaler consists of a mouthpiece and a cartridge containing a nicotine-impregnated plug. The smoker inhales through the mouthpiece, using either shallow or deep puffs. The inhaled air becomes saturated with nicotine, which is absorbed mainly through the tissues of the mouth. The inhaler releases less nicotine per puff than a cigarette and does not contain a cigarette's harmful tars, carbon monoxide, and smoke. Treatment is recommended for 3 months, with a gradual reduction over the next 6 to 12 weeks. Total treatment should not exceed 6 months.

Electronic Cigarettes

As described earlier in the chapter, e-cigarettes are compact, battery-powered devices that allow users to inhale a vaporized liquid nicotine solution instead of tobacco. They simulate the act of smoking and provide smokers with a nicotine "fix" without exposing themselves and others to the toxins in tobacco smoke. Most electronic cigarettes resemble traditional cigarettes and are reusable, with replaceable and refillable components. Although research on their long-term efficacy is limited, e-cigarettes seem as effective as nicotine patches in helping smokers quit.[109] Some people continue to smoke both traditional and e-cigarettes.[110]

As e-cigarettes have gained popularity, they have triggered considerable debate about their potential harms and the distinction between "bad" nicotine in cigarettes and "good" nicotine in devices used to stop smoking. Researchers have found that puffing on e-cigarettes produces airway constriction and inflammation, which might lead to respiratory symptoms and serious lung diseases such as emphysema.[111] Other potential risks include headache, cough, dizziness, sore throat, nose bleeds, chest pain or other cardiovascular problems, and allergic reactions such as itchiness and swelling of the lips. There have been reports of e-cigarettes overheating, igniting, or exploding.

Some argue that using e-cigarettes, referred to as "vaping," may promote continued smoking by allowing smokers of conventional cigarettes to use these alternatives in no-smoking environments or by encouraging people to take up this "safe" form of smoking. On the other hand, their use appears to enhance quitting motivation and significantly reduce cravings in smokers and exposure to toxins for nonsmokers.[112] However, transitioning from cigarettes to the electronic versions may increase the risk for higher and more hazardous patterns of alcohol use.[113]

Medications and Other Treatments

Medications also can help smokers quit. In a study that followed smokers for six weeks, varenicline (brand name Chantix) helped the highest percentage of smokers to quit, followed by bupropion (Zyban), originally developed to treat depression. The most common side effects of Chantix include nausea, insomnia, and abnormal dreams. Combining nicotine replacement products (such as a patch and lozenges) can be as effective as Chantix alone, but requires adherence to two treatments rather than just one.[114]

Hypnosis may help some people quit smoking. Hypnotherapists use their techniques to create an atmosphere of strict attention and give smokers in a mild trance positive suggestions for breaking their cigarette habit.

A form of acupuncture, in which a circular needle or staple is inserted in the flap in front of the opening to the ear, has also had some success. When smokers feel withdrawal symptoms, they gently move the needle or staple, which may increase the production of calming chemicals in the brain.

Combined Treatments

While counseling and medication are each beneficial, the combination is more effective than either alone. In a study of community college students, a computer-assisted interactive smoking cessation program helped almost one in five students stop. One campus-based program that employed peer facilitators to help smokers quit and avoid relapse reported a success rate of 88 percent. Being in the group was the single most powerful contributor to quitting, and participants said their sense of connectedness helped them quit and stay smoke-free. Community-based programs, such as initiatives for a smoke-free environment, also have proven effective, particularly for low-income urban populations.[115]

Quitting and the Risks Associated with Smoking

Not smoking another cigarette is a gift to your body and your life; however, it is not a guarantee that there will be no consequences of the cigarettes you've already smoked (see Health Now!).

Within a year of quitting, an ex-smoker's risk of heart disease drops to half that of active smokers. After 15 years, it approaches that of people who've never smoked. This is great news because the risk of dying prematurely from heart disease is far greater than that of dying from cancer (see Table 13.5).

The risk of lung cancer from smoking fades more slowly, perhaps because of permanent DNA damage to lung cells. Even 10 to 15 years after quitting, an ex-smoker is several times more likely to die of lung cancer than someone who has never smoked. Former smokers are also more vulnerable to the effects of secondhand smoke in the workplace, even if they haven't lit up for the last 10 years.

Does the lung cancer risk ever go away? That may depend partly on how old you are when you quit. Women who quit before age 30 are no more likely to die from lung cancer than those who never smoked. However, a study of American veterans started in the 1950s showed that, even 40 years later, former smokers had a 50 percent greater chance of dying from lung cancer than lifetime nonsmokers.

While quitting sooner is better than later, later is better than never. Even smokers who quit in their 60s significantly reduce their lung cancer risk— and add several years to their life expectancy.

Environmental Tobacco Smoke

Maybe you don't smoke—never have, never will. That doesn't mean you don't have to worry about the dangers of smoking, especially if you live or work with people who smoke. **Environmental tobacco smoke**, or secondhand cigarette smoke, the most hazardous form of indoor air pollution, ranks behind cigarette smoking and alcohol as the third-leading preventable cause of death.

On average, a smoker inhales what is known as **mainstream smoke** eight or nine times with each cigarette, for a total of about 24 seconds. However, the cigarette burns for about 12 minutes, and everyone in the room (including the smoker) breathes in what is known as **sidestream smoke**.

According to the American Lung Association, incomplete combustion from the lower temperatures of a smoldering cigarette makes sidestream smoke dirtier and chemically different from mainstream smoke. It has twice as much tar and nicotine, five times as much carbon monoxide, and 50 times as much ammonia. And because the particles in sidestream smoke are small, this mixture of irritating gases and carcinogenic tar reaches deeper into the lungs and poses a greater threat, especially to infants and children. If you're a nonsmoker sitting next to someone smoking seven cigarettes an hour, even in a ventilated room, you'll take in almost twice the maximum amount of carbon monoxide set for air pollution in industry—and it will take hours for the carbon monoxide to leave your body.

Even a little secondhand smoke is dangerous. As a cancer-causing agent, secondhand smoke may be twice as dangerous as radon gas and more than 100 times more hazardous than outdoor pollutants regulated by federal law. Secondhand smoke also increases the sick leave rates among employees.

environmental tobacco smoke Secondhand cigarette smoke; the third-leading preventable cause of death.

mainstream smoke The smoke inhaled directly by smoking a cigarette.

sidestream smoke The smoke emitted by a burning cigarette and breathed by everyone in a closed room, including the smoker; contains more tar and nicotine than mainstream smoke.

Health Effects of Secondhand Smoke

Environmental tobacco smoke is both dangerous and deadly. A proven culprit in the development of lung cancer, secondhand smoke leads to an estimated 3,000 deaths among adult nonsmokers every year (see Figure 13.7). Here are some of its dangers:

- Living with a smoker increases a nonsmoker's chances of developing lung cancer by 20 to 30 percent.

- Both smoking and secondhand smoke increase a postmenopausal woman's risk of breast cancer.

- Secondhand smoke may increase the risks of cancer of the nasal sinus cavity and of the pharynx in adults, and it may increase the risks of leukemia, lymphoma, and brain tumors in children.

- Exposure to tobacco smoke irritates the airways and contributes to respiratory diseases such as asthma.

- Because of its toxic effects on the heart and blood vessels, it may increase the risk of heart disease by an estimated 25 to 30 percent.

- In the United States, secondhand smoke is thought to cause about 46,000 heart disease deaths a year.

- Secondhand smoke may increase the risk of developing Alzheimer's disease or other dementias.

- Children are particularly vulnerable to secondhand smoke, beginning before birth. Prenatal exposure to tobacco can affect a child's growth, cognitive development, and behavior both before and after birth. Birth weight decreases in direct proportion to the number of cigarettes a mother smoked. As they grow, children of smokers tend to be shorter and weigh less than those of non-smokers. They also may be at higher risk of atherosclerosis.[116]

✓**check-in** How would you describe your lifetime exposure to secondhand smoke?

Thirdhand Smoke

Thirdhand smoke is the nicotine residue that is left behind on furniture, walls, and carpet after a cigarette has been smoked in a room. According to scientists, particulates made up of ozone and nicotine can become airborne a second time and, because they are so small, easily penetrate into

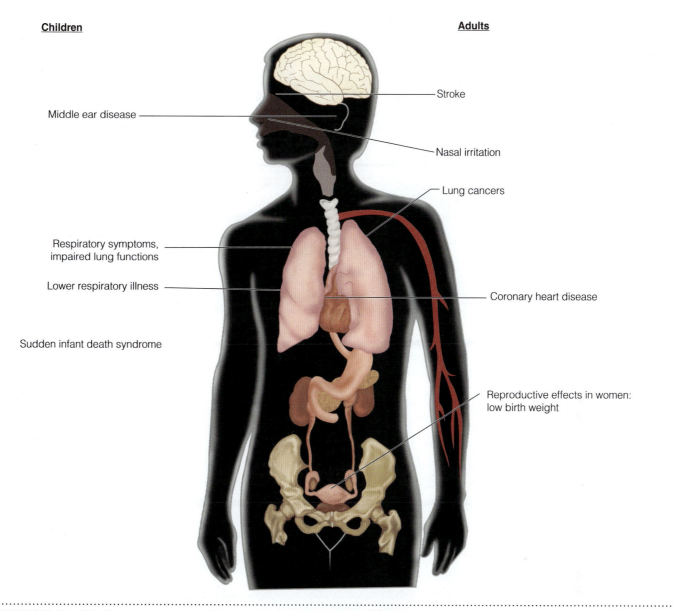

Children

Adults

Stroke

Middle ear disease

Nasal irritation

Lung cancers

Respiratory symptoms, impaired lung functions

Lower respiratory illness

Coronary heart disease

Sudden infant death syndrome

Reproductive effects in women: low birth weight

FIGURE 13.7 Health Consequences of Exposure to Secondhand Smoke

Source: The *Health Consequences of Smoking—50 Years of Progress: A Report of the Surgeon General.* Atlanta, GA: U.S. Department of Health and Human Services, Centers for Disease Control and Prevention, National Center for Chronic Disease Prevention and Health Promotion, Office on Smoking and Health, 2014.

the deepest parts of the lung. Over time, they could contribute to breathing problems such as asthma or possibly even cancer.

Hookah or water-pipe smoking raises levels of secondhand and thirdhand smoke even higher than cigarette smoke in the room where smoking occurs as well as adjacent rooms.[117]

Recent research has documented that third-hand smoke causes DNA damage in human cells. Because ozone can continue to pull nicotine off surfaces and back into the air for months, exposure to thirdhand smoke may continue long after smoking in the area has ceased. The danger may be greatest to infants, children, pregnant women, and the elderly.[118]

Secondhand smoke is the most common and hazardous form of indoor air pollution.

✓**check-in** How would you describe your lifetime exposure to thirdhand smoke?

Thirdhand smoke remains in houses, apartments, and hotel rooms even after smokers move out. The toxins it contains can enter the body by breathing, ingestion, or skin absorption.[119] Among the effects on nonsmokers is an increased risk of breathing problems and cancer.[120] The danger may be greatest to infants, children, pregnant women, and the elderly.

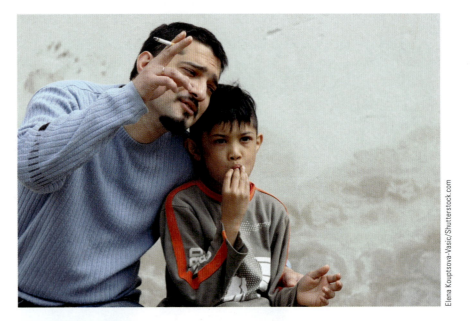

Secondhand smoke can be harmful to a child's growth and health.

Elena Kouptsova-Vasic/Shutterstock.com

WHAT DID YOU DECIDE?

- Why do people smoke even when they're aware of the risks?

- What are the short- and long-term effects of tobacco on health?

- Why are secondhand and thirdhand smoke dangerous to nonsmokers' health?

- Do you agree with experts who see alcohol as the greatest single threat to college students' health?

- What are the most dangerous forms of campus drinking?

- Are "emerging tobacco products" like electronic cigarettes safe to use?

Reflection

The majority of college students have never smoked. Are you among them? If not, reflect on what led you to try your first tobacco or e-cigarette. Do you still smoke? Reflect on the impact tobacco may have on your health now and in the years to come.

TAKING CHARGE OF YOUR HEALTH

Taking Charge of Alcohol and Tobacco

If you use alcohol, develop a defensive drinking program. Check the steps that you have taken or will take in the future to stay in control of your alcohol intake.

____ Finding alternative ways to soothe stress. Daily sessions of meditation have proven effective in helping high-risk student drinkers relax.

____ Setting a limit on how many drinks you're going to have ahead of time—and sticking to it.

____ Always measuring alcohol when you're mixing a drink.

____ Alternating nonalcoholic and alcoholic drinks.

____ Drinking slowly rather than guzzling a beer or tequila shooter.

____ Eating before and while drinking.

____ Avoiding tasks that require skilled reactions during or after drinking.

____ Not encouraging or reinforcing others' irresponsible behavior.

____ Checking out community resources. Are there chapters of AA and Al-Anon on campus? Find out more about the BACCHUS (Boosting Alcohol Consciousness Concerning the Health of University Students) network, including programs in your area. Do these groups offer volunteer opportunities that interest you?

____ Talking to your dorm mates, fraternity brothers, sorority sisters, or roommates about steps you could take collectively, such as restricting drinking in rooms or setting up a "Seize the Keys" policy to prevent drunk driving.

If you smoke—even just a few cigarettes a few times a week—you are at risk of nicotine addiction. Check the steps you will take to get back into control:

____ **Delaying tactics.** Have your first cigarette of the day 15 minutes later than usual, then 15 minutes later than that the next day, and so on.

____ **Distracting yourself.** When you feel a craving for a cigarette, talk to someone, drink a glass of water, or get up and move around.

____ **Establishing nonsmoking hours.** Instead of lighting up at the end of a meal, for instance, get up immediately, brush your teeth, wash your hands, or take a walk.

____ **Never smoking two packs of the same brand in a row.** Buy cigarettes only by the pack, not by the carton.

____ **Making it harder to get to your cigarettes.** Lock them in a drawer, wrap them in paper, or leave them in your coat or car.

____ **Changing the way you smoke.** Smoke with the hand you don't usually use. Smoke only half of each cigarette.

____ **Stopping completely for just one day at a time.** Promise yourself 24 hours of freedom from cigarettes; when the day's over, make the same commitment for one more day. At the end of any 24-hour period, you can go back to smoking and not feel guilty.

____ **Spending more time in places where you can't smoke.** Take up bike riding or swimming. Shower often. Go to movies or other places where smoking isn't allowed.

____ **Going cold turkey.** If you're a heavily addicted smoker, try a decisive and complete break. Smokers who quit completely are less likely to light up again than those who gradually decrease their daily cigarette consumption, switch to low-tar and low-nicotine brands, or use special filters and holders.

If these tactics don't work, talk to your doctor about nicotine replacement options or prescription medications.

SELF-SURVEY

Are You Addicted to Nicotine?

	Yes	No
1. Do you smoke every day?	____	____
2. Do you smoke because of shyness and to build up self-confidence?	____	____
3. Do you smoke to escape from boredom and worries or while under pressure?	____	____
4. Have you ever burned a hole in your clothes, carpet, furniture, or car with a cigarette?	____	____
5. Have you ever had to go to the store late at night or at another inconvenient time because you were out of cigarettes?	____	____
6. Do you feel defensive or angry when people tell you that your smoke is bothering them?	____	____
7. Has a doctor or dentist ever suggested that you stop smoking?	____	____
8. Have you ever promised someone that you would stop smoking, then broken your promise?	____	____
9. Have you ever felt physical or emotional discomfort when trying to quit?	____	____
10. Have you ever successfully stopped smoking for a period of time, only to start again?	____	____
11. Do you buy extra supplies of tobacco to make sure you won't run out?	____	____
12. Do you find it difficult to imagine life without smoking?	____	____
13. Do you choose only those activities and entertainments during which you can smoke?	____	____
14. Do you prefer, seek out, or feel more comfortable in the company of smokers?	____	____
15. Do you inwardly despise or feel ashamed of yourself because of your smoking?	____	____
16. Do you ever find yourself lighting up without having consciously decided to?	____	____
17. Has your smoking ever caused trouble at home or in a relationship?	____	____
18. Do you ever tell yourself that you can stop smoking whenever you want to?	____	____
19. Have you ever felt that your life would be better if you didn't smoke?	____	____
20. Do you continue to smoke even though you are aware of the health hazards posed by smoking?	____	____

Scoring

If you answered yes to one or two of these questions, there's a chance that you are addicted or are becoming addicted to nicotine. If you answered yes to three or more of these questions, you are probably already addicted to nicotine.

Source: Nicotine Anonymous World Services, San Francisco.

REVIEW QUESTIONS

(LO 13.1) 1. Which of the following statements is true about alcohol consumption in America?
   a. White men and women are less likely to drink than other adults.
   b. Married men and women are more likely to drink than their single or divorced counterparts.
   c. Nonstudents consume more alcohol more often than college students of the same age.
   d. More Americans are choosing not to drink, and alcohol consumption is at its lowest level in decades.

(LO 13.1) 2. The most common reason people drink alcohol is to _____.
   a. appear older than they look
   b. feel less tense
   c. treat medical conditions
   d. engage in skilled activities

(LO 13.2) 3. Which of the following statements is true of influences on student drinking?
   a. Students with symptoms of depression are least likely to report risky drinking behavior.
   b. Students who never join a fraternity or sorority report less risky drinking behavior.
   c. Students who live in on-campus housing drink the least.
   d. Students with parents who communicate zero-tolerance messages to alcohol drink the most.

(LO 13.2) 4. Which of the following has been found to be FALSE regarding college binge drinkers?
   a. Most are under the age of 24.
   b. They are likely to be satisfied with their bodies.
   c. They are likely to be involved in social activities.
   d. Binge drinking among college females has increased.

(LO 13.3) 5. The standard definition of "one drink" is based on _____.
   a. volume
   b. amount of alcohol
   c. blood alcohol concentration
   d. a serving

(LO 13.3) 6. Which of the following statements regarding blood-alcohol concentration is true?
   a. Martinis get alcohol into the bloodstream faster than beer or table wine.
   b. Chilled alcohol moves more quickly into the bloodstream than warm alcohol.
   c. Alcohol moves more slowly into the bloodstream when it is mixed with carbon dioxide.
   d. One drink for a man has the impact that two drinks have for a woman.

(LO 13.4) 7. Which of the following statements about alcohol's impact on the body is true?
   a. Alcohol slows down the elimination of fluid from the body.
   b. Alcohol strengthens the heart muscle and decreases the risk of heart diseases.
   c. Alcohol reduces appetite.
   d. Alcohol lowers the body temperature.

(LO 13.4) 8. The leading alcohol-related cause of death is _____.
   a. cancer
   b. liver dysfunction
   c. hepatitis
   d. injury

(LO 13.5) 9. Which of the following statements about sex differences in alcohol consumption is true?
   a. Women tend to have more irregular patterns of drinking than men.
   b. Female alcoholics are less likely to suffer from liver damage than men.
   c. Women absorb about 30 percent more alcohol into their bloodstream than men.
   d. Women have a higher amount of a stomach enzyme that helps digest alcohol than men.

(LO 13.5) 10. Which of the following statements is true about racial factors associated with alcohol consumption?
   a. Cases of cirrhosis of the liver among African Americans are extremely rare as compared with cases among whites.
   b. Hispanic men have a low rate of alcohol-induced cirrhosis of the liver.

c. American-born Hispanic men drink less than Hispanic men born in other countries.

d. Native Americans have three times the general population's rate of alcohol-related injury.

(LO 13.6) 11. _____ is defined by a need for markedly increased amounts of alcohol or a drug to achieve the desired effect or a markedly diminished effect with continued use of a substance.

a. Tolerance
b. Withdrawal
c. Allergy
d. Hypersensitivity

(LO 13.6) 12. Which of the following statements is true about alcoholism?

a. It is mainly caused by insufficient willpower.
b. It rarely has fatal consequences.
c. It can be influenced by heredity.
d. It has declined among women in recent years.

(LO 13.6) 13. Which of the following is true regarding alcohol and pregnancy?

a. It is extremely rare for a woman who drinks alcohol to give birth to a child with fetal alcohol syndrome or who suffers from fetal alcohol effects.
b. Light consumption of alcohol while pregnant cannot lead to fetal alcohol effects.
c. Drinking in the last couple months of pregnancy is likely to cause the child to exhibit the physical characteristics of fetal alcohol effects.
d. Woman who drink during pregnancy put their child at risk for having mental impairment.

(LO 13.7) 14. Which of the following statements is true about tobacco consumption in the United States?

a. Smoking rates are lowest among the poor.
b. Asian and Hispanic women have the lowest smoking rates.
c. Most smokers smoked daily when they first started smoking.
d. Tobacco dependence is more prevalent among individuals age 65 or older.

(LO 13.8) 15. Tobacco use on college campuses _____.

a. is higher among black students than among others
b. continues to increase despite no-smoking policies by all schools
c. is reported to be a way of managing stress
d. occurs primarily with college men

(LO 13.8) 16. Social smokers _____.

a. experience no effects as long as they do not inhale
b. have a higher risk of cancer than nonsmokers, even if they use less than a pack of cigarettes per week

c. sometimes smoke more frequently and intensely than regular smokers and are more dependent on tobacco
d. are more motivated to quit and make more committed attempts to do so

(LO 13.9) 17. Women smokers _____.

a. are less fertile than nonsmokers
b. are more likely to die from breast cancer than lung cancer
c. tend to be more hyperactive than women who do not smoke
d. tend to have a higher physical nicotine dependence

(LO 13.9) 18. Which of the following is one of the differences in smoking behaviors between various racial and ethnic groups?

a. Asian American and Hispanic women have the highest rates of smoking.
b. The proportion of women who smoke has continually increased.
c. Among adults, Native Americans and Alaska Natives have the lowest rates of tobacco use.
d. Tobacco use is significantly higher among white college students than among other students.

(LO 13.10) 19. Which of the following is an effect of nicotine?

a. Release of serotonin in the brain
b. Increased urination
c. Stimulation of the adrenal glands
d. Increased hunger

(LO 13.10) 20. Which of the following is an effect of the carbon monoxide in cigarette smoke?

a. Increased risk of cancer
b. Impairment of normal functioning of the nervous system
c. Constriction of the blood vessels
d. Damaged mucus and cilia in the bronchial tubes

(LO 13.11) 21. The health effects of cigarette smoking include _____.

a. psychological problems
b. earlier onset of dementia among males
c. a more rapid decline in brain function as they age among female smokers as compared with male smokers
d. lowered blood pressure

(LO 13.12) 22. Research conducted so far indicates that e-cigarettes _____.

a. can lead to airway constriction and inflammation
b. have no link to blood pressure
c. are not related to allergic reactions in users
d. do not contribute to thirdhand smoke

(LO 13.12) 23. As compared with other nicotine inhalation methods, water pipe smoking _____.
a. is not associated with lung cancer
b. helps a person avoid many negative effects of smoking tobacco
c. produces a much greater volume of smoke that is inhaled in a single puff
d. involves more puffs to get the same effect as cigarettes

(LO 13.12) 24. Which of the following statements is true about forms of tobacco other than cigarettes?
a. The use of smokeless tobacco is an acceptable alternative to help avoid nicotine dependence.
b. Water pipe smoking has considerably fewer health risks than cigarette smoking.
c. The tobacco in bidis is unprocessed and more potent than the tobacco in cigarettes.
d. Clove cigarettes have not been found to cause any lung injuries.

(LO 13.13) 25. Smokers who try to quit _____.
a. are often successful
b. usually substitute smokeless tobacco
c. typically require several tries to be successful
d. are successful only when they use nicotine replacement therapy

(LO 13.13) 26. Nicotine gum is best used _____.
a. with smokeless tobacco products
b. in conjunction with nicotine patches
c. to simulate the effects of smoking
d. to diminish withdrawal symptoms

(LO 13.14) 27. Secondhand tobacco smoke is _____.
a. the smoke inhaled by a smoker
b. more hazardous than outdoor pollution as a cancer-causing agent
c. not related to breast cancer
d. less likely to cause serious health problems in children than in adults

(LO 13.14) 28. Sidestream smoke is _____.
a. dirtier than mainstream smoke
b. free of the tar particles and carbon monoxide found in mainstream smoke
c. not a cause of serious health problems in small amounts
d. not harmful in a well-ventilated room

Answers to these questions can be found on page 531.

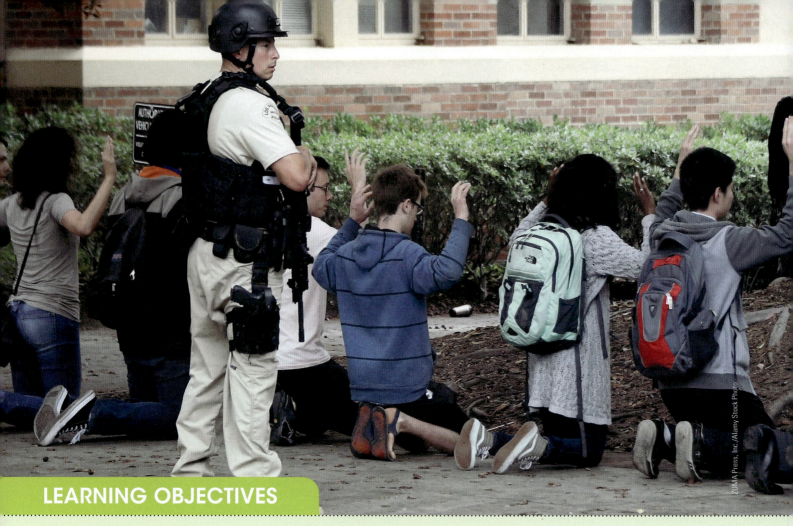

ZUMA Press, Inc./Alamy Stock Photo

LEARNING OBJECTIVES

After reading this chapter, you should be able to:

14.1 Discuss the threats posed by unintentional injuries.

14.2 Outline the best practices for road safety.

14.3 Examine the statement that violence is a significant public health problem.

14.4 Discuss the consequences of campus violence on students.

14.5 Assess the impact of sexual victimization and violence.

14.6 Analyze the relationship between individual health and the health of our environment.

14.7 Assess the impact of pollutants on the surrounding environment.

14.8 Enumerate the health threats posed by polluted air.

14.9 Explain the importance of safe drinking water.

14.10 Explain the importance of breathing clean air when indoors.

14.11 Review the ways that exposure to toxic chemicals can be harmful.

14.12 Describe the threats to health from radiation.

14.13 Enumerate the factors that lead to hearing loss.

WHAT DO YOU THINK?

- What puts college students at high risk for unintentional injury?
- How do campus crime and violence affect students?

- Does climate change pose a risk to health?
- Are you jeopardizing your hearing health?

14

Protecting Yourself and Your Environment

C.J. just wanted to send his friends a quick text to let them know he would be a few minutes late. When he glanced back at the road, all he could see were the headlights of an oncoming car. Then he heard the sickening sound of metal hitting metal and felt a terrible crushing pain shoot up his legs.

"You were lucky," the doctors told C.J. after his surgery.

During his long recovery, C.J. decided that he wanted to get involved with something bigger than his personal ambitions and desires. On campus, C.J. found an environmental action group that needed help with online networking—one of his skills. The more he learned about environmental issues, the more committed he became. When C.J. was able to return to full-time studies, he moved into a "green" residence hall, where he could practice the principles he embraced every day.

Accidents, injuries, assaults, crimes, toxic threats, and contaminated water—all may seem like things that happen only to other people, only in other places. But no one, regardless of how young, healthy, or strong, is immune to danger, both personally and as a citizen of Earth. Ultimately, we have to take responsibility both for our own well-being and for that of the planet we inhabit.

This chapter is a primer in self-protection that can help safeguard, or perhaps even save, your life—on the road, on campus, and in potentially violent situations. It also explores the complex interrelationships between your world and your well-being, including major environmental threats such as air, water, and noise pollution. By realizing that you have a personal responsibility for the health of your environment, you are also helping to safeguard your own well-being. <

Unintentional Injury

The major threat to the lives of college students isn't illness but injury. Almost 75 percent of deaths among Americans 15 to 24 years old are caused by "unintentional injuries" (a term public health officials prefer), suicides, and homicides.[1] Accidents, especially motor vehicle crashes, kill more college-age men and women than all other causes combined; the greatest number of lives lost to accidents is among those 25 years of age.[2] As many as a quarter of college students report suffering a nonfatal accidental injury; most occur during sports activities.[3]

YOUR STRATEGIES FOR PREVENTION

What to Do in an Emergency

Life-threatening situations rarely happen more than once or twice in any person's life. When they happen to you, you must think and act quickly to prevent disastrous consequences:

- **Stop, look, and listen.** Your immediate response to an emergency may be overwhelming fear and anxiety. Take several deep breaths. Start by assessing the circumstances. Look for any possible dangers to yourself or another victim, such as a live electrical wire or a fire. Listen for sounds, such as a cry for help or a siren. Don't attempt rescue techniques, such as cardiopulmonary resuscitation (CPR), unless you're trained.

- **Don't wait for symptoms to go away or get worse.** If you suspect that someone is having a heart attack or stroke, or has ingested something poisonous, *phone for help immediately*. A delay could jeopardize the person's life.

- **Don't move a victim.** The person may have a broken neck or back, and attempting to move him or her could cause extensive damage or even death.

- **Don't drive.** Even if the hospital is just 10 minutes away, you're better off waiting for a well-equipped ambulance with trained paramedics who can deliver emergency care on the spot.

- **Don't do too much.** Often well-intentioned good Samaritans make injuries worse by trying to tie tourniquets, wash cuts, or splint broken limbs. Also, don't give an injured person anything to eat or drink.

- **At home, keep a supply of basic first-aid items in a convenient place.** Beyond the emergency number 911, make sure that telephone numbers for your doctor and neighbors are handy.

The factors that increase the risk of car accidents in young adults include the following: lower economic status, male sex, smoking, binge drinking, drunk driving, illicit drug use, short sleep duration, inadequate sleep, psychological distress (depression and anxiety), danger or risk seeking, type A behavior pattern (irritable, easily angered), low social support.[4]

Life can never be risk-free, but you can do more than anyone else to avoid unnecessary hazards and to maximize your ability to cope with potentially dangerous situations. According to research on survivors of various types of disasters, those who respond well in a crisis tend to have three underlying psychological attributes:

- They believe that they can influence events. (See the discussion of self-efficacy in Chapter 1.)

- They are able to find meaningful purpose in turmoil and trauma. (See the discussion on spirituality in Chapter 2.)

- They know that they can learn from both positive and negative experiences.

✓**check-in** Do you think of yourself as accident-prone? Why or why not?

Safety on the Road

An estimated 40,000 people die in car crashes in the United States every year; about 4.5 million are seriously injured.[5] Alcohol use is a factor in about 40 percent of these crashes; speeding, in about one-third.

Teenage drivers and their passengers are at highest risk of vehicular accidents. Most accidents involving young drivers are due to three all-too-common errors:

- Failing to scan the environment by looking ahead and to the left and the right while driving.

- Going too fast for road conditions (even if under the speed limit).

- Being distracted by something inside or outside the vehicle.

College students aren't necessarily safer drivers than others their age. According to national data, full-time college students drink and drive more often than part-time students and other young adults, but they are also more likely to wear seat belts while driving and riding in cars.[6] (See Table 14.1.) Young women who drink and drive have closed the gender gap in recent years and are at increasing risk of being in fatal accidents.[7]

✓**check-in** Have you ever had a car accident? What happened?

Avoid Distracted Driving

Distracted driving refers to any nondriving activity a person engages in that has the potential to distract him or her from the primary task of driving: eating, drinking, reaching for the phone, texting, talking to a passenger, and so on. According to a study using video technology and in-vehicle sensors, drivers take their eyes off the road about 10 percent of the time they are behind the wheel.[8] Distracted driving contributes to about 6,000 deaths and more than half a million injuries every year.[9]

There are different types of distractions:

- **Visual.** Taking your eyes off the road—to read a text, check a navigation device, watch a video, look in the mirror, glance at something off to the side, etc.

- **Manual.** Taking your hands off the wheel to change a station or playlist, text, make a call, eat or drink something, etc.
- **Cognitive.** Taking your mind off what you're doing—to listen to lyrics, chat with a friend, place a call, pay attention to a podcast, think about what you have to do that day, etc.
- **Social.** Driving with passengers can be distracting—and dangerous. Young male drivers, at greater risk of automobile accidents than female and older drivers, drive faster when they have a friend in the car, particularly if in a happy mood.

The U.S. Department of Transportation offers the following safety precautions:

- Never text or talk on your cell phone while you're behind the wheel.
- Turn off the ringer on your phone and set the phone out of reach while you're driving.
- Never eat, drink, primp, focus on a GPS device, read, or surf through radio stations or playlists while you drive.
- If you happen to call someone who is driving, suggest that the driver call you back when he or she is done driving.

✓**check-in** What is most likely to distract you while driving?

Don't Text or Talk

Even if your cell phone is a hands-free model, using it while driving is as dangerous as driving drunk. Driving while dialing a cell phone makes the risk of a crash or near-crash three times more likely than if a driver were not distracted; texting increases the risk twentyfold.

What makes talking or texting while driving so dangerous?

- These activities distract the brain as well as the eyes—much more so than talking to another person in the vehicle. Conversations between drivers and passengers tend to slow down or stop as driving conditions change.
- Conversation on any type of phone leads to what researchers call "inattention blindness," the inability to recognize objects encountered in the driver's visual field. This form of cognitive impairment may distract drivers for up to 2 minutes after a phone conversation has ended.
- Cell phone use delays a driver's reactions as much as having a blood-alcohol concentration (BAC) at the legal limit of 0.08 percent.

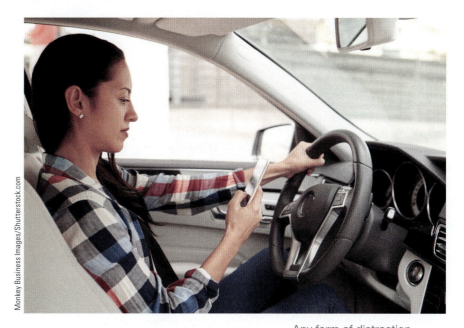

Any form of distraction, including texting on a cell phone, can put you and others at risk.

Many states have passed laws banning use of a cell phone to text or talk while driving. You can check the laws in your state at www.distraction.gov/content/get-the-facts/state-laws.html. Such bans have significantly reduced visits to emergency departments following a collision.[10]

✓**check-in** Have you ever texted while driving? Would you take a pledge never to text and drive?

Stay Alert

The number of fatalities caused by drunk driving, particularly among young people, has dropped. The National Highway Traffic Safety Administration (NHTSA) attributes this decline to several factors:

- Increases in the drinking age.
- Educational programs aimed at reducing nighttime driving by teens.

TABLE 14.1 Student Safety Strategies

	Percent (%)		
	Never	Rarely or sometimes	Mostly or always
Wear a seat belt when you ride in a car	0.4	2.7	97.0
Wear a helmet when you ride a bicycle	36.1	24.9	39.0
Wear a helmet when you ride a motorcycle	9.1	6.6	84.3
Wear a helmet when you are inline skating	50.6	14.7	34.8

Source: American College Health Association. American College Health Association-National College Health Assessment II: Reference Group Executive Summary Spring 2018. Silver Spring, MD: American College Health Association, 2018.

CONSUMER ALERT

Bicycle Helmet Heads-Up

When will you fall off your bike? According to the Bicycle Helmet Safety Institute, the average careful bike rider can expect to crash about every 4,500 miles.

Facts to Know

- Bike helmets can prevent 85 percent of cyclists' head injuries, which cause 75 percent of bicycle-related deaths.
- Even a low-speed fall on a bicycle path can result in a head injury.
- Laws in 22 states and at least 192 localities require helmets.

Steps to Take

- Always look inside a helmet for a Consumer Product Safety Commission (CPSC) sticker before purchasing.

- Check the fit. A helmet should sit level on your head, touching all around, comfortably snug but not tight. The helmet should not move more than about an inch in either direction, regardless of how hard you tug at it.
- Pick a bright color for visibility. Avoid dark colors, thin straps, or a rigid visor that could snag in a fall.
- Look for a smooth plastic outer shell, not one with alternating strips of plastic and foam.
- Watch out for excessive vents, which put less protective foam in contact with your head in a crash.

- The formation of Students Against Destructive Decisions (SADD; originally called Students Against Drunk Driving) and similar groups.
- Changes in state laws to lower the legal BAC level for young drivers. (Some states have a zero-tolerance blood-alcohol level for drivers under age 21.)

Falling asleep at the wheel is second only to alcohol as a cause of serious motor vehicle accidents. About half of drivers in the United States drive while drowsy. Men and young adults between the ages of 18 and 29 are at the highest risk for driving while drowsy or falling asleep at the wheel. Even after a night's sleep, the use of sleeping pills can impair driving ability, particularly in women and those who take extended-release formulations. In a study of college students, those who believed drowsiness would not impair their driving were more likely to get behind the wheel when tired.[11]

✓**check-in** Have you ever driven while drowsy?

Buckle Up

Seat belts save an estimated 9,500 lives in the United States each year, and their use has reached an all-time high, with three in four Americans buckling up. States with seat belt laws have even higher rates of use: 80 percent. However, young people, especially men between the ages of 19 and 29, are less likely than others to use seat belts.

Here's what you need to know about buckling up:

- By official estimates, two-thirds of 15- to 20-year-olds killed in motor vehicle accidents were not wearing seat belts (see Table 14.1).
- When lap–shoulder belts are used properly, they reduce the risk of fatal injury to front-seat passengers by 45 percent and the risk of moderate to critical injury by 50 percent.
- Because an unrestrained passenger can injure others during a crash, the risk of death is lowest when all occupants wear seat belts, according to federal analysts. Seat belt use by everyone in a car may prevent about one in six deaths that might otherwise occur in a crash.

✓**check-in** Do you always buckle up when driving? Do you do the same as a passenger?

Check for Air Bags

An air bag, either with or without a seat belt, has proved the most effective means of preventing adult death, somewhat more so for women than for men. The combination of air bags and seat belts affords the best protection against spine fractures; an air bag alone decreases this risk but to a lesser extent.

Because there is controversy over the potential hazard air bags pose to children, the American Academy of Pediatrics recommends that children sit in the backseat, whether or not the car is equipped with a passenger air bag.

Rein in Road Rage

Emotional outbursts known as road rage are a factor in half of all fatal and nonfatal accidents, according to the NHTSA. The primary triggers are drivers cutting in or weaving, speeding, and exhibiting hostile behaviors.

Some strategies for reducing road rage include:

- Lower the stress in your life. Take a few moments to breathe deeply and relax your shoulders before putting the key in the ignition.
- Consciously decide not to let other drivers get to you. Tell yourself that whatever happens, it's not going to make your blood pressure go up.
- Slow down. If you're going 5 or 10 miles over the speed limit, you won't have the time you need to react to anything that happens.

- Modify bad driving habits one at a time. If you tend to tailgate slow drivers, spend a week driving at twice your usual following distance. If you're a habitual horn-honker, silence yourself.

- Be courteous—even if other drivers aren't. Don't dawdle in the passing lane. Never tail-gate or switch lanes without signaling. Don't use your horn or high beams unless absolutely necessary.

- Never retaliate. Whatever another driver does, keep your cool. Count to 10. Take a deep breath. If you yell or gesture at someone who's upset with you, the conflict may escalate.

- If you do something stupid, show that you're sorry. On its website, the AAA Foundation for Traffic Safety solicited suggestions for automotive apologies. The most popular: slapping yourself on your forehead or the top of your head to indicate that you know you goofed. Such gestures can soothe a miffed motorist—and make the roads a slightly safer place for all of us.

Cycle Safely

Per vehicle mile, motorcyclists are 35 times more likely to die in a crash than passenger-car occupants. The most common motorcycle injury is head trauma, which can lead to physical disability, including paralysis and general weakness, as well as problems reading and thinking. It can also cause personality changes and psychiatric problems, such as depression, anxiety, uncontrollable mood swings, and anger. Complete recovery from head trauma can take 4 to 6 years, and the costs can be staggering. Head injury can also result in permanent disability, coma, and death.

After years of steady increases, motorcycle deaths have begun to fall. Much of the credit goes to helmets, which are required in most states and dramatically reduce the risk not just of death but of head injury and spinal trauma that could otherwise lead to paralysis (see Consumer Alert).

More than 80 million people ride bicycles, about half for basic transportation rather than recreation. Each year, bicycle crashes kill about 700 of these individuals and send 450,000 to 587,000 to emergency rooms. The number of bicyclist fatalities in the United States has increased dramatically in recent years as more Americans commute to school or work by bike. Two-thirds of the deaths occurred in riders who were not wearing helmets.

Only about half of cyclists wear helmets. On college campuses, even fewer students—12 to 25 percent—opt for helmets. Yet in a study of students requiring emergency care for a

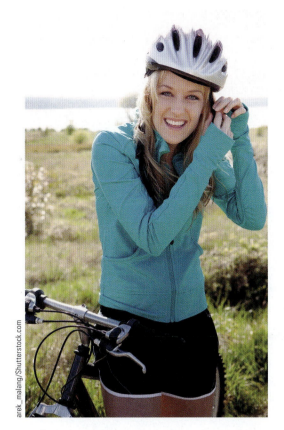

arek_malang/Shutterstock.com

A helmet can significantly reduce your risk of a bicycle-related head injury.

bicycle-related head injury, only 4 percent were wearing helmets. Among the reasons college students give for not wearing helmets are:

- Physical discomfort.
- Cost.
- Biking only a short distance.
- Inconvenience.
- Vanity.
- Concerns about ridicule.
- Impaired vision when wearing a helmet.

✓**check-in** Do you always wear a helmet when on a motorcycle or bicycle?

Violence in America

The World Health Organization (WHO) defines violence as "the intentional use of physical force or power, threatened or actual, against oneself, another person, or a group or community, that

TABLE 14.2 Warning Signs of Violence

Some signs of potential for violence may be historical or static (unchangeable) factors, such as the following:

- A history of violent or aggressive behavior
- Young age at first violent incident
- Having been a victim of bullying
- A history of discipline problems or frequent conflicts with authority
- Early childhood abuse or neglect
- Having witnessed violence at home
- Family or parent condones use of violence
- A history of cruelty to animals
- Having a major mental illness
- Being callous or lacking empathy for others
- A history of vandalism or property damage

Other signs of potential violence may escalate or contribute to the risk of violence given a certain event or activity:

- Serious drug or alcohol use
- Gang membership or strong desire to be in a gang
- Access to or fascination with weapons, especially guns
- Trouble controlling feelings like anger
- Withdrawal from friends and usual activities
- Regularly feeling rejected or alone
- Feeling constantly disrespected

Some signs of potential violence may be new or active:

- Increased loss of temper
- Frequent physical fighting
- Increased use of alcohol or drugs
- Increased risk-taking behavior
- Declining school performance
- Acute episode of major mental illness
- Planning how to commit acts of violence
- Announcing threats or plans for hurting others
- Obtaining or carrying a weapon

Adapted from materials developed by the American Psychological Association, www.apa.org.

TABLE 14.3 Incidences of Firearms Use

Firearms are involved in:

- 68 percent of homicides.
- 52 percent of suicides.
- 43 percent of robberies.
- 21 percent of aggravated assaults.
- 85 percent of fatal suicide attempts.

Source: Federal Bureau of Investigation.

either results in, or has a high likelihood of resulting in, injury, death, psychological harm, maldevelopment, or deprivation." A simpler way of putting it is that "violence is anything you wouldn't want someone to do to you." Although anyone is capable of violent crime, being aware of certain behaviors in a person may keep you safer (see Table 14.2).

Violence, a significant public health problem in this country, kills 55,000 people in the United States every year. The rate of violent injuries and deaths in the United States far exceeds that in any other high-income "peer" nation.

There are ethnic and racial differences in patterns of violence. African Americans are at greater risk of victimization by violent crime than whites or persons of other racial groupings. Hispanics are at greater risk of violent victimization than non-Hispanics.

There is little difference between white women and nonwhite women in rape, physical assault, or stalking. Native American and Alaska Native women are significantly more likely than white women or African American women to report being raped. Mixed-race women also have a significantly higher incidence of rape than white women. Native American and Alaska Native men report significantly more physical assaults than Asian and Pacific Islander men.

There is no simple answer to explain why a person becomes violent and punches, kicks, stabs, or fires a gun at someone else. Among the motives identified by psychologists are:

- **Expression.** Some people use violence to release feelings of anger or frustration.
- **Manipulation.** For some, violence is a way of controlling others or getting something they want.
- **Retaliation.** Individuals may use violence to get back at those who have hurt them or their loved ones.[12]

Gun Violence

More than half a million people died by firearms in the first two decades of the twenty-first century. In 2017, gun violence claimed 38,949 lives, and the age-adjusted death rate rose to 12 per 100,000 people (see Table 14.3).[13] Suicide, which accounts for about 60 percent of these fatalities, and homicide are the leading causes of violent death. Globally, the United States, home to 4.3 percent of the world's population, is second only to Brazil in the total number of firearm deaths.[14]

Firearms also cause nonfatal injuries. During the past 20 years, there have been more than 1.3 million nonfatal injuries by firearms, mostly from assaults. Gun violence shatters lives beyond those who are physically wounded, encompassing friends, family members, and communities. The economic burden of gun violence is enormous. Hospital emergency department and inpatient charges related to shootings are estimated to be almost $3 billion annually.[15]

Black non-Hispanic males have the highest age-adjusted rates of firearm homicide (29.8 firearm homicides per 100,000), followed by white Hispanic males (7) and American Indian, Eskimo, and Aleut non-Hispanic males (6.7). Men commit 94 percent of firearms homicides.[16]

States with the lowest gun ownership have the lowest rates of firearm homicide and suicide among white men. States with the highest gun ownership rates are among those with the highest rates of firearm homicide. States with more restrictive laws have lower rates of firearm death than those with more permissive laws.[17]

One in five Americans reported knowing a victim of gun violence—a family member, a friend, or even themselves. Young people between the ages of 18 and 20 are among those most likely to know a gun violence victim; those between the ages of 15 and 24 are most likely to be targets of gun violence.[18]

✓**check-in** Do you or does anyone in your family own a gun?

Mass Shootings

Mass murder—the killing of four or more people at a single location—has emerged as a national concern, with far too many tragic shootings occurring at schools, college campuses, movie theaters, and public events in recent years.

Although mass shootings had occurred in the past, the Columbine High School shooting in 1999 marked a turning point. Between Columbine and the mass shootings in Las Vegas and Parkland, Florida (in 2017 and 2018, respectively), there were more than 70 such events that killed a total of 620 people and wounded more than 1,000.[19]

Researchers have identified underlying psychosocial issues in mass shooters, including:

- Social alienation.
- Problems with self-esteem.
- Persecutory/paranoid outlook.
- Narcissism.
- Depression.
- Suicidality.
- Family dysfunction.

Mass shootings often reinforce common misconceptions, including the assumptions that mental illness causes gun violence, that psychiatrists can predict gun crime, that shootings represent the deranged acts of mentally ill loners, and that gun control won't prevent other mass shootings. Yet surprisingly little research-based evidence supports these notions[20]:

- Less than 3 to 5 percent of crimes involve people with mental illness, and the percentage for gun-related crimes committed by those with mental illness is lower than the national average for persons not diagnosed with mental illness.

- Although mental illness is strongly associated with increased risk of suicide, the large majority of people with serious mental illness are never violent.[21] A variety of risk factors—including drugs, alcohol, binge drinking, childhood abuse, male sex, and availability of firearms—correlate more strongly with gun violence than mental illness alone.

- Mass shootings represent distortions of, rather than depictions of, the actions of mentally ill people as a whole.

- The vast majority of people diagnosed with psychiatric disorders do not commit violent acts. Only about 4 percent of violence in the United States can be attributed to people diagnosed with mental illness.

✓**check-in** Has your life ever been touched by violence? In what way?

A Public Health Approach

Gun control remains one of the most controversial political issues, with intense disagreement about Second Amendment interpretations of the right to bear arms. However, medical groups are focusing on violence as a public health challenge involving sociocultural, educational, behavioral, and product safety issues rather than solely gun ownership.[22] As they point out, this sort of multidimensional approach has led to great success in reducing smoking rates by more than half since 1966 and in saving thousands of lives by making cars and roads safer.

In order to prevent gun violence, many public health initiatives have been proposed, including the following:[23]

- Prohibiting the purchase and possession of firearms by people with multiple criminal convictions related to alcohol abuse.

How Safe Do Students Feel?

	Percentage Feeling "Very Safe"		
	Male	**Female**	**Average**
On their campus (daytime)	86.0	79.1	80.8
On their campus (nighttime)	53.8	23.1	32.2
In the community surrounding their school (daytime)	59.0	47.1	50.4
In the community surrounding their school (nighttime)	32.1	12.8	18.6

Source: American College Health Association. American College Health Association-National College Health Assessment II: Reference Group Executive Summary Spring 2018. Silver Spring, MD: American College Health Association, 2018.

✓**check-in** Do you give much thought to your day-to-day safety? What do you think is the greatest threat to your well-being? Are there steps you could take to reduce the potential danger? Have you shared your concern with others?

- Prohibiting firearm purchase by people convicted of violent misdemeanor crimes, such as assault and battery.
- Requiring background checks on recipients to help prevent prohibited people from acquiring firearms anonymously and illegally from private parties, including via the Internet.[24]

✓**check-in** Which public policy changes do you think might help lessen the toll of gun violence in the United States?

Violence and Crime on Campus

Most college students feel safe on campus, especially during the daytime, but less so at night and in the community surrounding their school.[25] (See Snapshot: On Campus Now.) According to the Bureau of Justice Statistics, college students are victims of almost half a million violent crimes a year, including assault, robbery, sexual assault, and rape.

Although this number may seem high, the overall violent crime rate has dropped from 88 to 41 victimizations per 1,000 students in the past decade. You can take steps to lower your risk—at little or no financial cost.

College students ages 18 to 24 are less likely to be victims of violent crime, including robbery and assault, than nonstudents of the same age. However, fatalities and injuries from violent crimes are increasing on university campuses.[26]

More than half (58 percent) of crimes against students are committed by strangers. More than 9 in 10 occur off campus, most often in an open area or street, on public transportation, in a place of business, or at a private home. In about two-thirds of the crimes, no weapon is involved. Most off-campus crimes occur at night, while on-campus crimes are more frequent during the day (see Table 14.4).

✓**check-in** Do you feel safe on your campus? Why or why not?

Male college students are twice as likely as female students to be victims of violence overall. White undergraduates have higher rates of violent victimization than students of other races. Simple assault accounts for two-thirds of violent crimes against students; sexual assault or rape accounts for around 6 percent.[27]

Substance use increases the risk of sexual and physical victimization of college students. College women are more likely to report sexual violence associated with most forms of substance use, while college men are more likely to be victims of physical violence.

About three in four campus crimes are never reported to the police. The main reasons students give for not reporting crimes are that they are too minor or private or they are not certain that the action was a crime. Individuals also may be ashamed or too emotionally overwhelmed to contact authorities.

According to researchers, only 2 percent of victimized college women report crimes to the police. The most frequent reason for not reporting sexual and physical incidents is that they didn't seem serious enough. However, women who were sexually victimized also felt ashamed, feared that they would be held responsible, or didn't want anyone to know what happened. Nonwhite women were significantly more likely than white women to say that they did not report an incident to the police because they thought they would be blamed or because they did not want the police involved.

The Jeanne Clery Disclosure of Campus Security Policy and Campus Crime Statistics Act, originally known as the Student Right-to-Know and Campus Security Act, requires colleges to publish annual crime statistics for their campuses. However, the act excludes certain offenses, such as theft, threats, harassment, and vandalism, so the picture it presents may not be complete. The most recent crime statistics for the nation's colleges, universities, and career schools are posted online at http://ope.ed.gov/security.

✓**check-in** How would you rate safety at your school?

Campuses have implemented dozens of programs to halt violence, and many have proven effective. Some use posters to raise awareness of dating violence. Others have designed sexual violence prevention programs for members of fraternities, sororities, and intercollegiate athletic teams. Many have established codes of conduct barring the use of alcohol and drugs, fighting, and sexual harassment and have instituted policies requiring suspension or expulsion for students who violate the codes. Some schools are experimenting with social media messages and training bystanders to intervene to prevent problems such as violence against women.

Hazing

Hazing refers to any activity that humiliates, degrades, or poses a risk of emotional or physical harm for the sake of joining a group or maintaining full status in that group. This behavior may occur in fraternities and sororities, athletic teams, or other campus organizations. Its forms include verbal ridicule and abuse, forced consumption

TABLE 14.4 Violence, Abusive Relationships, and Personal Safety

Within the past 12 months, college students reported experiencing the following:			
	Percent %		
	Male	Female	Total
A physical fight	6.4	2.1	3.5
A physical assault (not sexual assault)	2.9	2.7	2.9
A verbal threat	21.2	15.8	17.7
Sexual touching without their consent	4.6	12.4	10.2
Sexual penetration attempt without their consent	1.0	5.0	3.9
Sexual penetration without their consent	0.7	3.2	2.5
Stalking	2.6	6.7	5.6
An emotionally abusive intimate relationship	6.5	10.7	9.6
A physically abusive intimate relationship	1.7	1.9	1.9
A sexually abusive intimate relationship	1.1	3.0	2.5

Source: American College Health Association. American College Health Association-National College Health Assessment II: Reference Group Executive Summary Spring 2018. Silver Spring, MD: American College Health Association, 2018.

of alcohol or ingestion of vile substances, sexual violation, sleep deprivation, paddling, beating, burning, and branding.

Hate or Bias Crimes

The term *hate crime* generally refers to a criminal offense committed against a person or property that is motivated, in whole or in part, by bias or prejudice against race, national or ethnic origin, religion, sexual orientation, or disability. In the last decade, there have been reports of more acts of hate on college campuses, such as vandalism of minority students' meeting places or painting of swastikas or racist words on walls. To counteract this trend, many schools have set up programs and classes to educate students about each other's backgrounds and to make campuses less alienating and more culturally and emotionally accessible to all.

Racism and prejudice can be hard to deal with individually. By banding together, however, those who experience discrimination can take action to protect themselves, challenge the ignorance and hateful assumptions that fuel bigotry, and promote a healthier environment for all. Beyond the immediate victims, hate crimes affect the psychological and emotional well-being of entire groups, with individuals of similar backgrounds or orientations reporting depression, anxiety, pain, and anger that, for some, result in feelings of inadequacy and low self-worth.

hazing Any activity that humiliates, degrades, or poses a risk of emotional or physical harm for the sake of joining a group or maintaining full status in that group.

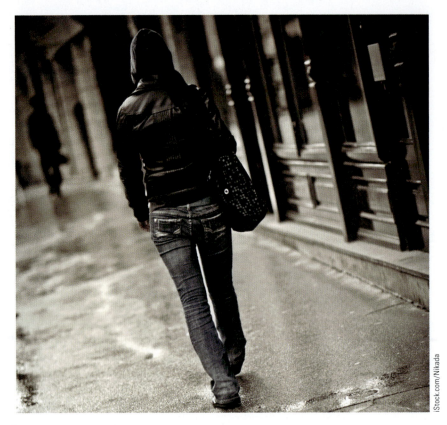
iStock.com/Nikada

Does your campus have regular security patrols, surveillance cameras, or late-night escorts? Have you taken advantage of these services?

The perpetrators of microaggressions may be unaware of the hidden messages that they transmit and that, even when inadvertent, foster negative stereotypes. In classic experiments, African Americans and women performed worse on academic tests when primed with stereotypes about race or sex. Women told that many females have poor math aptitude, for instance, typically do worse on math tests than those given positive encouragement. African Americans' intelligence test scores may plunge when they're primed with messages of inferior intelligence.[29]

✓**check-in** Do you know of hate or bias crimes on your campus? Have they ever been directed at you or your friends?

Campus Shootings

A study of 190 shootings at 142 two- and four-year colleges found an increase in shootings over time, with the greatest increase on campuses with greater access to guns. The causes of the shootings, in order of frequency, included:

- Disputes.
- Robbery.
- Drugs.
- Targeted students or staff.
- Domestic violence.
- Rampages with mass casualties.
- Shooters denied entry or kicked out of a party.

The majority of the shooters were not associated with the college. About a third were students or former students. Almost two-thirds of the incidents happened in Southern states.[30]

Most state colleges ban guns on campus, but some schools have allowed concealed weapons. According to several studies, laws allowing students to carry guns have had no statistically significant impact on campus crime or gun violence.[31]

The American College Health Association has recommended various strategies to keep campuses safe, including:

- Enforcing codes of conduct.
- Imposing tougher sanctions, including expulsion, for serious misconduct.
- Implementing zero-tolerance policies for campus violence.
- Building a sense of community.
- Screening out students who pose a real threat.

Microaggressions

While many minority students say that overt prejudice is rare and relatively easy to deal with, everyday insults, indignities, and demeaning messages, called microaggressions, can undermine their academic confidence and their ability to bond with the university.[28] They take several forms:

- Microassaults: conscious and intentional actions or slurs, such as using racial or sexual epithets or showing preferential treatment to nonminority customers at shops and restaurants.
- Microinsults: verbal and nonverbal communications that subtly convey rudeness and insensitivity and demean a person's racial heritage or identity—for example, comments that a Hispanic student speaks English without an accent or that an individual doesn't look or dress "gay."
- Microinvalidations: communications that subtly exclude, negate, or nullify the thoughts, feelings, or experiential reality of an individual. For instance, white people may ask Asian Americans where they were born, conveying the message that they are perpetual foreigners in their own land, or may ask someone of mixed-race background "what" he or she is.

- Warning students about criminal activity at orientation, through the campus newspaper, in residence halls, and through campus Internet communications devices.

✓check-in What is your school doing to keep students, faculty, and staff safe?

Consequences of Campus Violence

Crime and violence take a great toll at colleges and universities. Violence can seriously injure people as well as claim lives. Moreover, victims of violent crime often suffer lasting psychological and emotional effects. Some victims take a leave of absence or transfer to another school. Those who remain in school may have problems concentrating, studying, and attending classes, and they may avoid academic and social activities. Some develop clinical symptoms that affect their mental and physical health (see Chapter 3 on stress).

Sexual Victimization and Violence

Sexual violence includes any sexual act committed against someone without consent. The National Intimate Partner and Sexual Violence Survey includes four types of sexual violence, which it defines in the following ways:

- **Rape.** Attempted or completed, unwanted vaginal (for women), oral, or anal penetration through the use of physical force (such as being pinned or held down or by the use of violence) or threats of physical harm and includes any time when a victim is drunk, high, drugged, or passed out and unable to consent. This survey identifies three types of rape: completed forced penetration, attempted forced penetration, and completed alcohol- or drug-facilitated penetration.

  Among women, rape includes vaginal, oral, or anal penetration by a male using his penis. It also includes vaginal or anal penetration by a male or female using their fingers or an object. Among men, rape includes oral or anal penetration by a male using his penis. It also includes anal penetration by a male or female using their fingers or an object.

- **Forced penetration.** Forcing a person to penetrate someone else by use of physical force, threats of violence, or while they are under the influence of alcohol or drugs. Among women, this behavior reflects a female being made to orally penetrate another female's vagina or anus or a male's anus. Among men, being made to penetrate someone else can occur in multiple ways: being made to vaginally penetrate a female using one's own penis, orally penetrating a female's vagina or anus, anally penetrating a male or female, or being made to receive oral sex from a male or female. It also includes male and female perpetrators attempting to force male victims to penetrate them, even though it did not happen.

- **Sexual coercion.** Pressure to engage in an unwanted sexual activity. Sexual coercion involves unwanted vaginal, oral, or anal sex after being pressured in ways that include being worn down by someone who repeatedly asks for sex or shows they are displeased, feeling pressured by being lied to, being promised something that is untrue, having someone threaten to end a relationship or spread rumors, and sexual pressure due to someone using their influence or authority.

- **Unwanted sexual contact:** Unwanted sexual behaviors that do not involve penetration, such as being kissed in a sexual way or having sexual body parts fondled, groped, or grabbed.[32]

Sexual Violence against Women

- In the United States, 43.6 percent of women (nearly 52.2 million) have experienced some form of sexual violence in their lifetime, with 4.7 percent of women experiencing this violence in the 12 months preceding the survey.

- Approximately 1 in 5 (21.3 percent, or an estimated 25.5 million) experience completed or attempted rape at some point in their lifetime.

- About 13.5 percent of women experience completed forced penetration, 6.3 percent experience attempted forced penetration, and 11 percent experience completed alcohol/drug-facilitated penetration at some point in their lifetime.

- 1.2 percent of women (approximately 1.5 million) reported completed or attempted rape in the 12 months preceding the survey.

- Approximately 1.2 percent of women (nearly 1.4 million) have been made to penetrate someone else in their lifetime.

- Approximately 1 in 6 women (16 percent, or an estimated 19.2 million) experience sexual coercion at some point in their lifetime.

- More than a third of women (37 percent, or approximately 44.3 million) reported unwanted sexual contact (such as groping) in their lifetime.[33]

Sexual Violence against Men

- Nearly a quarter of men (24.8 percent, or 27.6 million) in the United States experience some form of sexual violence in their lifetime, with 3.5 percent of men experiencing sexual violence in the 12 months preceding the survey.

- About 1 in 14 men (7.1 percent, or nearly 7.9 million) in the United States have been made to penetrate someone else (attempted or completed) at some point in their lifetime.

- Approximately 1.6 percent of men were made to penetrate someone else through completed forced penetration, 1.4 percent experienced situations in which attempts were made to make them penetrate someone else through use of force, and 5.5 percent were made to penetrate someone else through completed alcohol/drug facilitation at some point in their lifetime.

- An estimated 0.7 percent of men (827,000) reported being made to penetrate someone else (attempted or completed) in the 12 months preceding the survey.

- About 2.6 percent of men (an estimated 2.8 million) experience completed or attempted rape victimization in their lifetime.

- Approximately 1 in 10 men (9.6 percent, or an estimated 10.6 million) experience sexual coercion in their lifetime.

- Almost one-fifth of men (17.9 percent, or approximately 19.9 million) reported unwanted sexual contact (such as groping) at some point in their lifetime.[34]

Cyberbullying and Sexting

The Internet, which brings friends and fans together to share common interests, also has given rise to new forms of victimization, including online stalking, false identities, and harassment. (See Chapter 3 for more on social networking.) One is cyberbullying, defined as an aggressive, intentional act carried out by a group or individual using electronic forms of contact repeatedly and over time against a victim who cannot easily defend oneself. Here is what we have learned about this behavior:

- As many as 20 percent of adolescents and young adults have reported being cyber-victims or cyberbullies; some describe themselves as both.

- Both cyberbullies and their victims are likely to experience psychiatric and psychosomatic problems. One in four of those who had been victimized reported fearing for his or her safety.[35]

- Male and female undergraduates agreed that cyberbullying is easier than face-to-face bullying because it is less personal and more indirect. Many students minimized it as a problem and argued that simply using technology—signing up for Facebook, for instance—qualifies as consent.

- Undergraduates with learning disabilities are more likely to experience cyber-victimization, especially if they are female and have low self-perception and little social support.[36]

Sexting is defined as "the sharing of images or videos of sexually explicit content." In the United States, about 7 in 10 adolescents (ages 12 to 18) reported having received sexually oriented material, while two-thirds reported having sent it.[37]

A photo that may be sent as a joke or intended for only one person can quickly make its way to countless viewers. Such violations of privacy can be emotionally devastating. In some states they are also illegal, and tough new laws are cracking down on cyberbullying and the transmission of sexual materials.

Sexual Harassment

Sexual harassment has been defined as "a form of gender-based maltreatment. . . . [It] may be 'sexual,' as with unwanted sexual attention or requests to engage in sexual acts. However, sexual harassment is more often gender-based, or 'nonsexual.' This includes derogating someone on the basis of their gender/sex or violations of their gender/sex norms, as with sexual minorities, nonsexual heterosexual men, or sexually agentic women, etc., and gender-based insults, jokes, and discrimination. Sexual harassment may be physical or verbal, in-person or electronic, isolated or repeated."[38]

All forms of sexual harassment or unwanted sexual attention—from the display of pornographic photos to the use of sexual obscenities to a demand for sex by anyone in a position of power or authority—are illegal. They nonetheless occur on college campuses and elsewhere[39]:

- Nearly two-thirds of students experience sexual harassment at some point during college, including nearly one-third of first-year students.

- Nearly one-third of students say they have experienced physical harassment, such as being touched, grabbed, or pinched in a sexual way.

- Sexual comments and jokes are the most common form of harassment. More than half of female students and nearly half of male students say they have experienced this type of harassment.

- Lesbian, gay, bisexual, transgender, and questioning (LGBTQ) students, as well as those with physical disabilities such as deafness, are more likely than other students to be sexually harassed.

- Sexual harassment takes an especially heavy toll on female students, who often feel upset, self-conscious, embarrassed, or angry. Men are much less likely to admit to being very or somewhat upset. One-third of harassed college women say they have felt afraid; one-fifth say they have been disappointed in their college experience as a result of sexual harassment.

- About half of college men and one-third of women admit that they have sexually harassed someone on campus. Private college students are more likely than their public college peers to have ever done so. Students at large schools (population 10,000 or more) are more likely than students at small schools with fewer than 5,000 students to say they have experienced sexual harassment.

- The most common rationale for harassment is "I thought it was funny." Harassment occurs in dorms or student housing as well as outside on campus grounds and in classrooms or lecture halls.

✓**check-in** Have you ever experienced or observed sexual harassment on campus?

If you encounter sexual harassment as a student, report it to the department chair or dean. If you don't receive an adequate response to your complaint, talk with the campus representatives who handle matters involving affirmative action or civil rights. Federal guidelines prevent any discrimination against you in terms of grades or the loss of a job or scholarship if you report harassment. Schools that do not take measures to remedy harassment could lose federal funds.

Stalking

Stalking, the willful, repeated, and malicious following, harassing, or threatening of another

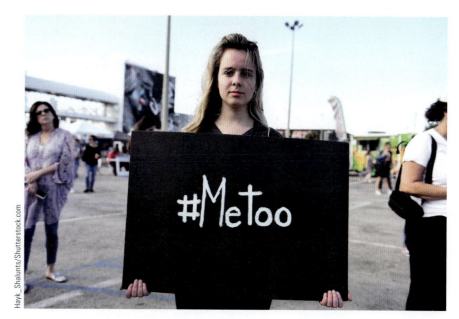

Hayk_Shalunts/Shutterstock.com

The #MeToo Movement has given a voice to thousands of women, including college students, who have experienced sexual harassment.

person, is common on college campuses—perhaps more so than in the general population.

Stalking is not a benign behavior and can result in emotional or psychological distress, physical harm, or sexual assault. The most common consequence is psychological, with victims reporting emotional or psychological distress. Simply because they are young and still learning how to manage complex social relationships, some individuals may not recognize their behavior as stalking or even as disturbing.

College students may be targeted for several reasons:

- College students tend to live close to each other and to have flexible schedules and large amounts of unsupervised time.

- Most college women know their stalkers. About half are acquaintances; a high percentage of them are classmates, boyfriends, or ex-boyfriends.

- In one study, about half of the women stalked on campus said they had not sought help from anyone. Those who did seek assistance turned to friends, parents, residence hall advisers, or police.

Intimate Partner (Dating) Violence

Intimate partner violence can occur between heterosexual, homosexual, or bisexual partners and can take different forms:

- **Physical violence.** The threat or the use of force, ranging from light pushes and slaps to punching and kicking.[40]

- **Sexual violence.** The threat or the use of force to engage a partner in sexual activity without consent, an attempted or completed sexual act without consent, or abusive sexual contact.

- **Psychological violence.** The use of threats, actions, or coercive tactics that cause trauma or emotional harm to a partner.

- **Social or intimate violence.** Establishing control over a partner by means of threats, restrictions on behavior, and social isolation from friends and family.[41]

All forms of intimate partner violence can have devastating psychological, physical, interpersonal, and occupational effects on the victim, his or her friends and family, and society in general. The negative impact can last for decades.

Young women ages 18 to 24, regardless of whether they are in college, are frequent targets of intimate partner violence. Almost one in three undergraduate women at a college in the United States was assaulted by a male dating partner in the past year. At varied sites worldwide, 17 to 49 percent of college students reported perpetrating physical assault against a dating partner in the past year. The median rate was 29 percent.[42]

Violent intimate relationships are often characterized by mutual aggression, and partners may be both victims and perpetrators. They are often also victims or perpetrators of other forms of violence. College students may be at greater risk for several reasons, including alcohol use, drug use, and risky sexual behaviors. Perpetrators may engage in a host of behaviors that prevent victims from fully engaging in college. This may increase the risk of dropping classes, scholastic failure, and school withdrawal, which can impair their academic performance.[43]

Risk Factors for Intimate Partner Violence

Factors that increase the likelihood of intimate partner violence include the following:

- **Sex.** Both men and women experience acts of violence and aggression by their partners, but the violence perpetrated against women by men is likely to be much more severe and potentially injurious.[44]

- **Sexual minority.** Compared with heterosexual students, male and female sexual-minority undergraduates (defined as having had any same-sex sexual experience) report significantly higher rates of physical sexual violence, sexual assault, and unwanted pursuit. Sexual-minority women (but not men) reported significantly higher rates of physical intimate partner violence than heterosexual students.[45]

- **Violence in the family of origin.** Childhood exposure to violence and abuse are risk factors for intimate partner violence, especially for women.

- **Emotional states and mental health.** Negative emotions, particularly anger, anxiety, and depression, are associated with intimate partner violence. Women who behave violently are more likely to be victims of partner violence and to have high levels of depression, anger, and hostility. Men who behave violently show more antisocial personality characteristics and have lower educational and economic status.

- **Substance use and abuse.** Drugs and alcohol reduce the ability to resist unwanted physical or sexual advances and/or may prevent a victim from being able to interpret warning cues of a potential assault.

- **Sexual risk taking.** Involvement with strangers and individuals who are close acquaintances may increase the risk for intimate partner violence.

Disclosure and Support

Most victims of intimate partner violence disclose what happened to at least one person, usually a friend, family member, classmate, coworker, or neighbor.[46] They are more likely to do so if they:

- Are female.
- Are white.
- Are younger.
- Are of higher socioeconomic status.
- Do not belong to a sexual minority.[47]
- Attach anger/jealousy motives to the violence.
- Feel less shame or fear regarding the violence.
- Experience psychological or stalking-related violence.
- Experience greater severity and frequency of violence.
- Had someone witness the violence.

Victims report that the most helpful reaction following disclosure is emotional support; the least helpful reactions are expressing disbelief and blaming the victim. Disclosure and social support following disclosure are associated with better mental health and psychological recovery. Innovative programs, such as Friends Helping Friends, train young adults ages 18 to 22 in skills that could help them recognize and intervene in intimate partner violence.[48]

Rape

Rape generally refers to sexual intercourse with an unconsenting partner under actual or threatened force. In 2012, the Justice Department updated the legal definition of *rape* as "the penetration, no matter how slight, of the vagina or anus with any body part or object, or oral penetration by a sex organ of another person, without the consent of the victim." Previously, it had been defined as "the carnal knowledge of a female forcibly and against her will."[49]

Sexual intercourse between a male over the age of 16 and a female under the age of consent (which ranges from 12 to 21 in different states) is called *statutory rape*. In *acquaintance rape*, or *date rape*, the victim knows the rapist. In *marital* or *spousal rape*, the perpetrator is the victim's spouse. In *stranger rape*, the rapist is an unknown assailant. Both acquaintance and stranger rapes are serious crimes that can have a devastating impact on their victims.

All states now recognize as rape the assault of a victim who is incapable of giving consent because of the influence of alcohol or other substances. However, many women who experience a sexual encounter that meets this legal definition do not label it as a rape or even as sexual victimization. Compared with stranger rapes, these assaults are typically less violent and involve less force by the assailant, less resistance by the victim, and less physical injury to the victim. Yet women who do not acknowledge an unwanted sexual experience as rape nonetheless suffer psychological consequences, including distress and other trauma symptoms.

For many years, the victims of rape were blamed for doing something to bring on the attack. This is one of several rape myths that remain prevalent on college campuses, particularly among male students and heavy drinkers.[50] However, researchers have shown that women are raped because they encounter sexually aggressive men, not because they look or act a certain way. Although no woman is immune to attack, many rape victims are children or adolescents.

Sexual Assault on Campus

According to its Campus Climate Survey Validation Study of more than 23,000 undergraduates at nine schools, 21 percent of female students have experienced a completed sexual assault since entering college. Rates at each of the schools varied significantly, from 12 to 38 percent.[51] In a survey of four-year residential colleges and universities, reported sexual assaults were higher in schools with a higher proportion of male students, a Greek life system, an alcohol policy, and religious affiliation.[52]

Victims of sexual assault often suffer physical and emotional trauma that can linger for years and stretch into nearly every area of their lives. In a federal survey, about one in five (19 percent) of female rape victims dropped or considered dropping classes, 7 percent changed where they lived, 31 percent said their academic performance suffered, and 22 percent considered taking time off or dropping out of school.[53]

Students who have experienced sexual violence are more vulnerable to what researchers call "revictimization," particularly if they identify as white and female and report trauma-related distress or increased symptoms of depression and alcohol use disorder.[54] Those who experienced sexual violence, including stranger assault and sexual coercion and/or engaged in binge drinking prior to college are also at great risk of revictimization as undergraduates.[55]

Changing the Campus Culture

Prevention of sexual violence begins with changes in attitudes by all members of a campus community. However, researchers are just beginning to investigate the nature of campus sexual assaults, evaluate existing institutional systems and processes, and promote effective approaches that respond to ongoing needs and challenges.[56]

The campaign to change how colleges address sexual violence dates back several decades. Title IX, a comprehensive federal law that prohibits discrimination on the basis of sex, requires that educational institutions address gender-based inequality concerning sexual harassment (including sexual assault), academics, and athletics.[57] In 1992, the U.S. Supreme Court recognized that sexual harassment could be considered gender discrimination as prohibited under Title IX.

The Obama administration implemented Title IX guidance and prevention initiatives, such as "It's On Us" and the White House Task Force to Protect Students from Sexual Assault. The Trump administration has proposed new Title IX regulations that increase protections for the accused, increase requirements for adjudications, restrict survivors' options for resolution, and narrow schools' latitude to act.

Many campuses have two pathways for reporting sexual assault: formal and confidential. The formal pathway usually begins when a survivor reports an assault to campus police, the Title IX office, or the dean of students' office. Schools then adopt a criminal justice–like approach. Few students use the formal pathway, often for reasons such as thinking it's "not serious enough" to report, fearing negative consequences, feeling ashamed, or lacking the resources to pursue a case against a wealthier student. The confidential pathway provides support and resources for survivors through campus health and sexual assault centers that "place survivors' needs and interests at the very center of their mission."[58]

Many schools have developed policies that emphasize gender equality, affirmative consent ("yes means yes"), consent at each step of sexual activity, and safe sex practices.[59] Classes on sexual victimization, often mandatory, increasingly focus not just on teaching women how to avoid being raped but also preventing potential perpetrators from acting and showing how students can help their friends, peers, or even strangers get out of potentially harmful situations.[60] Different colleges have taken different approaches, and researchers are investigating which programs are most effective.[61]

#MeToo

#MeToo has developed into a movement that encourages sexual abuse survivors to share their stories, offers support, and inspires activists to find solutions to sexual violence. Since the hashtag #MeToo went viral on social media in 2017, many prominent men have faced consequences for alleged sexual misconduct.[62]

Although policies and programs continue to evolve, the #MeToo movement has created greater openness on campuses. Rather than viewing sexual assault as a shameful secret, more young people are revealing that they have been victims of sexual assault and are initiating conversations about their experiences with their peers.[63]

Bystander Training Since many instances of sexual violence occur in party situations or public places, bystanders often are witnesses. Before the problem escalates, during an episode of threatened or actual sexual violence, or after the incident, they can choose to respond by doing nothing, stepping in and helping a victim, or making the situation worse by offering overt or tacit encouragement to the perpetrator. Undergraduates are most likely to intervene or, as sociologists put it, "engage in prosocial helping behavior" if they:

- Observe others doing the same.
- Perceive that there is a genuine problem.
- Feel it would be safe to intervene.
- Know the victim (students tend to feel more ambivalent if they know both parties or just the perpetrator).[64]

"Bystander training" is being offered on campuses to help community members become more sensitive to issues of interpersonal violence and to teach prevention and intervention skills. These include interrupting situations that could lead to assault before it happens, speaking out against social norms that tolerate sexual assault and violence, and becoming a supportive ally to survivors.[65]

✓**check-in** Have you encountered any form of sexual coercion?

Sexual Coercion

Nonvolitional sex is unwanted sexual behavior that violates a person's right to choose when and with whom to have sex and what sexual behaviors to engage in. The more extreme forms of this behavior include forced sex, childhood sexual abuse, and violence against people with nonconventional sexual identities. Other forms, such as engaging in sex to keep one's partner or to pass as heterosexual, are so common that many think of them as normal.

About 20 percent of students say they have coerced a partner into sex in the previous 12 months, and 24 percent of students report having been victims of sexual coercion. Men are more likely than women to engage in sexual coercion—for example, making a partner have sex without a condom or insisting on sex despite a partner's refusal. In a study of 387 college men, sexual arousal was significantly related to "overperception" of a woman's sexual interest and to sexually coercive behaviors.[66]

Incapacitated Sexual Assault and Date-Rape Drugs

Alcohol and drug use increase the risk of sexual assault. In a recent study of about 600 female undergraduates, incapacitated sexual assault was associated with higher perceived drinking norms (discussed in Chapter 13), more social drinking, more drinking before sexual activity, and more drinking to conform with peers.[67]

Drugs that can be mixed with drinks such as Rohypnol (flunitrazepam) and GHB (gammahydroxybutyrate) (discussed in Chapter 12) have been implicated in cases of incapacitated sexual assault. Since these drugs are odorless and tasteless, victims have no way of detecting them in their drinks. The subsequent loss of memory leaves victims with no explanation for where they've been or what's happened. Rohypnol—which can cause impaired motor skills and judgment, lack of inhibitions, dizziness, confusion, lethargy, very low blood pressure, coma, and death—has been outlawed in the United States. Deaths have also been attributed to GHB overdoses.

College women often aren't aware of the possibility that their drinks may be tampered with or that they may have been given a date-rape drug. As a result, many see no risk in leaving their drinks unattended. Even if they start feeling ill at a party, many do not suspect that a date-rape drug could be the cause. The victims of prior assaults tend to be slower at picking up on and responding to potentially dangerous dating situations, possibly because they feel that personal risks are unavoidable and beyond their control.

Many schools are alerting incoming female students about what researchers call "the red zone," a period of time early in one's first undergraduate year when women are at particularly high risk for unwanted sexual experiences. One university defines the red zone more precisely as "the time period between freshman move-in and winter break wherein there is a particularly high risk of victimization." Unwanted touching and attempted intercourse are the most common behaviors reported, although researchers have also documented sexual assaults and rapes.

Rape on Campus

Over the course of 5 years (the national average for a college career), including summers and vacations, one of every four or five female students is raped. In a single academic year, 3 percent of coeds are raped—35 rapes for every 1,000 women. According to the U.S. Department of Justice, a campus with 6,000 coeds averages one rape a day every day for the entire school year.

"Serial" perpetrators commit most college rapes. In a study of 12,624 men at community and four-year schools, nine in ten alcohol-involved sexual assaults were committed by men who had previously assaulted other women. Fraternity brothers and college athletes were significantly more likely to perpetrate such assaults than other male students.[68]

In nine surveys of male university students, between 3 and 6 percent had been raped by other men; up to 25 percent had been sexually assaulted.

Acquaintance or Date Rape
Approximately 35 percent of college students report experiencing some form of sexual violence, including rape and attempted rape, perpetrated by their dating partners. College women experience significantly higher rates of sexual violence in comparison with college men. Sexual violence and unwanted sexual contact are significantly more prevalent among heterosexual students than among LGBTQIA college students.[69]

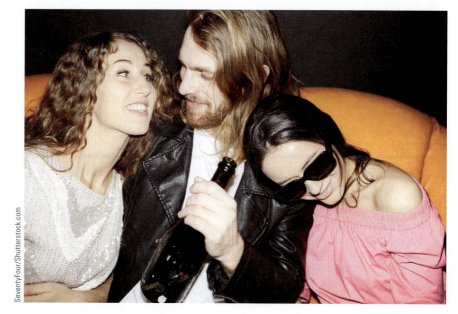

The same factors that lead to other forms of sexual victimization can set the stage for date rape. Socialization into an aggressive role, acceptance of rape myths, and a view that force is justified in certain situations increase the likelihood of a man's committing date rape (see Health Now! How to Avoid Date Rape).

✓**check-in** What steps do you take to prevent acquaintance rape? Compare your response with that of a classmate of the other sex.

Other factors that play a role in sexual aggression are as follows:

- **Personality and early sexual experiences.** These may include first sexual experience at a very young age, earlier and more frequent than usual childhood sexual experiences (both forced and voluntary), hostility toward women, irresponsibility, lack of social consciousness, and a need for dominance over sexual partners.

- **Situational variables (what happens during the date).** Men who initiate a date, pay all expenses, and provide transportation are more likely to be sexually aggressive, perhaps because they feel they can call all the shots.

- **Rape myths.** As several studies have confirmed, college men hold more rape-tolerant attitudes than do college women. For example, college men are significantly more likely than college women to agree with statements such as "Some women ask to be raped and

Acquaintance rape and alcohol use are very closely linked. Both men and women may find their judgment impaired or their communications unclear as a result of drinking.

How to Avoid Date Rape

For Men:

- Remember that it's okay not to "score" on a date.

- Don't assume that a sexy dress or casual flirting is an invitation to sex.

- Be aware of your partner's actions. If she pulls away or tries to get up, understand that she's sending you a message—one you should acknowledge and respect.

- Restrict drinking, drug use, or other behaviors that could affect your judgment and ability to act responsibly.

- Never assume consent. "No" means "no." Make sure your partner consents to every phase of sexual activity.

For Women:

- If the man pays for all expenses, he may think he's justified in using force to get "what he paid for." If you're concerned that this might be the case, insist on paying your share.

- Back away from a man who pressures you into other activities you don't want to engage in on a date.

- Be direct—with your words, your behavior, and, if necessary, physical force.

- Do not use alcohol or other drugs when you want to avoid sexual intimacy.

may enjoy it" and "If a woman says 'no' to having sex, she means 'maybe' or even 'yes.'"

- **Social norms.** Some social groups, such as fraternities and athletic teams, may encourage the use of alcohol; reinforce stereotypes about masculinity; and emphasize violence, force, and competition. The group's shared values, including an acceptance of sexual coercion, may keep individuals from questioning their behavior. They also may keep bystanders from intervening to prevent a potential rape.[70]

- **Drinking.** Alcohol use is one of the strongest predictors of acquaintance rape. Men who have been drinking may not react to subtle signals, may misinterpret a woman's behavior as a come-on, and may feel more sexually aroused. At the same time, drinking may impair a woman's ability to effectively communicate her wishes or cope with a man's aggressiveness. In a study of freshman women, binge or heavy episodic drinking increased the risk of hookups resulting in sexual victimization; sober hookups did not increase this risk.[71]

- **Gender differences in interpreting sexual cues.** In research comparing college men and women, the men typically overestimated the woman's sexual availability and interest, seeing friendliness, revealing clothing, and attractiveness as deliberately seductive. In one study of date rape, the men reported feeling "led on," in part because their female partners seemed to be dressed more suggestively than usual.

Women who successfully escape rape attempts do so by resisting verbally and physically, usually by yelling and fleeing. Women who use forceful verbal or physical resistance (screaming, hitting, kicking, biting, and running) are more likely to avoid rape than women who try pleading, crying, or offering no resistance.

Stranger Rape
Rape prevention consists primarily of making it as difficult as possible for a rapist to make you a victim:

- Don't advertise that you're a woman living alone. Use initials on your mailbox. Install and use secure locks on doors and windows; change door locks after losing keys or moving into a new residence.

- Don't open your door to strangers. If a repairperson or public official is at your door, ask him to identify himself and call his office to verify that he is a reputable person on legitimate business.

- Lock your car when it is parked and drive with locked car doors. If your car breaks down, attach a white cloth to the antenna

and lock yourself in. If someone other than a uniformed officer stops to offer help, ask that person to call the police or a garage but do not open your locked car door.

- Avoid dark and deserted areas and be aware of your surroundings when you're walking. If a driver asks for directions when you're a pedestrian, avoid approaching his car. Instead, call out your reply from a safe distance.

- Have house or car keys in hand as you approach the door. Check the backseat before getting into your car.

- Carry a device for making a loud noise, like a whistle or, even better, a pint-sized compressed air horn available in many sporting goods and boat supply stores. Sound the noise alarm at the first sign of danger.

✓**check-in** How would you rate your safety awareness and personal protection skills?

Male Nonconsensual Sex and Rape

No one knows how common male rape is because men are even less likely to report such assaults than women. Researchers estimate that the victims in about 10 percent of acquaintance rape cases are men. These hidden victims often keep silent because of embarrassment, shame, or humiliation, as well as their own feelings and fears about homosexuality and conforming to conventional sex roles.

Although many people think men who rape other men are always homosexuals, most male rapists consider themselves to be heterosexual. Young boys aren't the only victims. The average age of male rape victims is 24. Rape is a serious problem in prison, where men may experience brutal assaults by men who usually resume sexual relations with women once they're released.

Impact of Rape
Rape-related injuries include unexplained vaginal discharge, bleeding, infections, multiple bruises, and fractured ribs. Victims of sexual violence often develop chronic symptoms, such as headaches, backaches, high blood pressure, sleep disorders, pelvic pain, and sexual fertility problems. But sexual violence has both a physical and a psychological impact. The psychological scars of a sexual assault take a long time to heal. Therapists have linked sexual victimization with sexual dysfunction, hopelessness, low self-esteem, high levels of self-criticism, and self-defeating relationships.[72] An estimated 30 to 50 percent of women develop posttraumatic stress disorder (see Chapter 3) following a rape. Many do not seek counseling until a year or more after

an attack, when their symptoms have intensified or become chronic.

Acquaintance rape may cause fewer physical injuries but greater psychological torment. Often too ashamed to tell anyone what happened, victims may suffer alone, without skilled therapists or sympathetic friends to reassure them. Women raped by acquaintances blame themselves more, see themselves less positively, question their judgment, have greater difficulty trusting others, and have higher levels of psychological distress. Nightmares, anxiety, and flashbacks are common. The women may avoid others, become less capable of protecting themselves, and continue to be haunted by sexual violence for years. A therapist can help these victims begin the slow process of healing.

What to Do in Case of Sexual Assault and Rape

According to data from the National Sexual Assault Hotline, only one in five female student victims between ages 18 and 24 report sexual violence to law enforcement. The reasons women do not report these crimes include:

- Belief that it is a personal matter (26 percent).
- Fear of reprisal (20 percent).
- Belief that it is not important enough to report (12 percent).
- Not wanting to get the perpetrator in trouble (10 percent).
- Belief that the police will not or cannot do anything to help (9 percent).
- Reported, but not to law enforcement (4 percent).[73]

Many victims may remain in an abusive relationship for various reasons, including fear of the perpetrator, self-blame, minimization of the crime, loyalty or love for the perpetrator, and social or religious stigma.

Crisis hotlines or campus helplines can provide immediate assistance and referrals to sexual assault or domestic violence programs that provide shelter, counseling, support groups, legal assistance, and medical services. University and college health centers often offer counseling services. Campus police or school judicial programs can provide sanctions for on-campus violations.

Women who are raped should call a friend or a rape crisis center. A rape victim should not bathe or change her clothes before calling. Semen, hair, and material under her fingernails or on her apparel all may be useful in identifying the man who raped her. A rape victim who chooses to go to a doctor or hospital should remember that she may not necessarily have to talk to police. However, a doctor can collect the necessary evidence, which will then be available if she later decides to report the rape to police. All rape victims should talk with a doctor or health-care worker about testing and treatment for sexually transmitted infections and postintercourse conception.

Even an unsuccessful rape attempt should be reported because the information a woman may provide about the attack—the assaulter's physical characteristics, voice, clothes, and car, or even an unusual smell—may prevent another woman from being assaulted.

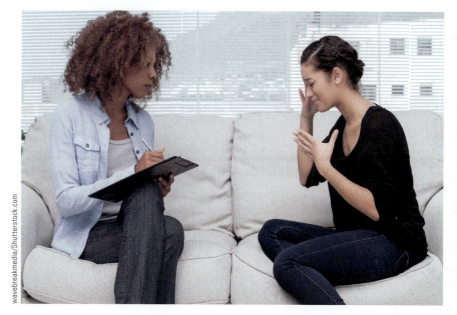
wavebreakmedia/Shutterstock.com

Counseling from a trained professional can help ease the trauma suffered by a rape victim.

From Personal to Planetary Threats: The Environment and Your Health

Ours is a planet in peril. Glaciers are melting. Sea levels are rising. Forests are being destroyed. Droughts have become more frequent and more intense. Heat waves have killed tens of thousands of people. Hurricanes and floods have ravaged cities. Millions have died from the effects of air pollution and contaminated water.

The planet Earth—once taken for granted as a ball of rock and water that existed for our use for all time—is a single, fragile **ecosystem** (a community of organisms that share a physical and chemical environment). Our environment is a closed ecosystem, powered by the sun. The materials needed for the survival of this planet must be

ecosystem A community of organisms sharing a physical and chemical environment and interacting with each other.

recycled over and over again. The health of this ecosystem is to our own well-being and survival.

Awareness of and concern about the environment vary. In a national survey of about 4,000 Americans, 6 in 10 respondents (58 percent) reported concerns about health risks from environmental pollutants. Four in 10 said they were aware of government efforts to combat them. Nearly as many felt that none of the health impacts listed in the survey were related to environmental issues. Among those most likely to express concern about the environment's impact on health were non-Hispanic blacks, women, people with a college degree or higher, and individuals living in the Midwest or South.[74] In a survey at one public midwestern university, the percentage of students who believed in climate change and were concerned about its impact was much higher than in national surveys.[75]

For good or for ill, we cannot separate our individual health from that of the environment in which we live. The lifestyle choices we make, the products we use, and the efforts we undertake to clean up a beach or save wetlands affect the quality of our environment.

✓**check-in** What do you see as the greatest environmental threat?

Climate Change

The Intergovernmental Panel on Climate Change of the United Nations, made up of leading scientists from around the world, has reported with absolute certainty that the world's climate is changing in significant ways and will continue to do so in the foreseeable future. These experts predict an increase in extreme weather events (such as hurricanes and heat waves), greater weather variability, and rising water temperatures.[76] The panel concluded that we need to reduce global greenhouse gas emissions by 2030 and cut them entirely by 2040 to avoid the most catastrophic effects of climate change. Recent research suggests the need for an even more ambitious approach to avert significant risks to human health, livelihoods, food and water supplies, security, and economic growth. Yet these emissions hit a record high in 2018.[77]

As numerous recent scientific assessments have confirmed, the health threats of climate change are no longer just a future threat but a current reality.[78] These dangers include illness, injuries, and deaths from increasingly dangerous weather (including extreme heat, precipitation, and flooding), worsening air pollution, the spread of infectious diseases, increases in foodborne and waterborne illnesses, and severe mental health impairments caused or worsened by traumatic climate events.[79]

Physicians have declared climate change a "health emergency" and called upon health care professionals to take a leading role "in confronting climate change with the urgency that it demands."[80] Even small changes by ordinary citizens can make a difference, but combined actions by governments, businesses, and scientists are critically important.[81] (See Strategies for Change: Protecting the Planet.)

Global Warming

Earth's average temperature increased about 1 to 2 degrees in the 20th century to approximately 59 degrees, but the rate of warming in the last three decades has been three times the average rate since 1900. Seas have risen about 6 to 8 feet globally over the last century and continue to rise at an increasing rate.

Why is our planet getting warmer? Figure 14.1 shows the normal greenhouse effect: Certain gases in Earth's atmosphere trap energy from the sun and retain heat somewhat like the glass panels of a greenhouse. These greenhouse gases include carbon dioxide, methane, and nitrous oxide. Human activities, scientists now say with 90 percent certainty, have increased the greenhouse gases in our atmosphere. We burn fossil fuels (oil, natural gas, and coal) and wood products, which release carbon dioxide into the atmosphere. We produce coal, natural gas, and oil, which emit methane. Livestock and the decomposition of organic wastes also produce methane. Agricultural and industrial processes emit nitrous oxide. These emissions enhance the normal greenhouse effect, trapping more heat and raising the temperature of the atmosphere and Earth's surface.

The Health Risks

The Global warming and related changes can imperil health indirectly through the following:

- More frequent and intense heat waves.
- Flooding.
- More extreme weather, such as hurricanes, tornadoes, cyclones, and tsunamis.
- More severe droughts.

All of these could jeopardize physical and psychological well-being, particularly among the most vulnerable members of society, such as children and older adults.[82]

Global warming also affects health indirectly by changing the patterns of infectious diseases, supplies of fresh water, and food availability. For example, as the planet continues to warm, infectious

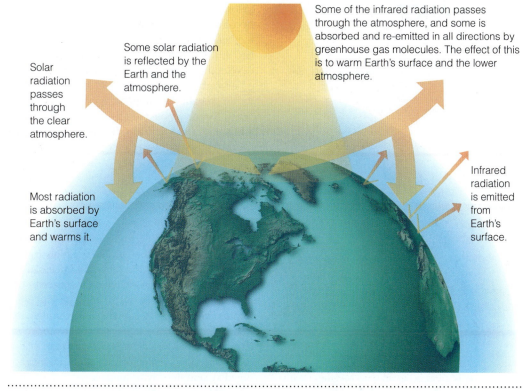

FIGURE 14.1 The Greenhouse Effect

The normal greenhouse effect warms Earth to a hospitable temperature. An increase in greenhouse gases intensifies the greenhouse effect, trapping more heat and raising Earth's temperature.

Image labels:

Solar radiation passes through the clear atmosphere.

Some solar radiation is reflected by the Earth and the atmosphere.

Some of the infrared radiation passes through the atmosphere, and some is absorbed and re-emitted in all directions by greenhouse gas molecules. The effect of this is to warm Earth's surface and the lower atmosphere.

Most radiation is absorbed by Earth's surface and warms it.

Infrared radiation is emitted from Earth's surface.

---

diseases—particularly mosquito-borne illnesses such as malaria, dengue fever, yellow fever, and encephalitis—may spread to more regions. Already in the United States, mosquitoes and other insects that carry diseases such as West Nile virus, Rocky Mountain spotted fever, and Lyme disease are spreading to areas once considered too cold for these insects to survive.[83] The rise in global temperatures has already led to a greater pollen load and more allergies among more people.

✓**check-in** How concerned are you about climate change as a threat to your health? To others on the planet? To the next generation?

The Impact of Pollution

Any change in the air, water, or soil that could reduce its ability to support life is a form of **pollution**. Natural events, such as smoke from fires triggered by lightning, can cause pollution. However, most sources of pollution are human

made. There are now about 10 times as many cars around the world as there were 50 years ago. The number of people living in cities has increased by more than a factor of four, and global energy consumption by nearly a factor of five.

The effects of pollution depend on the concentration (amount per unit of air, water, or soil) of the **pollutant**, how long it remains in the environment, and its chemical nature. An *acute effect* is a severe, immediate reaction, usually after a single, large exposure. For example, pesticide poisoning can cause nausea, dizziness, and even death. A *chronic effect* may take years to develop or may be a recurrent or continuous reaction, usually after repeated exposure. Years of exposure to traffic pollution, for instance, has been linked to an increase in blood pressure.

Environmental agents that trigger changes, or *mutations*, in the genetic material (the DNA) of living cells are called **mutagens**. The changes that result can lead to the development of cancer. A substance or agent that causes cancer is a **carcinogen**. All carcinogens are mutagens; most mutagens are carcinogens. Furthermore, when a mutagen affects an egg or a sperm cell, its effects can be passed on to future generations. Mutagens that can cross the placenta of a pregnant woman and cause a spontaneous abortion or birth defects in the fetus are called *teratogens*.

pollution Any change in the air, water, or soil that could reduce its ability to support life.

pollutant A substance or agent in the environment, usually the by-product of human industry or activity, that is injurious to human, animal, or plant life.

mutagens Agents that cause alterations in the genetic material of living cells.

carcinogen A substance or agent that causes cancer.

YOUR STRATEGIES FOR CHANGE

Protecting the Planet

Here are some recommendations from the Environmental Defense and World Wildlife Fund:

- Wash laundry in warm or cold water, not hot. *Average annual CO_2 reduction: up to 500 pounds for two loads of laundry a week.*

- Buy products sold in the simplest possible packaging. Carry a tote bag or recycle shopping bags. *Average annual CO_2 reduction: 1,000 pounds because garbage is reduced 25 percent.*

- Switch from standard lightbulbs to energy-efficient fluorescent ones. *Average annual CO_2 reduction: about 500 pounds per bulb.*

- Bike, carpool, or take mass transit whenever possible. *Average annual CO_2 reduction: 20 pounds for each gallon of gasoline saved.*

- Drive a car that gets high gas mileage and produces low emissions. Keep your speed at or below the speed limit.

- Keep your tires inflated and your engine tuned. Recycle old batteries and tires. (Most stores that sell new ones will take back old ones.)

- Turn off your engine if you're going to be stopped for more than a minute.

Pollution is a hazard to all who breathe. Deaths caused by air pollution exceed those from motor vehicle injuries. Those with respiratory illnesses and other chronic health problems are at greatest risk during days when smog or allergen counts are high. However, even healthy college students suffer impairments in their heart and circulatory systems as a result of urban air pollution. The effects of carbon monoxide are much worse in smokers, who already have higher levels of the gas in their blood.

Pollution can even pose a threat to unborn children. One recent study linked exposure in the womb to chemicals commonly found in plastics

Air pollution endangers the well-being of more than half of Americans, including many city dwellers.

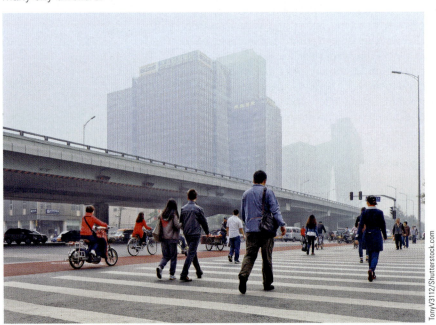

TonyV3112/Shutterstock.com

to lower IQs and to poorer learning skills at age 7. According to other reports, children born to mothers exposed to high levels of air pollution late in pregnancy may have an increased risk of developing autism spectrum disorder.[84]

As carbon dioxide levels in the air rise due to the greenhouse effect, air quality will worsen. Gases found in polluted air—such as ozone, sulfur dioxide, and nitrogen dioxide—contribute to heart disease and worsen the health of individuals who already have heart conditions. Poor air quality also contributes to breathing difficulties and may be responsible for the dramatic increase in asthma in recent decades. Elevated carbon dioxide levels can trigger asthma attacks and allergies by increasing ragweed pollen. Greater carbon dioxide in the air also stimulates the growth of poison ivy and other nuisance plants.

Toxic substances in polluted air can enter the human body in three ways: through the skin, through the digestive system, and through the lungs. The combined interaction of two or more hazards can produce an effect greater than that of either one alone. Pollutants can affect an organ or organ system directly or indirectly.

Among the health problems that have been linked with pollution are:

- Headaches and dizziness.
- Decline in cognitive functioning.
- Eye irritation and impaired vision.
- Nasal discharge.
- Cough, shortness of breath, and sore throat.
- Constricted airways.
- Constriction of blood vessels and increased risk of heart disease.
- Increased risk of stroke and of dying from a stroke.
- Chest pains and aggravation of the symptoms of colds, pneumonia, bronchial asthma, emphysema, chronic bronchitis, lung cancer, and other respiratory problems.
- Birth defects and reproductive problems including lower success with in-vitro fertilization.
- Nausea, vomiting, and stomach cancer.
- Allergies and asthma from diesel fumes in polluted air.

The Air You Breathe

Remember the last time you stood at a busy intersection as a bus or truck spewed brownish fumes in your face? Maybe your eyes stung or your throat burned. But breathing polluted air can do more than irritate: It can take months or even years off your life, particularly among the underprivileged who live in areas with dangerous levels of air pollution.[85] As traffic increases, so does pollution—and the risk to health.[86]

Air pollution is recognized as one of the leading causes of pulmonary, respiratory and skin diseases across the globe.[87] Researchers attribute approximately 4 million deaths a year to air pollution, mostly from cardiovascular and respiratory diseases.[88]

As pollutants destroy the hairlike cilia that remove irritants from the lungs, individuals may suffer chronic bronchitis, characterized by excessive mucus flow and continuous coughing. Emphysema may develop or worsen, as pollutants constrict the bronchial tubes and destroy the air sacs in the lungs, making breathing more difficult. Long-term exposure to air pollution may speed up the process of atherosclerosis (discussed in Chapter 10). Children are especially vulnerable to pollution's harmful effects.[89]

Breathing in polluted air can increase the risk for heart attack by nearly 5 percent. Among those at increased risk are individuals:

- Who have had a heart attack or angioplasty.
- Who have angina, heart failure, some types of heart rhythm problems, or diabetes.
- Who have asthma.
- With known risk factors for heart disease, such as smoking cigarettes.
- With high blood pressure or high blood cholesterol.
- With a family history of stroke or early heart disease (father or brother diagnosed before 55 years of age; mother or sister diagnosed before 65 years of age).
- Who are older than 65 years of age.[90]

Air pollution also poses a risk to healthy young individuals who exercise outdoors. In a study of 30 healthy runners (mean age, 20.6 years), those who ran on a polluted route showed higher levels of toxic black carbon and ozone as well as higher systolic blood pressure readings after their workouts.[91] A meta-analysis of studies of air pollution exposure on outdoor exercise found increased risk of airway inflammation, diminished lung function, and changes in blood pressure and circulation. The combination of air pollution and exercise was associated with increased risk to cardiopulmonary function, immune function, and exercise performance.[92]

The Water You Drink

The WHO estimates that 1.1 billion people lack access to sufficient water supplies and 2.6 billion lack adequate sanitation. The adverse health effects of drinking contaminated water range from acute gastrointestinal diseases to long-term outcomes, such as cancer and physical and neurodevelopmental delays in children. Millions of deaths, especially among children, are associated with water-related diseases and infections worldwide every year. The Environmental Protection Agency (EPA) has reported that as many as 63 million persons in the United States are exposed to potentially unsafe water.[93]

Fears about the public water supply have led many Americans to turn off their taps. About two-thirds take steps to drink purer water, either by using filtration and distillation methods or by drinking bottled water. Home filters can block certain pathogens that can cause diarrhea and other gastrointestinal problems, but they do not seem to remove most chemical contaminants. If you decide to use a filter, clean it regularly to prevent a buildup of bacteria.

The EPA has set standards for some 80 contaminants. These include many toxic chemicals and heavy metals—including lead, mercury, cadmium, and chromium—that can cause kidney and nervous system damage and birth defects. Each year the Centers for Disease Control and Prevention (CDC) reports an average of 7,400 cases of illness related to the water people drink.

Unsafe drinking water has become a serious health threat in a growing number of communities across the United States.

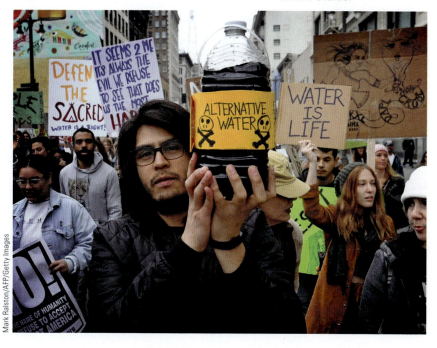

Mark Ralston/AFP/Getty Images

❗ CONSUMER ALERT

What Difference Does a Lightbulb Make?

Facts to Know

- Not all lightbulbs are the same. Incandescent bulbs use electricity to heat a metal filament until it becomes white hot or incandescent. In a compact fluorescent bulb (CFL), an electric current flows between electrodes at each end of a tube containing gases, producing ultraviolet (UV) light that is transferred into visible light when it strikes a phosphor coating on the inside of the bulb. In LED (light emitting diode) products, an electrical current passes through semiconductor material, which illuminates the tiny diodes.

- A CFL bulb that qualifies for the government's Energy Star symbol lasts about ten times longer and saves about $30 or more in electricity over an incandescent bulb. Because of its even higher efficiency and lower power usage, an LED bulb is 80 percent cheaper to run than a conventional bulb.

- LEDs, which cost significantly more to purchase, are more environmentally friendly and economical in the long run. They last longer, don't produce heat and carbon dioxide emissions like incandescent bulbs do, and normally don't contain any toxic materials like the mercury vapor in CFLs.

Steps to Take

- When shopping for a lightbulb, look for the federal Energy Star label. This indicates that the bulb uses about 70 to 90 percent less energy than traditional incandescent bulbs, lasts 10 to 25 times longer, saves $30 to $80 in electricity costs over its lifetime, and produces about 70 to 90 percent less heat so it is safer to operate.

- If you buy CFL bulbs be careful when removing them from their packaging and unscrewing them because they are made of glass and contain mercury. Screw and unscrew bulbs by their bases, not the glass. Never forcefully twist a CFL into a light socket.

- Some LED bulbs may look like familiar lightbulbs and some may not, but they can outperform traditional lightbulbs—if they carry an Energy Star label. A general-purpose LED bulb that does not qualify for the Energy Star label may not distribute light in all directions and therefore not work well in a table lamp.

The most common culprits include parasites, bacteria, viruses, chemicals, and lead. Medications and illicit drugs disposed in water and making their way into streams and rivers add to the health dangers.

The problem of lead-contaminated water in Flint, Michigan, made national headlines when researchers found that river water had corroded the city's pipes so that lead leached into the water. Some homes exceeded 100 parts per billion, well above the WHO's lead limit for safe drinking water of 10 parts per billion. Lead is especially toxic to fetuses, babies, and children, affecting every organ system, including the developing brain with a lifelong impact on IQ, learning, focus, and behavior.[94]

✓**check-in** Do you use a water filter? If so, clean or replace it regularly to prevent buildup of bacteria.

Is Bottled Water Better?

Consumers seem convinced that bottled water is purer than tap. The market for bottled water in the United States has been growing by 10 percent per year, making it second only to soft drinks as America's favorite beverage. On average we drink about 25 gallons of bottled water every year, compared to 51.5 gallons of soft drinks and 21 gallons of beer.

However, medical researchers have not found a scientific reason to recommend bottled water over tap water. Dentists report an increase in cavities among children and teenagers who drink bottled water rather than fluoridated tap water. Recent studies found a "negligible" risk of exposure to chemicals in plastic products for young children.[95] Despite images of mountain streams and glacier peaks on the labels, most bottled water comes from urban water supplies.

✓**check-in** Did you know that an estimated 25 to 30 percent of bottled water sold in this country is, in fact, tap water, sometimes further treated and sometimes not?

Portable Water Bottles

The simplest, safest, most eco-friendly water container is a glass. If you want to carry water with you, you have plenty of alternatives, but some portable drinking containers may pose risks to you or to the environment.

Most disposable water bottles are made with lightweight polyethylene terephthalate (PET). Reusing these bottles may pose some health dangers, although there is little scientific agreement on how serious these risks may be. Your mouth leaves a residue of bacteria when you drink from a bottle, and these bacteria may accumulate with repeated use. Disposable bottles also pose a risk to the environment. The manufacture of the estimated 30 billion PET water bottles sold annually in the United States requires about 17 million barrels of oil. About 86 percent of these bottles become waste.

✓**check-in** Did you know that it may take as long as 400 to 1,000 years for some disposable water bottles to degrade once dumped in a landfill?

Many consumers have switched to harder bottles made with polycarbonate plastic (known by brand names such as Camelbak and Nalgene). Portable metal containers are another option.

$ HEALTH ON A BUDGET

No- and Low-Cost Ways to Green Your Space

Whether you live in a dorm, apartment, or house, you can take simple, inexpensive steps to create a greener personal environment. Here are some ways to get started:

- **Buy furniture and household items secondhand, or recycle your parents' things.** If you can't find everything you need in the attic or basement, try a website such as **www.freecycle .com**, where you can barter your way to greener furnishings.

- **Choose recycled notebooks and printer paper and ecofriendly shampoos, conditioners, and lotions.**

- **Rather than relying on air-conditioning or central heat, use a space heater or fan, depending on the season, to regulate the temperature around you.**

- **Buy a stainless steel or coated aluminum water bottle instead of using disposable bottles.**

- **Use green cleaning products like vinegar and baking soda instead of expensive and potentially harmful chemicals.**

- **Tote books and groceries in canvas bags rather than paper or plastic ones.**

- **Chip in with roommates or friends so you can buy in bulk, which saves money and requires less packaging.**

- **Don't throw anything out before asking yourself if it can be recycled, donated, or simply used in another way.**

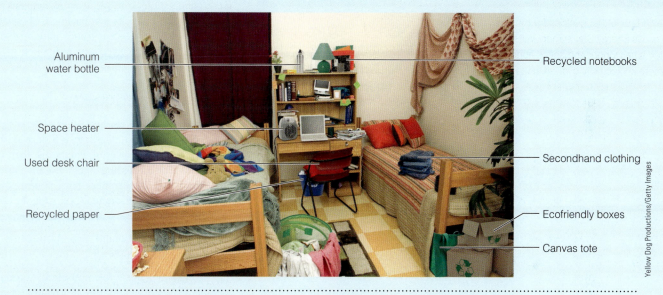

Aluminum water bottle

Space heater

Used desk chair

Recycled paper

Recycled notebooks

Secondhand clothing

Ecofriendly boxes

Canvas tote

Yellow Dog Productions/Getty Images

FIGURE 14.2 Greening Your Space

Some bottles are aluminum with a nontoxic liner; others are simply made of stainless steel.

Indoor Pollutants: The Inside Story

You may think of pollution as primarily a threat when you're outdoors, but people in industrialized societies spend more than 90 percent of their time inside buildings. Think of how much time you spend in your dorm, apartment, or home and in classrooms, dining halls, movie theaters, offices, stores, and shops. The quality of the air you breathe inside these places can have an even greater impact on your well-being than outdoor pollution (see Health on a Budget).

Household air pollution has emerged as a growing global environmental and public health issue. Its potential dangers include reducing lung function and contributing to respiratory illness, asthma, pneumonia, tuberculosis, eye diseases, pregnancy complications, cardiovascular diseases, and cancer.[96] Some sources—such as building materials and household products such as air fresheners—release pollutants more or less continuously. Other sources—such as tobacco smoke, solvents in cleaning products, and pesticides—can produce high levels of pollutants that remain in the air for long periods after their use.

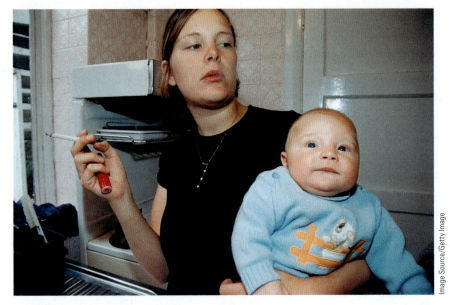
Infants and children face the greatest health risks from secondhand smoke.

Image Source/Getty Image

radioactive gas enters homes through dirt floors, cracks in concrete walls and floors, floor drains, and sumps. When radon becomes trapped in buildings and concentrations build up indoors, exposure to the gas becomes a concern.

Molds and Other Biological Contaminants

Bacteria, mildew, viruses, animal dander, cat saliva, house dust mites, cockroaches, and pollen can all pose a threat to health. One of the oldest and most widespread substances on Earth, mold—a type of fungus that decomposes organic matter and provides plants with nutrients—has emerged as a major health concern. Common molds include *Aspergillus*, *Penicillium*, and *Stachybotrys*, a slimy, dark green mold that has been blamed for infant deaths and various illnesses, from Alzheimer's disease to cancer, in adults that breathe in its spores. Faulty ventilation systems and airtight buildings have been implicated as contributing to the increased mold problem.

Household Products

The liquids, foams, gels, and other materials you use to clean, disinfect, degrease, polish, wax, and preserve contain powerful chemicals that can pollute indoor air during and for long periods after their use. Researchers have found levels of some 55 common organic pollutants in common products such as soaps, lotions, detergents, cleaners, sunscreens, air fresheners, kitty litters, shaving creams, vinyl shower curtains, cosmetics, and perfumes.

The health effects of household products include eye, nose, and throat irritation; headaches, loss of coordination, and nausea and damage to the liver, kidney, and central nervous system. In women they also may lower estrogen and lead to earlier menopause. Exposure to bisphenol A (BPA), a controversial chemical commonly used to make plastics such as that used to hold packaged food and drinks, may increase a healthy person's risk of developing heart disease later in life.

✓**check-in** Have you ever had an adverse reaction to a cleaning product or a cosmetic?

Formaldehyde

Some indoor pollutants come from the various materials that buildings are made of and from the appliances inside them. Formaldehyde is commonly used in building materials, carpet backing, furniture, foam insulation, plywood, and particle

Wood-burning fireplaces and stoves also pose a risk to both indoor and outdoor air quality because the smoke contains fine particles that, as discussed earlier in this chapter, can injure the lungs, blood vessels, and heart.[97] House dust can contain chemicals from outdoor and indoor air as well as from occupants and their pets. Exposure to airborne dust can affect the immune system and may trigger genetic changes over time.[98]

Environmental Tobacco Smoke

Environmental tobacco smoke (ETS) and its sequelae are among the largest economic and healthcare burdens in the United States and worldwide.[99]

The mixture of smoke from the burning end of a cigarette, pipe, or cigar and a smoker's exhalations contains over 4,000 compounds, more than 40 of which are known to cause cancer in humans or animals. More than half of U.S. states have enacted smoking bans in private worksites, restaurants, bars, airports, schools, hospitals, and many other locations. However, some states, mainly in the South and parts of the West, have resisted comprehensive bans. As a result, about 88 million nonsmokers in the United States are still exposed to environmental tobacco smoke.

Radon

Created by the breakdown of uranium in rocks, soil, and water, radon is the second-leading cause of lung cancer. Colorless and odorless, this

board. This chemical can cause nausea, dizziness, headaches, heart palpitations, stinging eyes, and burning lungs. Formaldehyde gas, which is colorless and odorless, has been shown to cause cancer in animals. Most manufacturers have voluntarily quit using it, but many homes already contain materials made with urea-formaldehyde, which can seep into the air.

Pesticides

According to a recent survey, 75 percent of U.S. households used at least one pesticide product indoors during the past year. Products used most often are insecticides and disinfectants.

The EPA requires manufacturers to put information on the label about when and how to use a pesticide. Remember that the -cide in pesticides means "to kill." Pesticides are also made up of ingredients that are used to carry the active agent. These carrier agents are called "inerts," because they are not toxic to the targeted pest; nevertheless, some inerts are capable of causing health problems.

Asbestos

This mineral fiber has been used commonly in a variety of building construction materials for insulation and as a fire retardant. The government has banned several asbestos products, and manufacturers have also voluntarily limited use of asbestos. Today asbestos is most commonly found in older homes, pipe and furnace insulation materials, asbestos shingles, millboard, textured paints, and floor tiles.

Lead

People are exposed to lead, a long-recognized health threat, through air, drinking water, food, contaminated soil, deteriorating paint, and dust. Airborne lead enters the body when an individual breathes or swallows lead particles or dust. Before its risks were known, lead was used in paint, gasoline, water pipes, and many other products. Although lead exposure has declined, about 2.6 percent of children ages 1 to 5 still have dangerous levels of lead in their blood. Boys are at greater risk than girls because female hormones may protect the brain against lead's harmful effects.[100]

Carbon Monoxide and Nitrogen Dioxide

Carbon monoxide (CO) gas—which is tasteless, odorless, colorless, and nonirritating—can be deadly. Produced by the incomplete combustion of fuel in space heaters, furnaces, water heaters, and engines, CO reduces the delivery of oxygen

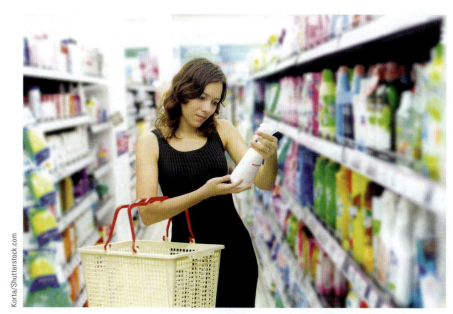

Korta/Shutterstock.com

Read the labels on common cleaning products and follow instructions for use and storage to avoid possible health risks.

in the blood. Every year an estimated 10,000 Americans seek treatment for CO inhalation; at least 250 die because of this silent killer. Those most at risk are the chronically ill, older adults, pregnant women, and infants.

Chemical Risks

Various chemicals, including benzene, asbestos, and arsenic, have been shown to cause cancer in humans. Probable carcinogens include DDT and PCB. Risks can be greatly increased with simultaneous exposures to more than one carcinogen—for example, tobacco smoke and asbestos.

According to the CDC, the levels of potentially harmful chemicals, including pesticides and lead, in Americans' blood have declined. Still, an estimated 50,000 to 70,000 U.S. workers die each year of chronic diseases related to past exposure to toxic substances, including lung cancer, bladder cancer, leukemia, lymphoma, chronic bronchitis, and disorders of the nervous system. Endocrine disruptors, chemicals that act as or interfere with human hormones, particularly estrogen, may pose a different threat. Scientists are investigating their impact on fertility, falling sperm counts, and cancers of the reproductive organs. Exposure to toxic chemicals causes about 3 percent of developmental defects.

Heavy metals, such as arsenic, chromium, and lead, can leach into groundwater or run off into surface water and soil, eventually making their way into the food chain. All have proven toxic effects on animals and humans.[101] Plastic materials can break down into extremely small "nanoparticles," called nanoplastics, that may pose a new environmental threat—although their potential danger to humans has not yet been extensively studied.[102]

Invisible Threats

Among the unseen threats to health are various forms of *radiation*, energy radiated in the form of waves or particles.

Electromagnetic Fields

Any electrically charged conductor generates two kinds of invisible fields: electric and magnetic. Together they're called **electromagnetic fields (EMFs)**. For years, these fields, produced by household appliances, home wiring, lighting fixtures, electric blankets, and overhead power lines, were considered harmless. However, epidemiological studies have revealed a link between exposure to high-voltage lines and cancer (especially leukemia, a blood cancer) in electrical workers and children. Exposure to EMFs can break DNA chains, damage proteins, disturb sleep, cause fatigue, impair memory and concentration, and affect brain and hormonal development.[103]

Researchers have documented increases in breast cancer deaths in women who worked as electrical engineers, electricians, or in other high-exposure jobs, and a link between EMF exposure and increased risk of leukemia and possibly brain cancer.

The National Institute of Environmental Health Sciences has concluded that the evidence of a risk of cancer and other human disease from the electric and magnetic fields around power lines is "weak." This finding applies to the extremely low-frequency electric and magnetic fields surrounding both the big power lines that distribute power and the smaller but closer electric lines in homes and appliances. However, the researchers also noted that EMF exposure "cannot be recognized as entirely safe."

Cell Phones

Since cellular phone service was introduced in the United States in 1984, mobile and handheld phones have become ubiquitous, and concern has grown about their possible health risks. The federal government sets upper limits for exposure to electromagnetic energy from cell phones, known as the specific absorption rate (SAR). A phone emits the most radiation during a call, but it also emits small amounts periodically whenever it's turned on.

Excessive use of mobile devices has been linked to poorer sleep in children and may also affect their physical activity and weight as well as cause musculoskeletal pain or discomfort.[104] There also is concern about the impact of electromagnetic radiation from cell phones on both adults and children, although its effects on health are not yet clear.[105]

Researchers have found that a 1-hour cell phone conversation stimulates the areas of the brain closest to the phone's antenna, but they do not know if these effects pose any long-term risk. More than 70 research papers on the potentially harmful effects of cell phone use have raised concerns about cancer, neurological disorders, sleep problems, or headaches; others have shown no association or have been inconclusive.[106]

Other adverse effects of cell phone use include changes in brain activity, reaction times, exercise duration and intensity,[107] and sleep patterns.[108] Drivers using cell phones, whether handheld or hands-free, have a three to four times greater chance of an accident because of the distraction.

The Food and Drug Administration (FDA) and Federal Communications Commission (FCC) have stated that "the available scientific evidence does not show that any health problems are associated with using wireless phones. There is no proof, however, that wireless phones are absolutely safe." Additional studies are under way.

✓**check-in** How much time do you spend talking on your cell phone every day?

Microwaves

Microwaves (extremely high-frequency electromagnetic waves) increase the rate at which molecules vibrate; this vibration generates heat. There's no evidence that existing levels of microwave radiation encountered in the environment pose a health risk to people, and all home microwave ovens must meet safety standards for leakage.

A concern about the safety of microwave ovens stems from the chemicals in plastic wrapping and plastic containers used in microwave ovens. Chemicals may leak into food. In high concentrations, some of the chemicals (such as DEHA, which makes plastic more pliable) can cause cancer in mice. Consumers should be cautious about using clingy plastic wrap when reheating leftovers, and plastic-encased metal "heat susceptors" included in convenience foods such as popcorn and pizza. Although these materials seem safe when

electromagnetic fields (EMFs) The invisible electric and magnetic fields generated by an electrically charged conductor.

microwaves Extremely high-frequency electromagnetic waves that increase the rate at which molecules vibrate, thereby generating heat.

tested in conventional ovens at temperatures of 300 degrees, microwave ovens can boost temperatures to 500 degrees Fahrenheit.

Ionizing Radiation

Radiation that possesses enough energy to separate electrons from their atoms, leaving charged ions, is called **ionizing radiation**. Its effects on health depend on many factors, including the amount, length of exposure, type, part of the body exposed, and the health and age of the individual.

We're surrounded by low-level ionizing radiation every day. Most comes from cosmic rays and radioactive minerals, which vary according to geography. (Denver has more than Atlanta, for instance, because of its altitude.) Human-made sources, including medical and dental X-rays, account for approximately 18 percent of the average person's lifetime exposure. Exposure to some dental X-rays performed in the past, when radiation levels were higher, may increase the risk of meningioma, a common type of brain tumor.

Your Hearing Health

Worldwide, 466 million people live with disabling hearing loss; of these, 34 million are children. In addition, 1.1 billion young people are at risk of hearing loss due to exposure to noise in recreational settings and through personal audio devices.[109]

Hearing loss is the third most common chronic health problem, after high blood pressure and arthritis, among older Americans. Noise-induced hearing loss is the most frequent preventable disability. Regular use of over-the-counter painkillers can also lead to hearing loss, especially in younger men. Road traffic noise has been linked with hearing loss, thinking, annoyance,[110] and increased heart attack risk.[111]

How Loud Is That Noise?

Loudness, or the intensity of a sound, is measured in **decibels (dB)**. A whisper is 20 dB; a conversation in a living room is about 50 dB. On this scale, 50 isn't 2.5 times louder than 20, but 1,000 times louder: Each 10-dB rise in the scale represents a tenfold increase in the intensity of the sound. Very loud but short bursts of sounds (such as gunshots and fireworks) and quieter but longer-lasting sounds (such as power tools) can induce hearing loss.

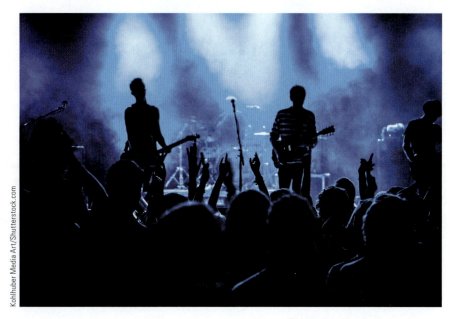

Kohlhuber Media Art/Shutterstock.com

The noise level at a rock concert can be as loud as an air-raid siren.

Sounds under 75 dB don't seem harmful. However, prolonged exposure to any sound over 85 dB (the equivalent of a power mower or food blender) or brief exposure to louder sounds can harm hearing. The noise level at rock concerts can reach 110 to 140 dB, about as loud as an air-raid siren.

ionizing radiation A form of energy emitted from atoms as they undergo internal change.

decibels (dB) Units for measuring the intensity of sounds.

YOUR STRATEGIES FOR PREVENTION

How to Protect Your Ears

- **If you must live or work in a noisy area, wear hearing protectors to prevent exposure to blasts of very loud noise.** Don't think cotton or facial tissue stuck in your ears can protect you; foam or soft plastic earplugs are more effective. Wear them when operating lawn mowers, weed trimmers, or power tools.

- **Give your ears some quiet time.** Rather than turning up the volume on your personal music player to blot out noise, look for truly quiet environments, such as the library, where you can rest your ears and focus your mind.

- **Soundproof your home by using draperies, carpets, and bulky furniture.** Put rubber mats under washing machines, blenders, and other noisy appliances. Seal cracks around windows and doors.

- **Beware of large doses of aspirin.** Researchers have found that 8 aspirin tablets a day can aggravate the damage caused by loud noise; 12 tablets a day can cause ringing in the ears (tinnitus).

- **Don't drink in noisy environments.** Alcohol intensifies the impact of noise and increases the risk of lifelong hearing damage.

- **When you hear a sudden loud noise, press your fingers against your ears.** Limit your exposure to loud noise. Several brief periods of noise seem less damaging than one long exposure.

Note: The maximum exposure allowed on the job by federal law, in hours per day: 90 decibels, 8 hours; 100 decibels, 2 hours; 110 decibels, 0.5 hour.

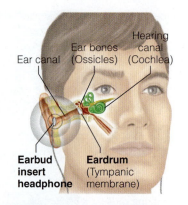

Ear canal · Ear bones (Ossicles) · Hearing canal (Cochlea)

Earbud insert headphone · **Eardrum** (Tympanic membrane)

Decibels	Example	Zone
0	The softest sound a typical ear can hear	Safe
10 dB	Just audible	
20 dB	Watch ticking; leaves rustling	
30 dB	Soft whisper at 16 feet	
40 dB	Quiet office; suburban street (no traffic)	
50 dB	Interior of typical urban home; rushing stream	1,000 times louder than 20 dB
60 dB	Normal conversation; busy office	
70 dB	Vacuum cleaner at 10 feet; hair dryer	
80 dB	Alarm clock at 2 feet; loud music; average daily traffic	1,000 times louder than 50 dB
90 dB	Motorcycle at 25 feet; jet 4 miles after takeoff	Risk of injury
100 dB	Video arcade; loud factory; subway train	
110 dB	Car horn at 3 feet; symphony orchestra; chain saw	1,000 times louder than 80 dB
120 dB	Jackhammer at 3 feet; boom box; nearby thunderclap	**Injury**
130 dB	Rock concert; jet engine at 100 feet	
140 dB	Jet engine nearby; amplified car stereo; firearms	**1,000 times louder than 110 dB**

FIGURE 14.3 Louder and Louder

The human ear perceives a 10-decibel increase as a doubling of loudness. Thus, the 100 decibels of a subway train sound much more than twice as loud as the 50 decibels of a rushing stream.

Effects of Noise

Noise-induced hearing loss is 100 percent preventable—and irreversible. Hearing aids are the only treatment, but they do not correct the problem; they just amplify sound to compensate for hearing loss.

The healthy human ear can hear sounds within a wide range of frequencies (measured in hertz), from the low-frequency rumble of thunder at 50 hertz to the high-frequency overtones of a piccolo at nearly 20,000 hertz. High-frequency noise damages the delicate hair cells that serve as sound receptors in the inner ear. Damage first begins as a diminished sensitivity to frequencies around 4,000 hertz, the highest notes of a piano.

Early symptoms of hearing loss include difficulty understanding speech and *tinnitus* (ringing in the ears). Brief, very loud sounds, such as an explosion or gunfire, can produce immediate, severe, and permanent hearing loss. Longer exposure to less intense but still hazardous sounds, such as those common at work or in public places, can gradually impair hearing, often without the individual's awareness.[112]

Are Earbuds Hazardous to Hearing?

Although there is limited research, audiologists (who specialize in hearing problems) report seeing greater noise-induced hearing loss in young people. One probable culprit is extended use of earbuds, the tiny earphones used with portable music players that deliver sound extremely close to the eardrum. Hearing loss can be temporary or permanent.[113]

✓**check-in** How often do you use earbuds?

The dangers to your hearing depend on how loud the music is and how long you listen. Because personal music players have long-lasting rechargeable batteries, people—especially young people—both listen for long periods and turn up the volume because they feel "low personal vulnerability" to hearing loss. As long as the sound level is within safety levels (see Figure 14.3), you can listen as long as you'd like. If you listen to music so loud that someone else can hear it 2 or 3 feet away, it's too loud.

For safe listening, limit listening to a portable music player with earphones or earbuds at 60 percent of its potential volume to 1 hour a day. At the very least, take a 5-minute break after an hour of listening and keep the volume low.

Ask yourself the following questions to determine if you should have your hearing checked:

- Do you frequently have to ask people to repeat themselves?
- Do you have difficulty hearing when someone speaks in a whisper?
- Do people complain that you turn up the volume too much when watching television or listening to music?
- Do you have difficulty following conversation in a noisy environment?
- Do you avoid groups of people because of hearing difficulty?
- Have your friends or family suggested you might have hearing loss?

Hearing Loss

More than 30 million U.S. adults have hearing loss. This condition is underrecognized, and hearing aids and other hearing enhancement technologies are underused. Age-related sensorineural hearing loss is the most common type in adults.[114]

Hearing loss is not just for seniors. About one in five 6- to 19-year-olds has impaired hearing. As many as one-quarter of college students may suffer mild hearing loss, including some who believe their hearing is normal.[115] This loss could be the result of use of personal music devices such as smartphones. Exposure to urban noise, such as the sounds of subways and ferries, also increases the risk of hearing problems.

WHAT DID YOU DECIDE?

- How are college students at high risk for unintentional injury?
- How do campus crime and violence affect students?
- Does climate change pose a risk to health?
- Are you jeopardizing your hearing health?

Reflection
Accidents and injuries put one person or a few people in danger, while other threats—such as climate change—imperil larger populations. Reflect on the ways you take responsibility to safeguard your personal safety and that of the entire planet.

TAKING CHARGE OF YOUR HEALTH

Creating a Safer World

Like other aspects of your health, you are responsible for protecting yourself and Mother Earth from harm.

Taking Care of Yourself

Are you as safe as you can be? Answer the questions below by providing a numerical score between 0 and 10 to describe to what extent you usually behave this way:

_____ I am alert to my surroundings.

_____ I do not pursue relationships with people out of a feeling that I should rescue them.

_____ I am careful to observe others long and well before allowing them into an intimate position in my life.

_____ If someone behaves strangely, I move away and keep my distance.

_____ I do not let people "guilt" or pressure me into situations that make me feel uncomfortable or unsafe.

_____ I do not lend money.

_____ I avoid Internet scams.

_____ I keep a close eye on my credit and identification cards.

_____ I get the sleep I need.

_____ I wear a seat belt whenever I'm in a vehicle.

_____ I wear a helmet when biking or skateboarding.

_____ I practice safe sex.

_____ I lock the doors and windows to my car, room, apartment, or dormitory.

_____ I do not let strangers enter my car or residence.

_____ I know where fire alarms and fire extinguishers are located.

_____ I control my alcohol intake so I can keep my wits about me in any situation.

Taking Care of Mother Earth

As a citizen of this planet, you are responsible for its well-being. Check the steps you have taken or plan to take in the future.

_____ Limit your driving. If you usually drive to campus, check out alternatives, such as carpooling and public or campus transportation.

_____ Precycle. Surf the Web for sites that sell products made from recycled materials. Click on *www.ecomall.com* for listings.

_____ Save the juice. Plug your appliances and e-gadgets, which drain electricity even when turned off, into a power strip. Whenever you leave, flicking off the switch effectively unplugs them.

_____ Integrate a new "green" habit into your life every week. Turn the thermostat down in winter and up in summer. Spend a few minutes less in the shower. Use both sides of printer paper.

_____ Avoid using disposables. Use a mug instead of a paper or foam cup, a sponge instead of a paper towel, a cloth napkin instead of a paper one.

Review your responses. Which behaviors could you improve? Make a to-do list of the changes you will implement today, in the coming week, and by the end of the term.

SELF-SURVEY

Are You Doing Your Part for the Planet?

You may think that there is little you can do, as an individual, to save Earth. But everyday acts can add up and make a difference in helping or harming the planet on which we live.

	Almost Never	Sometimes	Always
1. Do you walk, cycle, carpool, or use public transportation as much as possible to get around?	_____	_____	_____
2. Do you recycle?	_____	_____	_____
3. Do you reuse plastic and paper bags?	_____	_____	_____
4. Do you try to conserve water by not running the tap as you shampoo or brush your teeth?	_____	_____	_____
5. Do you use products made of recycled materials?	_____	_____	_____
6. Do you drive a car that gets good fuel mileage and has up-to-date emission control equipment?	_____	_____	_____
7. Do you turn off lights, televisions, and appliances when you're not using them?	_____	_____	_____
8. Do you avoid buying products that are elaborately packaged?	_____	_____	_____

	Almost Never	Sometimes	Always
9. Do you use glass jars and waxed paper rather than plastic wrap for storing food?	_____	_____	_____
10. Do you take brief showers rather than baths?	_____	_____	_____
11. Do you use cloth towels and napkins rather than paper products?	_____	_____	_____
12. When listening to music, do you keep the volume low?	_____	_____	_____
13. Do you try to avoid any potential carcinogens, such as asbestos, mercury, or benzene?	_____	_____	_____
14. Are you careful to dispose of hazardous materials (such as automobile oil or antifreeze) at appropriate sites?	_____	_____	_____
15. Do you follow environmental issues in your community and write your state or federal representatives to support green legislation?	_____	_____	_____

Scoring

Count the number of items you've checked in each column. If you've circled 10 or more in the "Always" column, you're definitely helping to make a difference. If you've mainly circled "Sometimes," you're moving in the right direction, but you need to be more consistent and more conscientious. If you've circled 10 or more in the "Never" column, carefully read this chapter and identify steps you can take to improve.

REVIEW QUESTIONS

(LO 14.1) 1. Unintentional injury is the leading cause of death for people who _____.
   a. are older
   b. are younger
   c. have unpredictable lives
   d. engage in criminal activities

(LO 14.1) 2. Which of the following tends to be one of the underlying psychological attributes exhibited by individuals who respond well in a crisis?
   a. Having learned from positive experiences
   b. Believing that all injuries are unintentional
   c. Believing that they can influence events
   d. Confidence that nothing bad will happen to them

(LO 14.2) 3. A majority of motor vehicle crashes are due to _____.
   a. speeding
   b. alcohol use
   c. distracted driving
   d. rollovers

(LO 14.2) 4. he second most common cause of motor vehicle accidents is _____.
   a. poor weather
   b. alcohol use
   c. distracted driving
   d. falling asleep at the wheel

(LO 14.3) 5. Which of the following is true of mass shootings?
   a. They are defined as the killing of four or more people at a single location.
   b. Psychiatrists can predict when someone is likely to be homicidal.
   c. It is a public health issue mainly in terms of gun ownership.
   d. They are often perpetrated by people diagnosed with mental illnesses.

(LO 14.3) 6. Which of the following are among the leading causes of violent death?
   a. Rape and relationships
   b. Cancer and emphysema
   c. Drugs and vaping
   d. Suicide and homicide

(LO 14.4) 7. Which of the following statements is true about violence on college campuses?
   a. Most crimes against students occur on campus.
   b. Men are more likely than women to be victims of physical violence.
   c. On-campus crimes are more frequent at night than during the day.
   d. Incidents of violence are always reported to higher authorities.

(LO 14.4)   8. _____ refers to any activity that humiliates, degrades, or poses a risk of emotional or physical harm for the sake of joining a group or maintaining full status in that group.
a. Discrimination
b. Bragging
c. Hazing
d. Hate

(LO 14.6)   9. Which of the following is NOT a health risk attributable to climatic changes?
a. Air pollution
b. Severe droughts
c. Spread of infectious diseases
d. Plastic pollution

(LO 14.6)   10. Which of the following greenhouse gases is released into the atmosphere when fossil fuels are burned?
a. Carbon dioxide
b. Methane
c. Nitrous oxide
d. Propane

(LO 14.7)   11. Which of the following is an example of a chronic effect caused by traffic pollution?
a. Dizziness
b. Nausea
c. Increased blood pressure
d. Death

(LO 14.7)   12. Mutagens are environmental agents that trigger changes in the _____.
a. composition of pollutants
b. genetic material of living cells
c. average temperature of the atmosphere
d. impact of greenhouse gases

(LO 14.8)   13. _____ is a health risk caused by pollutants destroying the air sacs in the lungs.
a. High blood pressure
b. Heart failure
c. Stroke
d. Emphysema

(LO 14.8)   14. Air pollution can increase the risk for heart attack by nearly _____ percent.
a. 1
b. 5
c. 10
d. 18

(LO 14.9)   15. Water bottles made with lightweight polyethylene terephthalate may take as long as _____ years to degrade.
a. 7 to 10
b. 100 to 140
c. 400 to 1,000
d. 100,000 to 200,000

(LO 14.9)   16. Consumers in the United States prefer to use bottled water over tap water because of _____.
a. fears about the public water supply
b. scientific recommendations of medical researchers
c. reports of decreased cavities among children drinking bottled water
d. the proven purity of the bottled water

(LO 14.12)   17. According to scientific researches, electromagnetic fields _____.
a. can be recognized as entirely safe
b. can be linked to cancer in children
c. are harmless irrespective of the level of exposure
d. are visible fields threatening to health

(LO 14.13)   18. Which of the following is true of noise-induced hearing loss?
a. It is irreversible.
b. It is not preventable.
c. It is an issue mainly for older people.
d. It is due to intensity of sound rather than length of exposure.

(LO 14.13)   19. Which of the following is NOT linked to hearing loss?
a. Large doses of aspirin
b. Giving your ears some quiet time
c. Road traffic noise
d. Brief, very loud sounds

Answers to these questions can be found on page 531.

After reading this chapter, you should be able to:

15.1 Distinguish between life expectancy and health-adjusted life expectancy in the United States.

15.2 Examine the factors that influence successful aging and the characteristics of old age.

15.3 Explain the physiological changes involved in aging.

15.4 Assess different ways to prepare for medical crises and the end of life.

15.5 Discuss the emotional and psychological responses to dying.

15.6 Describe the process of dying.

15.7 Analyze the reasons why people commit suicide.

15.8 Summarize the effects of grief at the death of a loved one.

WHAT DO YOU THINK?

- Can your health choices and behaviors affect how long you live?

- What is the greatest challenge you expect to face in old age?

- Are you prepared for medical crises that may affect you or your family?

- How do people respond to the loss of a loved one?

15

A Lifetime of Health

Stephanie decided to do something different for her term project for her Personal Health course. Unlike other students, who analyzed their diets or launched fitness programs, she assembled three generations of her family—some in person, some on phones or computers—on the annual National Healthcare Decisions Day to talk about a subject most people avoid: planning for illness, aging, and death.

The oldest generation—Stephanie's two surviving grandparents—had already completed advance directives that gave her mother a health-care power of attorney and spelled out the type of medical treatments they did or did not want at the end of life. Yet her parents, both in their 60s, had never disclosed their preferences. Stephanie and her husband, just turning 30, had never discussed their own wishes.

Talking about the inevitable challenges that aging brings wasn't easy, but it brought Stephanie and her family closer and made them more appreciative of each other. It also served as a reality check. Stephanie, noting some of the medical complications affecting her parents and grandparents, realized that the health choices she was making every day would affect not only how long she might live but also how she might feel and fare as she aged.

This chapter provides a preview of the changes age brings, the steps you can take to age healthfully, and the ways you can make the most of all the years of your life.

To many students, the prospect of their own death seems unthinkable. Yet the rates of death caused by unintentional injuries (including drug overdoses) and by suicide have increased among Americans between the ages of 15 and 44.[1]

Invariably, no one gets out of this life alive. Death is the natural completion of things, as much a part of the real world as life itself. In time we all lose people we cherish: grandparents, aunts and uncles, parents, friends, neighbors, coworkers, and siblings. With each loss, part of us may seem to die, yet each loss also reaffirms how precious life is.

This chapter explores the meaning of death, describes the process of dying, provides information on end-of-life issues, and offers advice on comforting the dying and helping their survivors. <

Quality and Quantity of Life

Within just 10 years, there will be 1 billion more older people around the globe.[2] By 2030 the number of Americans over age 65 will more than double to 70.3 million (20 percent of the total population). At age 65, women can expect to live an average of 20.5 more years; men, another 18 years.[3] The number of Americans age 85 and over, the fastest-growing cohort in the country, is projected to grow from 5.8 million today to 19 million in 2050.[4]

Yet the United States lags behind other countries in life expectancy, which has decreased in recent years to an average of 78.6 years. American males now have an average life expectancy at birth of 76.1 years, while life expectancy for female newborns is 81.1 years.[5] By comparison, all high-income countries combined have an average 78.1 years of life expectancy for men and 83.4 years for women. Among all nations, life expectancy has increased from 61.7 years in 1980 to 71.8 years today.[6]

Americans today experience more injuries and illnesses than people in other high-income countries. Almost 9 in 10 people over age 65 suffer at least one chronic illness; the majority of these men and women have two or more ongoing health conditions.

Although no one can turn back the clock, a healthy lifestyle can increase an individual's years of "able life" without need for assistance in daily living. The keys to boosting your healthy life expectancy include:

- Not smoking.

- Regular physical activity.

- A nutritious diet.

- Maintaining a healthy weight.

- Limited alcohol consumption.

- Social support.

Healthy habits can increase longevity as well as health. In a recent analysis based on tens of thousands of individuals, those who didn't smoke, exercised regularly, ate a nutritious diet, consumed only moderate amounts of alcohol, and maintained a healthy weight added years to their lifespans—an average of 12 years for men and 14 years for women.[7] Physicians describe the benefits of healthful living as a "rejuvenation" for the body.[8] And it's never too late to begin. Changing health behaviors in midlife greatly increases the likelihood of living fully and independently throughout the lifespan.[9]

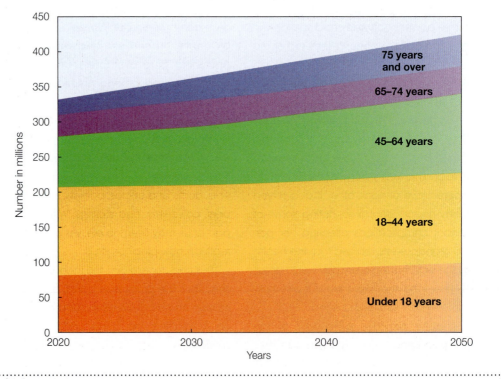

FIGURE 15.1 The Age Boom

As the generation of baby boomers (born between 1946 and 1964) age, the number of older people will increase dramatically. The older population in 2030 is projected to be twice as large as in 2000.

✓**check-in** How old is the oldest person you know? Do you expect to live as long as that person? Do you think you will be more or less healthy? Why?

Will You Live to 50?

If you're in your 20s or 30s, the question may strike you as absurd. Yet, you are less likely to hit the half-century mark than your peers in other affluent countries (see Figure 15.1).

What can you do to improve your odds? Stay in school. White Americans with no more than a high school education are more likely to die at younger ages than their college-educated peers. The most frequent causes are drug overdoses, smoking-related diseases, accidents, and injuries.[10] A growing number of people are using opioids, and the drugs themselves have become more deadly.[11] Overdoses now kill more younger Americans than guns, car crashes, or HIV.[12] Chapter 12 provides in-depth information on the opioid epidemic.

You can also increase your odds of staying alive by paying attention to four factors: blood pressure, blood sugar, weight, and smoking. Here is the difference in life expectancy each of these can make in lowering life expectancy:

- High blood pressure: 1.5 fewer years for men and 1.6 years for women.
- Obesity: 1.3 years for both men and women.
- High blood sugar: 0.5 year for men, and 0.3 year for women.
- Smoking: 10 years for both men and women, but those who quit before age 35 can gain back these years.

✓**check-in** What do you think is the biggest threat to your reaching age 50? What can you do to avoid or overcome it?

Aging Well

Although **aging**—the characteristic pattern of normal life changes that occurs as humans, plants, and animals grow older—remains inevitable, you can do a great deal to influence the impact that the passage of time has on you. But there is more than one way to age well.

"Successful" aging is defined as "freedom from disease or disease-related disability, high cognitive and physical functioning, and active engagement with life." "Effective" aging describes the experience of older adults who are not necessarily

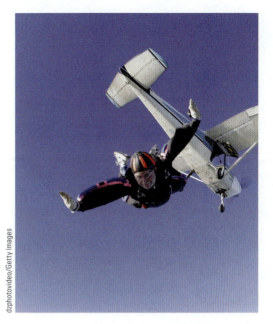

dzphotovideo/Getty Images

free of disease but are able to adapt to related challenges and sometimes transcend them. "Optimal" aging encompasses several dimensions of well-being, including autonomy, environmental mastery, personal growth, positive relations with others, purpose in life, and self-acceptance.[13]

According to research on "exceptional longevity" (survival to at least age 90), the key factors to living long and well are maintaining a healthy lifestyle (including regular exercise, weight management, and smoking avoidance) and avoiding or delaying chronic illnesses. Genetic factors contribute to healthy aging and exceptional longevity, but researchers have not been able to pinpoint specific "aging" genes. Older individuals who see themselves as isolated and disconnected from others consistently report lower levels of physical health.[14]

Whether you're in your teens, 20s, 30s, or older, now is the time to take the steps that will add healthy, active, productive years to your life.

Physical Activity: It's Never Too Late

Lack of physical activity, dangerous even for the young, becomes deadly among the old. As discussed in Chapter 6, simply sitting for prolonged periods increases "all-cause mortality," the risk of dying for any reason, in both sexes and all age groups, regardless of general health, body mass index (BMI), and physical activity levels. For seniors, gardening, dancing, and brisk walking, as well as more intense exercise, can delay chronic physical disability and cognitive decline. In fact, the effects of ongoing activity are so profound that gerontologists sometimes refer to exercise as "the closest thing to an anti-aging pill."

Exercise slows many changes associated with advancing age, such as loss of lean muscle tissue,

Staying active and seeking new adventures can add many vital years to your life.

aging The characteristic pattern of normal life changes that occur as living things grow older.

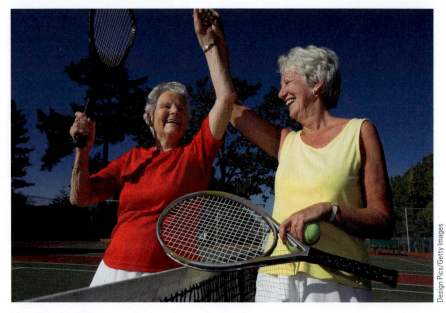

Keeping both brain and body active can enhance physical health, cognitive ability, and emotional well-being as we age.

increase in body fat, and decrease in work capacity. Consistent lifelong exercise preserves heart muscle in older adults to levels that match or even exceed those of healthy young sedentary individuals. High-intensity training is especially effective in improving fitness in both younger and older adults.[15]

Physical activity offers older Americans many other benefits, including:

- Greater ability to live independently.
- Reduced risk of frailty.
- Enhanced mental well-being, reduced stress and anxiety, and increased self-esteem.
- Healthier bones, muscles, and joints.
- Reduced risk of falling and fracturing bones.
- Protection against many health problems, including cardiovascular disease; cancers of the colon, breast, lung, and prostate; type 2 diabetes; and musculoskeletal disorders such as arthritis and osteoporosis.
- Reduced risk of dying from coronary heart disease and of developing high blood pressure, colon cancer, and diabetes.
- Reduced blood pressure in some people with hypertension.
- Fewer symptoms of anxiety and depression.
- Improvements in mood and feelings of well-being.
- Lower health-care costs (see Health on a Budget).

No one is ever too old to get in shape. The American College of Sports Medicine (ACSM) recommends that older adults develop a fitness plan with a health professional to manage risks and take into account health conditions. Its basics should consist of:

- Moderately intense aerobic exercise 30 minutes a day, 5 days a week

    or

- Vigorously intense aerobic exercise 20 minutes a day, 3 days a week

    and

- Eight to 10 strength-training exercises, with 10 to 15 repetitions of each exercise, two or three times a week

    and

- Balance exercises

✓**check-in** Are you active enough to keep your body "young" as long as possible?

Nutrition and Obesity

The most common nutritional disorder in older people is obesity. Overweight men and women over age 65 face increased risk of diabetes, heart disease, stroke, and other health problems, including arthritis. The Mediterranean diet (discussed in Chapter 4)—rich in whole grains, vegetables, legumes, nuts, fish, and olive oil—is associated with better heart health as well as lower risk for chronic disease and premature death. In addition, a low intake of vitamins can increase the risk of frailty; supplements may help.[16]

✓**check-in** What effects do you think your weight may have on the way you age?

The Aging Brain

Scientists used to think that the aging brain, once worn out, could never be fixed. Now they know that the brain can and does repair itself. When neurons (nerve cells) in the brain die, the surrounding cells develop "fingers" to fill the gaps and establish new connections, or synapses, between surviving neurons. Although self-repair occurs more quickly in young brains, the process continues in older brains. Even victims of Alzheimer's disease, the most devastating form of dementia, have enough healthy cells in the diseased brain to regrow synapses. Scientists hope to develop drugs that someday may help the brain repair itself.

The brain, like the rest of the body, may begin to show signs of aging in middle age. Researchers have documented dips in memory, reasoning, and other cognitive functions beginning at age 45, although the declines are greater in older people. However, just as exercise can maintain physical health, mental workouts

$ HEALTH ON A BUDGET

Reduce Your Future Health-Care Costs

Seniors with several chronic health problems can incur more than five times as much in health-care costs compared to older adults with no chronic conditions. You may be able to reduce your expenses by following four basic steps:

- **Keep your arteries young.** If your arteries are clear and healthy, you're more likely to have a healthy heart and a sharper brain and less likely to develop high blood pressure, high cholesterol, kidney problems, and memory impairment. For your arteries' sake, exercise regularly, avoid high-fat foods, watch your weight, and find ways to manage daily stress (see Chapter 3).

- **Avoid illness.** Most individuals who live to see 100 don't suffer from chronic diseases. Defend yourself by eating a healthy diet, not smoking, avoiding weight gain in middle age, recognizing and treating conditions like high blood pressure and elevated cholesterol, and keeping up with immunizations.

- **Stay strong.** As landmark studies with frail nursing home residents in their 80s and 90s have shown, strength training at any age builds muscle and bone, speeds up metabolic rate, improves sleep and mobility, boosts the spirit, and enhances self-confidence.

- **Maintain your zest for living.** Just as with muscles, the best advice to keep your brain strong is "use it or lose it." Keep challenging yourself, asking questions, and pursuing new passions. Individuals who are optimistic, sociable, and happy generally outlive their more pessimistic, grumpier peers.

can benefit our brains. Individuals who engage in activities such as reading and playing mind-engaging games may lower a protein in the brain linked with Alzheimer's disease. The higher the level of cognitive stimulation in young and middle-aged adults, the lower the risk of Alzheimer's later in life.[17]

Cognitive Aging Older people who remain mentally and physically healthy think just as sharply as college students. Wisdom increases because more mature minds can better see multiple points of view, search for compromise, and solve social conflicts. However, older adults may find it more difficult to multitask and split their focus between two tasks. The ability to remember newly learned information also declines with age. The reason may be that structural changes in the brain interfere with sleep quality, which in turn impairs memory. Sleeping well earlier in life may lead to better mental functioning as people age.

✓**check-in** Did you realize that people who live to age 85 may have slept nearly 250,000 hours—the equivalent of more than 10,000 full days?

Memory According to data from a National Institute on Aging survey, memory loss and cognitive problems are becoming less common among older Americans. The reasons may be that today's seniors have more formal education, higher economic status, and better health care for problems such as high blood pressure and high cholesterol that can jeopardize brain function. Higher education does not prevent cognitive decline over time,

but schooling does yield an advantage: Individuals with more education continue to have a higher level of cognitive functioning into old age, so they remain independent for a longer period.

Using your brain as you age—by reading, playing games, solving crossword puzzles, and doing crafts such as pottery or quilting—can decrease the risk of memory loss. Even work helps—if it involves the mind as well as the body. Jobs requiring intellectually challenging tasks have proven to help preserve thinking skills and memory as empoyees get older.[18]

✓**check-in** How do you exercise your brain to keep it healthy?

Women at Midlife

In the next two decades some 40 million American women will end their reproductive years. Medical specialists have identified several stages that characterize the aging of the female reproductive system:

- **Late reproductive stage.** Declines in fertility and changes in the menstrual cycle.

- **Early menopausal transition.** Increased variability in menstrual cycles.

- **Late menopausal transition.** Hormonal changes and amenorrhea, or lack of menstrual bleeding, for 60 days or longer.

- **Early postmenopause.** Five to eight years after the final menstrual period, when hormones fluctuate and then stabilize.

- **Late postmenopause.** Limited changes in reproductive hormones.

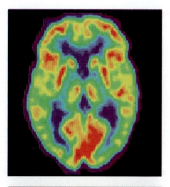
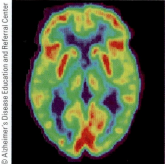

In these PET scans, the red and yellow show greater neuron activity in the young adult. The brain of the older person shows less activity and more dark areas, indicating that the fluid-filled ventricles have grown larger.

© Alzheimer's Disease Education and Referral Center

While the average age of **menopause**—defined as the complete cessation of menstrual periods for 12 consecutive months—is 51.5, a woman's reproductive system begins changing more than a decade earlier. Genes may determine the age at which women begin the transition to menopause.

For many women, **perimenopause**—the 4- to 10-year span before a woman's last period—can be more baffling and bothersome than the years after. During this time the egg cells, or oocytes, in a woman's ovaries start to senesce, or die off, at a faster rate. Eventually, the number of egg cells drops to a tiny fraction of the estimated 2 million packed into her ovaries at birth. Trying to coax some of the remaining oocytes to ripen, the pituitary gland churns out extra follicle-stimulating hormone (FSH). This surge is the earliest harbinger of menopause, occurring 6 to 10 years before a woman's final period. Eventually, the other menstrual messenger, luteinizing hormone (LH), also increases, but at a slower rate.

These hormonal shifts can trigger an array of symptoms. The most common is night sweats (a *subdromal hot flash*, in medical terms), which can be intense enough to disrupt sleep. The drop in estrogen levels also may cause hot flashes (bursts of warmth and perspiration that last from a few seconds to 15 minutes).

A woman's habits and health history also have an impact. Women with a lifelong history of depression are more likely to experience early perimenopause. Women without a history of depression or anxiety also are at greater risk of symptoms of anxiety and depression during perimenopause.[19] Smokers experience more symptoms at an earlier age than nonsmokers. Heavier women also tend to have more severe symptoms.

··
✓check-in If you are a woman, do you know the age your mother entered perimenopause or went through menopause? Have you ever talked with her about her experience?
··

Menopause

About 10 to 15 percent of women breeze through this transition with only trivial symptoms. Another 10 to 15 percent are virtually disabled. The majority fall somewhere in between these extremes. Women who undergo surgical or medical menopause (the result of removal of their ovaries or chemotherapy) often experience abrupt symptoms, including flushing, sweating, sleeplessness, early-morning awakenings, involuntary urination, changes in libido, mood swings, perception of memory loss, and changes in cognitive function.

Race and ethnicity profoundly affect women's experience. African American women report more hot flashes and night sweats but have more positive attitudes toward menopause. Japanese and Chinese women experience more muscle stiffness and fewer hot flashes but view menopause more negatively. Hispanic women reach menopause a year or two earlier than Caucasian women; Asian women reach menopause a year or two later.

Dwindling levels of estrogen subtly affect many aspects of a woman's health, from her mouth (where dryness, unusual tastes, burning, and gum problems can develop) to her skin (which may become drier, itchier, and overly sensitive to touch). With less estrogen to block them, a woman's androgens, or male hormones, may have a greater impact, causing acne, hair loss, and, according to some anecdotal reports, surges in sexual appetite. (Other women, however, report a drop in sexual desire.)

At the same time, a woman's clitoris, vulva, and vaginal lining begin to shrivel, sometimes resulting in pain or bleeding during intercourse. Since the thinner genital tissues are less effective in keeping out bacteria and other pathogens, urinary tract infections may become more common. Some women develop breast or ovarian cysts, which usually go away on their own. Eventually, a woman's ovaries don't respond at all to her pituitary hormones. After the last ovulatory cycle, progesterone is no longer secreted, and estrogen levels decrease rapidly. A woman's testosterone level also falls.

In the United States, the average woman who reaches menopause has a life expectancy of about 30 more years. However, she faces risks of various diseases, including an increased risk of obesity, metabolic syndrome, heart disease, stroke, and breast cancer. Women can reduce these risks through exercise, good nutrition, and weight control both before and after menopause. Those with low levels of vitamin D may benefit from supplements.[20]

Hormone Therapy

Medical thinking on **hormone therapy (HT)**, long believed to prevent heart disease and stroke and help women live longer, has changed, particularly related to the combination of estrogen and progestin. Based on the Women's Health Initiative (WHI)—a series of clinical trials begun in 1991 on postmenopausal women—HT now is recommended for fewer than 5 years as "a reasonable option" for the relief of moderate to severe symptoms such as hot flashes. As various studies have confirmed, longer-term combination therapy increases the risk of breast cancer, heart disease, blood clots, stroke, and ovarian cancer.[21] Although exercise can reduce the risk of breast cancer, it does not have the same preventive effects in women who have ever used HT.

Middle-aged women who undergo hormone therapy are not at increased risk of heart attack, memory loss, or dementia years down the road. Earlier research had raised alarms that hormone therapy might increase the risk of these health problems. Many of the women in these studies

menopause The complete cessation of ovulation and menstruation for 12 consecutive months.

perimenopause The period from a woman's first irregular cycles to her last menstruation.

hormone therapy (HT) The use of supplemental hormones during and after menopause.

were older than age 65 and had started taking hormones 20 years past menopause.[22]

In its most recent practice guidelines, the American College of Obstetricians and Gynecologists recommended the following options for relief of hot flashes and night sweats:

- Minimal doses of hormone therapy, with estrogen alone or estrogen plus progestin.
- Low doses of certain antidepressants, such as Prozac or Paxil.
- The antiseizure drug gabapentin.
- The blood pressure medication clonidine.

Black cohosh, soy supplements, and acupuncture have not been shown to reduce hot flashes or improve a woman's quality of life during menopause.[23]

Men at Midlife

Although men don't experience the dramatic hormonal upheaval that women do, they do experience a decline by as much as 30 to 40 percent in their primary sex hormone, testosterone, between the ages of 48 and 70. This change, sometimes called *andropause*, may cause a range of symptoms, including decreased muscle mass, greater body fat, loss of bone density, flagging energy, lowered fertility, and impaired virility. As they age, men who smoke may lose more Y chromosomes from their cells, a change that has been correlated with a shorter lifespan and an increased risk of dying from cancer.[24]

Low Testosterone
As men age, they produce somewhat less testosterone, especially compared to the years of peak testosterone production during adolescence and early adulthood. Although the media have popularized the concepts of male menopause and "low T" (low testosterone), there is little scientific evidence that normally decreasing testosterone levels are responsible for many changes that take place in older men. Testosterone supplements have not been proven effective and pose serious risks to middle-aged and older men. In a study of 48,000 middle-aged men with previous histories of heart disease, testosterone almost tripled the risk of heart attacks within 90 days of beginning treatment.[25]

✓**check-in** If you are a man, would you ever consider taking supplemental testosterone? Why or why not?

Prostate Problems
After age 40, the prostate gland, which surrounds the urethra at the base of the bladder, enlarges. This condition, called *benign prostatic hypertrophy*, occurs in every man. By age 50, half of all men have some enlargement of the gland; after 70, three-quarters do. As it expands, the prostate tends to pinch the urethra, decreasing urinary flow and creating a sense of urinary urgency, particularly at night. Other warning signs of prostate problems include difficult urination, blood in the urine, painful ejaculation, or constant lower-back pain.

Medical treatments for benign prostate hypertrophy include drugs that improve urine flow and reduce obstruction of the bladder outlet as well as medications that partially shrink the enlarged prostate by lowering the level of the major male hormone inside the prostate. In some cases, surgical treatment is necessary.

Sexuality and Aging

Health and sexuality interact in various ways as we age. When they are healthy and have a willing partner, a substantial number of older men remain sexually active. The fittest men and women report more frequent sexual activity. Better health translates into a better sex life. Healthy people are more likely to express an interest in sex, engage in sex, and enjoy sex.

On average, 55-year-old men can expect to remain sexually active for another 15 years, while women the same age can expect about 11 more sexually active years. Women with partners remain sexually active longer. Being in good health may provide men with an additional 5 to 7 years of sexual life expectancy.[26]

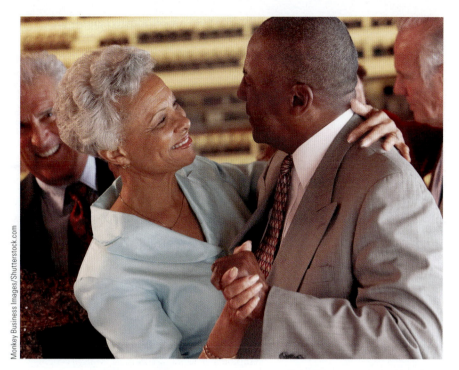

For older couples, sexual desire and pleasure can be enhanced by years of intimacy and affection.

Monkey Business Images/Shutterstock.com

Aging does cause some changes in sexual response. Women produce less vaginal lubrication. An older man needs more time to achieve an erection or orgasm and to attain another erection after ejaculating. Both men and women experience fewer contractions during orgasm. However, none of these changes reduces sexual pleasure or desire.

The Challenges of Age

No matter how well we eat, exercise, and take care of ourselves, some physical changes are inevitable as we age. Figure 15.2 shows some of these changes, but most of them are not debilitating, and most

people can remain active and vital into extreme old age. Aging brains and bodies do become vulnerable to diseases such as Alzheimer's disease and osteoporosis. The immune system declines over time, which increases vulnerability to infectious diseases.[27] Specially targeted approaches, such as high-dose flu vaccines, have proven effective in protecting older individuals.[28]

Other common life problems, such as depression, substance misuse, and safe driving, become more challenging as we age. Nearly 40 percent of Americans over the age of 65 live with at least one disability that affects their hearing, sight, walking, thinking, self-care, or independent living, according to a government report. The most common—reported by two-thirds of seniors with a disability—is difficulty walking or climbing stairs.[29] This increases the risk of falls, which pose a greater risk of injury and death in older individuals.[30]

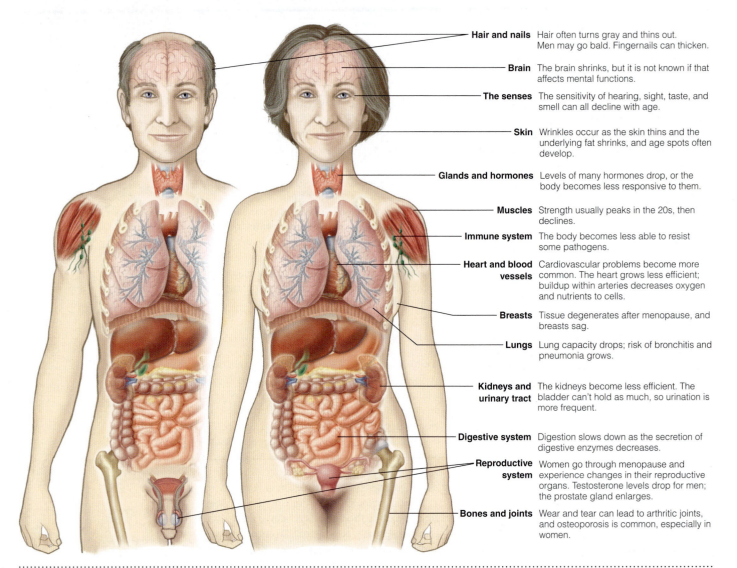

Hair and nails Hair often turns gray and thins out. Men may go bald. Fingernails can thicken.

Brain The brain shrinks, but it is not known if that affects mental functions.

The senses The sensitivity of hearing, sight, taste, and smell can all decline with age.

Skin Wrinkles occur as the skin thins and the underlying fat shrinks, and age spots often develop.

Glands and hormones Levels of many hormones drop, or the body becomes less responsive to them.

Muscles Strength usually peaks in the 20s, then declines.

Immune system The body becomes less able to resist some pathogens.

Heart and blood vessels Cardiovascular problems become more common. The heart grows less efficient; buildup within arteries decreases oxygen and nutrients to cells.

Breasts Tissue degenerates after menopause, and breasts sag.

Lungs Lung capacity drops; risk of bronchitis and pneumonia grows.

Kidneys and urinary tract The kidneys become less efficient. The bladder can't hold as much, so urination is more frequent.

Digestive system Digestion slows down as the secretion of digestive enzymes decreases.

Reproductive system Women go through menopause and experience changes in their reproductive organs. Testosterone levels drop for men; the prostate gland enlarges.

Bones and joints Wear and tear can lead to arthritic joints, and osteoporosis is common, especially in women.

FIGURE 15.2 The Effects of Aging on the Body

✓**check-in** Do you have concerns about the health of an aging relative? Why?

Mild Cognitive Impairment

An estimated 10 to 20 percent of those age 65 and older may suffer **mild cognitive impairment (MCI)**, which causes a slight but noticeable and measurable decline in cognitive abilities, including memory and thinking skills. The changes are not severe enough to interfere with independent living, but people with MCI have an increased risk of developing Alzheimer's disease or another type of dementia.

According to the American Psychiatric Association's *Diagnostic and Statistical Manual of Mental Disorders, Fifth Edition* (*DSM-5*), MCI can affect one or more cognitive abilities, including complex attention, executive functions, learning and memory, language, perceptions, movement, and social cognition.[31] There are no tests to diagnose MCI conclusively. Physicians evaluate patients on the basis of a medical history, neuropsychological testing, assessment of mental status, input from family, and laboratory tests.

No medications are currently approved to treat mild cognitive impairment. Vitamins or folic acid supplements, contrary to previous studies, do not have any effect on thinking and memory and do not reduce the risk of Alzheimer's disease as people age. Drugs that treat symptoms of Alzheimer's disease have not shown any lasting benefit in delaying or preventing progression of MCI to dementia.

The following coping strategies may help slow decline in thinking skills:

- Exercise to benefit blood vessels, including those that nourish the brain.

- Reduce cardiovascular risk factors (see Chapter 12) to protect the heart and the blood vessels that support brain function.

- Participate in mentally stimulating and socially engaging activities. Cognitive training that focuses on memory, reasoning, and everyday problem solving has proven to significantly improve mental acuity and performance.[32]

Alzheimer's Disease

About 15 percent of older Americans lose previous mental capabilities, a brain disorder called **dementia**.[33] Sixty percent of these—an estimated 2.4 to 4.5 million—suffer from the type of dementia called **Alzheimer's disease**, a progressive deterioration of brain cells that results in a gradual loss of cognitive function and, eventually, dementia. In addition to its physical and psychological benefits, physical activity may reduce the risk of dementia.

Age is the top risk factor for Alzheimer's, but cognitive decline may begin up to 6 years before it is evident. Someone in America develops Alzheimer's every 72 seconds; by 2050 the rate will increase to every 33 seconds. The percentage of people with Alzheimer's doubles for every 5-year age group beyond 65. By age 85, nearly half of men and women have Alzheimer's. A person with the disease typically lives 8 years after the onset of symptoms, but some live as long as 20 years.

People whose parents have been diagnosed with Alzheimer's disease or dementia may be more likely to experience memory loss themselves in middle age. Scientists have identified multiple genes that make people more likely to develop Alzheimer's. Women are at higher risk than men, and women with Alzheimer's perform significantly worse than men in various visual, spatial, and memory tests. Black Americans are about two times more likely to develop Alzheimer's than whites; Hispanics face about 1.5 times the risk. Older adults who report feeling lonely are more likely to develop dementia, regardless of other risk factors.

The early signs of dementia are usually subtle and insidious. They include:

- Sleep problems.

- Irritability.

- Increased sensitivity to alcohol and other drugs.

- Decreased energy.

- Lower tolerance of frustration.

- Depression.

Diagnosis requires a comprehensive assessment of an individual's medical history, physical health, and mental status, often involving brain scans and a variety of other tests.

Cholesterol-lowering statin drugs, discussed in Chapter 10, and low-dose daily aspirin may reduce the risk of Alzheimer's, regardless of a person's genetic risk for the disease. Vitamins C, D, and E, as well as calcium supplements, once touted as possible memory preservers, have not proven to lower the risk of dementia or Alzheimer's in older adults.

Many factors—genetic, medical, social, and environmental—can affect the progression of Alzheimer's disease.[34] Although medical science cannot restore a brain that is in the process of being destroyed by an organic brain disease such as Alzheimer's, medications can control difficult behavioral symptoms and enhance or partially restore cognitive ability. Often physicians find other medical or psychiatric problems, such as

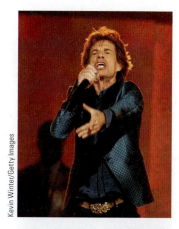

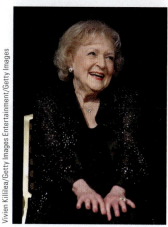

What life after 70 can look like.

mild cognitive impairment (MCI) A slight but noticeable and measurable decline in cognitive abilities, including memory and thinking skills.

dementia Deterioration of mental capability.

Alzheimer's disease A progressive deterioration of intellectual powers due to physiological changes within the brain; symptoms include diminishing ability to concentrate and reason, disorientation, depression, apathy, and paranoia.

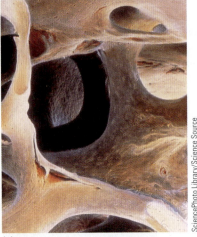
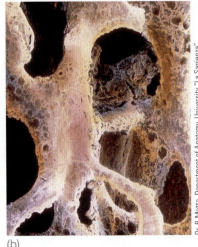

(a)

(b)

ScitencePhoto Library/Science Source

Dr. P. Motta, Department of Anatomy, University "La Sapienza" Rome/Science Photo Library/Science Source

The effect of osteoporosis on bone density. (a) Normal bone tissue. (b) After the onset of osteoporosis, bones lose density and become hollow and brittle.

depression, in these patients; recognizing and treating these conditions can have a dramatic impact. The FDA has approved several prescription drugs for people with mild to moderate dementia that do not cure or halt the progression of Alzheimer's but may improve cognitive and daily functioning.[35]

✓**check-in** Have any of your close relatives developed cognitive impairment or Alzheimer's? Would you be able to recognize the early signs?

Osteoporosis

Another age-related disease is *osteoporosis*, a condition in which losses in bone density become so severe that a bone will break with even slight trauma or injury. A chronic disease, osteoporosis is silent for years or decades before a fracture occurs. Each year more than one-third of Americans age 65 and older experience falls, and nearly 16,000 die as a result of their injuries. Even a low-trauma fracture increases the risk of dying during the subsequent 5 years, and a hip fracture heightens this risk for 10 years.[36]

Women, who have smaller skeletons, are more vulnerable to osteoporosis than men; in extreme cases, their spines may become so fragile that just bending causes severe pain. But although commonly seen as an illness of women, osteoporosis occurs frequently in men. One in every two women and one in four men over age 50 will have an osteoporosis-related fracture in their lifetimes.

As discussed in Chapter 6, regular exercise can help maintain and improve bone density. As studies of postmenopausal women have shown, high levels of cardiovascular fitness are associated

with reduced risk of low bone density. Daily calcium, between 700 and 1200 mg, from diet or supplements, may also reduce the risk of fractures. Higher doses can be potentially harmful.[37]

Earlier research had concluded that the adverse risks of hormone therapy, which include breast cancer and coronary artery disease, outweighed its benefits in preventing osteoporosis. However, newer studies indicate that lower doses and hormonal patches (rather than pills) pose less risk and should be used on an individualized basis.[38]

✓**check-in** Are you taking steps now to prevent future bone problems?

Preparing for Medical Crises and the End of Life

This book has presented many ways in which you can determine how well and how long you live. You can also make decisions about the end of your life. When facing a serious, potentially life-threatening illness, people typically have practical, realistic goals, such as maintaining their quality of life, remaining independent, being comfortable, and providing for their families (see Health Now!).

Most Americans—40 percent in a national sample of Medicare beneficiaries—do not express their preferences for dealing with end-of-life issues.[39] Women, whites, married people, and those with a college degree or postgraduate training are more likely to prepare advance directives ("living wills"), while black and Hispanic respondents and low-income Americans, regardless of education, are less likely to do so.[40] Their reasons include lack of awareness and poor social support.

Various racial and ethnic groups have different preferences for their end-of-life wishes. Many Arab Americans prefer not to go to nursing homes as they near the end of their lives, while many African Americans are comfortable with nursing homes and hospitals. Hispanic individuals express strong concerns about dying with dignity. Many white people don't want their families to take care of them, although they—like members of most other racial and ethnic groups—want their families nearby as they live out their last days.

Advance Directives

Advance directives enable individuals to specify the kind of medical treatment they want in case of a medical crisis. These documents are important because, without clear indications of a person's preferences, hospitals and other institutions often make decisions on an individual's behalf, particularly if family members are not available or disagree among themselves.

The two most common advance directives are health-care proxies and living wills. Each state has different legal requirements for these forms. You can find state-specific forms at www.caringinfo.org. Once the forms are completed, make copies of your advance directives and give them to anyone who might have input into decisions on your behalf. Also give copies to your physician or health-care organization and ask that they be made part of your medical record.

Health-Care Proxies A *health-care proxy* is an advance directive that gives someone else the power to make health decisions on your behalf. This advance directive is also called medical power of attorney or health-care power of attorney. People typically name a relative or close friend as their agent. Let family members and friends know that you have completed a health-care proxy. You should tell your primary physician, but you should not designate your doctor as your agent. Many states prohibit this. Even when allowed, it is not a good idea because your doctor's primary responsibility is to administer care.

Living Wills Individuals can use a **living will** (also called health-care directive or physician's directive) to indicate whether they want or don't want all possible medical treatments and technology used to prolong their lives. Living wills are most effective when they focus on priorities and goals rather than on how to achieve them. Most states recognize living wills as legally binding, and a growing number of health-care professionals and facilities offer patients help in drafting living wills.

The Five Wishes An innovative document called "Five Wishes" helps aged and seriously ill people, as well as their loved ones and caregivers, prepare for medical crises. Written with the help of the American Bar Association's Commission on the Legal Problems of the Elderly, the Five Wishes document has a health-care

YOUR STRATEGIES FOR PREVENTION

Keep Your Bones Healthy

- **Get adequate calcium.** Increased calcium intake, particularly during childhood and the growth spurt of adolescence, can produce a heavier, denser skeleton and reduce the risk of the complications of bone loss later in life. College-age women can also strengthen their bones and reduce their risk of osteoporosis by increasing their calcium intake and physical activity.

- **Drink alcohol only moderately.** More than two or three alcoholic beverages a day impairs intestinal calcium absorption.

- **Don't smoke.** Smokers tend to be thin and enter menopause earlier.

- **Let the sunshine in (but don't forget your sunscreen).** Vitamin D, a vitamin produced in the skin in reaction to sunlight, boosts calcium absorption.

- **Exercise regularly.** Both aerobic exercise and weight training can help preserve bone density.

proxy, a health-care directive, and three other "wishes." People using this document can specify the following:

- Which person they want to make health-care decisions for them when they are no longer able to do so.

- Which kinds of medical treatments they do or don't want.

- How comfortable they want to be made.

- How they want people to treat them.

- What they want loved ones to know.

The Five Wishes document (available at https://fivewishes.org/) is legally valid in almost all states. Churches, synagogues, hospices, hospitals, physicians, social service agencies, and employers are also distributing the document to help people plan for their own care or that of aging parents.

DNR Orders You can sign an advance directive specifying that you want to be allowed to die naturally—that you do not want to be resuscitated when your heart stops beating. **Do-not-resuscitate (DNR)** orders apply mainly to hospitalized, terminally ill patients and must be signed by a physician. However, in some states, it is possible to complete a *nonhospital DNR* form that specifies an individual's wish not to be resuscitated at home. Patients in the final

advance directives Documents that specify an individual's preferences regarding treatment in a medical crisis.

living will An advance directive that provides instructions for the use of life-sustaining procedures in the event of terminal illness or injury.

do-not-resuscitate (DNR) orders An advance directive that expresses an individual's preference that resuscitation efforts not be made during a medical crisis.

Preparing for a Medical Crisis in an Aging Relative

As your parents, grandparents, and other relatives get older, here is what you can do in advance:

- Watch for warning signals.
- Suggest a surrogate.
- Talk to loved ones.
- Focus on values.
- Involve the person's primary physician.
- Investigate alternative living options.
- Make sure you know where to find key documents.

holographic will A will wholly in the handwriting of its author.

coma A state of total unconsciousness.

persistent vegetative state A state of being awake and capable of reacting to physical stimuli, such as light, while being unaware of pain or other environmental stimuli.

---

stages of advanced cancer or AIDS may choose to use such forms to protect their rights in case paramedics are called to their homes.

Holographic Wills Perhaps you think that only wealthy or older people need to write wills. However, if you're married, have children, or own property, you should either hire a lawyer to draw up a will or at least write a **holographic will** yourself, specifying who should inherit your possessions. If you die *intestate* (without a will), the state will make these decisions for you. Even a modest estate can be tied up in court for a long period of time, depriving family members of money when they need it most.

A holographic will is a handwritten (not typed) statement that some states will recognize. You can

- **Name a family member or friend** as the executor, the person who sees that your wishes are carried out.

- **List the things you own** and to whom you want them to go; include addresses and telephone numbers, if possible.

- **Select a guardian for your children** (if any), presumably someone whose ideas about raising children are similar to your own. Be sure that any named guardians are willing and able to accept this responsibility before writing them into your will.

- **Specify any funeral arrangements.**

Be sure to keep the will in a safe place, where your executor, family members, or closest beneficiary can find it quickly and easily; tell them where it is.

Ethical Dilemmas

Modern medicine can do more to delay or defy death than was once thought possible. However, the ability to sustain life in patients with no hope of recovery has created wrenching medical and moral dilemmas. Increasingly, lawyers, ethicists, and consumer advocates are arguing that health-care providers must recognize a fundamental right of patients: the right to die.

Health economists, noting that more than half of U.S. health-care dollars are spent in the last year of life, have questioned "heroic" measures to prolong the life of chronically ill elderly patients or those with fatal diseases. Policies on such aggressive measures vary from hospital to hospital and state to state; often medical staff are not aware of patients' wishes.

Some health-care facilities require that staff members try to resuscitate any patient whose heart stops unless a do-not-resuscitate (DNR) order has been written, usually with the family's permission.

Families may demand aggressive medical care near the end of life on the basis of religious grounds, such as a conviction that every moment of life is a gift from God worth preserving at any cost. However, doctors are not obliged to provide a treatment they consider medically inappropriate or inhumane simply because of the family's religious beliefs. Ideally, doctors and family members, perhaps with the aid of a chaplain, work together to reach a consensus on the appropriate limits to life-sustaining treatment.

Another major ethical concern is the fate of an estimated 5,000 to 10,000 unconscious Americans who are being kept alive by artificial means. Some are in a **coma**, a state of total unconsciousness. They may have no sense of where they are, no memory, and no experience of pain. Others are in a **persistent vegetative state**, in which they're awake and yet unaware. They open their eyes; their brain waves show the characteristic patterns of waking and sleep. They can usually breathe on their own after a few weeks on artificial respiration; they can cough; the pupils of their eyes respond to light; but they do not respond to pain.

The Gift of Life

If you're at least 18 years old, you can fill out a donor card agreeing to designate, in the event of your death, any organs or tissues needed for transplantation (see Figure 15.3). Corneas may help a blind person see, for example. Kidneys, or even a heart, may be transplanted. The donation takes effect upon your death and is a generous way of giving others the possibilities for life that you have had yourself. The card should be filled out and signed; some must be signed in the presence of two witnesses. Attach the donor card to the back of your driver's license or I.D. card. (Whole-body donations may require other arrangements.)

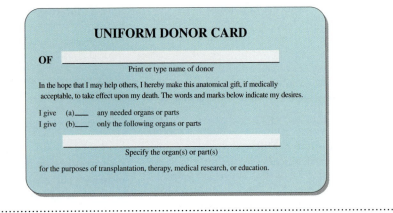

UNIFORM DONOR CARD

OF _____
Print or type name of donor

In the hope that I may help others, I hereby make this anatomical gift, if medically acceptable, to take effect upon my death. The words and marks below indicate my desires.

I give (a)____ any needed organs or parts
I give (b)____ only the following organs or parts

_____
Specify the organ(s) or part(s)

for the purposes of transplantation, therapy, medical research, or education.

FIGURE 15.3 Example of a Uniform Donor Card

Persons Ages 15–24 Years	Persons Ages 25–44 Years
Unintentional Injury (including overdose)	Unintentional Injury (including overdose)
Suicide	Cancer
Homicide	Suicide
Cancer	Heart disease
Heart disease	Homicide
Congenital malformations (birth defects)	Chronic liver disease

What have been the primary causes of death among young adults in your community?

Source: National Center for Health Statistics. *Health, United States, 2017: With special feature on mortality.* Hyattsville, MD. 2018.

✓**check-in** Have you signed up to be an organ donor? Why or why not?

Death and Dying

Some 2.7 million people die in the United States each year.[41] According to medical statisticians, your risk of death doubles every 8 years after about age 20 or 30. Although previously thought to level off at about age 80, the death rate continues to rise at about the same rate until at least age 106.

The causes of death vary with both gender and age. For both men and women, heart disease and cancer ranked as the first and second leading causes of death, respectively. Unintentional injury is the third leading cause of death for men, but ranks sixth among causes of female deaths.[42]

Unintentional injury is the leading cause of death for young adults between the ages of 15 and 34 (see Snapshot: On Campus Now). This includes fatal drug overdoses, two-thirds of which involve opioids. Recent increases in drug use have been especially pronounced among men between ages 25–34 and women between ages 15–24 (see Chapter 12).[43]

Death Literacy and Education

Death used to be such a taboo subject that people for a long time avoided even mentioning it, let alone treating it as a subject worthy of study and discussion. This attitude is changing as communities and individuals develop greater "death literacy," defined as the knowledge and skills that make it possible to understand and act upon end-of-life and death care options.[44] "Death education," which consists of a variety of educational activities and experiences related to death, dying, and bereavement, becomes more widespread in colleges and schools for health professionals.

Formal death education may involve courses, independent research, and clinical experiences, offered at every educational level, from elementary to graduate school, or seminars or workshops for health professionals and the public. Informal death education can take place whenever and wherever a "teachable moment" occurs, whether it's the death of a family pet or media coverage of a mass shooting. The goal is to challenge individuals to acknowledge their personal mortality so they can create a more meaningful life.

✓**check-in** Do you think that learning about death can reduce fears of dying?

Defining Death

In our society, death isn't a part of everyday life, as it once was. Because machines can now keep people alive when they would have died in the past, the definition of death has become more complex. Death has been broken down into the following categories:

- **Functional death.** The end of all vital functions, such as heartbeat and respiration.
- **Cellular death.** The gradual death of body cells after the heart stops beating. If placed in a tissue culture or, as is the case with various organs, transplanted to another body, some cells can remain alive indefinitely.

YOUR STRATEGIES FOR CHANGE

Learning about Death

College students enrolled in death education classes have passed along some of the lessons they've learned from the experience:

- **If you have anyone you need to forgive, do it now.** If that person is you, write yourself a letter absolving yourself of blame for whatever wrong you feel that you did.

- **Write a letter to someone, dead or alive, to say thank you.** This could be a grandparent who cherished you as a child or a friend you lost touch with long ago. Reflect on your gratitude for their gifts to you.

- **Don't assume that it's ever too late for love.** Until their final breath, people find strength and solace in expressing their feelings, touching and being touched, and reaching out to others.

- **Accept the prospect of death but don't focus on it.** People of every age—from the very young to the extremely old—die every day. The point is to live life to the fullest no matter how much is left.

- **Death.** The moment the heart stops beating.

- **Brain death.** The end of all brain activity, indicated by an absence of electrical activity (confirmed by an electroencephalogram [EEG]) and a lack of reflexes. The notion of brain death is bound up with what we consider to be the actual person, or self. The destruction of a person's brain means that his or her personality no longer exists; the lower brain centers controlling respiration and circulation no longer function.

- **Spiritual death.** The moment the soul, as defined by many religions, leaves the body.

When does a person actually die? The traditional legal definition of death is failure of the lungs or heart to function. However, because respiration and circulation can be maintained by artificial means, most states have declared that an individual is considered dead only when the brain, including the brain stem, completely stops functioning. Brain-death laws prohibit a medical staff from "pulling the plug" if there is any hope of sustaining life.

Denying Death

Most of us don't quite believe that we are going to die. A reasonable amount of denial helps us focus on the day-to-day realities of living. However, excessive denial can be life-threatening. Some drivers, for instance, refuse to buckle their seat belts because they refuse to acknowledge that a drunk driver might collide with them. Similarly, cigarette smokers deny that lung cancer will ever strike them, and people who eat high-fat meals deny that they'll ever suffer a heart attack.

One important factor in denial is the nature of the threat. It's easy to believe that death is at hand when someone's pointing a gun at you; it's much harder to think that cigarette smoking might cause your death 20 or 30 years down the road. The late Elisabeth Kübler-Ross, a psychiatrist who extensively studied the process of dying, described the downside of denying death in *Death: The Final Stage of Growth*:

> It is the denial of death that is partially responsible for people living empty, purposeless lives; for when you live as if you'll live forever, it becomes too easy to postpone the things you know that you must do. You live your life in preparation for tomorrow or in the remembrance of yesterday—and meanwhile, each today is lost. In contrast, when you fully understand that each day you awaken could be the last you have, you take the time that day to grow, to become more of who you really are, to reach out to other human beings.

Emotional Responses to Dying

Kübler-Ross identified five typical stages of reaction that a person goes through when facing death (see Figure 15.4).

1. Denial ("No, not me"). At first knowledge that death is coming, a terminally ill patient rejects the news. The denial overcomes the initial shock and allows the person to begin to gather together his or her resources. Denial, at this point, is a healthy defense mechanism. It can become distressful, however, if it's reinforced by the relatives and friends of the dying patient.

2. Anger ("Why me?"). In the second stage, the dying person begins to feel resentment and rage regarding imminent death. The anger may be directed at God or at the patient's family and caregivers, who can do little but try to endure any expressions of anger, provide comfort, and help the patient on to the next stage.

3. Bargaining ("Yes, me, but . . ."). In this stage, a patient may try to bargain, usually with God, for a way to reverse or at least postpone dying. The patient may promise, in exchange for recovery, to do good works or to see family members more often. Alternatively, the patient may say, "Let me live long enough to see my grandchild born" or "to see the spring again."

4. Depression ("Yes, it's me"). In the fourth stage, the patient gradually realizes the full consequences of his or her condition. This may begin as grieving for health that has been lost and then become anticipatory grieving for the loss that is to come of friends, loved ones, and life itself. This stage is perhaps the most difficult; the dying person should not be left alone during this period. Neither should loved ones try to cheer up the patient, who must be allowed to grieve.

5. Acceptance ("Yes, me; and I'm ready"). In this last stage, the person has accepted the reality of death. The moment looms as neither frightening nor painful, neither sad nor happy—only inevitable. The person who waits for the end of life may ask to see fewer visitors, to separate from other people, or perhaps to turn to just one person for support.

Several stages may occur at the same time and some may happen out of sequence. Each stage may take days or only hours or minutes. Throughout, denial may come back to assert itself unexpectedly, and hope for a medical breakthrough or a miraculous recovery is forever present.

Some experts dispute Kübler-Ross's basic five-stage theory as too simplistic and argue that not all people go through such well-defined stages in the dying process. The way a person faces death is often a mirror of the way he or she has faced other major stresses in life. Those who have had the most trouble adjusting to other crises will have the most trouble adjusting to the news of their impending death.[45]

An individual's will to live can postpone death for a while. In a study of elderly Chinese women, researchers found that their death rate decreased before and during a holiday during which the senior women in a household play a central role; it increased after the celebration. A similar temporary drop occurs among Jews at the time of Passover. However, different events may have different effects. The prospect of an upcoming birthday postpones death in women but hastens it in men. The will to live typically fluctuates in terminal patients, varying along with depression, anxiety, shortness of breath, and a sense of well-being.

The family of a dying person experiences a spectrum of often wrenching emotions. Family members, too, may deny the verdict of death, rage at the doctors and nurses who can't do more to save their loved one, bargain with God to give up their own health if necessary, sink into helplessness and depression, and finally accept the reality of their anticipated loss.

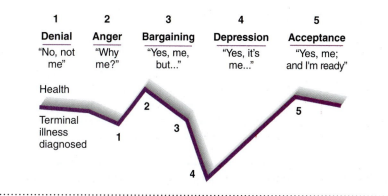

1	2	3	4	5
Denial	**Anger**	**Bargaining**	**Depression**	**Acceptance**
"No, not me"	"Why me?"	"Yes, me, but..."	"Yes, it's me..."	"Yes, me; and I'm ready"

FIGURE 15.4 Kübler-Ross's Five Stages of Adjustment to Facing Death

Dying can be seen from different perspectives. The Renz model, for example, views it as a process of maturation consisting of pretransition, transition, and posttransition. The initial response is an upsurge of emotions, including anger, grief, feelings of personal emptiness, and despair. These may emerge again and again.

However, as patients confront reality, they eventually can "let go and let be." As one researcher observed, "There is happiness and well-being in the midst of illness. In the course of the dying process spiritual experiences of such intensity often happen more than just once. After a shorter or longer struggle, patients reach a new mental state, a gift of grace beyond human endeavor and power."

How We Die

Life can end in very different ways. Sudden death, by accident or assault, for instance, brings an abrupt end to life in individuals who may have been in optimal health. A **terminal illness**, such as an aggressive and fatal cancer, can lead to a steep drop in functioning prior to death. When organs such as the kidneys fail, a patient's well-being tends to plummet and then recover but in a downward pattern. The frailty of old age leads to a gradual decline to ever lower levels of functioning and eventual death.

Most people who have a fatal or terminal illness prefer to know the truth about their health and chances for recovery. Even when they're not officially informed by a doctor or relative, most fatally ill people know or strongly suspect that they're dying. Dying people usually make it clear whether they want to talk about death and to what extent. The most frequent concern is how much time is left. Usually physicians can give only a rough estimate, such as "several weeks or months."

terminal illness An illness in which death is inevitable.

A "Good" Death

Many health-care professionals as well as citizens and social organizations have begun to demand a better way of caring for those who are dying. The Center to Improve Care of the Dying, in Washington, D.C., has set goals for reintegrating dying within living, thus enhancing the prospect for growth at the end of life. These experts talk of "dying well," "living while dying," and "physician-assisted living." They aim to change our way of thinking about dying so that we view the end of life as a time of love and reconciliation and a transcendence of suffering.

The qualities of a good death are more similar than different across cultures.[46] Psychological factors affect those approaching the end of life. Elderly people who lack hope in the future are much more likely to die within the next few years. Researchers speculate that hopelessness may lead to biochemical and nervous system abnormalities or that hopeless individuals may not eat well, take medications as prescribed, or follow a doctor's recommendations.

Spirituality plays a major role. In various surveys, many patients say they want their doctors and nurses to address their spiritual concerns. Even nonreligious patients say that physicians should inquire politely about patients' spiritual needs. However, some worry that such queries may be inappropriate or detract from their primary mission as healers.

Many people say they would prefer to die in their own homes, but most Americans die elsewhere—in emergency rooms, hospitals, nursing homes, or hospices. Older persons, who may have greater opportunity to plan for their deaths, are more likely to die at home.[47]

Caregiving

When someone becomes terminally ill, a woman—usually the patient's wife, daughter, or sister—is most likely to provide day-to-day care, often for periods longer than a year. Caregiving takes a different toll on men and women. In one study of adult daughters and husbands caring for terminally ill breast cancer patients, the daughters experienced more symptoms of anxiety and depression and greater family strain.

The impact of caregiving continues even after the death of an ill spouse. In one study, the health of older caregivers who had experienced strain prior to a spouse's death did not deteriorate. They showed no increase in depressive symptoms or use of antidepressant drugs and did not lose weight. Those who had not been caregivers were more likely to experience depression and weight loss.

hospice A homelike health-care facility or program committed to supportive care for terminally ill people.

transcendence The sense of passing into a foreign region or dimension, often experienced by a person near death.

Hospice: Caring When Curing Isn't Possible

A **hospice** helps dying men and women live their final days to the fullest, as free as possible from disabling pain and mental anguish. Race and ethnicity affect the use of hospice. In a study of patients over age 65 (and all covered by Medicare) with terminal cancer, Asian American and black patients were less likely to enroll in a hospice program than whites and Hispanics. They also were more likely to be hospitalized in an intensive care unit at least twice during their last month of life.

Hospice workers generally work in teams, usually consisting of a nurse, physician, social worker, chaplain, and trained volunteers. Other professionals, such as a physical therapist, may join the team when needed. These workers provide the comfort, support, and care dying patients need until they die.

Hospice programs offer a combination of medical and emotional care that involves not only the patient but also the family members or others concerned with caring for the patient. Most hospice patients have life expectancies of 6 months or less and are no longer receiving treatments aimed at curing their diseases. When someone is available to provide care, patients remain in their own homes. Hospice nurses regularly visit all home patients and are available around the clock. For patients requiring care that the family cannot provide, round-the-clock care is available at a hospice facility. Unlike a traditional hospital, where the focus is on diagnosis, cure, and treatment, a hospice works to make what is left of life pain-free and comfortable. Visiting hours for relatives and friends are flexible, with no restrictions on visits by children and grandchildren. Hospice services are covered, in full or in part, by most private and government insurance.

Near-Death Experiences

Interest in near-death experiences has grown, thanks largely to popular books such as *Proof of Heaven* by neurosurgeon Eben Alexander. Most accounts are remarkably similar, whether they occur in children or adults, whether they're the result of accidents or illnesses, even whether the individuals actually are near death or only think they are. Some individuals who have survived a close brush with death report autoscopy (watching, from several feet in the air, resuscitation attempts on their own bodies) or **transcendence** (the sense of passing into a foreign region or dimension). Some see light, often at the end of a tunnel. Their vision seems clearer; their hearing, sharper. Some recall scenes from their lives or feel the presence of loved ones who have died. Many report profound feelings of joy, calm, and peace. Fewer than 1 percent of those who've reported near-death experiences described them as frightening or distressing, although a larger number recall transitory feelings of fear or confusion.

Many near-death experiences occur in individuals who've been sedated or given other medications; however, many others do not. Several studies have shown that individuals who received medication or anesthesia were actually less likely to remember near-death experiences than those who hadn't had any drugs. Some scientists have speculated that lack of oxygen, changes in blood gases, altered brain functioning, or the release of neurotransmitters (messenger chemicals in the brain) may play a role in near-death experiences. However, there's little solid evidence that physiological events are responsible. There's also no proof that wishful thinking, cultural conditioning, posttraumatic stress, or other psychological mechanisms may be at work. For now, the most that scientists can say for sure about this medical mystery is that it needs further study.

Suicide

Suicide increases with age and is most common in persons age 65 and older. Elderly men, particularly non-Hispanic white men, have much higher suicide rates than women. However, suicide rates have increased among children aged 14 and under as well as young adults from ages 15 to 44.[48] For every completed suicide, there are 10 to 40 unsuccessful attempts. As discussed in Chapter 3, an estimated 1 in 10 college students seriously considers suicide, and nearly half suffer from significant depression. Other factors that may place a college student at risk for suicide include substance abuse, a family history of suicide, impulsive and aggressive behavior, and relationship difficulties. (Chapter 2 presents a detailed discussion of the risk factors and warning signs of suicide.)

One of the main factors leading to suicide is illness, especially terminal illness. Simply receiving a diagnosis of cancer increases the danger of suicide. A great deal of debate centers on quality of life, yet there is no reliable or consistent way to measure this. Patients who are dying may feel some quality of life, even when others do not recognize it, or their evaluations of the quality of their lives may fluctuate. Dying patients who say their lives are not worth living may be suffering from depression; hopelessness is one of its characteristic symptoms.

"Rational" Suicide

An elderly widow suffering from advanced cancer takes a lethal overdose of sleeping pills. A young man with several AIDS-related illnesses shoots himself. A woman in her 50s, diagnosed as having Alzheimer's disease, asks a doctor to help her end her life. Are these suicides "rational" because these individuals used logical reasoning in deciding to end their lives?

Advocates of the right to "self-deliverance" argue that individuals in great pain or faced with the prospect of a debilitating, hopeless battle against an incurable disease can and should be able to decide to end their lives. As legislatures and the legal system tackle the thorny questions of an individual's right to die, mental health professionals worry that, even in those with fatal diseases, suicidal wishes often stem from undiagnosed depression.

Because depression may indeed warp the ability to make a rational decision about suicide, mental health professionals urge physicians and family members to make sure individuals with chronic or fatal illnesses are evaluated for depression and given medication, psychotherapy, or both. It is also important for everyone to allow enough time—an average of 3 to 8 weeks—to see if treatment for depression will make a difference in their desire to keep living.

Euthanasia and Assisted Suicide

Euthanasia, the administration of a lethal medication by a physician or another person, is illegal in the United States. **Assisted suicide**, in which a health professional gives a patient the means to end his or her life, has been legalized by several states for patients of sound mind with a confirmed terminal illness.

Right-to-Die Laws

If patients have a right to die, should doctors help them end their lives? Physicians could stop any extraordinary efforts to sustain life (for example, by withholding oxygen or ending intravenous feedings); such actions are referred to as passive *euthanasia*, or *dyathanasia*. Euthanasia, the active form of so-called mercy killing, has generally been viewed as illegal and unethical. Euthanasia is tolerated and legally pardoned in the Netherlands in cases of hopeless and unbearable suffering, but remains illegal in all European countries. The demand for physician-assisted death in the Netherlands has not risen, and patients and physicians have become more reluctant to ask for or offer this option over the past few years.

euthanasia The painless killing of a patient with an incurable fatal disease or in an irreversible coma.

assisted suicide Providing the means to end life to a patient by a health professional.

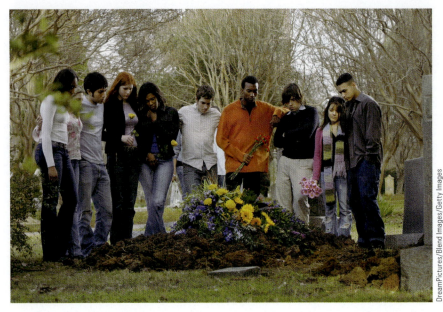

Funerals and memorial services help those in mourning to honor the deceased and to come to terms with their loss.

The Practicalities of Death

At a time of great emotional pain, grieving family members must cope with medical, legal, and practical concerns, including obtaining a medical certificate of the cause of death, registering the death, and making funeral arrangements. They also may want to arrange for organ donations and, in some circumstances, an autopsy.

Funeral Arrangements

A body can be either buried or cremated. Burial requires the purchase of a cemetery plot, which many families do decades before death. A burial is typically one of the most expensive investments of a lifetime. The average national costs range as high as $6,000, although they vary considerably. Memorial societies are voluntary groups that help people plan in advance for death. They obtain services at moderate cost, keep the arrangements simple and dignified, and—most important, perhaps—ease the emotional and financial burden on the rest of the family when death finally does come.

If the body is to be cremated, you must comply with some additional formalities, with which the funeral director can help you. After a *cremation* (incineration of the remains), you can either collect the ashes to keep, bury, or scatter yourself, or ask the crematorium to dispose of them.

The tradition of a funeral may help survivors come to terms with the death, enabling them to mourn their loss and to celebrate the dead person's life. Funerals are usually held two to four days after the death. Many have two parts: a religious ceremony at a church or funeral home, and a burial ceremony at the grave site.

Alternatively, the body may be disposed of immediately, through burial, cremation, or bequeathal to a medical school, and a memorial service held later. In a memorial service, the body is not present, which may change the focus of the service from the person's death to a celebration of his or her life.

Autopsies

An **autopsy** is a detailed examination of a body after death, also called a postmortem exam. There are two types:

- **Medicolegal.** This type of autopsy is performed to establish the cause of death and to gather information about the death for use as evidence in any legal proceedings. It is done to detect any crimes and to help identify the proper person for prosecution, to investigate possible industrial hazards or contagious diseases that may endanger the public health, or to establish the cause of death for insurance purposes.

- **Medical/educational.** This type of autopsy is performed, usually in the hospital where the person died, to increase medical knowledge and to determine a more exact cause of death. It may be requested by the attending physician or the family, but it cannot be performed without the family's permission.

Autopsies can be extremely valuable in establishing an accurate cause of death, revealing a different diagnosis that might have led to a change in therapy and prolonged survival in about 10 percent of cases. Thirty years ago about 50 percent of patients who died in hospitals were autopsied. However, the autopsy rate in the United States has been steadily declining, and today about 10 to 20 percent of deaths in teaching hospitals are autopsied.

Grief

More than 8 million Americans lose a member of their immediate family each year. Each death leaves an average of five people bereaved. Such loss may be the single most upsetting and feared

autopsy A detailed examination of a body after death.

DreamPictures/Blend Images/Getty Images

event in a person's life. It produces a wide range of reactions, including anxiety, guilt, anger, and financial concern.

Many may see the death of an old person as less tragic than the death of a child or young person. A sudden death is more of a shock than one following a long illness. A suicide can be particularly devastating because family members may wonder whether they could have done anything to prevent it. The cause of death can also affect the reactions of friends and acquaintances. Some people express less sympathy and support when individuals are murdered or take their own lives.

According to the stage theory of grief, individuals respond to the loss of a loved one by progressing through several steps, just like people facing death. These consist of:

- Shock-numbness.
- Yearning-searching.
- Disorganization-despair.
- Reorganization.

All these reactions can occur simultaneously, although most peak within 6 months. Acceptance continues to increase over time. The most common and one of the most painful experiences is the death of a parent. When both parents die, even adult individuals may feel like orphaned children. They mourn not just for the father and mother who are gone but also for their lost role of being someone's child.

Grief's Impact on Students

Bereavement is not a rare occurrence on college campuses. In a recent survey, 22 to 30 percent of students reported experiencing the death of a family member or close friend in the previous 12 months. Another multicampus study found that 47 percent of participants identified an unexpected death as the most traumatic event they had experienced.[49]

The grief process is particularly challenging for students, in part because college life typically centers on work and play rather than coping with death and loss. After the loss of a loved one or a close friend, college students may be at risk for poor academic performance, disengaging from campus life, and ultimately dropping out of school. Friends may pull away from them, not out of malice but because of their own discomfort with loss.

Among the problems that grieving students report are:

- Insomnia.
- Lack of motivation.

YOUR STRATEGIES FOR CHANGE

How to Cope with Grief

- **Accept your feelings—sorrow, fear, emptiness, whatever—as normal.** Don't try to deny emotions such as anger, guilt, despair, or relief.

- **Let others help you—by bringing you food, taking care of daily necessities, providing companionship and comfort.** (It will make them feel better, too.)

- **Face each day as it comes.** Let yourself live in the here-and-now until you're ready to face the future. Give yourself time—perhaps more than you ever imagined—for the pain to ebb, the scars to heal, and your life to move on.

- **Don't think there's a right or wrong way to grieve.** Mourning takes many forms, and there's no set timetable for working through the various stages of grief.

- **Seek professional counseling if your grief does not ease over time.** Therapy can help prevent potentially serious physical and psychological problems.

- Difficulty concentrating.
- Depression.
- Emotional problems.
- Relationship concerns.[50]

Counselors have called upon universities to help students who have lost a loved one through initiatives such as training students untouched by grief to provide peer support and raising consciousness about bereavement. Students who have coped with grief suggest the colleges should display greater sensitivity, more flexibility in completion of coursework, and easier access to counseling and psychological support.

✓**check-in** If you have suffered the loss of a loved one, how did you experience grief?

Grief's Effects on Health

Men and women who lose partners, parents, or children endure so much stress that they're at increased risk of serious physical and mental illness, and even of premature death. Studies of the health effects of grief have found the following:

- Grief produces changes in the respiratory, hormonal, and central nervous systems and may affect functions of the heart, blood, and immune systems.

- Grieving adults may experience mood swings between sadness and anger, guilt, and anxiety.

- Grievers may feel physically sick, lose their appetites, sleep poorly, or fear that they're going crazy because they "see" the deceased person in different places.

- Friendships and remarriage offer the greatest protection against health problems.

- Some widows may have increased rates of depression, suicide, and death from cirrhosis of the liver. The greatest risk factors are poor previous mental and physical health and a lack of social support.

- Grieving parents, partners, and adult children are at increased risk of serious physical and mental illness, suicide, and premature death.

Sometimes grief progresses from an emotionally painful but normal experience to a more persistent problem, called *complicated grief*. Individuals who experience very long-lasting or severe symptoms, including inability to accept a loved one's death, persistent thoughts about the death, and preoccupation with the lost loved one, can benefit from professional treatment.[51] Cognitive behavioral therapy (discussed in Chapter 2), whether face-to-face or Internet-based, has proven most effective.[52]

WHAT DID YOU DECIDE?

- Can your health choices and behaviors affect how long you live?

- What is the greatest challenge you expect to face in old age?

- Are you prepared for medical crises that may affect you or your family?

- How do people respond to the loss of a loved one?

Reflection

Consider how your answers changed after reading this chapter. Can you identify one way you might apply what you've learned to your life now or in the future?

TAKING CHARGE OF YOUR HEALTH

Staying Alive and Well

"Every man desires to live long," wrote Jonathan Swift, "but no man would be old." We all wish for long lives, yet we want to avoid the disease and disability that can tarnish our golden years. Which of the following steps will you take to ensure a lifetime of health?

____ Exercise regularly. By improving blood flow, staving off depression, warding off heart disease, and enhancing well-being, regular workouts help keep mind and body in top form.

____ Don't smoke. This habit can take an estimated 10 years off a lifespan. Even light smokers (one to nine cigarettes a day) are twice as likely to die as nonsmokers.

____ Watch your weight and blood pressure. Increases in these vital statistics can increase your risk of hypertension, cardiovascular disease, stroke, and other health problems.

____ Eat more fruits and vegetables. These foods, rich in vitamins and protective antioxidants, can reduce your risk of cancer and damage from destructive free radicals.

____ Cut down on fat. Fatty foods can clog the arteries and contribute to various cancers.

____ Limit drinking. Alcohol can undermine physical health and sabotage mental acuity.

____ Cultivate stimulating interests. Elderly individuals with complex and interesting lifestyles are most likely to retain sharp minds and memories beyond age 70.

____ Don't worry; be happy. At any age, emotional turmoil can undermine well-being. Relaxation techniques, such as meditation, help by reducing stress.

____ Reach out. Try to keep in contact with other people of all ages and experiences. Make the effort to invite them to your home or go out with them. On a regular basis, do something to help another person.

____ Make the most of your time. Greet each day with a specific goal—to take a walk, write letters, visit a friend.

In your online journal, describe the life you envision for yourself at ages 50, 60, 75, and 100.

SELF-SURVEY

What is Your Aging IQ?

Use the National Institute for Aging website to test your knowledge about aging, https://www.nia.nih.gov. Answer True or False.

1. **True** or **False**: Everyone becomes "senile" sooner or later, if he or she lives long enough.

2. **True** or **False**: More than 60 percent of Americans 65 years and older have more than one chronic health condition.

3. **True** or **False**: Depression is a normal part of aging.

4. **True** or **False**: The numbers of older people are growing.

5. **True** or **False**: Walking speed at age 45 is associated with future physical and brain health.

6. **True** or **False**: Mental confusion is an inevitable, incurable consequence of old age.

7. **True** or **False**: All adults over the age of 65 should follow a calorie restriction and fasting diet pattern.

8. **True** or **False**: Sexual urges and activity normally cease around ages 55 to 60.

9. **True** or **False**: If a person has been smoking for 30 or 40 years, it does no good to quit.

10. **True** or **False**: Older people should stop exercising and rest.

11. **True** or **False**: Only children need to be concerned about calcium for strong bones and teeth.

12. **True** or **False**: As you grow older, you may need more vitamins and minerals to stay healthy.

13. **True** or **False**: Extremes of heat and cold can be particularly dangerous to old people.

14. **True** or **False**: Many older people are hurt in accidents that could have been prevented.

15. **True** or **False**: More men than women survive to old age.

16. **True** or **False**: Stroke is the top cause of serious adult disability in the United States.

17. **True** or **False**: Older people on average take more medications than younger people.

18. **True** or **False**: There are several effective supplements available that prevent Alzheimer's disease.

19. **True** or **False**: It's normal for older adults to have an increased difficulty finding words and recalling names.

20. **True** or **False**: Sight changes with age.

Scoring

1. **False.** While everyone loses some neurons as they age, most people with dementia experience much greater loss. Up to half of all people that are 85 or older may have some form of dementia. Even though dementia is more common as people grow older, it is not a normal part of aging. Many people live into their 90s and beyond without any signs of dementia.

2. **True.** Sixty-one percent of American's 65 years and older live with multiple chronic conditions. Although Americans now live longer than their grandparents, they may not be in better health. There are many older adults who live with more than one chronic condition. About 79 percent of those 70 years of age and older have at least one of seven potentially disabling chronic conditions (arthritis, hypertension, heart disease, diabetes, respiratory diseases, stroke, and cancer). These chronic diseases can affect their quality of life.

3. **False.** Though depression is a common problem for older adults, it is not a normal part of aging. Studies show that as we age, older adults feel satisfied with their lives even though they may experience more illness and physical challenges. As we age, there can be stress and sadness caused by life events. The good news is that depression can be treated.

4. **True.** Americans are growing older as a population. By 2030, it is estimated that those who are over 65 or older will have more than doubled the number from 2000.

5. **True.** How fast someone walks (gait speed) is used to test older adults' physical capacity and to predict risk of future disease. Studies published in 2019 indicate a positive association of gait speed in midlife (45 years of age) and their rate of aging and their future brain health. Gait speed is an accepted indicator of health risk in late life, including risk of hospitalization, disability, dementia, and mortality.

6. **False.** Mental confusion and serious forgetfulness in old age can be caused by Alzheimer's disease or other conditions that cause incurable damage to the brain, but many other problems can cause the same symptoms. A minor head injury, certain vitamin deficiencies, drinking too much

alcohol, emotional problems, delirium, thyroid problems, a high fever, poor nutrition, adverse drug reactions, and depression are among the many problems that can all be treated and reversed.

7. **False.** The current recommendation is that there are no firm conclusions about the benefits for human health.

8. **False.** Most older people can lead an active, satisfying sex life. Our bodies do change as we age. There is help for many of the things that can cause sexual problems in older adults. Many older couples are more satisfied with their sex lives compared to when they were younger.

9. **False.** It's never too late to quit smoking. Stopping smoking at any age not only reduces the risk of cancer and heart disease but also leads to healthier lungs.

10. **False.** Exercise helps support emotional and mental health. Exercise and physical activity aren't just good for the mind and body, they can help you stay active and mobile as you age. Exercise is an important way to stay healthy as you age, it can even improve some chronic health conditions. Certain exercises can help prevent falls in older people. If an older adult has a chronic condition, this does not mean they have to rest all day. For older people with chronic disease, it's recommended they ask their doctor if there are exercises they should avoid.

11. **False.** Older people may require fewer calories, but adequate intake of calcium for strong bones can become more important as they age. This is particularly true for women, because after menopause their risk of osteoporosis increases. Milk and cheese are rich in calcium, as are cooked dried beans, collards, and broccoli. Some people need calcium supplements as well. Your doctor or a dietitian can tell you whether you need to change your diet or add additional calcium to your diet.

12. **True.** Older adults may have different vitamin and mineral needs than younger adults. For most older adults, they need the same amounts of most vitamins and minerals as younger people. Though some people over age 50 may need more of some vitamins and minerals than younger adults do. Your doctor or a dietitian can tell you whether you need to change your diet or take a vitamin or mineral supplement to get enough of these: calcium, vitamin D, vitamin B6 or vitamin B12. The Dietary Guidelines for Americans, 2015–2020, recommend how much of each vitamin and mineral men and women of different ages need. It's important to note that certain vitamins and supplements can adversely affect how certain medications work.

13. **True.** With age the body's thermostat tends to function less efficiently, and the older person's body may be less able to adapt to heat or cold. Most people who die from hyperthermia are over 50 years old. It doesn't have to be 100°F+ to put them at risk for a heat-related illness.

14. **True.** Balance problems, along with falls, are common as we age. Good safety habits, include staying physically active, knowing medication side effects, standing up slowly, using a walker device if needed, and wearing non-skid shoes are among good safety habits for older adults.

15. **False.** Overall women live longer than men. Women are more at risk of developing osteoporosis, becoming depressed, or having functional problems. Men are more likely to develop cancer, heart disease, or diabetes.

16. **True.** Stroke causes more serious long-term disabilities than any other disease and is the fourth leading cause of death in the United States.

17. **True.** The elderly consume 25 percent of all medications and, as a result, have many more problems with adverse drug reactions.

18. **True.** There are currently NO supplements or "quick cures" to help prevent Alzheimer's disease.

19. **True.** There are some changes in thinking that are common as we age. Increased difficulty finding words, having more problems multitasking, and mild decreases in the ability to pay attention are normal.

20. **True.** As we age, changes can occur that affect eyesight. Some are serious changes. As you age it's important to have regular eye exams to spot problems early. Low vision means a person cannot fix eyesight with glasses, contact lenses, medicine, or surgery. Low vision affects some people as they age. If problems are found early, often there are treatments that can help.

Identify at least one change or behavior that you can initiate now that may affect how long and how well you live. What is the first step you are willing to take? When and how will you begin?

Source: National Institute on Aging, https://www.nia.nih.gov.

REVIEW QUESTIONS

(LO 15.1) 1. The difference between life expectancy and health-adjusted life expectancy is that health-adjusted life expectancy _____.
   a. is based on the average health of people at a certain age
   b. factors in illnesses a person is likely to die from
   c. is the amount of healthy years a person is likely to live
   d. assumes that a person will not have disabilities later in life

(LO 15.1) 2. Which of the following is true of current life expectancies in the United States?
   a. They are lower than in other high-income countries.
   b. Men now have about as high a life expectancy as women do.
   c. Life expectancy has stabilized and is not expected to change much in the near future.
   d. The degree to which life expectancies are shortened by injuries and accidents is about the same as it was in the past.

(LO 15.2) 3. What is the single factor that contributes the most to healthy aging?
   a. Exercise
   b. Having friends
   c. Reduced stress
   d. Lack of illnesses

(LO 15.2) 4. Which of the following is true of men older than 40?
   a. Their prostate glands decrease in size.
   b. They produce greater amounts of testosterone.
   c. Their prostate glands enlarge.
   d. They experience more contractions during orgasm.

(LO 15.3) 5. Bone density can be maintained by _____.
   a. stretching
   b. taking vitamin supplements
   c. taking care to prevent falls
   d. regular exercise

(LO 15.3) 6. What is the most common disability experienced by Americans over the age of 65?
   a. Osteoporosis
   b. Mild cognitive impairment (MCI)
   c. Low levels of sex hormones
   d. Difficulty walking or climbing stairs

(LO 15.4) 7. Which of the following is an early sign of dementia?
   a. Sleep problems
   b. Insensitivity to alcohol
   c. Increased energy
   d. Craving for fatty foods

(LO 15.4) 8. A health-care proxy _____.
   a. indicates who should have your property in the event that you die
   b. gives someone else the power to make health decisions on your behalf
   c. can specify your desires related to the use of medical treatments and technology to prolong your life
   d. designates your doctor as your health agent by default

(LO 15.4) 9. What is the purpose of a DNR order?
   a. It designates, in the event of your death, any organs or tissues needed for transplantation.
   b. It gives someone else the power to make health decisions on your behalf.
   c. It specifies how comfortable you need to be made in case of a terminal illness.
   d. It specifies that you do not want to be resuscitated in the event of a medical crisis.

(LO 15.5) 10. The first stage a person goes through when facing death is _____.
   a. anger
   b. denial
   c. bargaining
   d. depression

(LO 15.6) 11. An absence of electrical activity and a lack of reflexes are indicators of _____.
   a. cellular death
   b. functional death
   c. brain death
   d. spiritual death

(LO 15.6) 12. Which of the following is true of hospice care?
   a. It is done primarily by nurses.
   b. It must be done in special hospice facilities.
   c. It helps people who are dying to live their final days to the fullest, as free as possible from disabling pain and mental anguish.
   d. It involves using experimental treatments to cure a disease when other methods have failed.

(LO 15.7) 13. Which of the following statements is true of suicide?
   a. Suicide is most common in people ages 35 and younger.
   b. Elderly women have much higher suicide rates than men.
   c. A family history of suicide increases a person's risk for suicide.
   d. Being diagnosed with a terminal illness does not increase the danger of suicide.

(LO 15.7) 14. Which of the following factors can place a college student at risk for suicide?
a. Rash driving
b. Passive behavior
c. Substance abuse
d. Minority status

(LO 15.8) 15. Which of the following offers the greatest protection against health problems that result from grief?
a. Medication
b. Low alcohol intake
c. Regular exercise
d. Friendships and remarriage

(LO 15.8) 16. What is the first stage that individuals go through in the process of responding to the death of a loved one?
a. Yearning-searching
b. Shock-numbness
c. Disorganization-despair
d. Reorganization

Answers to these questions can be found on page 531.

Answers to Review Questions

Chapter 1

1. d; 2. b; 3. c; 4. a; 5. c; 6. a; 7. d; 8. a; 9. d

Chapter 2

1. d; 2. d; 3. c; 4. d; 5. b; 6. b; 7. d; 8. c; 9. c; 10. c;
11. b; 12. c; 13. d; 14. c; 15. d

Chapter 3

1. b; 2. b; 3. b; 4. c; 5. b; 6. d; 7. d; 8. c; 9. b; 10. d; 11. d;
12. b; 13. a; 14. b; 15. d; 16. c; 17. d; 18. c; 19. c

Chapter 4

1. c; 2. d; 3. c; 4. c; 5. b; 6. a; 7. d; 8. d; 9. a; 10. b; 11. b;
12. d; 13. c; 14. b

Chapter 5

1. b; 2. a; 3. a; 4. d; 5. a; 6. d; 7. a; 8. c; 9. a; 10. b; 11. d;
12. c; 13. a; 14. c; 15. b; 16. d

Chapter 6

1. a; 2. b; 3. b; 4. c; 5. b; 6. b; 7. c; 8. c; 9. b; 10. d;
11. b; 12. b; 13. a; 14. c; 15. d; 16. c; 17. a; 18. b;
19. d; 20. a; 21. c

Chapter 7

1. d; 2. b; 3. a; 4. b; 5. b; 6. c; 7. a; 8. d; 9. d; 10. a; 11. c;
12. b; 13. b; 14. d; 15. b; 16. d; 17. a

Chapter 8

1. a; 2. d; 3. a; 4. b; 5. d; 6. c; 7. d; 8. b; 9. d; 10. c; 11. d;
12. c; 13. b; 14. a; 15. a; 16. c; 17. b; 18. b; 19. c;
20. c; 21. b; 22. a; 23. d; 24. b; 25. a; 26. c

Chapter 9

1. b; 2. a; 3. d; 4. b; 5. d; 6. d; 7. c; 8. d; 9. a; 10. b;
11. c; 12. d; 13. b; 14. b

Chapter 10

1. a; 2. b; 3. b; 4. a; 5. a; 6. d; 7. c; 8. a; 9. d; 10. c;
11. d; 12. c; 13. a; 14. b; 15. c; 16. d; 17. d; 18. c;
19. b; 20. a; 21. c; 22. d; 23. d; 24. d; 25. b; 26. b;
27. d; 28. b; 29. b; 30. a; 31. d

Chapter 11

1. c; 2. d; 3. c; 4. b; 5. a; 6. c; 7. c; 8. d; 9. c; 10. b; 11. a;
12. d; 13. d; 14. c; 15. a; 16. b; 17. d

Chapter 12

1. c; 2. b; 3. b; 4. d; 5. a; 6. d; 7. c; 8. d; 9. c; 10. c; 11. d;
12. c; 13. c; 14. a; 15. d; 16. d; 17. b; 18. d

Chapter 13

1. d; 2. b; 3. b; 4. b; 5. b; 6. a; 7. d; 8. d; 9. c; 10. d;
11. a; 12. c; 13. d; 14. b; 15. c; 16. b; 17. a; 18. d;
19. c; 20. b; 21. b; 22. a; 23. c; 24. c; 25. c; 26. d;
27. b; 28. a

Chapter 14

1. b; 2. c; 3. b; 4. d; 5. a; 6. d; 7. b; 8. c; 9. d; 10. a; 11. c;
12. b; 13. d; 14. b; 15. c; 16. a; 17. b; 18. a; 19. b

Chapter 15

1. c; 2. a; 3. a; 4. c; 5. d; 6. d; 7. a; 8. b; 9. d; 10. b; 11. c;
12. c; 13. c; 14. c; 15. d; 16. b

Glossary

12-Step program Self-help group program based on the principles of Alcoholics Anonymous.

absorption The passage of substances into or across membranes or tissues.

abstinence Voluntarily refraining from sexual intercourse.

acquired immune deficiency syndrome (AIDS) The final stages of HIV infection, characterized by a variety of severe illnesses and decreased levels of certain immune cells.

active stretching A technique that involves stretching a muscle by contracting the opposing muscle.

acupuncture A Chinese medical practice of puncturing the body with needles inserted at specific points to relieve pain or cure disease.

acute time-limited stressor A temporary anxiety-provoking situation.

addiction A behavioral pattern characterized by compulsion, loss of control, and continued repetition of a behavior or an activity in spite of adverse consequences.

additive Characterized by a combined effect that is equal to the sum of the individual effects.

adoption The legal process for becoming the parent to a child of other biological parents.

advance directives Documents that specify an individual's preferences regarding treatment in a medical crisis.

aerobic exercise Physical activity in which sufficient or excess oxygen is continually supplied to the body.

aging The characteristic pattern of normal life changes that occur as living things grow older.

alcoholism A chronic, progressive, potentially fatal disease characterized by impaired control of drinking, a preoccupation with alcohol, continued use of alcohol despite adverse consequences, and distorted thinking—most notably denial.

alcohol use disorder Problematic pattern of alcohol use leading to significant impairment or distress.

altruism Acts of helping or giving to others without thought of self-benefit.

Alzheimer's disease A progressive deterioration of intellectual powers due to physiological changes within the brain; symptoms include diminishing ability to concentrate and reason, disorientation, depression, apathy, and paranoia.

AmED (alcohol mixed with energy drinks) Any combination of alcohol with caffeine and other stimulants.

amenorrhea The absence or suppression of menstruation.

amino acids Organic compounds containing nitrogen, carbon, hydrogen, and oxygen; the essential building blocks of proteins.

amnion The innermost membrane of the sac enclosing the embryo or fetus.

amphetamines Any of a class of stimulants that trigger the release of epinephrine, which stimulates the central nervous system; users experience a state of hyperalertness and energy, followed by a crash as the drug wears off.

anaerobic exercise Physical activity in which the body develops an oxygen deficit.

angina Chest pain.

anorexia nervosa A psychological disorder in which refusal to eat and/or an extreme loss of appetite leads to malnutrition, severe weight loss, and possibly death.

antagonistic Opposing or counteracting.

antidepressants Drugs used primarily to treat symptoms of depression.

antioxidants Substances that prevent the damaging effects of oxidation in cells.

anxiety disorders A group of psychological disorders involving episodes of apprehension, tension, or uneasiness, stemming from the anticipation of danger and sometimes accompanied by physical symptoms, which cause significant distress and impairment.

aorta The main artery of the body, arising from the left ventricle of the heart.

APR (annual percentage rate) The amount of interest a credit card company charges each year on the unpaid balance.

arteriosclerosis Any of a number of chronic diseases characterized by degeneration of the arteries and hardening and thickening of arterial walls.

artificial insemination The introduction of viable sperm into the vagina by artificial means for the purpose of inducing conception.

asexual Without sexual feelings or desires.

assisted suicide Providing the means to end life to a patient by a health professional.

atherosclerosis A form of arteriosclerosis in which fatty substances (plaque) are deposited on the inner walls of arteries.

atrium Either of the two upper chambers of the heart, which receive blood from the veins.

attention-deficit/hyperactivity disorder (ADHD) A spectrum of difficulties in controlling motion and sustaining attention, including hyperactivity, impulsivity, and distractibility.

autism spectrum disorder (ASD) A neurodevelopmental disorder that causes social and communication impairments.

autopsy A detailed examination of a body after death.

aversion therapy A treatment that attempts to help a person overcome a dependence or bad habit by making the person feel disgusted or repulsed by that habit.

Ayurveda A traditional Indian medical treatment involving meditation, exercise, herbal medications, and nutrition.

bacterial vaginosis (BV) A common vaginal infection caused by an imbalance of normal bacteria in the vagina.

ballistic stretching Rapid bouncing movements.

barbiturates Anti-anxiety drugs that depress the central nervous system, reduce activity, and induce relaxation, drowsiness, or sleep; often prescribed to relieve tension and treat epileptic seizures or as a general anesthetic.

barrier contraceptives Birth control devices that block the meeting of egg and sperm, either by physical barriers, such as condoms, diaphragms, or cervical caps, or by chemical barriers, such as spermicide, or both.

basal metabolic rate (BMR) The number of calories required to sustain the body at rest.

behavioral therapy A technique that emphasizes application of the principles of learning to substitute desirable responses and behavior patterns for undesirable ones.

benzodiazepine An antianxiety drug that depresses the central nervous system, reduces activity, and induces relaxation, drowsiness, or sleep; often prescribed to relieve tension, muscular strain, sleep problems, anxiety, and panic attacks; also used as an anesthetic and in the treatment of alcohol withdrawal.

bidis Skinny, sweet-flavored cigarettes.

binge For a man, having five or more alcoholic drinks at a single sitting; for a woman, having four or more drinks at a single sitting.

binge eating The rapid consumption of an abnormally large amount of food in a relatively short time.

binge-eating disorder Chronic or repeated episodes of uncontrollable binge eating.

biofeedback A technique of becoming aware, with the aid of external monitoring devices, of internal physiological activities in order to develop the capability of altering them.

bipolar disorder Severe depression alternating with periods of manic activity and elation.

bisexual Sexual attraction to both males and females.

bisexuality Sexual attraction to both males and females.

blastocyst In embryonic development, a ball of cells with a surface layer and an inner cell mass.

blended families Families formed when one or both of the partners bring children from a previous union to the new marriage.

blood-alcohol concentration (BAC) The amount of alcohol in the blood, expressed as a percentage.

body composition The relative amounts of fat and lean tissue (bone, muscle, organs, and water) in the body.

body mass index (BMI) A mathematical formula that correlates with body fat; the ratio of weight to height squared.

brief stressor A more serious and extended challenge.

bulimia nervosa Episodic binge eating, often followed by forced vomiting or laxative abuse, and accompanied by a persistent preoccupation with body shape and weight.

burnout A state of physical, emotional, and mental exhaustion resulting from constant or repeated emotional pressure.

calorie balance The relationship between calories consumed from foods and beverages and calories expended in normal body functions and through physical activity. If the calories consumed equal calories expended, you will have calorie balance.

calories The amount of energy required to raise the temperature of 1 gram of water by 1 degree Celsius. In everyday usage related to the energy content of foods and the energy expended in activities, a calorie is actually the equivalent of a thousand such calories, or a kilocalorie.

cannabinoids A group of closely related compounds that include cannabinol and the active constituents of cannabis (marijuana).

capillaries Minute blood vessels that connect arteries to veins.

carbohydrates Organic compounds, such as starches, sugars, and glycogen, that are composed of carbon, hydrogen, and oxygen and are sources of bodily energy.

carbon monoxide A colorless, odorless gas produced by the burning of gasoline or tobacco; it displaces oxygen in the hemoglobin molecules of red blood cells.

carcinogen A substance or agent that causes cancer.

cardiometabolic Referring to the heart and to the biochemical processes involved in the body's functioning.

cardiopulmonary resuscitation (CPR) Emergency treatment to maintain circulation in a person whose heart has stopped or who is no longer breathing.

cardiorespiratory fitness The ability of the heart and blood vessels to circulate blood through the body efficiently.

cathinone An amphetamine-like stimulant derived from the khat plant.

celibacy Abstention from sexual activity; can be partial or complete, permanent or temporary.

certified organic Foods that meet strict criteria set by the U.S. Department of Agriculture.

cervical cap A thimble-size rubber or plastic cap that is inserted into the vagina to fit over the cervix and prevent the passage of sperm into the uterus during sexual intercourse; used with a spermicidal foam or jelly, it serves as both a chemical and a physical barrier to sperm.

cervix The narrow, lower end of the uterus that opens into the vagina.

cesarean delivery A surgical procedure in which an infant is delivered through an incision made in the abdominal wall and uterus.

challenge response A physiological response that strengthens connections between the parts of the brain that suppress fear and enhance learning and positive motivation so as to prepare and enable a person to face a stressor directly.

chancroid A soft, painful sore or localized infection usually acquired through sexual contact.

chiropractic A method of treating disease, primarily through manipulating the bones and joints to restore normal nerve function.

chlamydia A common sexually transmitted infection caused by bacteria known as *Chlamydia trachomatis*.

cholesterol An organic substance found in animal fats; it is linked to cardiovascular disease, particularly atherosclerosis.

chronic stressor Unrelenting demands and pressures that go on for an extended time.

club drugs A variety of drugs including MDMA, GHB, GBL, ketamine, fentanyl, Rohypnol, and nitrites that first became popular at nightclubs, bars, and raves.

circumcision The surgical removal of the foreskin of the penis.

cisgender A person whose sense of personal identity and gender corresponds with the individuals birth sex.

clitoris A small erectile structure on the female, corresponding to the penis on the male.

cocaine A white crystalline powder extracted from the leaves of the coca plant that stimulates the central nervous system and produces a brief period of euphoria followed by a depression.

codependency An emotional and psychological behavioral pattern in which the spouses, partners, parents, children, and friends of individuals with addictive behaviors allow or enable their loved ones to continue their self-destructive habits.

cognitive therapy A technique used to identify an individual's beliefs and attitudes, recognize negative thought patterns, and educate in alternative ways of thinking.

cohabitation Two people living together as a couple, without official ties such as marriage.

coitus interruptus The removal of the penis from the vagina before ejaculation.

coma A state of total unconsciousness.

combination oral contraceptives (COCs) Combination oral contraceptives are birth control pills that consist of two hormones, synthetic estrogen and progestin, which play important roles in controlling ovulation and the menstrual cycle.

complementary and alternative medicine (CAM) A term applied to all health-care approaches, practices, and treatments not widely taught in medical schools, not generally used in hospitals, and not usually reimbursed by medical insurance companies.

complementary protein Incomplete proteins that, when combined, provide all the amino acids essential for protein synthesis.

complete protein Proteins that contain all the amino acids needed by the body for growth and maintenance.

complex carbohydrates Starches, including cereals, fruits, and vegetables.

conception The merging of a sperm and an ovum.

condoms Latex or polyurethane sheaths worn over the penis during sexual acts to prevent conception and/or the transmission of disease; the female condom lines the walls of the vagina.

contraception The prevention of conception; birth control.

Cowper's glands Two small glands that discharge into the male urethra; also called bulbourethral glands.

cyberbullying Deliberate, repeated, and hostile actions that use information and communication technologies, including online Web pages and text messages, with the intent of harming others by means of intimidation, control, manipulation, false accusations, or humiliation.

cyberstalking A form of cyberbullying that uses online sites, Twitter, e-mail messages, and social media to harass victims and try to damage their reputation or turn others against them.

culture The set of shared attitudes, values, goals, and practices of a group that are internalized by an individual within the group.

cunnilingus Sexual stimulation of a woman's genitals by means of oral manipulation.

decibels (dB) Units for measuring the intensity of sounds.

dementia Deterioration of mental capability.

designer drugs Illegally manufactured psychoactive drugs that have dangerous physical and psychological effects.

diabetes mellitus A disease in which the inadequate production of insulin leads to failure of the body tissues to break down carbohydrates at a normal rate.

diaphragm A bowl-like rubber cup with a flexible rim that is inserted into the vagina to cover the cervix and prevent the passage of sperm into the uterus during sexual intercourse; used with a spermicidal foam or jelly, it serves as both a chemical and a physical barrier to sperm.

diastole The period between contractions in the cardiac cycle, during which the heart relaxes and dilates as it fills with blood.

diastolic blood pressure Lowest blood pressure, which occurs between contractions of the heart.

dietary fiber The nondigestible form of carbohydrates found in plant foods, such as leaves, stems, skins, seeds, and hulls.

distant stressor Traumatic experience that occurred long ago yet continues to have an emotional or psychological impact.

distress A negative stress that may result in illness.

do-not-resuscitate (DNR) An advance directive that expresses an individual's preference that resuscitation efforts not be made during a medical crisis.

dopamine A brain chemical associated with feelings of satisfaction and euphoria.

drug Any substance, other than food, that affects bodily functions and structures when taken into the body.

drug abuse The excessive use of a drug in a manner inconsistent with accepted medical practice.

drug dependence Continued substance use even when its use causes cognitive, behavioral, and physical symptoms.

drug diversion The transfer of a drug from the person for whom it was prescribed to another individual.

drug misuse The use of a drug for a purpose (or person) other than that for which it was medically intended.

dynamic flexibility The ability to move a joint quickly and fluidly through its entire range of motion with little resistance.

dynamic stretching Stretching that increases the range of motion around a joint or group of joints by using active muscular effort, momentum, and speed.

dysfunctional Characterized by negative and destructive patterns of behavior between partners or between parents and children.

dysmenorrhea Painful menstruation.

eating disorders Unusual, often dangerous patterns of food consumption, including anorexia nervosa and bulimia nervosa.

ecosystem A community of organisms sharing a physical and chemical environment and interacting with each other.

ectopic pregnancy A pregnancy in which the fertilized egg has implanted itself outside the uterine cavity, usually in the fallopian tube.

ejaculation The expulsion of semen from the penis.

ejaculatory ducts The canal connecting the seminal vesicles and vas deferens.

electromagnetic fields (EMFs) The invisible electric and magnetic fields generated by an electrically charged conductor.

embryo An organism in its early stage of development; in humans, the embryonic period lasts from the second to the eighth week of pregnancy.

emergency contraception (EC) Types of oral contraceptive pills, usually taken after unprotected intercourse or failed birth control, that can prevent pregnancy.

emotional health The ability to express and acknowledge one's feelings and moods and exhibit adaptability and compassion for others.

emotional intelligence The ability to monitor and use emotions to guide thinking and actions.

enabling factors The skills, resources, and physical and mental capabilities that shape our behavior.

endometrium The mucous membrane lining the uterus.

environmental tobacco smoke Secondhand cigarette smoke; the third-leading preventable cause of death.

epididymis The portion of the male duct system in which sperm mature.

erogenous Sexually sensitive.

essential nutrients Nutrients that the body cannot manufacture for itself and must obtain from food.

ethyl alcohol The intoxicating agent in alcoholic beverages; also called ethanol.

eustress Positive stress, which stimulates a person to function properly.

euthanasia The painless killing of a patient with an incurable fatal disease or in an irreversible coma.

evidence-based medicine The choice of a medical treatment on the basis of large randomized, controlled research trials and large prospective studies.

exercise A type of physical activity that requires planned, structured, and repetitive bodily movement with the intent of improving one or more components of physical fitness.

fallopian tubes The pair of channels that transport ova from the ovaries to the uterus; the usual site of fertilization.

families Groups of people united by marriage, blood, or adoption—each residing in the same household; maintaining a common culture; and interacting with one another on the basis of their roles within the group.

fellatio Sexual stimulation of a man's genitals by means of oral manipulation.

fertilization The fusion of sperm and egg nucleus.

fetal alcohol effects (FAE) Milder forms of FAS, including low birth weight, irritability in newborns, and permanent mental impairment as a result of the mother's alcohol consumption during pregnancy.

fetal alcohol syndrome disorder (FASD) A cluster of serious physical and mental defects linked with alcohol consumption during pregnancy.

fetus The human organism developing in the uterus from the ninth week until birth.

"fight-or-flight" response The body's automatic physiological response that prepares the individual to take action upon facing a perceived threat or danger.

fitness The ability to respond to routine physical demands, with enough reserve energy to cope with a sudden challenge.

fixed interest rate An interest rate that stays the same over time.

flexibility The range of motion allowed by one's joints; determined by the length of muscles, tendons, and ligaments attached to the joints.

folic acid A form of folate used in vitamin supplements and fortified foods.

functional fiber Isolated, nondigestible carbohydrates that have beneficial effects in humans.

functional fitness The ability to perform real-life activities, such as lifting a heavy suitcase.

gambling disorder Persistent and recurrent problematic gambling that leads to significant impairment or distress.

gamma butyrolactone (GBL) The main ingredient in gamma hydroxybutyrate (GHB); once ingested, GBL converts to GHB and can cause the ingestor to lose consciousness.

gamma hydroxybutyrate (GHB) A brain messenger chemical that stimulates the release of human growth hormone; commonly abused for its high and its alleged ability to trim fat and build muscles. Also known as "blue nitro" or the "date-rape drug."

gender identity An individual's perception of having a particular gender, which may or may not correspond with the person's birth sex.

generalized anxiety disorder (GAD) An anxiety disorder characterized as chronic distress.

generic A consumer product with no brand name or registered trademark.

gingivitis Inflammation of the gums.

gonorrhea A sexually transmitted infection caused by the bacterium *Neisseria gonorrhoeae*; symptoms include discharge from the penis; women are generally asymptomatic.

gum disease Infection of the gums and bones that hold teeth in place.

hallucinogens Drugs that cause hallucinations.

hashish A concentrated form of a drug derived from the cannabis plant that contains the psychoactive ingredient THC, which causes a sense of euphoria when inhaled or eaten.

hazing Any activity that humiliates, degrades, or poses a risk of emotional or physical harm for the sake of joining a group or maintaining full status in that group.

health A state of complete well-being, including physical, psychological, spiritual, social, intellectual, and environmental dimensions.

health belief model (HBM) A model of behavioral change that focuses on the individual's attitudes and beliefs.

health literacy Ability to understand health information and use it to make good decisions about health and medical care.

health promotion Any planned combination of educational, political, regulatory, and organizational supports for actions and conditions of living conducive to the health of individuals, groups, or communities.

herbal medicine An ancient form of medical treatment using substances derived from trees, flowers, ferns, seaweeds, and lichens to treat disease.

heterosexual Primary sexual orientation toward members of the other sex.

holistic A perspective that looks at health and an individual as a whole rather than part by part; also an approach to medicine that takes into account body, mind, emotions, and spirit.

holographic will A will wholly in the handwriting of its author.

home health care Provision of equipment and services to patients in their homes.

homeopathy A system of medical practice that treats a disease by administering dosages of substances that would in healthy persons produce symptoms similar to those of the disease.

homeostasis The body's natural state of balance or stability.

homosexual Those with primary sexual orientation toward members of the same sex.

hooking up An experience in which partners engage in intimate behaviors without explicit expectation of future romantic commitment.

hospice A homelike health-care facility or program committed to supportive care for terminally ill people.

hormone therapy (HT) The use of supplemental hormones during and after menopause.

human immunodeficiency virus (HIV) A virus that causes a spectrum of health problems, ranging from a symptomless infection to changes in the immune system, to the development of life-threatening diseases because of impaired immunity.

human papillomavirus (HPV) A pathogen that causes genital warts and increases the risk of cervical cancer.

hypertension High blood pressure that occurs when the blood exerts excessive pressure against the arterial walls.

hypothermia An abnormally low body temperature; if not treated appropriately, coma or death could result.

implantation The embedding of the fertilized ovum in the uterine lining.

incomplete protein Proteins that lack one or more of the amino acids essential for protein synthesis.

infertility The inability to conceive a child.

infiltration A gradual penetration or invasion.

informed consent Permission (to undergo or receive a medical procedure or treatment) given voluntarily, with full knowledge and understanding of the procedure or treatment and its possible consequences.

inhalants Substances that produce vapors having psychoactive effects when sniffed.

insulin resistance A condition in which the body produces insulin but does not use it properly.

integrative medicine An approach that combines traditional medicine with alternative/complementary therapies.

intercourse Sexual stimulation by means of entry of the penis into the vagina; coitus.

interpersonal therapy (IPT) A technique used to develop communication skills and relationships.

intimacy A state of closeness between two people, characterized by the desire and ability to share one's innermost thoughts and feelings with each other either verbally or nonverbally.

intoxication Maladaptive behavioral, psychological, and physiologic changes that occur as a result of substance abuse.

intramuscular Into or within a muscle.

intrauterine device (IUD) A device inserted into the uterus through the cervix to prevent pregnancy by interfering with implantation.

intravenous Into a vein.

introductory interest rate A rate that starts low but increases after a certain period of time.

ionizing radiation A form of energy emitted from atoms as they undergo internal change.

isokinetic Having the same force; exercise with specialized equipment that provides resistance equal to the force applied by the user throughout the entire range of motion.

isometric Of the same length; exercise in which muscles increase their tension without shortening in length, such as when pushing an immovable object.

isotonic Having the same tension or tone; exercise requiring the repetition of an action that creates tension, such as weightlifting or calisthenics.

labia majora The fleshy outer folds that border the female genital area.

labia minora The fleshy inner folds that border the female genital area.

labor The process leading up to birth: effacement and dilation of the cervix; the movement of the baby into and through the birth canal, accompanied by strong contractions; and contraction of the uterus and expulsion of the placenta after the birth.

laparoscopy A surgical sterilization procedure in which the fallopian tubes are observed with a laparoscope inserted through a small incision, and then cut or blocked.

life-change event An occurrence, planned or unplanned, that requires some degree of re-adjustment.

lipoproteins Compounds in blood that are made up of proteins and fat; high-density lipoproteins (HDL) pick up excess cholesterol in the blood; low-density lipoproteins (LDL) carry more cholesterol and deposit it on the walls of arteries.

living will An advance directive that provides instructions for the use of life-sustaining procedures in the event of terminal illness or injury.

locus of control An individual's belief about the sources of power and influence over his or her life.

long-acting reversible contraceptives (LARCs) Contraceptive devices that provide protection from pregnancy for an extended period without any action by users. Examples include intrauterine devices, injections, and implants.

LSD (lysergic acid diethylamide) A synthetic psychoactive substance originally developed to explore mental illness.

luteum A yellowish mass of tissue that is formed, immediately after ovulation, from the remaining cells of the follicle; it secretes estrogen and progesterone for the remainder of the menstrual cycle.

macronutrients Nutrients required by the human body in the greatest amounts, including water, carbohydrates, proteins, and fats.

mainstream smoke The smoke inhaled directly by smoking a cigarette.

major depressive disorder Sadness that does not end; ongoing feelings of utter helplessness.

marijuana The drug derived from the cannabis plant, containing the psychoactive ingredient THC, which causes a mild sense of euphoria when inhaled or eaten.

mastectomy The surgical removal of an entire breast.

masturbation Manual (or nonmanual) self-stimulation of the genitals, often resulting in orgasm.

MDMA/Ecstasy A synthetic compound, also known as methylenedioxymethamphetamine, that is similar in structure to methamphetamine and has both stimulant and hallucinogenic effects.

medical abortion Method of ending a pregnancy within 9 weeks of conception using hormonal medications that cause expulsion of the fertilized egg.

medical history Health-related information that a health-care professional collects while interviewing a patient.

meditation A group of approaches that use quiet sitting, breathing techniques, and/or chanting to relax, improve concentration, and become attuned to one's inner self.

menopause The complete cessation of ovulation and menstruation for 12 consecutive months.

menstruation Discharge of blood from the vagina as a result of the shedding of the uterine lining at the end of the menstrual cycle.

mental disorder A behavioral or psychological syndrome associated with distress or disability or with a significantly increased risk of suffering death, pain, disability, or loss of freedom.

mental health The ability to perceive reality as it is, respond to its challenges, and develop rational strategies for living.

metabolic fitness The reduction in risk for diabetes and cardiovascular disease, which can be achieved through a moderate-intensity exercise program.

metabolic syndrome A cluster of disorders of the body's metabolism that make diabetes, heart disease, or stroke more likely.

metastasize To spread to other parts of the body via the bloodstream or lymphatic system.

microaggressions Subtle racial expressions.

microassaults Conscious and intentional actions and slurs.

microinsults Verbal and nonverbal communications that subtly convey rudeness and insensitivity.

microinvalidations Communications that subtly exclude, negate, or nullify the thoughts, feelings, or experiential reality of a person of color.

micronutrients Vitamins and minerals needed by the body in very small amounts.

microwaves Extremely high-frequency electromagnetic waves that increase the rate at which molecules vibrate, thereby generating heat.

mild cognitive impairment (MCI) A slight but noticeable and measurable decline in cognitive abilities, including memory and thinking skills.

mindfulness A method of stress reduction that involves experiencing the physical and mental sensations of the present moment.

minerals Naturally occurring inorganic substances, small amounts of some being essential in metabolism and nutrition.

minipills Oral contraceptives containing a small amount of progestin and no estrogen, which prevent contraception by making the mucus in the cervix so thick that sperm cannot enter the uterus.

miscarriage A pregnancy that terminates before the 20th week of gestation; also called spontaneous abortion.

mons pubis The rounded, fleshy area over the junction of the female pubic bones.

mood A temporary state of mind or feeling.

muscular endurance The ability to withstand the stress of continued physical exertion.

muscular strength Physical power; the maximum weight one can lift, push, or press in one effort.

muscle dysmorphia A condition that affects mostly male bodybuilders in which they become obsessed with appearance and size of muscles.

mutagens Agents that cause alterations in the genetic material of living cells.

myocardial infarction (MI) A condition characterized by the dying of tissue areas in the myocardium, caused by interruption of the blood supply to those areas; the medical name for a heart attack.

naturopathy An alternative system of treatment of disease that emphasizes the use of natural remedies such as sun, water, heat, and air. Therapies may include dietary changes, steam baths, and exercise.

NEAT (nonexercise activity thermogenesis) Nonvolitional movement that can be an effective way of burning calories.

neustress Neutral stressors that do not affect us immediately or directly but may trigger stressful feelings.

nicotine The addictive substance in tobacco; one of the most toxic of all poisons.

nongonococcal urethritis (NGU) Inflammation of the urethra caused by organisms other than the *Gonococcus* bacterium.

nutrition The science devoted to the study of dietary needs for food and the effects of food on organisms.

obesity The excessive accumulation of fat in the body; class 1 obesity is defined by a BMI between 30.0 and 34.9; class 2 obesity is a BMI between 35.0 and 39.9; class 3, or severe obesity, is a BMI of 40 or higher.

obsessive–compulsive disorder (OCD) An anxiety disorder characterized by obsessions and/or compulsions that impair one's ability to function and form relationships.

opioids Drugs that have sleep-inducing and pain-relieving properties, including opium and its derivatives and nonopioid, synthetic drugs.

optimism The tendency to seek out, remember, and expect pleasurable experiences.

oral contraceptives Preparations of synthetic hormones that inhibit ovulation; also referred to as *birth control pills* or simply *the pill*.

orgasm A series of contractions of the pelvic muscles occurring at the peak of sexual arousal.

outcomes The ultimate impacts of particular treatments or absence of treatment.

overloading A method of physical training that involves increasing the number of repetitions or the amount of resistance gradually to work the muscle to temporary fatigue.

overload principle The idea that for the body to get stronger, you must provide a greater stress or demand on the body than it is normally accustomed to handling.

over-the-counter (OTC) Medications that can be obtained legally without a prescription from a medical professional.

overtrain Working muscles too intensely or too frequently, resulting in persistent muscle soreness, injuries, unintended weight loss, nervousness, and an inability to relax.

overweight A condition of having a BMI between 25.0 and 29.9.

ovulation The release of a mature ovum from an ovary approximately 14 days prior to the onset of menstruation.

ovum (plural, ova) The female gamete (egg cell).

panic attacks Short episodes characterized by physical sensations of light-headedness, dizziness, hyperventilation, and numbness of extremities, accompanied by an inexplicable terror, usually of a physical disaster such as death.

panic disorder An anxiety disorder in which the apprehension or experience of recurring panic attacks is so intense that normal functioning is impaired.

pap smear A test in which cells are removed from the cervix for microscopic examination for signs of cancer.

passive stretching A stretching technique in which an external force or resistance (your body, a partner, gravity, or a weight) helps the joints move through their range of motion.

pelvic inflammatory disease (PID) An inflammation of the internal female genital tract, characterized by abdominal pain, fever, and tenderness of the cervix.

penis The male organ of sex and urination.

perimenopause The period from a woman's first irregular cycles to her last menstruation.

perineum The area between the anus and vagina in the female and between the anus and scrotum in the male.

periodontitis Severe gum disease in which the tooth root becomes infected.

persistent vegetative state A state of being awake and capable of reacting to physical stimuli, such as light, while being unaware of pain or other environmental stimuli.

phencyclidine (PCP) A synthetic psychoactive substance that produces effects similar to those of other psychoactive drugs when swallowed, smoked, sniffed, or injected and also may trigger unpredictable behavioral changes.

phobias Anxiety disorders marked by an inordinate fear of an object, a class of objects, or a situation, resulting in extreme avoidance behaviors.

physical activity Any movement produced by the muscles that results in expenditure of energy.

physical dependence Physiological attachment to, and need for, a drug.

phytochemicals Chemicals such as indoles, coumarins, and capsaicin, which exist naturally in plants and have disease-fighting properties.

placenta An organ that develops after implantation and to which the embryo attaches, via the umbilical cord, for nourishment and waste removal.

plaque A sludgelike substance that builds up on the inner walls of arteries; also a sticky film of bacteria that forms on teeth.

pollutant A substance or agent in the environment, usually the by-product of human industry or activity, that is injurious to human, animal, or plant life.

pollution Any change in the air, water, or soil that could reduce its ability to support life.

polyabuse The misuse or abuse of more than one drug.

posttraumatic stress disorder (PTSD) The repeated reliving of a trauma through nightmares or recollection.

potentiating Making more effective or powerful.

practice guidelines Recommendations for diagnosis and treatment of various health problems, based on evidence from scientific research.

prediabetes A condition in which blood glucose levels are higher than normal but not high enough for a diagnosis of diabetes.

predisposing factors The beliefs, values, attitudes, knowledge, and perceptions that influence our behavior.

predrinking Consuming alcoholic beverages, usually with friends, before going out to bars or parties; also called pregaming, preloading, or front-loading.

premenstrual dysphoric disorder (PMDD) A disorder that causes symptoms of psychological depression during the last week of the menstrual cycle.

premenstrual syndrome A disorder that causes physical discomfort and psychological distress prior to a woman's menstrual period.

preterm labor Labor that occurs after the 20th week but before the 37th week of pregnancy.

prevention Information and support offered to help healthy people identify their health risks, reduce stressors, prevent potential medical problems, and enhance their well-being.

primary care Ambulatory or outpatient care provided by a physician in an office, an emergency room, or a clinic.

progestin-only pills Oral contraceptives containing a small amount of progestin and no estrogen, which prevent contraception by making the mucus in the cervix so thick that sperm cannot enter the uterus.

progressive overloading Gradually increasing physical challenges once the body adapts to the stress placed upon it to produce maximum benefits.

progressive relaxation A method of reducing muscle tension by contracting, then relaxing, certain areas of the body.

proof The alcoholic strength of a distilled spirit, expressed as twice the percentage of alcohol present.

prostate gland A structure surrounding the male urethra that produces a secretion that helps liquefy the semen from the testes.

protection Measures that an individual can take when participating in risky behavior to prevent injury or unwanted risks.

proteins Organic compounds composed of amino acids; one of the essential nutrients.

psychiatric drugs Medications that regulate a person's mental, emotional, and physical functions to facilitate normal functioning.

psychoactive Mind-affecting.

psychodynamic Interpreting behaviors in terms of early experiences and unconscious influences.

psychological dependence Strong craving for a drug because it produces pleasurable feelings or relieves stress and anxiety.

psychotherapy Treatment designed to produce a response by psychological rather than physical means, such as suggestion, persuasion, reassurance, and support.

quackery Medical fakery; unproven practices claiming to cure diseases or solve health problems.

range of motion The fullest extent of possible movement in a particular joint.

rating of perceived exertion (RPE) A self-assessment scale that rates symptoms of breathlessness and fatigue.

refractory period The period of time following orgasm during which a male cannot experience another orgasm.

reinforcing factors Rewards, encouragement, and recognition that influence our behavior in the short run.

relapse prevention An alcohol recovery treatment method that focuses on social skills training to develop ways of preventing a relapse.

reps (or repetitions) In weight training, multiple performances of a movement or an exercise.

reversibility principle The idea that the physical benefits of exercise are lost through disuse or inactivity.

rhythm method A birth control method in which sexual intercourse is avoided during those days of the menstrual cycle in which fertilization is most likely to occur.

rubella An infectious disease that may cause birth defects if contracted by a pregnant woman; also called German measles.

same-sex marriage Governmentally, socially, or religiously recognized marriage in which two people of the same sex live together as a family.

saturated fats A chemical term indicating that a fat molecule contains as many hydrogen atoms as its carbon skeleton can hold. These fats are normally solid at room temperature.

schizophrenia A general term for a group of mental disorders with characteristic psychotic symptoms, such as delusions, hallucinations, and disordered thought patterns during the active phase of the illness, and a duration of at least six months.

scrotum The external sac or pouch that holds the testes.

self-actualization A state of wellness and fulfillment that can be achieved once certain human needs are satisfied; living to one's full potential.

self-care Head-to-toe maintenance, including good oral care, appropriate screening tests, knowing your medical rights, and understanding the health-care system.

self-compassion A healthy form of self-acceptance in the face of perceived inadequacy or failure.

self-disclosure Sharing personal information and experiences with another that he or she would not otherwise discover; self-disclosure involves risk and vulnerability.

self-efficacy Belief in one's ability to accomplish a goal or change a behavior.

semen The viscous whitish fluid that is the complete male ejaculate; a combination of sperm and secretions from the prostate gland, seminal vesicles, and other glands.

seminal vesicles Glands in the male reproductive system that produce the major portion of the fluid of semen.

sets In weight training, multiples of repetitions of the same movement or exercise.

sex Maleness or femaleness, resulting from genetic, structural, and functional factors.

sexual health The integration of the physical, emotional, intellectual, social, and spiritual aspects of sexual being in ways that are positively enriching and that enhance personality, communication, and love.

sexuality The behaviors, instincts, and attitudes associated with being sexual.

sexually transmitted disease (STD) A disease that is caused by a sexually transmitted infection that produces symptoms.

sexually transmitted infection (STI) The presence in the human body of an infectious agent that can be passed from one sexual partner to another.

sexual orientation The direction of an individual's sexual interest, either to members of the opposite sex or to members of the same sex.

sidestream smoke The smoke emitted by a burning cigarette and breathed by everyone in a closed room, including the smoker; contains more tar and nicotine than mainstream smoke.

simple carbohydrates Sugars; like all other carbohydrates, they provide the body with glucose.

snus A smokeless tobacco product similar to snuff and chewing tobacco.

social anxiety disorder A fear and avoidance of social situations.

social contagion The process by which friends, friends of friends, acquaintances, and others in our social circle influence our behavior and our health—both positively and negatively.

social norm A behavior or an attitude that a particular group expects, values, and enforces.

sperm The male gamete produced by the testes and transported outside the body through ejaculation.

spermatogenesis The process by which sperm cells are produced.

spiritual health The ability to identify one's basic purpose in life and to achieve one's full potential.

spiritual intelligence The capacity to sense, understand, and tap into ourselves, others, and the world around us.

spirituality A belief in someone or something that transcends the boundaries of self.

static flexibility The ability to assume and maintain an extended position at one end point in a joint's range of motion.

static stretching A stretching technique in which a gradual stretch is held for a short time of 10–30 seconds.

sterilization A surgical procedure to end a person's reproductive capability.

stimulants Agents, such as drugs, that temporarily relieve drowsiness, help in the performance of repetitive tasks, and improve capacity for work.

stress The nonspecific response of the body to any demands made upon it; may be characterized by muscle tension and acute anxiety, or may be a positive force for action.

stressor A specific or nonspecific agent or situation that causes the stress response in a body.

stress response The cascade of internal changes that mobilize the body's resources for action.

stroke A cerebrovascular event in which the blood supply to a portion of the brain is blocked.

subcutaneous Under the skin.

suction curettage A procedure in which the contents of the uterus are removed by means of suction and scraping.

synergistic Characterized by a combined effect that is greater than the sum of the individual effects.

systole The contraction phase of the cardiac cycle.

systolic blood pressure Highest blood pressure, which occurs when the heart contracts.

tar A thick, sticky dark fluid produced by the burning of tobacco, made up of several hundred different chemicals, many of them poisonous, some of them carcinogenic.

tend-and-befriend model A behavioral response to stress characterized by increased feelings of trust.

terminal illness An illness in which death is inevitable.

testes (singular, testis) The male sex organs that produce sperm and testosterone.

tobacco use disorder A problematic pattern of tobacco use leading to clinically significant impairment or distress.

tolerance A need for markedly increased amounts of alcohol or a drug to achieve the desired effect or a markedly diminished effect with continued use of a substance.

toxicity Poisonousness; the dosage level at which a drug becomes poisonous to the body, causing either temporary or permanent damage.

toxic shock syndrome (TSS) A disease characterized by fever, vomiting, diarrhea, and often shock, caused by a bacterium that releases toxic waste products into the bloodstream.

transactional or cognitive-relational model A framework for evaluating the process of coping with a stressful event in four stages (primary appraisal, secondary appraisal, coping, and reevaluation); based on the theory that the level of stress that people experience depends on their assessment of a stressor and on the resources available to deal with it.

transcendence The sense of passing into a foreign region or dimension, often experienced by a person near death.

transgender Having a gender identity opposite one's biological sex.

trans fats Fat formed when liquid vegetable oils are processed to make table spreads or cooking fats; also found in dairy and beef products; considered to be especially dangerous dietary fats.

transtheoretical model A model of behavioral change that focuses on the individual's decision making; it states that an individual progresses through a sequence of six stages as he or she makes a change in behavior.

trauma The experience of a direct or perceived uncontrollable threat to the safety of individuals, their loved ones or their community.

triglycerides Fats that flow through the blood after meals and are linked to increased risk of coronary artery disease.

tubal ligation The suturing or tying shut of the fallopian tubes to prevent pregnancy.

tubal occlusion The blocking of the fallopian tubes to prevent pregnancy.

urethra The canal through which urine from the bladder leaves the body; in the male, also serves as the channel for seminal fluid.

urethral opening The outer opening of the thin tube that carries urine from the bladder.

uterus The female organ that houses the developing fetus until birth.

vagina The canal leading from the exterior opening in the female genital area to the uterus.

vaginal contraceptive film (VCF) A small dissolvable sheet saturated with spermicide that can be inserted into the vagina and placed over the cervix.

vaginal spermicide A substance that kills or neutralizes sperm, inserted into the vagina in the form of a foam, cream, jelly, suppository, or film.

values The criteria by which one makes choices about one's thoughts, actions, goals, and ideals.

variable interest rate A rate that changes over time and can be raised at any time, or in response to your credit behavior.

vas deferens Two tubes that carry sperm from the epididymis into the urethra.

vasectomy A surgical sterilization procedure in which each vas deferens is cut and tied shut to stop the passage of sperm to the urethra for ejaculation.

ventricles The two lower chambers of the heart, which pump blood out of the heart and into the arteries.

visualization or guided imagery An approach to stress control, self-healing, or motivating life changes by means of seeing oneself in the state of calmness, wellness, or change.

vital signs Measurements of physiological functioning—specifically temperature, blood pressure, pulse rate, and respiration rate.

vitamins Organic substances that the body needs in very small amounts and that carry out a variety of functions in metabolism and nutrition.

waist-to-hip ratio (WHR) The proportion of one's waist circumference to one's hip circumference.

wellness A deliberate lifestyle choice characterized by personal responsibility and optimal enhancement of physical, mental, and spiritual health.

withdrawal Development of symptoms that cause significant psychological and physical distress when an individual reduces or stops drug use.

zygote A fertilized egg.

Index